OPTICAL COHERENCE TOMOGRAPHY

RETINAL DISEASES - GLAUCOMA

OPTICAL COHERENCE TOMOGRAPHY
RETINAL DISEASES - GLAUCOMA

Chief Editor

George P. Theodossiadis MD
Emeritus Professor in Ophthalmology
University of Athens
Director of 2nd Department of Ophthalmology
Henry Dunant Hospital
Athens, Greece

Section Editors

Vlassis G. Grigoropoulos MD
Consultant Ophthalmologist
2nd Department of Ophthalmology
Henry Dunant Hospital
Athens, Greece

Ioannis G. Emfietzoglou MD, FEBO
Consultant Ophthalmologist
2nd Department of Ophthalmology
Henry Dunant Hospital
Athens, Greece

Panagiotis G. Theodossiadis MD
Associate Professor in Ophthalmology
University of Athens
2nd Department of Ophthalmology
Attikon Hospital
Athens, Greece

Pantelis P. Nikolaidis MD
Consultant Ophthalmologist
2nd Department of Ophthalmology
Henry Dunant Hospital
Athens, Greece

Paschalidis
P.M.P.
Medical Publications

NOTICE

Medicine is an ever-changing field. Standard safety precautions must be followed, but as new research and clinical experience broaden our knowledge, changes in treatment and drug therapy may become necessary or appropriate. Readers are advised to check the most current product information provided by the manufacturer of each drug to be administered to verify the recommended dose, the method and duration of administration, and contraindications. It is the responsibility of the treating physician, relying on experience and knowledge of the patient, to determine dosages and the best treatment for each individual patient. Neither the publisher nor the authors assume any liability for any injury and/or damage to persons or property arising from this publication.

PMP (Paschalidis Medical Publications, Ltd.).
14th, Tetrapoleos str., Athens, 115 27, Greece
Tel.: 0030-210-7789125, 0030-210-7793012, Fax: 0030-210-7759421,
e-mail: Paschalidis@Medical-Books.gr
orders: Paschalidis@Medical-Books.gr
© information: GP@Medical-Books.gr, CP@Medical-Books.gr
distributed by Elsevier U.K.

Dedicated to

Michael and Mary Jaharis

FOREWORD

The diagnosis and management of vitreoretinal disorders have been revolutionized over the last thirty years. The eye is a unique organ with transparent media, allowing the direct visualization and study of the retina and optic disc with unparalleled clarity that cannot be achieved in any other part of the body. The development of new instrumentation allows detailed examination of the whole fundus, and presently we have at our disposal a vast array of imaging modalities, including fundus photography, fluorescein angiography and ultrasonography. The recent development of Optical Coherence Tomography (OCT) provides detailed cross sectional images of the retina and vitreoretinal interface, and the information obtained helps us in establishing the diagnosis and developing rational therapeutic plans.

Professor George Theodossiadis and his collaborators have assembled a clear, timely, and highly informative book on the rapidly expanding imaging technique of OCT, which has especially revolutionized the diagnosis and management of macular disorders and glaucoma. The material covered in this book's fifteen chapters is comprehensive and authoritative, covering all common disorders of the posterior segment. The clinical information obtained with this relatively new imaging modality is meaningful, and has led to a better understanding of the pathogenesis of many vitreoretinal disorders. The extraordinary illustrations demonstrate the nature and extent of the pathology in not only the different layers of the retina, but also the vitreoretinal interface and subretinal space.

It is a special honor to write the forward for this excellent book. The authors deserve congratulations for their product, which will benefit both general ophthalmologists and vitreoretinal specialists. It is fascinating to observe these new developments in imaging of the posterior segment and as the authors have emphasized, refinement of this imaging modality will provide even more exciting and gratifying understanding of vitreoretinal pathology. The newer systems have a higher resolution in tissue, a much faster acquisition rate and produce dramatically improved image quality.

On a personal level, I congratulate Professor George Theodossiadis who continues to work with endless enthusiasm and produced this excellent and beautiful textbook for the ophthalmologist.

Evangelos Gragoudas
Professor of Ophthalmology
Harvard Medical School

PREFACE

In the last few years we have witnessed a very rapid progress in the diagnosis and treatment of vitreoretinal diseases, which are one of the main causes of severe visual loss. The diagnostic technique that changes dramatically the way that we look into the retina is Optical Coherence Tomography (OCT).

OCT is a noninvasive diagnostic imaging technique that can perform high-resolution, micron scale, cross-sectional or tomographic imaging by measuring the echo time delay and intensity of backscattered light. The technique, which provides images of the macula very similar to obtaining in vivo histopathological sections, is analogous to ultrasound, except that optical rather than acoustic reflectivity is measured.

OCT is an especially useful examination in diagnosing and in monitoring therapeutically a variety of macular diseases. The technique enables examination of epiretinal, intraretinal and subretinal macular morphology and it is particularly helpful in the study and management of vitreoretinal traction syndrome, macular holes, macular edema, neovascular age related macular degeneration and many other retinal diseases.

It is also useful for the early diagnosis of glaucoma since it provides quantitative and reproducible assessment of the peripapillary retinal nerve fiber layer helping in that way in the early diagnosis of the disease. The technique has the advantage to detect early losses of the retinal nerve fiber layer well in advance of the visual field changes and therefore is especially helpful in monitoring the disease progress.

The included material in this Atlas-book is divided into 15 chapters. Each of them is written in a comprehensive way that addresses the needs of residents in ophthalmology, retinal fellows and practicing ophthalmologists.

Each chapter begins with an overview of the clinical characteristics of the described disease and then progresses to fundus imaging which includes OCT scans and histograms that depict in detail the existing pathology. Fundus photographs and fluorescein angiograms are also included for most of the included cases.

The publication of the book would not have been possible without the help of my collaborators to whom I would like to express my sincere thanks. I have also to acknowledge with thanks the encouragement and support of Michael and Mary Jaharis. I would also like to express my appreciation and sincere thanks to Professor E. Gragoudas for writing the foreword of the book.

It is my hope that this book will help the experienced ophthalmologist, the student and the resident in ophthalmology in the better understanding of the macular diseases.

George P. Theodossiadis

Emeritus Professor in Ophthalmology
University of Athens

TABLE OF CONTENTS

CHAPTER 1

INTRODUCTION

VLASSIS GRIGOROPOULOS

Optical Coherence Tomography is a new imaging and diagnostic method for ocular diseases[6]. The instrument measures the time delay and intensity of backscattered or backreflected light from biological tissues in order to provide a tomographic imaging of their internal structure. This is achieved by scanning tissues with a resolution as high as 1 to 15μm. Contemporary imaging technologies such as magnetic resonance tomography, computer tomography or ultrasound have a considerably lower resolution compared to Optical Coherence Tomography.

Optical Coherence Tomography has been used in ophthalmology to visualize in detail the anterior segment and the retina of the eye. It has also been used in other areas of medicine such as cardiology, gastroenterology, pneumonology, oncology, dentistry etc. Optical Coherence Tomography enables real-time imaging of tissues in situ without the need of a biopsy and histological process, a unique characteristic and advantage of that method[3,11]. Optical Coherence Tomography can be used when traditional biopsy has a high possibility of wrong diagnosis (i.e. in cancer diagnosis, when tumor localization during biopsy is not precise, then we may have a false negative result and therefore Optical Coherence Tomography may be useful in order to direct the biopsy and reduce the possibility of diagnostic error). It can also be used in cases where conventional biopsy is dangerous or impossible (i.e. eye, heart or nervous tissues). Finally, Optical Coherence

Tomography can help in interventional procedures, such as blood vessel and nerve anastomosis or stent placement and atherectomy in cardiology, with its ability to identify structures beneath the surface of tissues.

Ophthalmology is the faculty of medicine where Optical Coherence Tomography has its main application due to the structure of the eye and its relation with light. Optical Coherence Tomography provides real-time, cross-sectional, non contact, high resolution images of the retina and the anterior segment of the eye providing information that, together with other imaging modalities, such as fundus photography, fluorescein and indocyanine green angiography, may assist in the accurate diagnosis of many ophthalmic conditions. Optical Coherence Tomography enables visualization of the retinal structure (macula, optic disc etc) as well as the internal retinal morphology (nerve fiber layer, ganglion cell layer, photoreceptor layer etc)[9]. It enables also visualization of the anterior segment of the eye (cornea, iris, angle of anterior chamber and lens). Optical Coherence Tomography may help in the detection and monitoring of a variety of macular diseases (macular edema, macular hole, central serous chorioretinopathy, retinal detachment, vitreoretinal traction, age - related macular degeneration, epiretinal membrane etc) and can also perform quantitative retinal measurements. Optical Coherence Tomography is also very useful in the diagnosis and monitoring of glaucoma. Acquired images can be analyzed with special algorithms to automatically calculate the retinal thickness or retinal nerve fiber layer thickness and can also perform an optic nerve head mapping without physician intervention. Finally, Optical Coherence Tomography can be used to monitor the progression of the disease and the effectiveness of treatment.

PRINCIPLES OF OPTICAL COHERENCE TOMOGRAPHY

Optical Coherence Tomography performs cross-sectional imaging by measuring the time delay and intensity of backscattered or backreflected light from the internal structure of tissues. It is similar to B-mode ultrasonography with the main difference being that it uses light instead of sound. Optical Coherence Tomography application has the disadvantage to be constrained to tissues that are optically accessible, which is something that makes it ideal for ophthalmology. Optical Coherence Tomography can be performed without the need of physical contact to the eye and by using light rather than sound it provides a much higher resolution compared to ultrasound. Optical Coherence Tomography has an axial resolution of about 10μm, almost 10–20 times higher than B-mode ultrasonography, thus permitting visualization of the individual retinal layers[7].

In Optical Coherence Tomography, the first step in obtaining a tomographic image is the measurement of the axial distance within the tissue. This is achieved by directing a continuous beam of low coherence light into the eye and measuring the time delay and intensity of backscattering or backreflection from the different structures in the eye. The boundaries and different optical properties of the ocular tissues backreflect or backscatter the light in a manner and intensity unique for each tissue. As a result, by measuring the light delay, we are able to obtain information regarding the distances and dimensions of several different tissues. Light has a velocity of almost a million times faster than sound and therefore, distance measurement by Optical Coherence Tomography has a much higher time resolution than B-mode ultrasonography.

Optical Coherence Tomography is based on an optical measurement method known as interferometry of low coher-

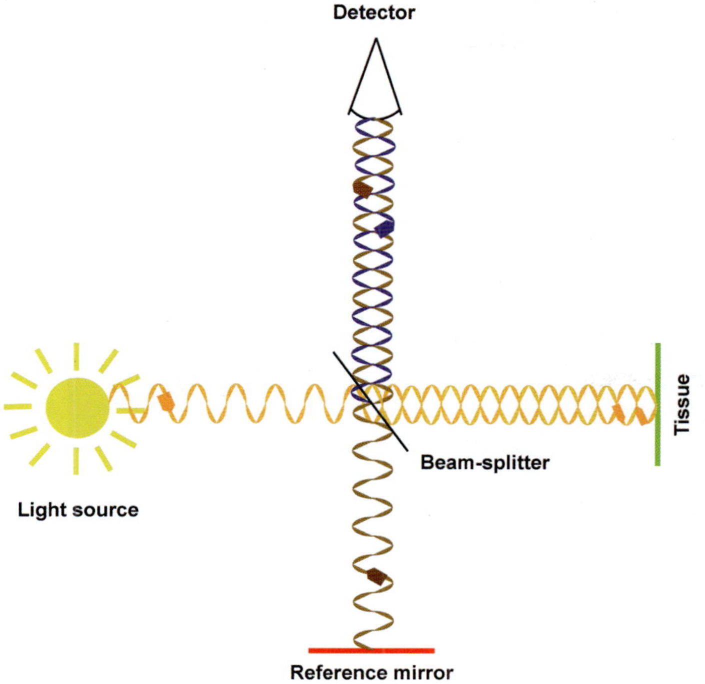

Fig. 1: The system that uses low coherence interferometry to calculate the tissue structure. An optical beam from a light source is directed onto a partially reflecting mirror (beam-splitter) that splits the light into two parts. The first is directed onto the eye and is reflected from the intraocular structures. The second is directed to a reference mirror at a known distance from which is reflected. The two light beams – the one backreflected from the eye and the one from the reference mirror – return to the beam-splitter, where they coincide only if both beams arrive at exactly the same time. This occurs only if the distance that light travels to and from the reference mirror is exactly the same with the distance that backreflected light travels to and from the study structure. They then produce a phenomenon known as interference, which can be measured by a light-sensitive detector. By varying the position of the reference mirror and comparing the reflected light beam from the mirror with the one backreflecting from the eye we are able to precisely measure the distance and thickness of the different ocular tissue structures.

ence, a technique that was first described by Isaac Newton. Interferometry compares one optical beam or light wave with another reference optical beam or light wave. This is achieved by directing the optical beam from the light source onto a partially reflecting mirror (beam-splitter) that splits the light into two parts. The first is directed onto the eye and is reflected from the intraocular structures. The second is directed to a reference mirror at a known distance from which is reflected. The two light beams – the one backreflected from the eye and the one from the reference mirror – return to the beam-splitter, where they coincide only if both beams arrive at exactly the same time. This occurs only if the distance that light travels to and from the reference mirror is exactly the same with the distance that backreflected light travels to and from the study structure. They then produce a phenomenon known as interference, which can be measured by a light-sensitive detector. By varying the position of the reference mirror and comparing the reflected light beam from the mirror with the one backreflecting from the eye we are able to precisely measure the distance and thickness of the different ocular tissue structures *(figure 1)*. Optical Coherence Tomography detects the output signal from the study tissue with the interferometer, processes it electronically (based on the different index of light refraction of each tissue) and displays it on a computer, acquiring information on tissue distance or thickness. Because the intensity of backreflected or backscattered light is extremely small (approximately -50 to -90 decibels [db] of the incident light), detectors of very high sensitivity are required for the detection of the extremely weak reflected echoes from the ocular tissues. Once the first axial scan has been made, then the optical beam moves transversally, making successive rapid axial scans and measuring the relative tissue position with high precision. A complete set of those measurements represents a cross-sectional image of the ocular tissue *(figure 2)*.

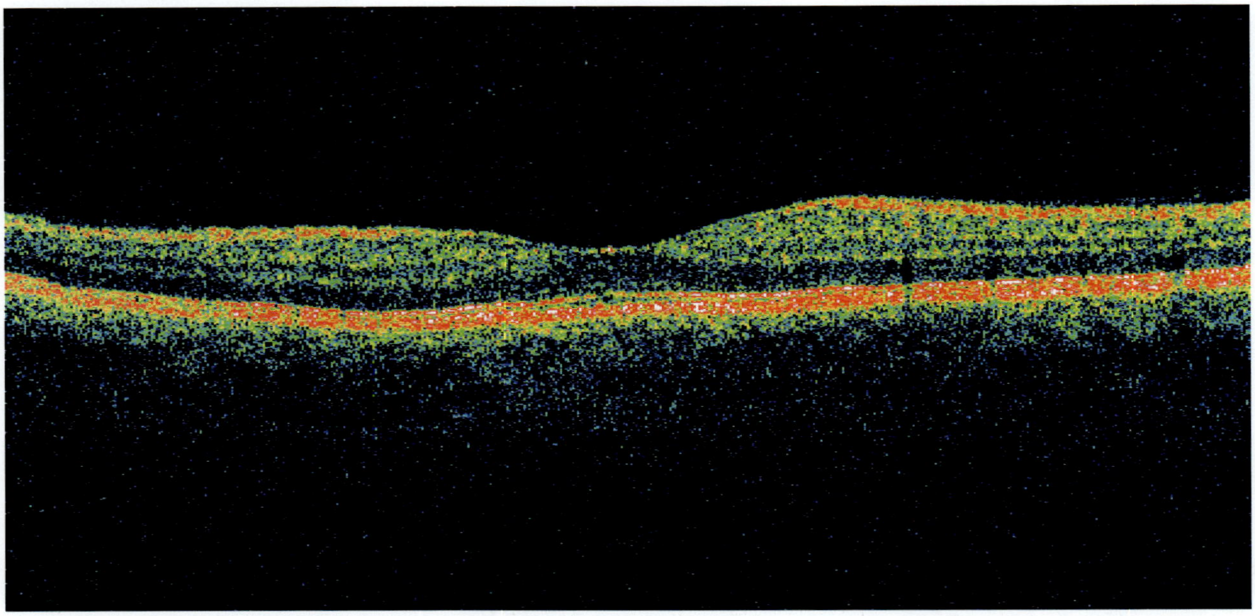

Fig. 2: Cross sectional image of the macula as shown on Optical Coherence Tomography.

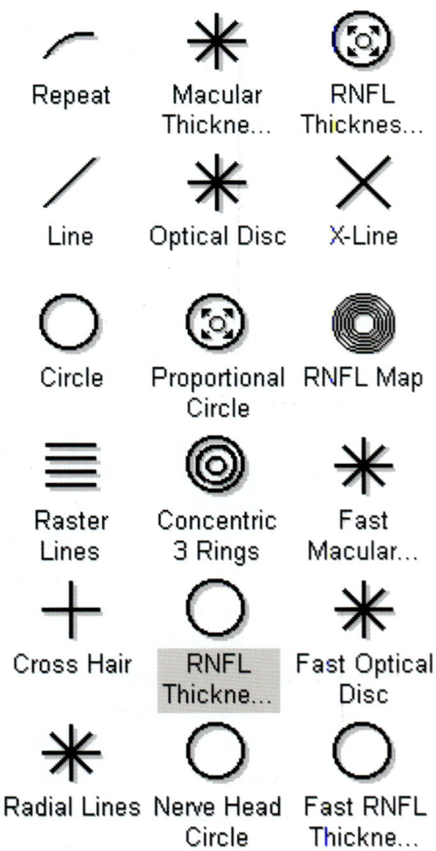

Fig. 3: The 18 examination protocols of the software of Optical Coherence Tomography.

Fig. 4: The 18 analysis protocols of the software of Optical Coherence Tomography.

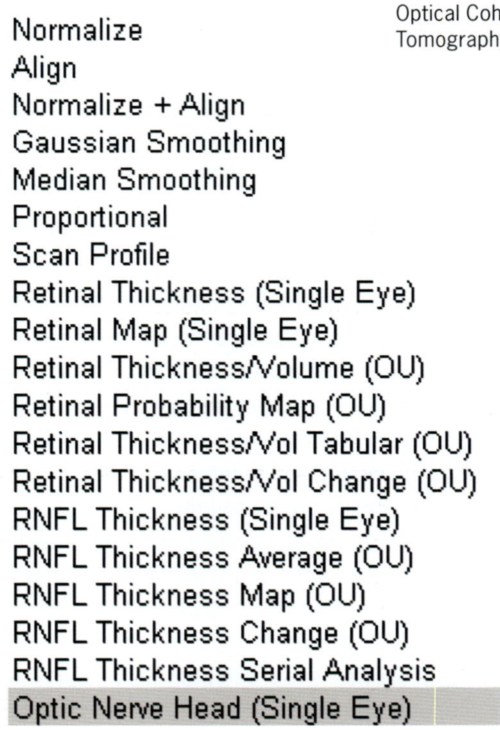

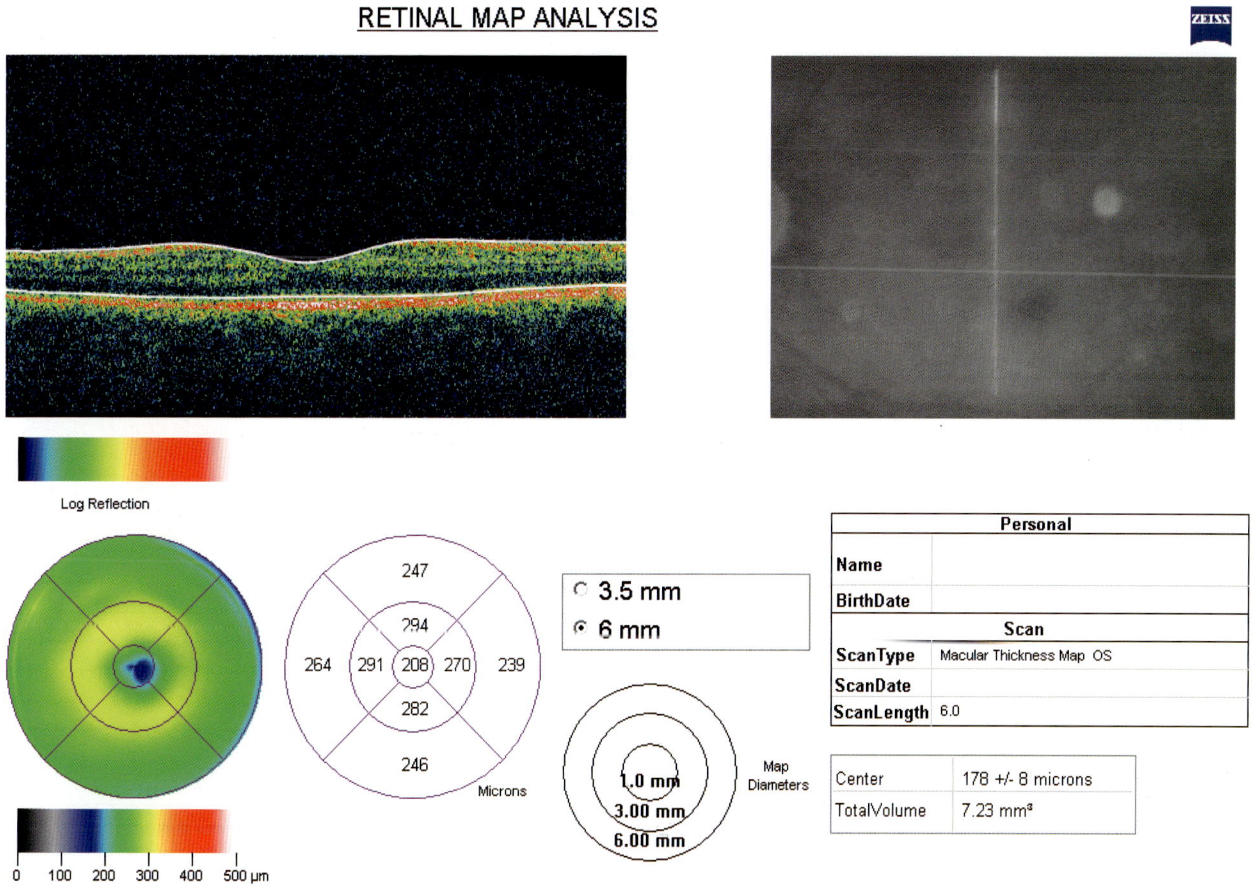

Fig. 5: The retinal map protocol of the macula that calculates the retinal thickness (in µm) in all 8 quadrants as well as in the central circle of 1mm diameter that corresponds to the foveola. The retinal thickness at the centre of the fovea, the total macular volume and the retinal map of the macula are also calculated.

Recent technological advances allow the use of laser diode light of low coherence with wave length 820nm, near the infrared spectrum. During each scanning, which lasts 1.28 – 1.92sec, 128 – 768 axial scans and on each scan 1024 focal measurements at a tissue depth of 2mm are realized. Therefore, Optical Coherence Tomography performs 131072 – 786432 focal scans in order to achieve a cross-sectional image of the retina. Optical Coherence Tomography scan is then stored by the instrument, together with the gray–scale retina video image that shows the direction of the scan *(figure 5)*. Scanning is performed by the software, using precise patterns and with the possibility of qualitative and quantitative image processing and topographic map display.

There are 18 acquisition protocols for retinal diseases and glaucoma. These protocols vary from simple linear scans to groups of parallel, crossing, radial and circular scans *(figure 3)*. In the fast protocols, the image quality as well as the time of each scanning is decreased, resulting in a more precise centering of central fixation for all scans and therefore, a more reliable analysis of each measurement.

The software offers 18 analysis protocols *(figure 4)*. There is the possibility of retinal mapping with calculation of the retinal thickness and volume and also comparison with previous tests in order to monitor disease progression *(figure 5)*. The software is able to also perform nerve fiber layer mapping around the optic disc *(figure 6)* and optic disc head mapping *(figure 7)*, calculating various parameters (cupping, diameter, thickness and volume of the optic disc rim etc) – without the need to manually define the borders of the optic disc – that are important for assessing and monitoring the

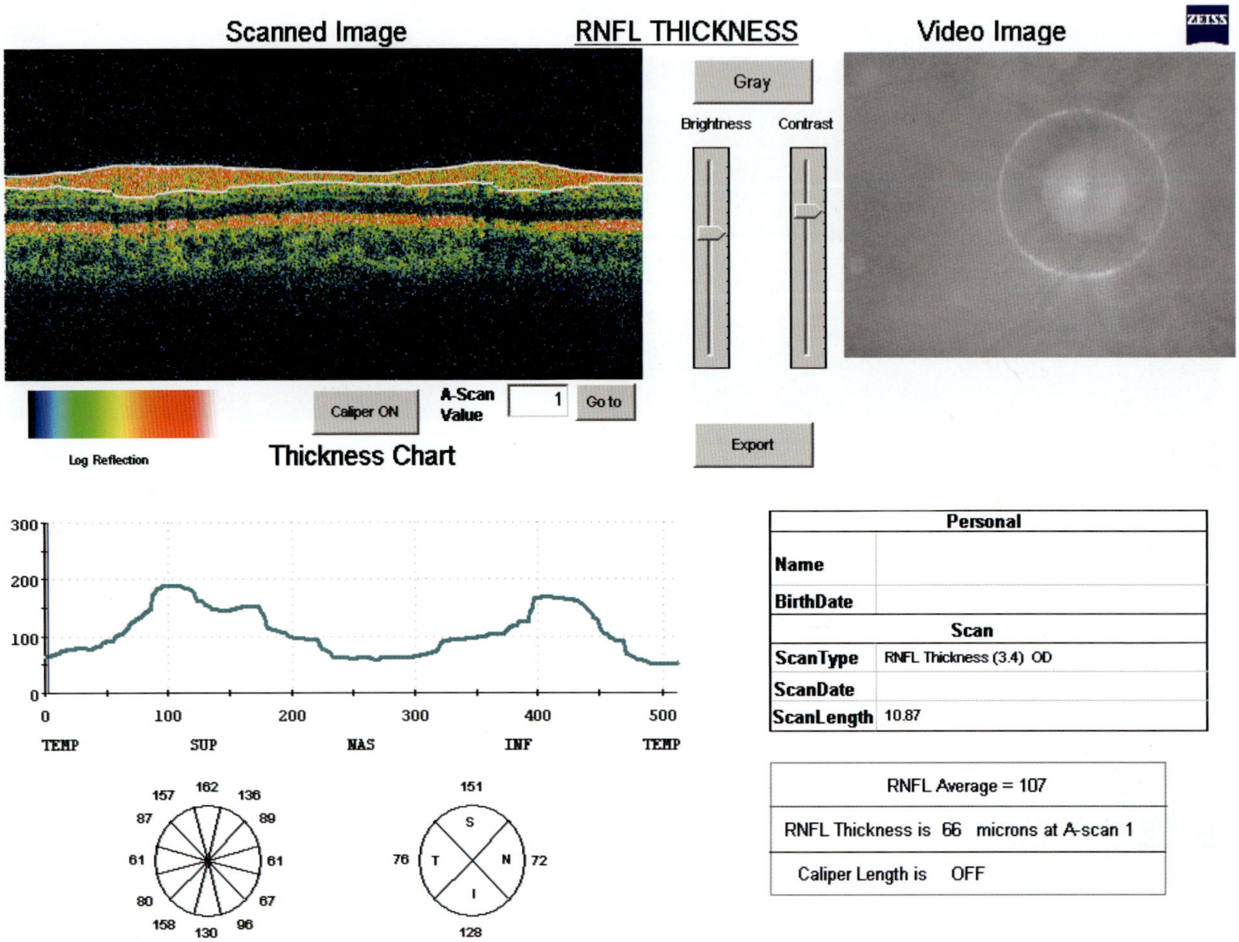

Fig. 6: The retinal nerve fiber layer thickness protocol that calculates the thickness (in μm) of the nerve fiber layer around the optic nerve head scanning in a circular fashion the entire peripapillary area with a diameter of 3.4mm. The retinal nerve fiber layer thickness is calculated in every quadrant and in 12 equal parts, while the mean nerve fiber layer thickness is computed and the nerve fiber layer thickness can be obtained at any given point of the scan.

glaucoma patient. The software has also image processing protocols in order to offer improved scanning interpretation. The "Normalize" protocol eliminates background noise and uses the whole color scale in the processed scan image. The "Align" protocol corrects the data for effects due to patient motion in the axial direction. The "Gaussian" and "Meridian" smoothing protocols average out noise and blend the colors of the scan image. Finally, the "Proportional" protocol processes the scan image so that it is true in its horizontal and vertical proportions and therefore, compared to the usual presentation of Optical Coherence Tomography scan images, the proportional scan image appears compressed vertically *(figure 8)*. The software contains a normative database for retinal nerve fiber layer thickness values around the optic disc, thus facilitating the evaluation of our measurements. There is also, a normative database for macular thickness values.

Optical Coherence Tomography images can be displayed into a gray–scale *(figure 9)* or false color scale *(figure 2)*. Gray level imaging is already used by ultrasound with a good image interpretation. White color corresponds to higher intensity optical signals while black color to weaker ones. When optical signal intensity falls below a certain limit, then it is displayed as black in an attempt to eliminate the background imaging noise. The disadvantage of color representation in gray–scale level consists in the decreased ability to differentiate between variations in intensity. Computer monitors display only 8-bit gray resolution or 256 levels of gray while the eye has a limited ability to distinguish different levels of

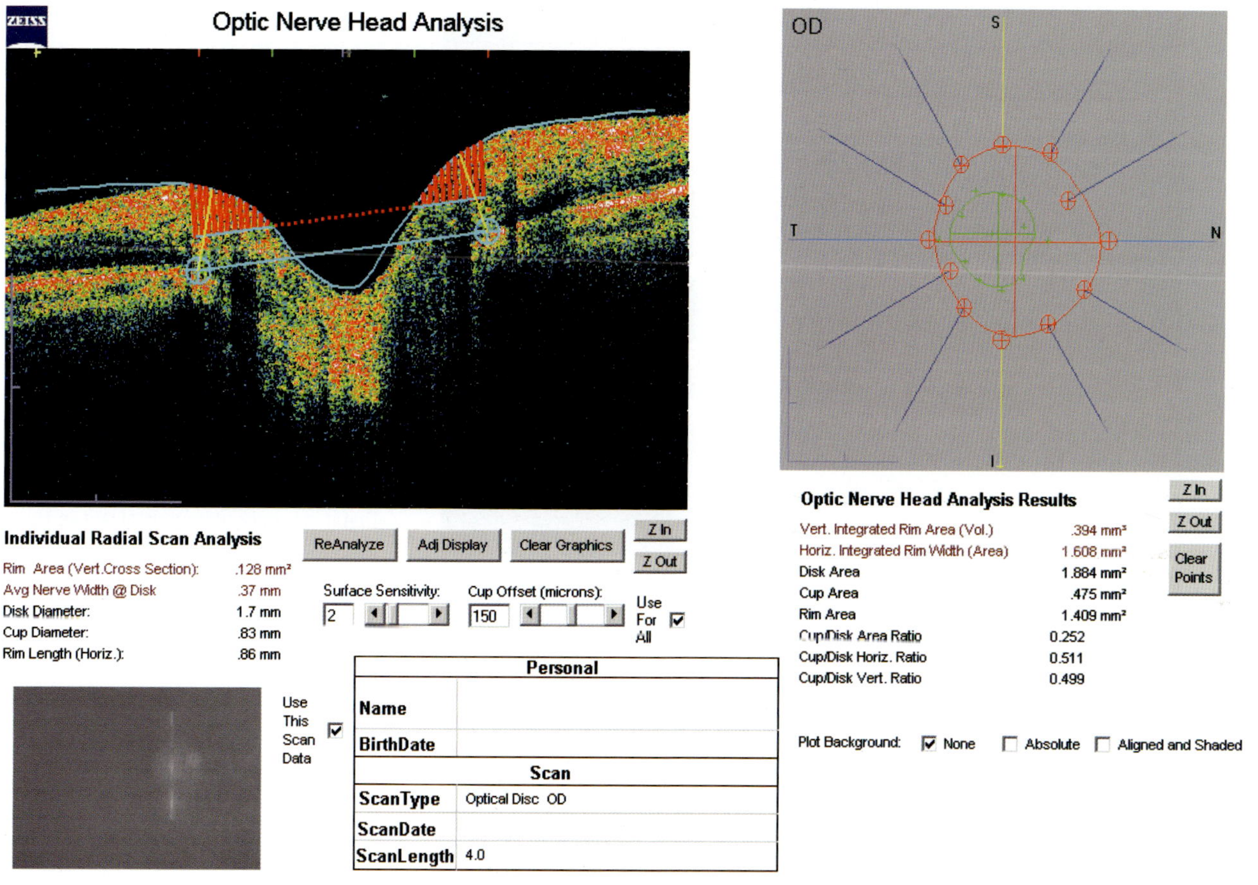

Fig. 7: The optic nerve head analysis protocol with the localization of the optic disc borders as calculated automatically by the software of Optical Coherence Tomography. The optic disc cupping, volume, diameter, rim and several other parameters are also calculated together with the topographic map of the optic nerve head.

---

grey. Therefore, gray scale images cannot correctly represent the color diversity that is offered by Optical Coherence Tomography. However, computer monitors have 32-bit or more color levels and the human eye can distinguish millions of different colors. Optical Coherence Tomography uses false colors in order to differentiate between different structures within human tissues. White and red colors correspond to the strongest signal (-50db) while black and blue colors correspond to the weakest signal (-95db). One disadvantage of false color representation is the generation of artifacts.

Tissues with different optical properties are represented with different colors. However, it is important to remember that while Optical Coherence Tomography displays real dimensions, different color imaging corresponds to different optical properties and not to different tissue morphologies. Areas with the same color in Optical Coherence Tomography don't correspond to the same tissue but rather to tissues with the same optical properties. Therefore, we should not interpret Optical Coherence Tomography images as histopathology specimens.

The axial resolution of Optical Coherence Tomography instrument for ophthalmology is about 10μm while new machines have an axial resolution of about 1-2μm (Ultra High Resolution Optical Coherence Tomography)[2]. The typical transverse resolution of Optical Coherence Tomography is 20-25 μm. Because of the high resolution of the Optical Coherence Tomography images they are very vulnerable to distortion due to every kind of movement (i.e. intraocular

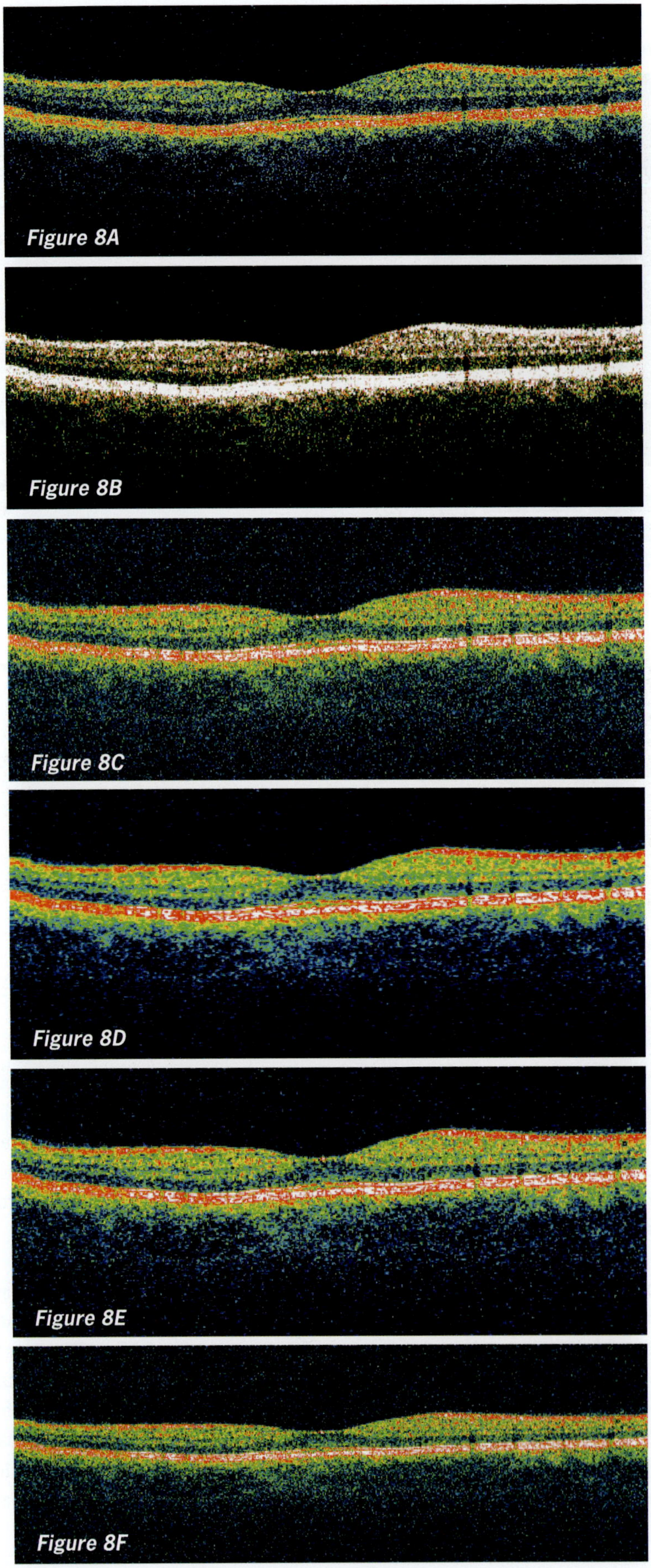

Fig. 8: The software of Optical Coherence Tomography has image processing protocols in order to offer improved scanning interpretation. The raw cross sectional image of the macula (A) as obtained by Optical Coherence Tomography without any processing. The "Normalize" protocol (B) eliminates background noise and uses the whole color scale in the processed scan image. The "Align" protocol (C) corrects the data for effects due to patient motion in the axial direction. The "Gaussian" (D) and "Meridian" (E) smoothing protocols average out noise and blend the colors of the scan image. Finally, the "Proportional" protocol (F) processes the scan image so that it is true in its horizontal and vertical proportions and therefore, compared to the usual presentation of Optical Coherence Tomography scan images, the proportional scan image appears compressed vertically.

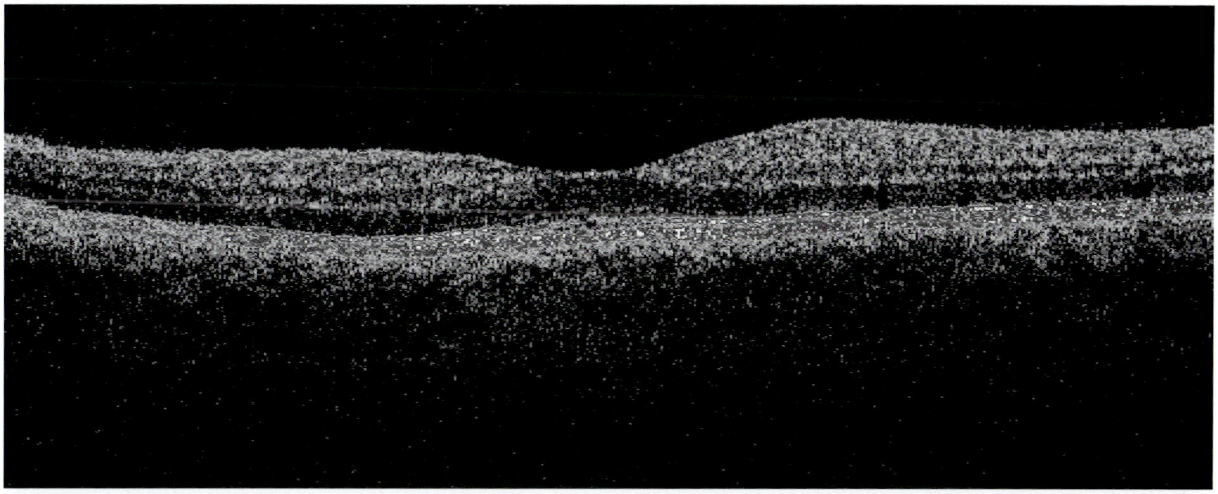

Fig. 9: The cross sectional image of the macula in gray scale as obtained by Optical Coherence Tomography.

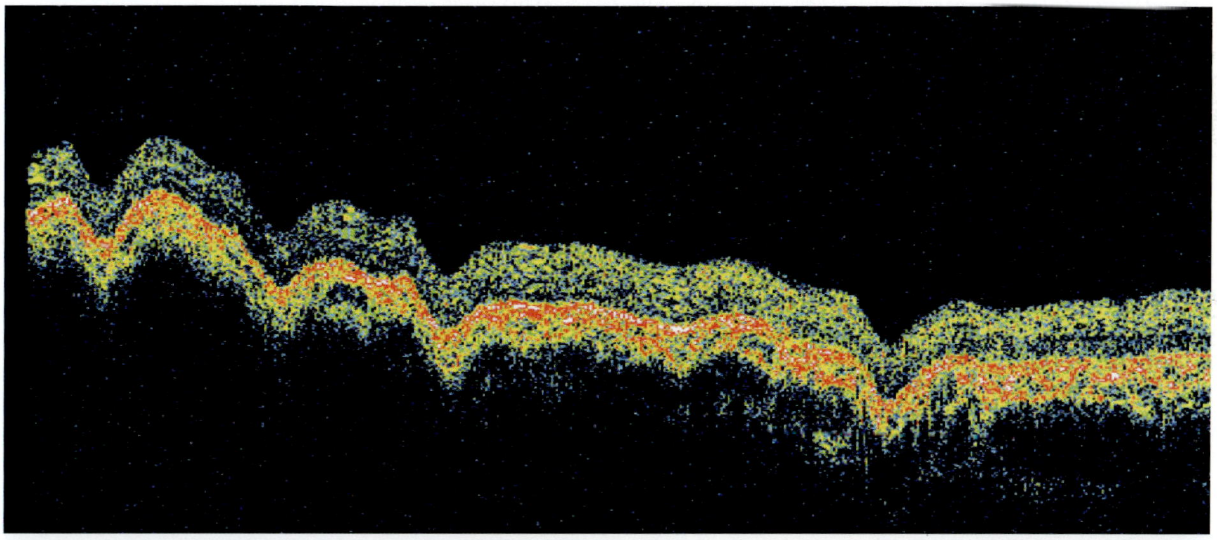

Fig. 10: Irregularities in the optic signal during retinal scanning may be attributed to intraocular pressure fluctuations, the circulation inside the retinal blood vessels, the microsaccades or loss of fixation.

pressure fluctuation, blood circulation in blood vessels, microsaccades, loss of fixation etc) resulting in image distortion *(figure 10)*. Optical Coherence Tomography is able, with special software, to correct image alterations due to axial movement and provide a clear image. Unfortunately, this cannot be done in the transverse axis, where loss of fixation or sudden movement can decrease image quality *(figures 11, 12)*. In these cases the high speed of successive image acquisition can improve image quality (High Speed Ultra High Resolution Optical Coherence Tomography).

INTERPRETATION

Light incident onto tissue is transmitted, absorbed or scattered. Transmitted light is free to penetrate deeper layers while absorbed light is essentially removed from the incident beam. Absorption takes place usually from tissue structures, such as hemoglobin or melanin, which have absorption spectra near the energy of the incident light. Optical scattering (backreflection) occurs with heterogeneous materials or homogeneous materials with different indices of refraction

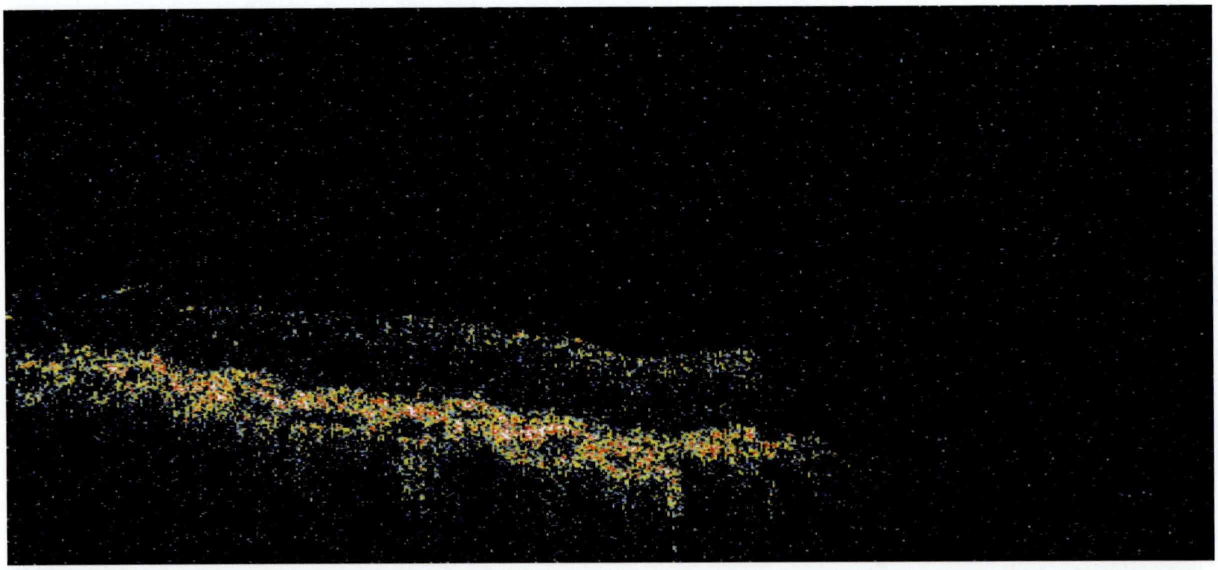

Fig. 11: Cataract or other media opacities can greatly reduce the quality of the image resulting in poor evaluation and interpretation of the scans obtained by Optical Coherence Tomography.

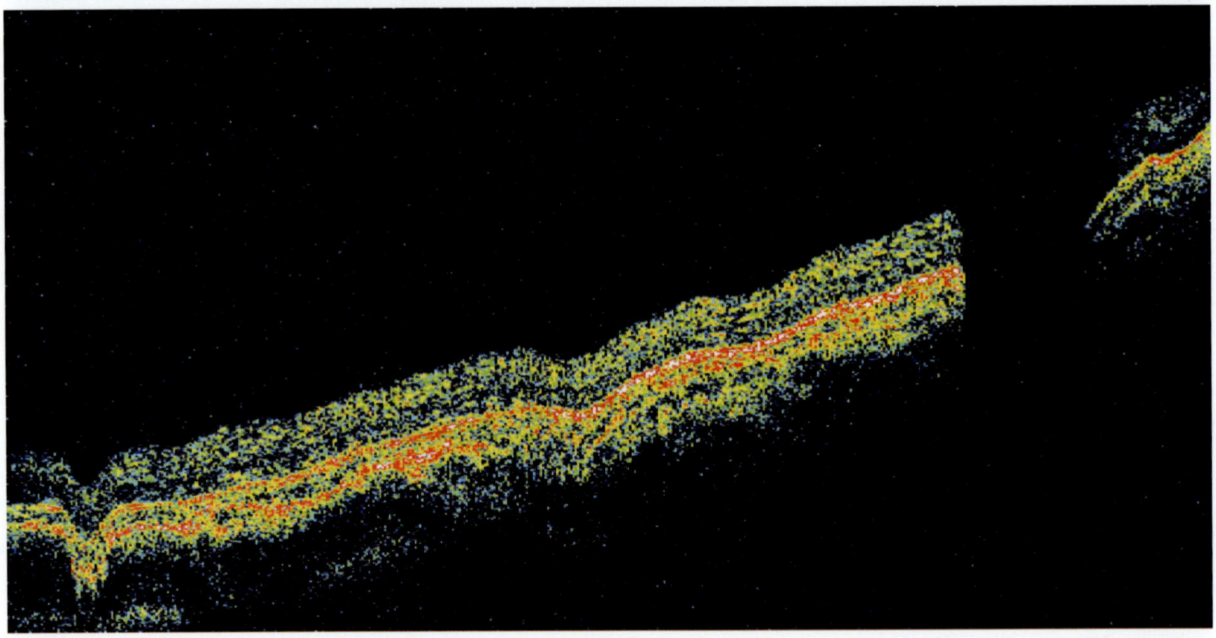

Fig. 12: Sudden movement or closing of the eyelids can cause loss of part or the whole of the image resulting in poor evaluation and interpretation of the scans obtained by Optical Coherence Tomography.

and is due to the different refractive index of the several tissue structures, such as nuclei, cytoplasm, cell membranes, nerve fibers, blood vessels etc. When the light reverses its direction completely, then it is called backscattered. When a light beam is incident onto tissue, initially loses part of its intensity by absorption and scattering as it travels into the tissue. Then, the light is backscattered by structures at different tissue depths. Finally, the light that returns to the Optical Coherence Tomography detector is further attenuated as it travels back out of the tissue. When light is strongly

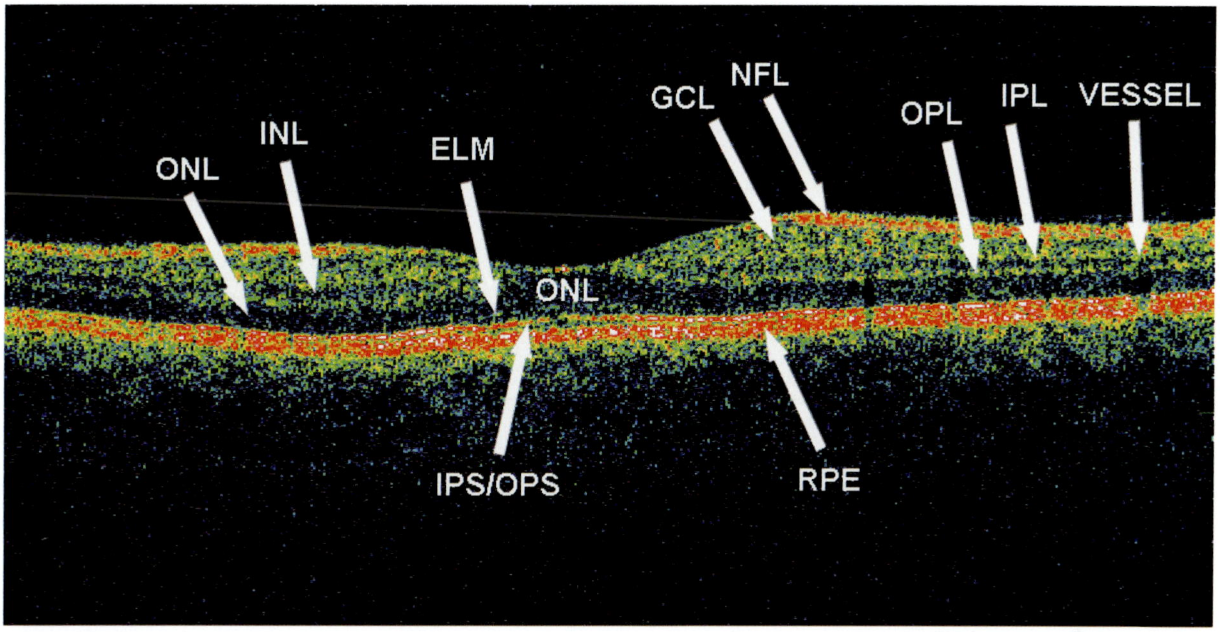

Fig. 13: The cross sectional image of the macula as obtained by Optical Coherence Tomography. The retinal layers* are indicated by the arrows.
*ONL: outer nuclear layer, INL: inner nuclear layer, OPL: outer plexiform layer, IPL: inner plexiform layer, NFL: nerve fiber layer, GCL: ganglion cell layer, ELM: external limiting membrane, IPS: inner photoreceptor segments, OPS: outer photoreceptor segments, RPE: retinal pigment epithelium.

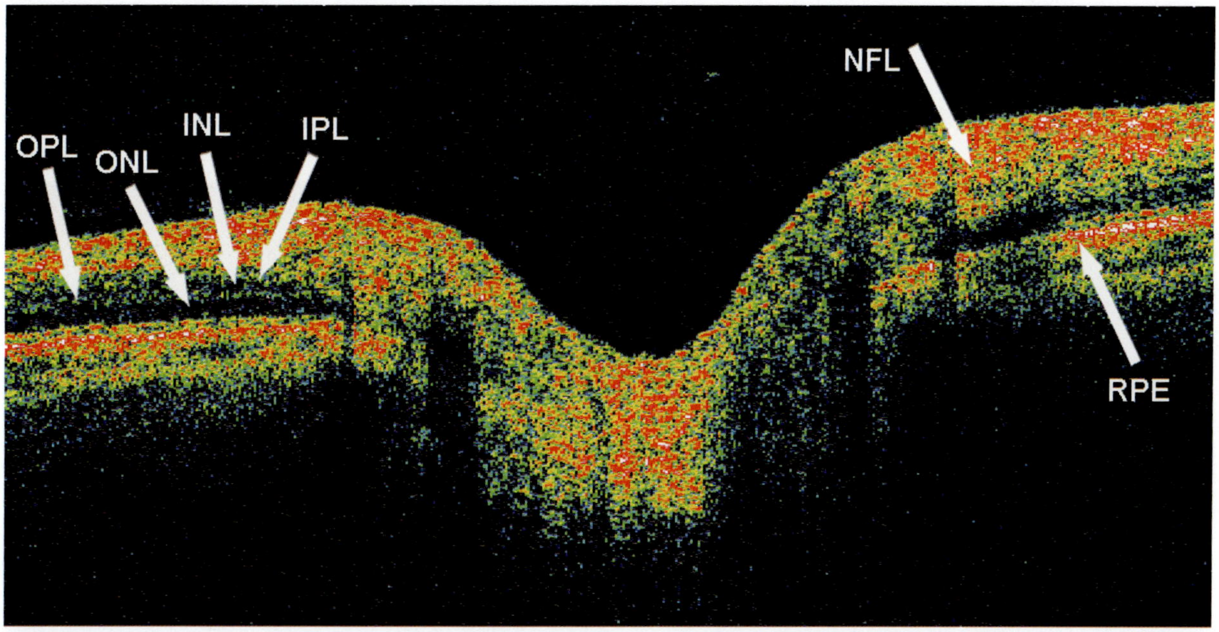

Fig. 14: The cross sectional image of the retina at the optic nerve head as obtained by Optical Coherence Tomography. The retinal layers* are indicated by the arrows.
*ONL: outer nuclear layer, INL: inner nuclear layer, OPL: outer plexiform layer, IPL: inner plexiform layer, NFL: nerve fiber layer, RPE: retinal pigment epithelium.

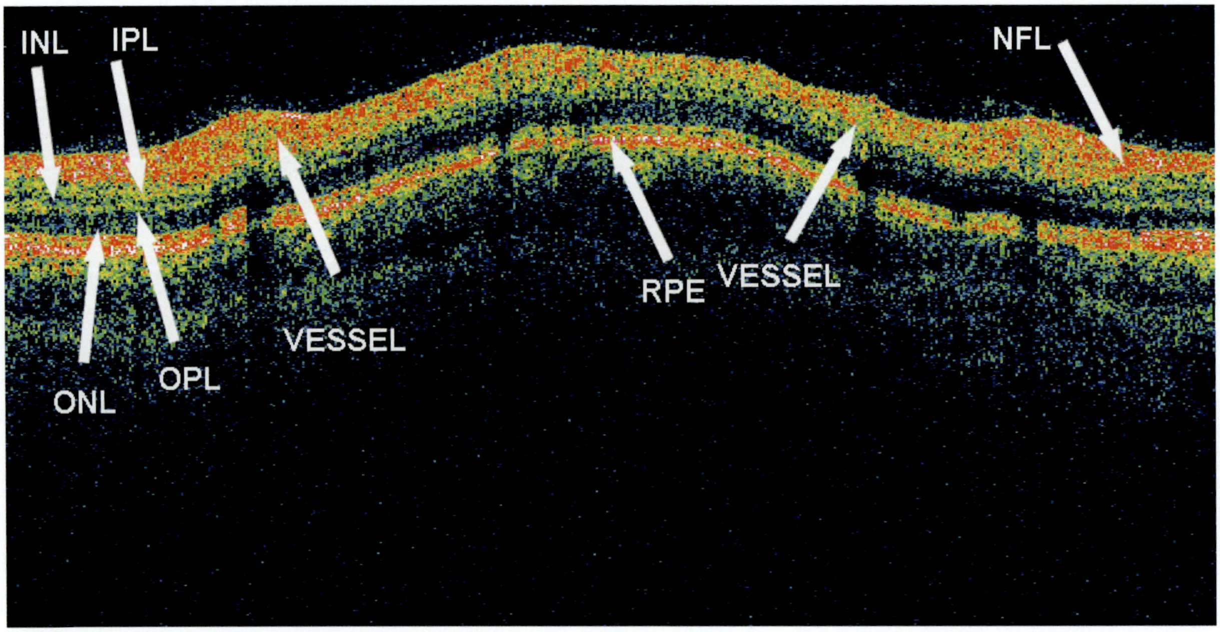

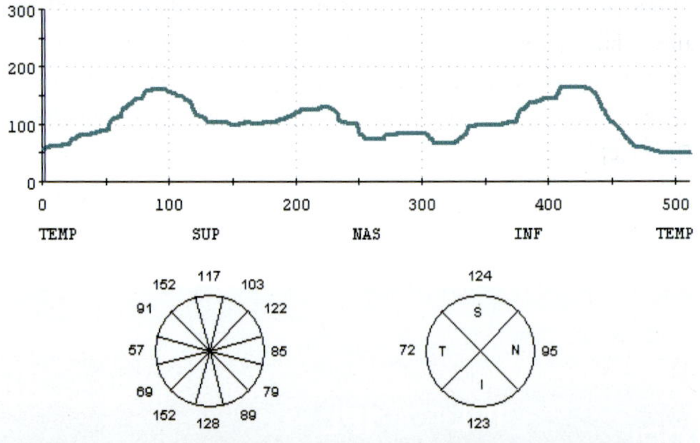

Fig. 15: The cross sectional image of the retina at the optic nerve head as obtained by Optical Coherence Tomography "unfolded", in a circle of 3.4mm diameter centered on the optic disc. The retinal layers* are indicated by the arrows. Also shown is the nerve fiber layer thickness in all quadrants as well as in 12 equal parts of the optic disc and its graphical representation. *ONL: outer nuclear layer, INL: inner nuclear layer, OPL: outer plexiform layer, IPL: inner plexiform layer, NFL: nerve fiber layer, RPE: retinal pigment epithelium.

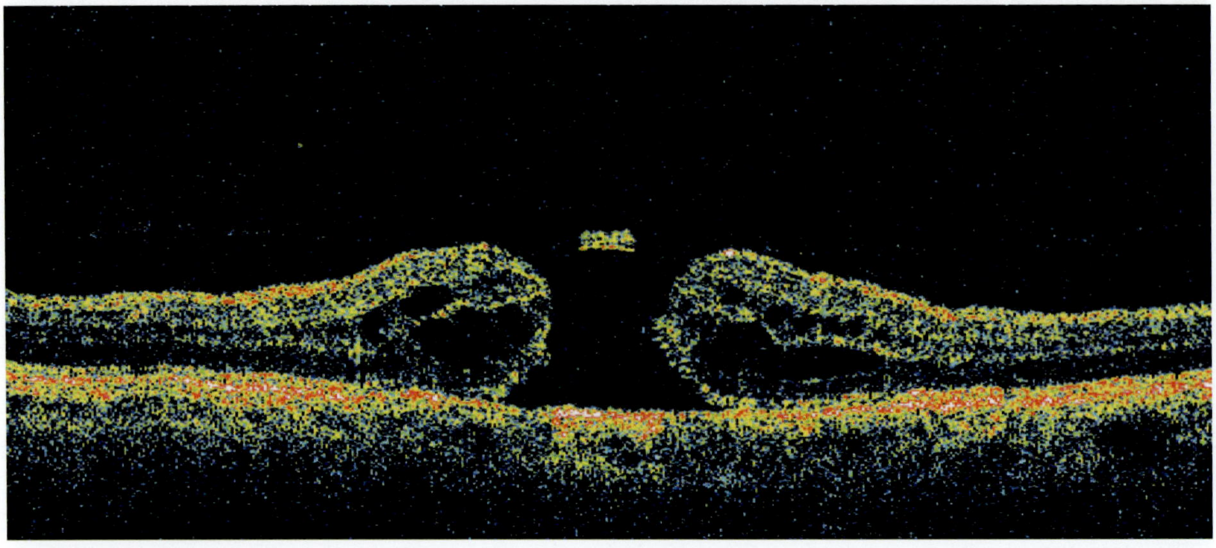

Fig. 16: Cross sectional image of a full thickness macular hole as obtained by Optical Coherence Tomography.

absorbed or scattered from tissues such as haemorrhage, then it loses a lot or all of its intensity and we observe a shadowing of the corresponding deeper structures.

PHYSIOLOGIC MACULA

Optical Coherence Tomography images reproduce retina morphology in total accordance with histopathology studies. The first, of variable thickness, high reflective red layer on the inner retina is the nerve fiber layer, which is thicker near the optic disc and thinner near the macula region *(figure 13)*. Due to low reflectivity the ganglion cell layer, the inner and the outer nuclear layers appear with black and blue color. The inner plexiform layer has mild reflectivity while the outer plexiform layer has increased reflectivity. The boundary between the photoreceptor inner and outer segments is shown as a thin red line of high reflectivity immediately anterior to the retinal pigment epithelium – choriocapillaries complex, probably because of the refractive index difference between the inner photoreceptor segment and the highly organized structure of the outer photoreceptor segment, which contains membranous discs rich in rhodopsin. The height of that line increases in the foveal region due to the increased length of the outer segments of the cones in this region. Sometimes, anterior to the retinal pigment epithelium and the boundary between the inner and outer photoreceptor segments, a thin line of mildly high reflectivity but weaker compared to that of the photoreceptors is detected, corresponding to the external limiting membrane. The red thick surface of high reflectivity, which is detected under the photoreceptors, represents the retinal pigment epithelium – choriocapillaries complex. Since the retinal pigment epithelium is in very close proximity to the choriocapillaries, it is often not distinguishable as a separate anatomical element. Under the choriocapillaries weak signals of black and blue color are detected (due to attenuation of the optical beam as it passes through the retina, retinal pigment epithelium and choriocapillaries) corresponding to the choroid. The foveola is detected with the characteristic thinner retinal layer and thicker photoreceptor layer. The vascular structures are of high reflectivity producing a shadowing of the deeper structures.

PHYSIOLOGIC OPTIC NERVE HEAD

Optic disc visualization is important for the evaluation of patients with glaucoma or neuro-ophthalmic disease. The normal cupping of the optic disc is evident *(figure 14)*. In the inner

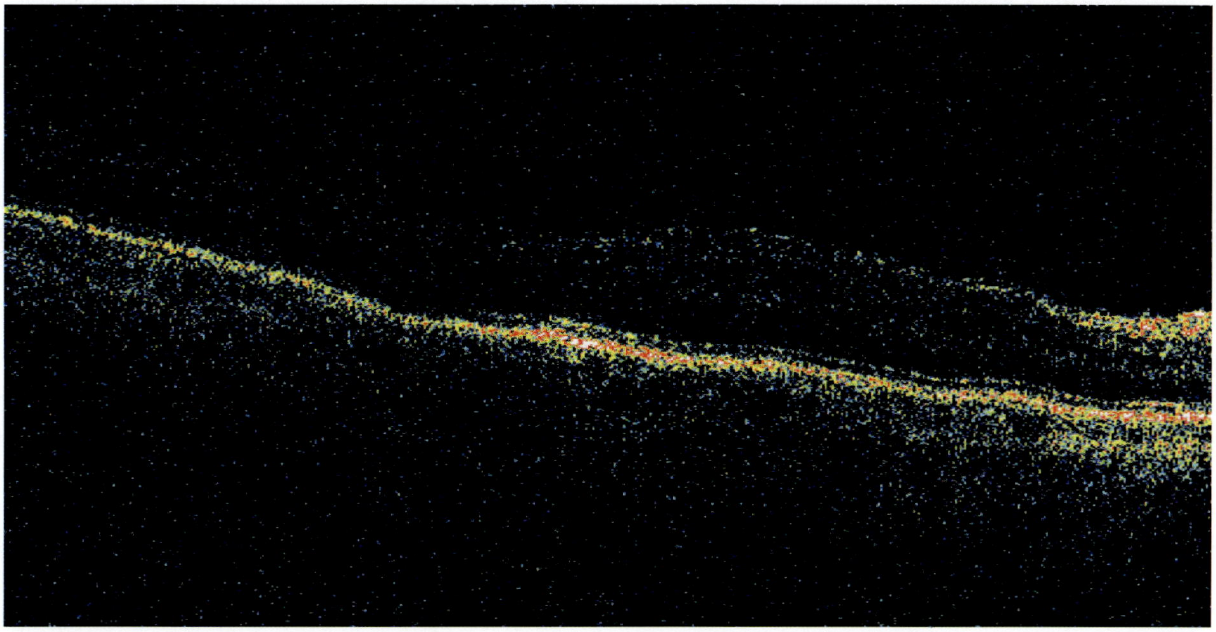

Fig. 17: Low signal due to media opacities leads to a weak representation of the retinal layers, even from structures with normally high reflectivity, such as the retinal pigment epithelium and the choriocapillaries.

retina around the optic disc a thick area of high reflectivity is detected, occupying almost the entire retinal thickness and corresponding to the nerve fiber layer. The retinal pigment epithelium and choriocapillaries can be seen as a highly reflective layer that terminates at the lamina cribrosa. The boundary between the photoreceptor inner and outer segments is shown as a thin red line of high reflectivity immediately anterior to the retinal pigment epithelium – choriocapillaries complex. The area where the photoreceptor, retinal pigment epithelium and choriocapillaries layers terminate as they approach the disc can be used as a landmark in order to define the optic disc margin. Between the nerve fiber layer and the photoreceptors, with black and blue color due to low reflectivity, appear the ganglion cell layer, the inner and the outer nuclear layers. The inner plexiform layer has mild reflectivity while the outer plexiform layer has increased reflectivity.

PHYSIOLOGIC PERIPAPILLARY REGION

Nerve fiber layer thickness evaluation in the peripapillary area is important for the diagnosis and management of the glaucoma patient. There is a special Optical Coherence Tomography protocol for nerve fiber layer scanning the peripapillary region. That consists of circumferential scans around the optic disc center with diameters of 2.3mm or 3.4mm. The image is displayed "unwrapped" with the superior, inferior, nasal and temporal quadrants clearly labeled. The nerve fiber layer is visible as a thick area of high reflectivity in the inner retina around the optic disc *(figure 15)*. The highest thickness of the nerve fiber layer is detected at the superior temporal and inferior temporal areas. The retinal pigment epithelium and the choriocapillaries are detected as a high reflectivity area under the nerve fiber layer, while the junction between the inner and outer photoreceptor segments is detected like a red thin line of high reflectivity exactly above the retinal pigment epithelium – choriocapillaries complex. The nerve fiber layer is automatically detected using special algorithms and its thickness is measured.

MACULAR HOLE

Optical Coherence Tomography imaging offers important diagnostic information and can assist fundus examination and fluorescein angiography in macular hole staging and its differentiation from lamellar macular hole[5]. Full thickness macular hole is characterized by a loss of normal fovea anatomy and discontinuation of normal retinal tissue throughout the full thickness of the retina in the fovea *(figure 16)*. Intraretinal edema and cystic changes are seen around the hole. The retinal pigment epithelium is intact at the base of the hole and the adjacent retina appears lifted away from the retinal pigment epithelium, forming the retinal detachment that is clinically observed as a ring around the hole (cuff). The vitreous often appears partially detached and is detected as a moderately reflective thin line inside the vitreous cavity and above the retina. Optical Coherence Tomography has greatly assisted in the understanding of the pathophysiology of macular hole. It also offers information about the hole diameter and the extent of either the intraretinal edema or the subretinal fluid. Finally, Optical Coherence Tomography is invaluable in assessing the effectiveness of the surgical treatment. A lamellar hole is detected as a partial thickness retinal defect in the fovea. A separation between the outer plexiform and outer nuclear layer is observed with preservation of the photoreceptor layer. The often coexisting epiretinal membrane is exerting traction on the retina creating a wrinkling appearance of the retinal surface.

VITREORETINAL INTERFACE ABNORMALITIES

The normal vitreous is highly transparent and therefore not visible in Optical Coherence Tomography imaging. Pathologies where the vitreous has inflammatory infiltrates, condensations or haemorrhage result in increased optical scattering and the vitreous becomes evident in the Optical Coherence Tomography image. Posterior vitreous detachment is detected as a thin mildly reflective line inside the vitreous cavity and above the inner retinal surface. This line is weak without continuity because the vitreous gel and the surrounding fluid have similar indices of refraction. Optical Coherence Tomography is often more sensitive in detecting posterior vitreous detachment than biomicroscopy. Optical Coherence Tomography can also be used to visualize epiretinal membrane. The epiretinal membrane can be distinguished from the posterior hyaloid from the epiretinal membrane's higher reflectivity, greater thickness and differences in shape. The epiretinal membrane may create a wrinkling appearance of the retinal surface by exerting traction on the retina. Optical Coherence Tomography can also be used to assess the outcome of surgical treatment for epiretinal membrane.

FLUID ACCUMULATION

Optical Coherence Tomography is very useful in detecting accumulation of fluid under or into the retina and under the retinal pigment epithelium. Subretinal fluid is shown as an area of low reflectivity (black or blue color) between the neurosensory retina and the retinal pigment epithelium. All retinal layers are intact and visible above the fluid. Optical Coherence Tomography is able to detect very small collections of subretinal fluid that are difficult to identify with biomicroscopy and can also monitor the state or resolution of subretinal fluid during treatment. Retinal pigment epithelium detachment has a more acute bell-like shape probably due to the tight junctions between the retinal pigment epithelium basement membrane and cells. The retinal pigment epithelium is presented like a red thin line at the roof of the detachment. Its high reflectivity produces shadowing of the choroid under the detachment. The retina loses its physiological shape but maintains its layers intact. In hemorrhagic detachment of the retinal pigment epithelium the fluid accumulation is not optically clear but presents mild reflectivity due to the combination of the highly reflective retinal pigment epithelium and haemorrhagic material, with increased, related to the hemorrhage density, shadowing of the underlying choroid. The differential diagnosis between a neurosensory retina and retinal pigment epithelium detachment is based on the signal strength (shadowing) under the fluid and the angle of the detachment. Confusion may also be caused between

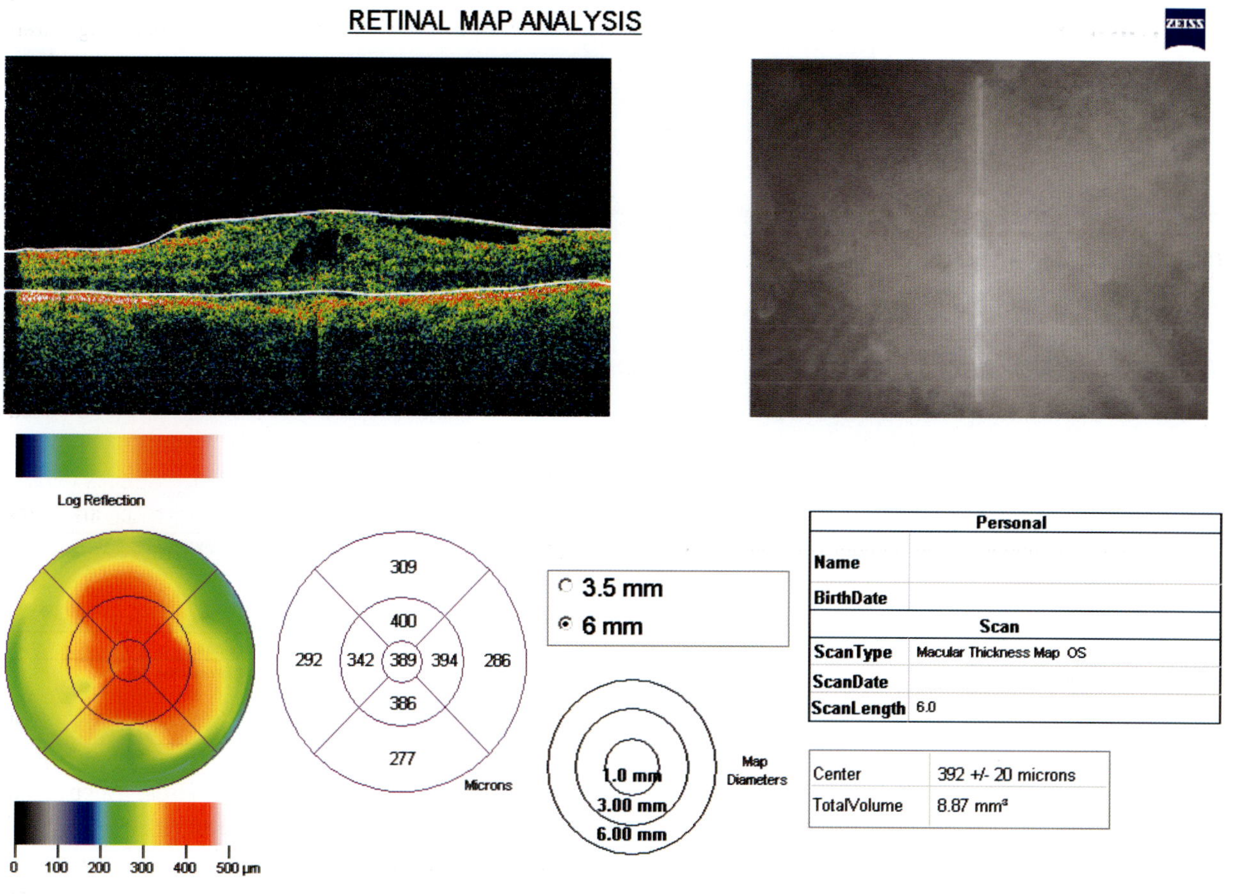

Fig. 18: In cases of epiretinal membrane, the membrane may be incorrectly identified by the software of Optical Coherence Tomography as the inner retinal surface, as shown here on both sides of the foveola, resulting in mistakes in the retinal thickness and in the retinal map calculations.

retinal detachment and severe diffuse retinal edema, the latter being usually located in the outer retinal layers. In these cases it is useful to detect the regular continuous smooth distinct line between the retina and the fluid, as a sign of a retinal detachment. Optical Coherence Tomography can also help in differentiating retinal detachment from retinoschisis, where splitting within the retinal layers occurs.

MACULAR EDEMA

Optical Coherence Tomography is very useful in detecting and evaluating macular edema. An increase of retinal thickness can be detected in diabetic retinopathy[4], vein occlusion or after cataract surgery and Optical Coherence Tomography can be proven invaluable in the follow-up of those patients. In cystoid macula edema large cysts of low reflectivity located within the nuclear retinal layers are detected. Several other abnormalities coexisting with macular edema can be detected, such as epiretinal membranes, lamellar holes, retinal exudates, neovascularization etc. We must remember that changes in retinal thickness in the macula don't always correlate with visual acuity.

RETINAL PIGMENT EPITHELIUM – CHORIOCAPILLARIES

Pigment accumulation in retinal pigment epithelium provides the high reflectivity of the retinal pigment epithelium – choriocapillaries complex causing shadowing of the underlying choroid. Scars and fibrosis in this layer appear like a highly reflective and thickened posterior reflective area. Hypopig-

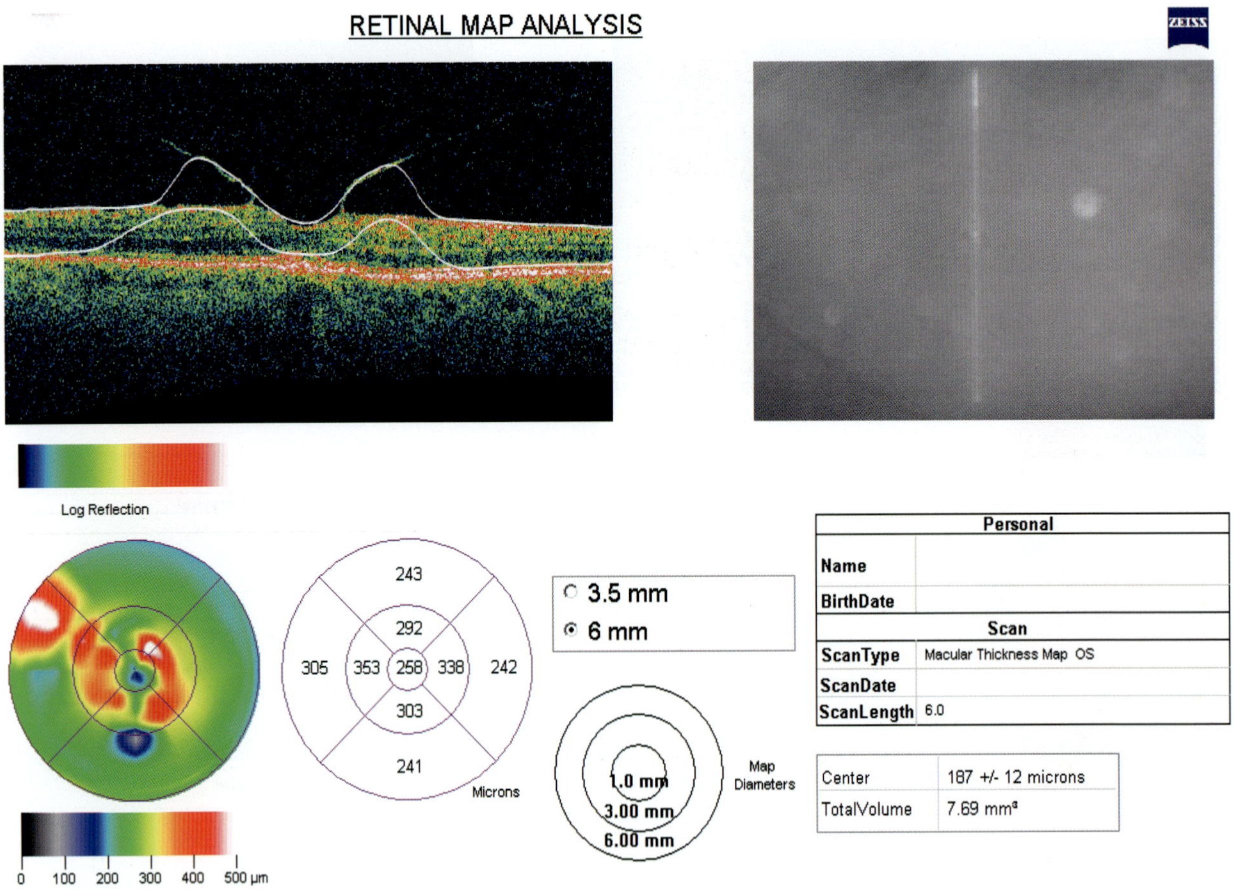

Fig. 19: In cases of vitreoretinal traction or strong signal from the vitreous, the posterior hyaloid may be incorrectly identified by the software of Optical Coherence Tomography as the inner retinal surface resulting in mistakes in the retinal thickness and in the retinal map calculations.

mentation and retinal pigment epithelium atrophy leads to decreased reflectivity, associated with window defect and high intensity signals from the deeper layers. Soft drusen are detected as highly reflective thickening of the photoreceptors – retinal pigment epithelium – choriocapillaries complex with shallow soft margins and lower reflectivity and shadowing of the underlying tissues compared to a retinal pigment epithelium detachment.

NERVE FIBER LAYER AND OPTIC DISC

Optical Coherence Tomography consists of an examination method capable in assisting in the diagnosis, management and follow-up of patients suffering from neurodegenerative diseases such as glaucoma[1]. The study of the nerve fiber layer around the optic disc is important for the diagnosis and follow-up of the glaucomatous patient. The nerve fiber layer is visible as a thick area of high reflectivity in the inner retina around the optic disc. It is automatically detected by the software using special algorithms, enabling the calculation of the nerve fiber layer thickness and performing mapping of the peripapillary area. Optical Coherence Tomography can also perform a topographic map of the optic nerve head[10]. Powerful algorithms calculate the cupping, dimensions, volume and area of the neuroretinal rim, diameter and other optic disc parameters that are important to the ophthalmologist in evaluating glaucoma progression[8].

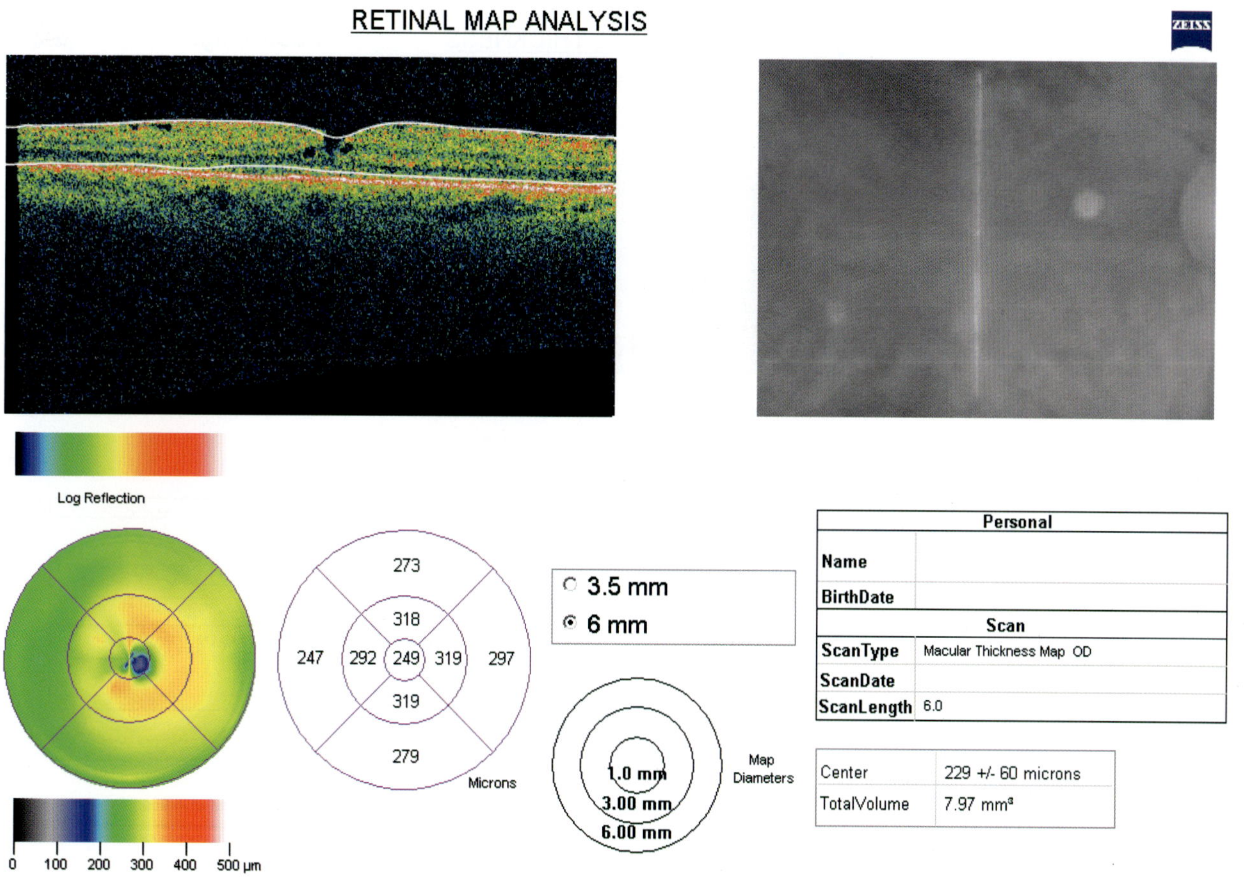

Fig. 20: In cases of lamellar macular hole the software of Optical Coherence Tomography often cannot correctly identify the abrupt and uneven foveal depression resulting in mistakes in the retinal thickness and in the retinal map calculations.

IMAGE QUALITY

Optical Coherence Tomography contains powerful algorithms to enable us to acquire quantitative information from its images. However, those images must be of good quality, because otherwise the calculations that Optical Coherence Tomography performs may be wrong. In cases of media opacities or out of focus images, we observe a weak detection with a low intensity signal backscattering from the retinal layers, even from those that normally would be of high reflectivity like the retinal pigment epithelium – choriocapillaries layer *(figure 17)*. The same happens when the pupil blocks part of the incident light *(figure 11)*. In that case we must reposition the light beam to coincide with the optical axis of the eye or repeat the scanning. When the patient loses fixation or closes his eyes during the examination then sharp image alterations or interruptions on the transverse axis are detected, which cannot be rectified *(figures 10, 12)*. Consequently, special attention is needed at the patient's fixation during scanning.

Attention is also needed when applying the several analysis protocols that are available by Optical Coherence Tomography. All calculations and topographic maps generated by the software are based on the automatic determination of tissue boundaries by the software. Most of the times the automatic determination by the software is correct and all calculations are precise. However, there are diseases that can create problems in automatically determining tissue boundaries. One such example is the epiretinal membrane because, by protruding from the retinal surface, it can incorrectly be identified by the software as the inner retinal surface *(figure 18)*, resulting in errors to the retinal thickness and topographic map calcula-

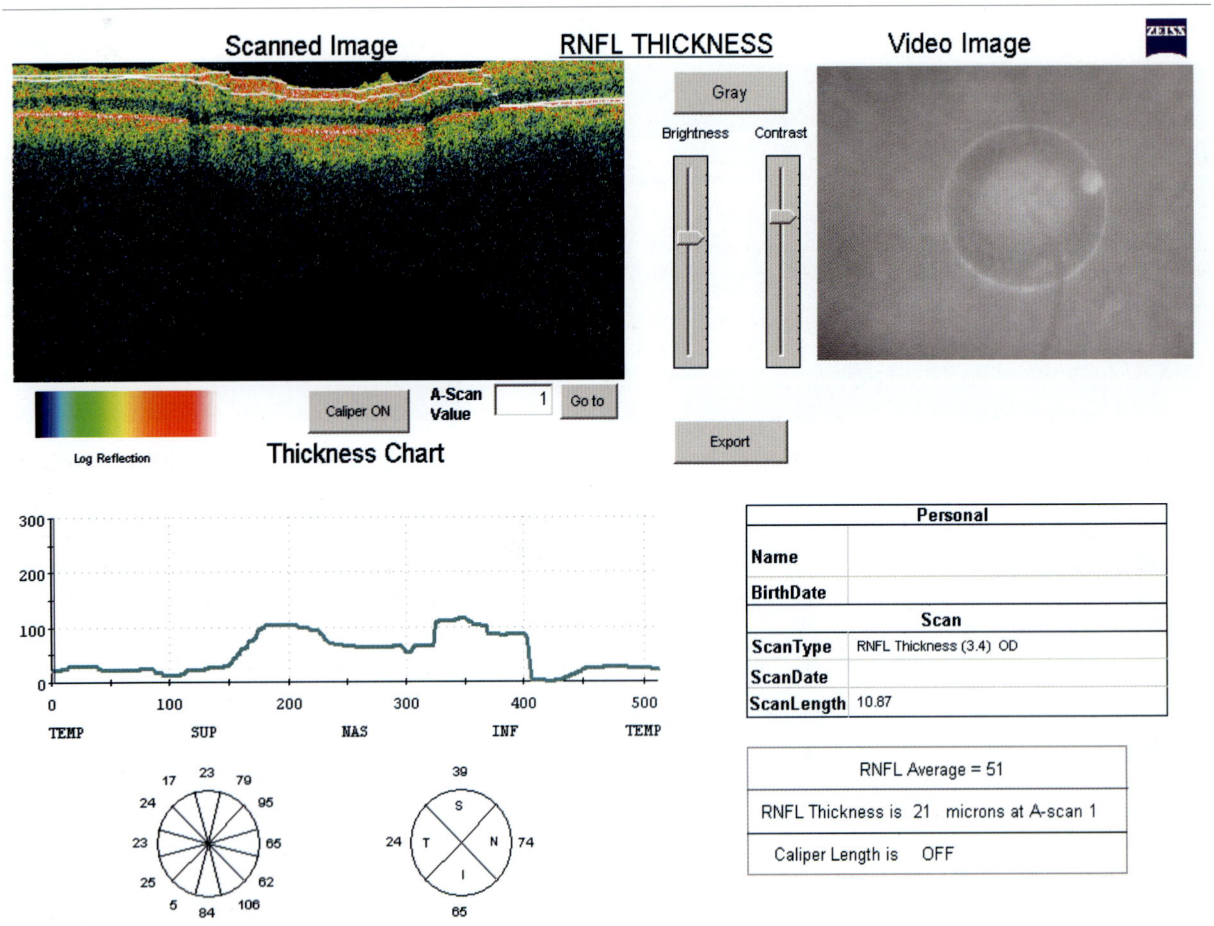

Fig. 21: In glaucoma the inner and outer limits of the nerve fiber layer around the optic disc may be incorrectly identified by the software of Optical Coherence Tomography resulting in mistakes in the peripapillary retinal nerve fiber layer thickness calculations.

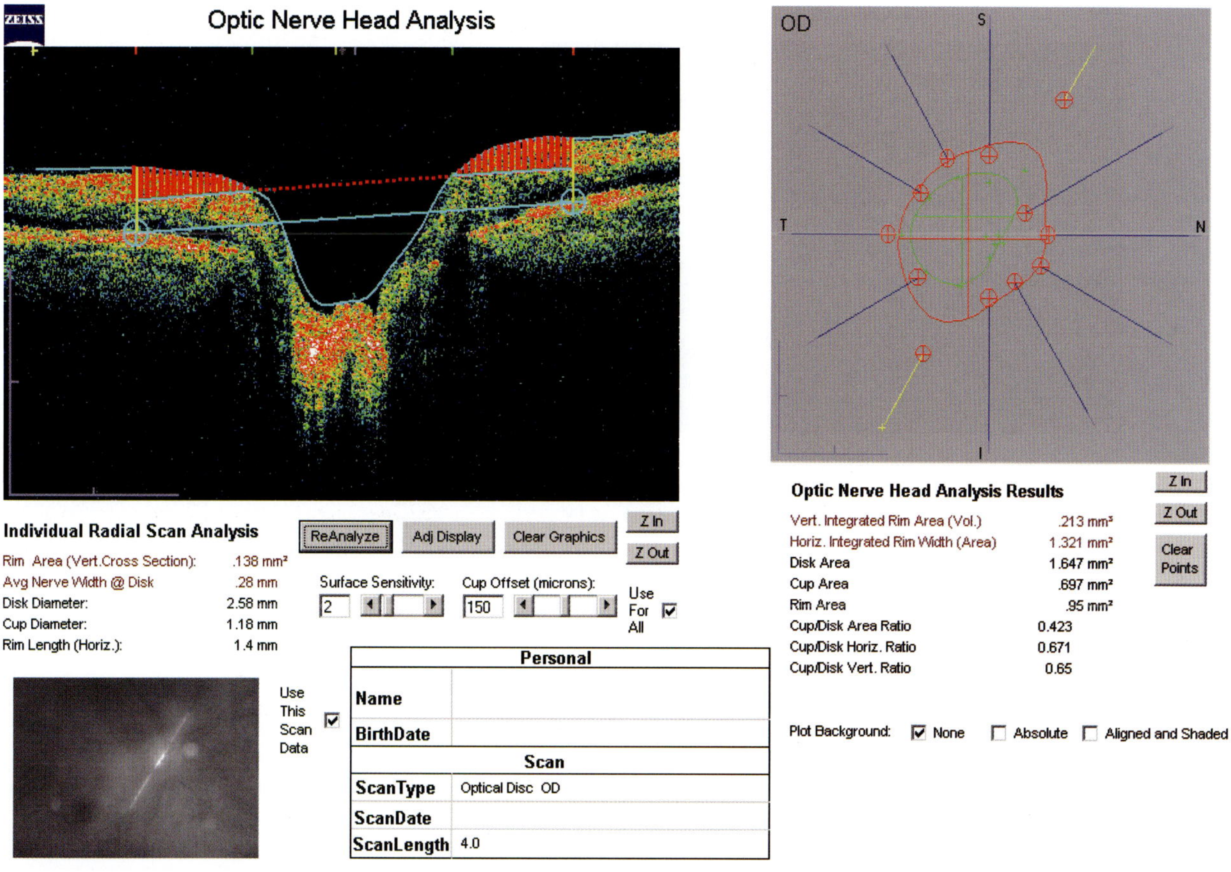

Fig. 22: The borders of the optic disc may be incorrectly identified by the software of Optical Coherence Tomography resulting in mistakes in all the parameters calculated by the optic nerve head analysis protocol.

tions. Additionally, in patients with vitreoretinal traction and a strong delineation of the posterior hyaloid, the vitreous can mistakenly be identified as the inner retinal surface *(figure 19)*. The same problem can appear in lamellar macular holes because the software cannot follow the irregular and deep foveal impression created by the membrane *(figure 20)*, resulting in errors in the determination of the retinal shape and thickness at the fovea.

The same errors can appear in the evaluation of the glaucomatous patient. The inner and outer boundaries of the nerve fiber layer around the optic disc can be incorrectly identified resulting in errors in the nerve fiber layer thickness measurement *(figure 21)*. Wrongly set optic disc margins can result in errors to the optic nerve head topographic map and the dimensions of the optic disc *(figures 22, 23)* and vitreous opacities may contribute to the miscalculation of the volume and area of the optic disc rim *(figure 24)*.

In some cases the examiner may be able to correct the software errors, as for example when there is an incorrect determination of the optic disc margins, by manually repositioning the margins to the correct position. However, in most cases this may not be possible and the examiner must be experienced enough to identify the errors made by the software. In those cases, the examiner must repeat the scanning until he is satisfied that the images are of good quality and properly delineated or if this is not possible, then he must be prepared to manually calculate the appropriate parameters. Finally, it must be noted that we cannot draw definitive conclusions regarding the correct diagnosis based only on one or two images of the software. In most cases a complete evaluation of the patient by an experienced examiner is required.

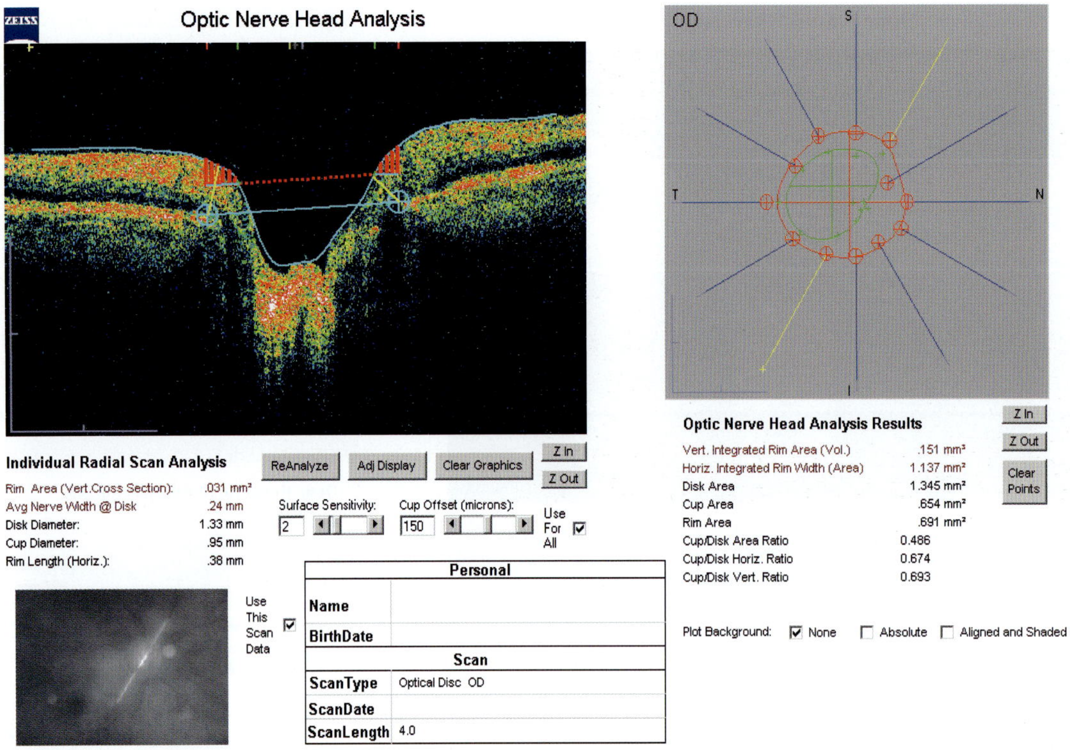

Fig. 23: By manually redefining the borders of the optic disc the software of Optical Coherence Tomography is able to correctly show all the parameters calculated by the optic nerve head analysis protocol.

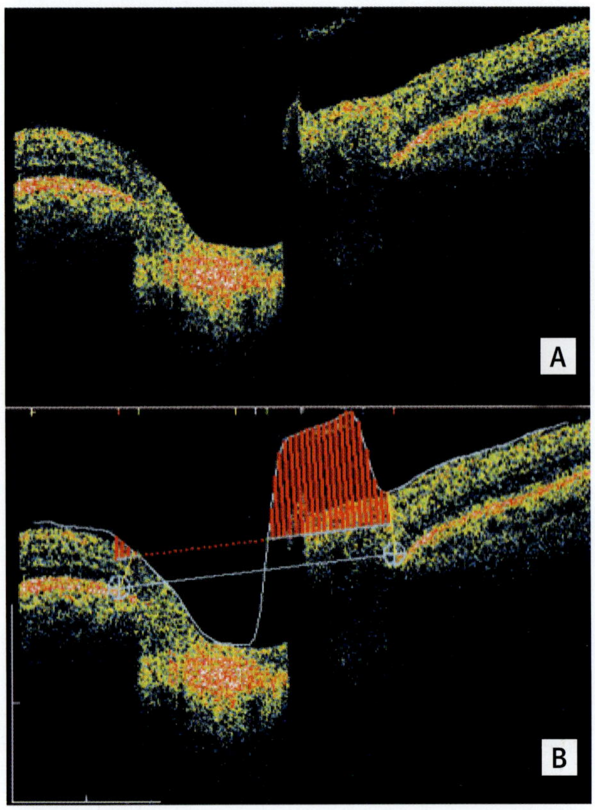

Fig. 24: (A) Cross sectional image of the optic nerve head as obtained by Optical Coherence Tomography. Note the vitreous floaters located in front of the optic disc. (B) The software of Optical Coherence Tomography incorrectly identifies the vitreous floaters as the inner retinal surface resulting in mistakes in all the parameters calculated by the optic nerve head analysis protocol.

INTRODUCTION

1. Bowd C, Zangwill LM, Berry CC, Blumenthal EZ, Vasile C, Sanchez-Galeana C, Bosworth CF, Sample PA, Weinreb RN. Detecting early glaucoma by assessment of retinal nerve fibre layer thickness and visual function. Invest Ophthalmol Vis Sci 2001;42(9):1993-2003.

2. Drexler W, Morgner U, Ghanta RK, Kartner FX, Schuman JS, Fujimoto JG. Ultrahigh-resolution ophthalmic optical coherence tomography. Nat Med. 2001;7(4):502-7.

3. Fujimoto JG, Brezinski ME, Tearney GJ, Boppart SA, Bouma B, Hee MR, Southern JF, Swanson EA. Optical biopsy and imaging using optical coherence tomography. Nat Med. 1995;1(9):970-2.

4. Hee MR, Puliafito CA, Duker JS, Reichel E, Coker JG, Wilkins JR, Schuman JS, Swanson EA, Fujimoto JG. Topography of diabetic macular edema with optical coherence tomography. Ophthalmology 1998;105(2):360-70.

5. Hee MR, Puliafito CA, Wong C, Duker JS, Reichel E, Schuman JS, Swanson EA, Fujimoto JG. Optical coherence tomography of macular holes. Ophthalmology 1995;102(5):748-56.

6. Huang D, Swanson EA, Lin CP, Schuman JS, Stinson WG, Chang W, Hee MR, Flotte T, Gregory K, Puliafito CA, et al. Optical coherence tomography. Science 1991;254(5035):1178-81.

7. Puliafito CA, Hee MR, Lin CP, Reichel E, Schuman JS, Duker JS, Izatt JA, Swanson EA, Fujimoto JG. Imaging of macular diseases with optical coherence tomography. Ophthalmology 1995;102(2):217-29.

8. Schuman JS, Pedut-Kloizman T, Hertzmark E, Hee MR, Wilkins JR, Coker JG, Puliafito CA, Fujimoto JG, Swanson EA. Reproducibility of nerve fibre layer thickness measurements using optical coherence tomography. Ophthalmology 1996;103(11):1889-98.

9. Schuman JS, Puliafito CA, Fujimoto JG. Optical Coherence Tomography of ocular diseases. Thorofare, NJ: SLACK Incorporated; 2004.

10. Schuman JS, Wollstein G, Farra T, Hertzmark E, Aydin A, Fujimoto JG, Paunescu LA. Comparison of optic nerve head measurements obtained by optical coherence tomography and confocal scanning laser ophthalmoscopy. Am J Ophthalmol 2003;135(4):504-12.

11. Tearney GJ, Brezinski ME, Bouma BE, Boppart SA, Pitris C, Southern JF, Fujimoto JG. In vivo endoscopic optical biopsy with optical coherence tomography. Science 1997;276(5321):2037-9.

CHAPTER 2

AGE-RELATED MACULAR DEGENERATION AND ALLIED DISEASES

Ioannis Emfietzoglou

Age-related macular degeneration constitutes the commonest cause of visual loss in individuals over 60 years of age in the developed countries. Many factors – smoking, sunlight exposure and decreased levels of antioxidants – have been incriminated, but the cause seems to be multifactorial. There are various clinical forms of age-related macular degeneration that are classified in two types: the dry or non-neovascular and the wet or neovascular age-related macular degeneration.

The **dry type** is the mildest form of age-related macular degeneration. It is characterized by: a) the presence of drusen, which are deposits of eosinophilic material between the basal lamina of the retinal pigment epithelium and Bruch's membrane and b) areas of focal atrophy of the retinal pigment epithelium – Bruch's membrane – choriocapillaries complex. These areas, if joined together, coalesce and form the geographic atrophy of the macula, which constitutes the latest stage of the dry type age- related macular degeneration.

In Optical Coherence Tomography *drusen* are illustrated as localized thickenings of the retinal pigment epithelium – Bruch's membrane – choriocapillaries complex with preservation of the architecture of the retinal layers and the foveal depression and absence of intraretinal or subretinal fluid. Several soft drusen may rarely get together to form a localized solid "drusenoid" detachment of the retinal pigment epithelium. This is illustrated as a smooth elevation of the retinal pigment epithelium that masks the high reflectivity of the drusen material.

In *geographic atrophy* both the retinal layers and the retinal pigment epithelium – Bruch's membrane – choriocapillaries complex are thin, allowing an increased penetration of the light in the deeper layers of the choroid, thus producing enhanced reflectivity from this layer. The borders of the geographic atrophy are well-defined[4-5].

The **wet or neovascular type** of age-related macular degeneration is characterized by a choroidal neovascular membrane under the retinal pigment epithelium (type I choroidal neovascularization) with or without a retinal pigment epithelium detachment.

Serous detachment of the retinal pigment epithelium due to age-related macular degeneration is present in 1.5% of newly diagnosed patients with exudative age-related macular degeneration. Optical Coherence Tomography shows a smooth, dome-shaped elevation of the retinal pigment epithelium that appears optically empty. The deeper choroidal layers are well illustrated, as opposed to cases of hemorrhagic retinal pigment epithelium detachment, where there is shadowing of the choroidal layers due to the obstruction of the light signal from the subretinal blood.

The choroidal neovascular membrane, which derives from the choriocapillaries, is initially located under the retinal pigment epithelium and finally infiltrates into the subretinal space through a dehiscence of the outer part of Bruch's membrane. According to the fluoroangiographic appearance choroidal neovascular membranes are divided in two patterns, the classic and the occult.

The minority of cases belong to the *classic choroidal neovascularization*, which is well delineated during the early phases of the angiogram and is characterized by a progressive leakage of dye in the middle and late phases of the angiogram. Optical Coherence Tomography reveals an irregular, fusiform or nodular enlargement of the retinal pigment epithelium – Bruch's membrane – choriocapillaries complex with relatively well defined borders that correspond to the borders of the choroidal neovascularization.

The *occult choroidal neovascularization*, which is not clearly delineated in fluorescein angiography, is distinguished in two subtypes, the fibrovascular retinal pigment epithelium detachment and the late leakage of undetermined source. The *fibrovascular retinal pigment epithelium detachment* is characterized by stippled hyperfluorescence within 1 to 2 minutes after the fluorescein injection and dye leakage in the late phase. Optical Coherence Tomography shows an elevation of the retinal pigment epithelium – Bruch's membrane – choriocapillaries with a mild reflection to the choroidal layers. Sometimes the occult choroidal neovascularization is located at the edges of the elevated retinal pigment epithelium[14]. The *late leakage of undetermined source* is characterized by fluorescein leakage at the retinal pigment epithelium level only in the late phase of fluorescein angiography. The Optical Coherence Tomography image of the late leakage of undetermined source is not typical. It is illustrated as a diffuse, irregular thickening of the retinal pigment epithelium – Bruch's membrane – choriocapillaries complex and, occasionally, as small retinal pigment epithelium detachments that are not visible in fluorescein angiography[3].

The presence of a choroidal neovascularization may be accompanied by other secondary retinal features. The serous leakage from a choroidal neovascularization produces an intraretinal or subretinal fluid accumulation. The *subretinal fluid* is illustrated as an optically empty space between the retinal layers and the retinal pigment epithelium – Bruch's membrane – choriocapillaries complex. The *intraretinal fluid* can be either diffuse, illustrated as thickening of the retinal layers, or cystoid, illustrated as round, optically empty spaces (cysts) within the retinal layers. Optical Coherence Tomography observations show a significant correlation between cystoid macular edema and classic choroidal neovascularization. The retinal layers' architecture and the physiologic foveal depression can be altered by the presence of choroidal neovascularization.

Haemorrhages are another usual finding in exudative age-related macular degeneration. These can be located under the retinal pigment epithelium or under the retina. In the first case the retinal pigment epithelium appears elevated but with normal thickness and with an underlying area of high reflectivity that corresponds to the haemorrhage. The choroidal signal is weaker because of the shadow to the underlying tissues. In the second case, the haemorrhage is illustrated as an area of high reflectivity between the elevated retinal layers and the retinal pigment epithelium, the latter appearing thin because of the shadowing effect from the high signal of the haemorrhage[17].
The *fibrous tissue*, which is a component of the choroidal

neovascularization, is illustrated as a hyperereflective thickening of the retinal pigment epithelium – Bruch's membrane – choriocapillaries complex.

Optical Coherence Tomography helps in determining the macular morphology in cases where choroidal neovascular membrane exists. It also contributes to the estimation of the response to treatment and to the follow-up of treated patients

In studying age-related macular degeneration cases fluorescein and indocyanine green angiography have also their specific roles. These techniques help in the diagnosis and differentiation of the various choroidal neovascular membrane types, such as retinal angiomatous proliferation and idiopathic polypoidal choroidal vasculopathy, which cannot be distinguished by Optical Coherence Tomography.

During the course of the disease the angiographic appearance of the macula may be confusing, mainly because of staining of scar tissues[2,12]. In such cases Optical Coherence Tomography is invaluable in detecting with accuracy the presence or not of intraretinal and subretinal fluid and therefore in deciding the continuation of further treatment[15].

Optical Coherence Tomography is very important in the follow-up of patients who have been treated with photodynamic therapy or intravitreous injections for choroidal neovascularization. In these cases repeated fluorescein angiograms are not so useful in detecting any remaining leakage because of the co-existing hyperfluorescence from the fibrous tissue staining and the presence or not of intraretinal or subretinal fluid can be revealed by Optical Coherence Tomography. In case of fluid detection, which is indicative of active choroidal neovascularization, Optical Coherence Tomography offers the possibility for quantitative comparison to previous examinations, which is very useful in determining the most appropriate therapeutic option. The absence of intraretinal or subretinal fluid indicates no choroidal neovascularization leakage[11,13].

IDIOPATHIC POLYPOIDAL CHOROIDAL VASCULOPATHY

This disease constitutes an age-related macular degeneration variant. Indocyanine green angiography has played a major role in idiopathic polypoidal choroidal vasculopathy determination, by illustrating a network of dilated vessels with polypoidal aneurysmatic endings, located at the inner choroidal layers that may be clinically visible as orange spherical polypoidal formations. A serous or haemorrhagic detachment of the retina or the retinal pigment epithelium is also often observed.
As the polyps are located in the choriocapillaries layer, it is often difficult for them to be illustrated on Optical Coherence Tomography, especially if a haemorrhagic or exudative detachment of the retina or the retinal pigment epithelium co-exists, because of the attenuation of the signal beyond the choriocapillaries. However, occasionally these orange choroidal polyps are visible as highly reflective structures through the choriocapillaries layer[10].

RETINAL ANGIOMATOUS PROLIFERATION

This is another age-related macular degeneration subcategory, in which the neovascular tissue is generated from the retina, not from the choroid, and it infiltrates the deeper layers at a later stage[1]. The following stages can be described:

Stage I: Intraretinal neovascularization. The vascular hyperplasia is located in the inner and medial retinal layers and can be accompanied by small retinal haemorrhages, retinal edema and/or retinal vessel anastomoses.

Stage II: Subretinal neovascularization. The neovascular tissue is extended under the photoreceptors' layer and a serous detachment of the retina or/and the retinal pigment epithelium can also be observed.

Stage III: Choroidal neovascularization. The neovascular issue infiltrates the retinal pigment epithelium and is extended into the choroid[7].

IDIOPATHIC CHOROIDAL NEOVASCULARIZATION

Idiopathic choroidal neovascular membrane is characterized by the absence of signs of age-related macular degeneration, intraocular inflammation, atrophic retinal scar, drusen, tumor or other abnormality[6].

The Macular Photocoagulation Study (MPS) - Idiopathic Neovascularization Study and the Idiopathic Neovascularization Study-Krypton showed that thermal laser therapy is effective on extrafoveal and parafoveal idiopathic choroidal neovascular membranes with regression rates of 34% and 22% respectively.

Photodynamic therapy in subfoveal idiopathic choroidal neovascularization has been studied retrospectively in 8 patients aged 25 to 53 years. In 75% of these cases the visual acuity remained the same or improved. According to the authors[15], the positive results may have been due to: a) the fact that idiopathic choroidal neovascular membranes are generally of the classic type, which respond better to photodynamic therapy and, as it has been observed, they can shrink under the macula b) the high tissue regeneration capability of the young people c) the fact that young people visit the ophthalmologist upon the first symptoms.

Encouraging results have also been observed after intravitreal injection of bevacizumab[8]. There have been reported 3 cases of children aged 11 to 13 years, treated with photodynamic therapy that had stabilization or improvement in their visual acuity[9].

AGE-RELATED MACULAR DEGENERATION

1. Brancato R, Introini U, Pierro L, Setaccioli M Forti M, Bolognesi G, Tremolada G. Optical coherence tomography (OCT) in retinal angiomatous proliferation (RAP). Eur J. Ophthalmol 2002; 12: 467-472.

2. Costa RA, Farah ME, Cardillo JA, Calucci D, Williams GA. Immediate indocyanine green angiography and optical coherence tomography evaluation after photodynamic therapy for subfoveal choroidal neovascularization. Retina 2003; 23: 159-165.

3. Costa RA, Calucci D, Paccola L, Jorge R, Cardillo JA, Castro JC, Scott IU. Occult chorioretinal anastomosis in age-related macular degeneration: a prospective study by optical coherence tomography. Am J Ophthalmol 2005; 140: 107-116.

4. Coscas G, Coscas F, Zourdani A, Soubrane G. Optical coherence tomography and ARMD. J Fr Ophthalmol 2004; 27: 3S7-30.

5. Hee MR, Baumal CR, Puliafito CA, Duker JS, Reichel E, Wilkins JR, Coker JG, Schuman JS, Swanson EA, Fujimoto JG. Optical coherence tomography in age-related macular degeneration and choroidal neovascularization. Ophthalmology 1996;103:1260-1270.

6. Ho A, Yannuzzi L, Pisicano K, DeRosa J: The natural history of idiopathic subfoveal choroidal neovascularization. Ophthalmology 1995; 102:782-789.

7. Hunter MA, Dunbar MT, Rosenfeld PJ. Retinal angiomatous proliferation: clinical characteristics and treatment options. Optometry 2004;75: 577-588.

8. Mandal S, Garq S, Venkatesh P, Mithal C, Vohra R, Mehrotra A. Intravitreal bevacizumab for subfoveal idiopathic choroidal neovascularization. Arch Ophthalmol 2007;125(11):1487-92.

9. Mimouni K, Bressler S, Bressler N: Photodynamic therapy with verteporfin for subfoveal neovascularization in children. Am J Ophthalmol 2003; 135:900-902.

10. Otsuji T, Takahashi K, Fukushima I, Uyama M. Optical coherence tomographic findings of idiopathic polypoidal choroidal vasculopathy. Ophthalmic Surg Lasers 2000; 31: 210-214.

11. Rogers AH, Martidis A, Greenberg PB, Puliafito Ca. Optical coherence tomography findings following photodynamic therapy of choroidal neovascularization. Am J Ophthalmol 2002; 134: 566-576.

12. Sahni J, Stanga P, Wong D, Harding S. Optical coherence tomography in photodynamic therapy for subfoveal choroidal neovascularization secondary to age related macular degeneration: a cross sectional study. Br J Ophthalmol 2005; 89: 316-320.

13. Salinas-Alaman A, Garcia-Layana A, Maldonado MJ, Sainz-Gomez C, Alvarez –Vidal A. Using optical coherence tomography to monitor photodynamic therapy in age related macular degeneration. Am J Ophthalmol 2005;140: 23-28.

14. Sato T, Iida T, Hagimure N, Koshi S. Correlation of optical coherence tomography with angiography in retinal pigment epithelial detachment associated with age-related macular degeneration. Retina 2004; 24: 910-914.

15. Spaide R, Martin M, Slakter J, Yannuzzi L, Sorenson J, Guyer D, Freund B: Treatment of idiopathic choroidal neovascular lesions using photodynamic therapy with verteporfin. Am J Ophthalmol 2002;134:62-68.

16. Spraul CW, Lang GE, Lang GK. Value of optical coherence tomography in diagnosis of age-related macular degeneration. Correlation of fluorescein angiography and OCT findings. Klin Monatsbl Augenheilkd 1998: 212: 141-148.

17. Theodossiadis GP, Panagiotidis D, Georgalas IG, Moschos M, Theodossiadis PG. Retinal hemorrhage after photodynamic therapy in patients with subfoveal choroidal neovascularization caused by age-related macular degeneration. Graefes Arch Clin Exp Ophthalmol 2003; 24: 13-18.

DRY TYPE AGE-RELATED MACULAR DEGENERATION

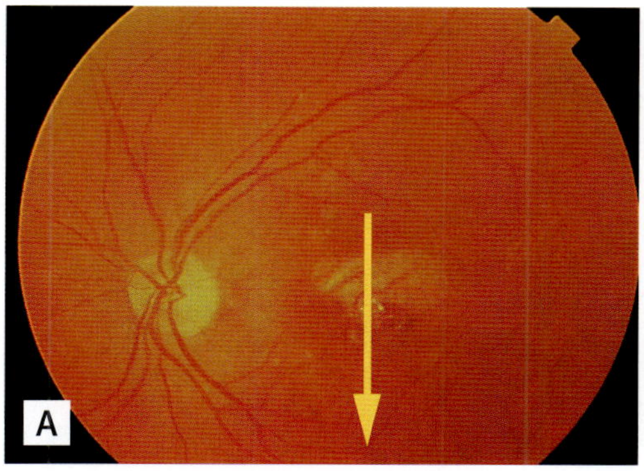

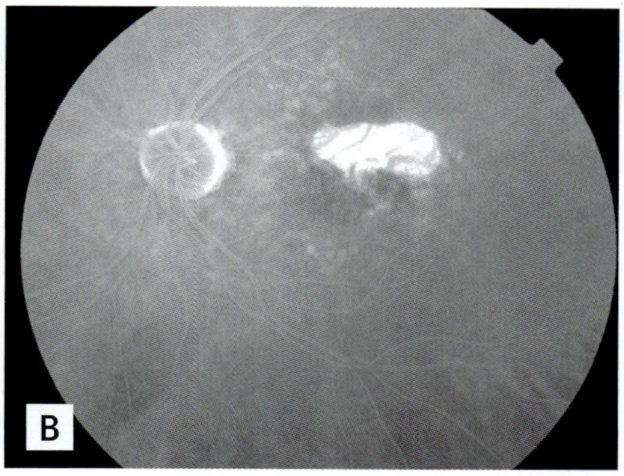

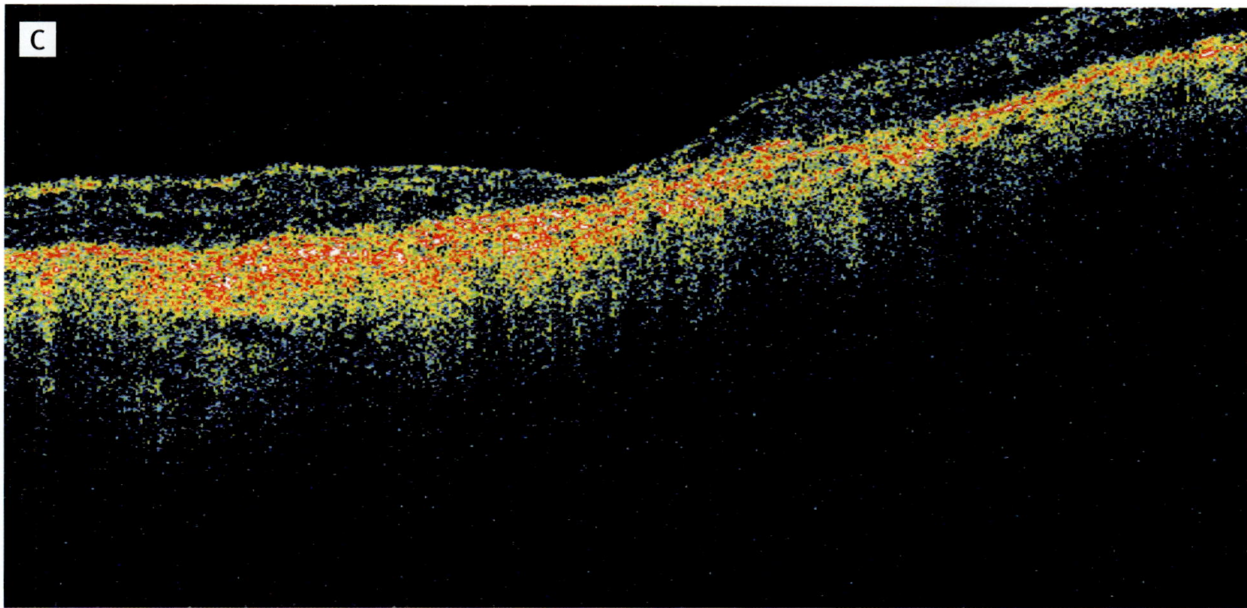

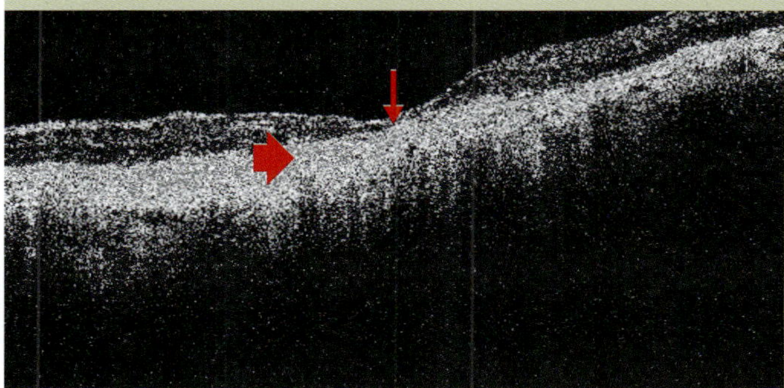

Patient with dry type age-related macular degeneration. A. Geographic atrophy of the macula (the arrow shows the scan direction). B. Window defect type hyperfluorescence corresponding to the area of atrophy. C. There is a diffuse decrease of retinal thickness in the area of the fovea and around it (small arrow). The increased reflectivity of the retinal pigment epithelium-choriocapillaries complex, that gives the impression of thickening, is due to the decreased light absorption by the thin retinal layers (thick arrow).

DRY TYPE AGE-RELATED MACULAR DEGENERATION

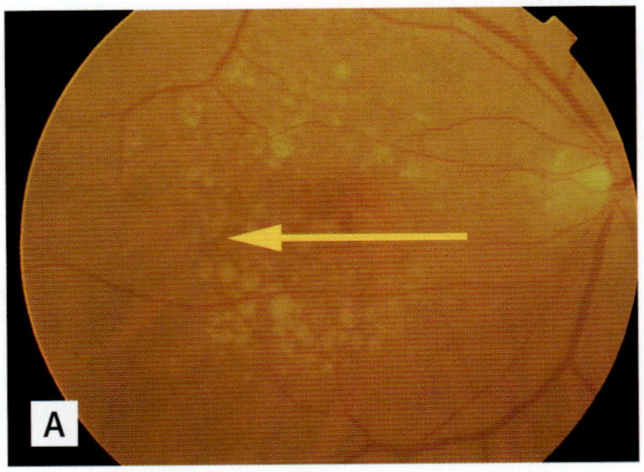

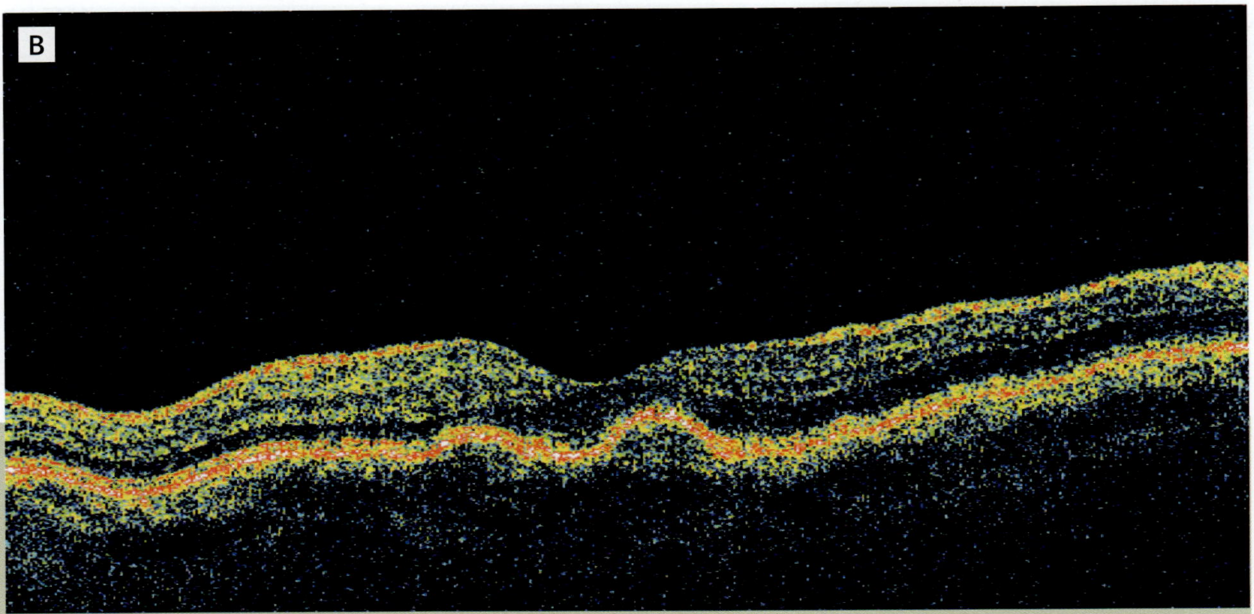

Patient with macular drusen. A. There are multiple soft coalescent drusen in the posterior pole (the arrow shows the scan direction). B. Nodular elevations of the retinal pigment epithelium-choriocapillaries complex, with an underlying high reflective tissue, are illustrated and correspond to drusen located in the fovea (arrows).

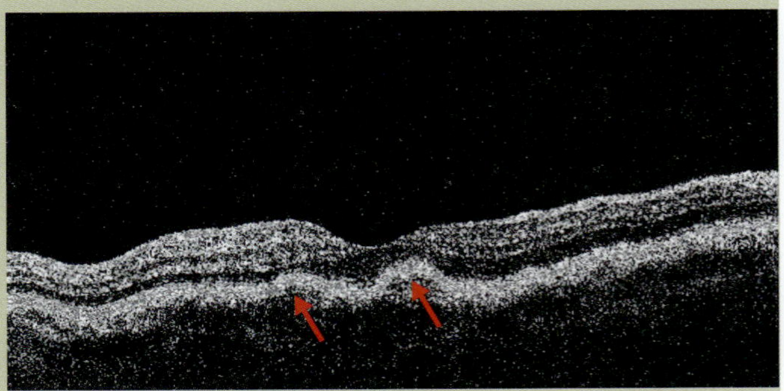

DRY TYPE AGE-RELATED MACULAR DEGENERATION

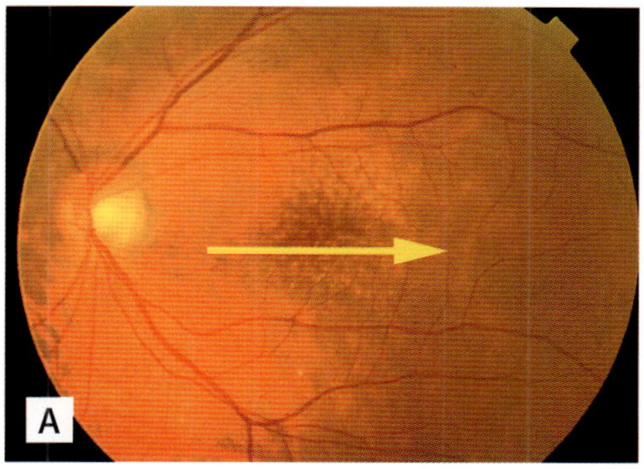

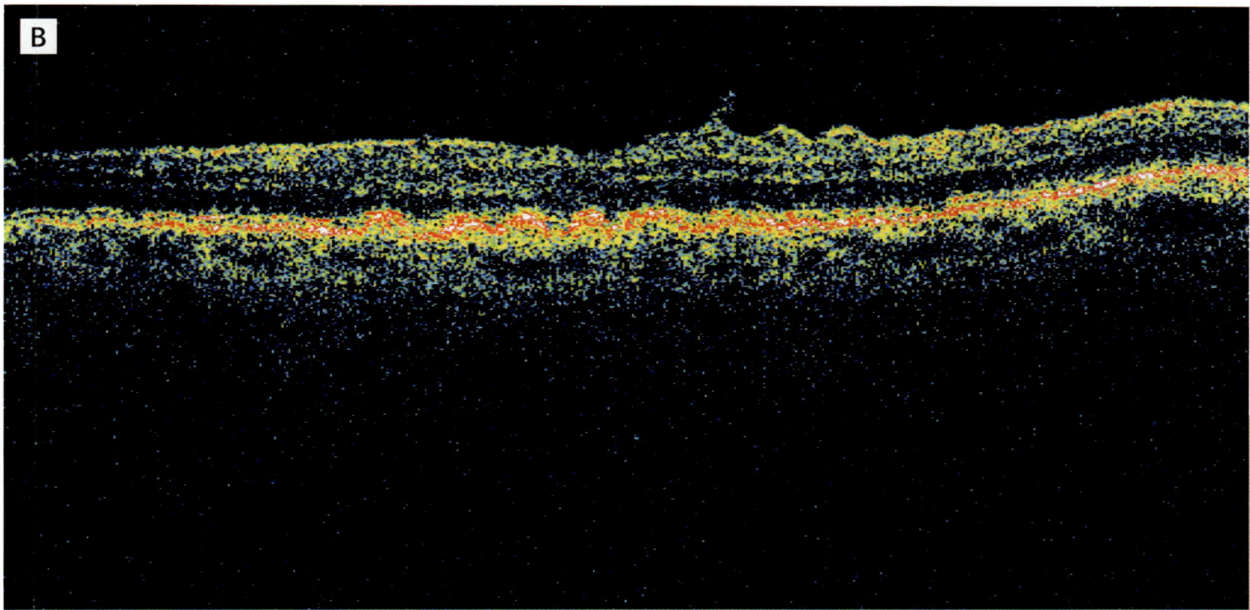

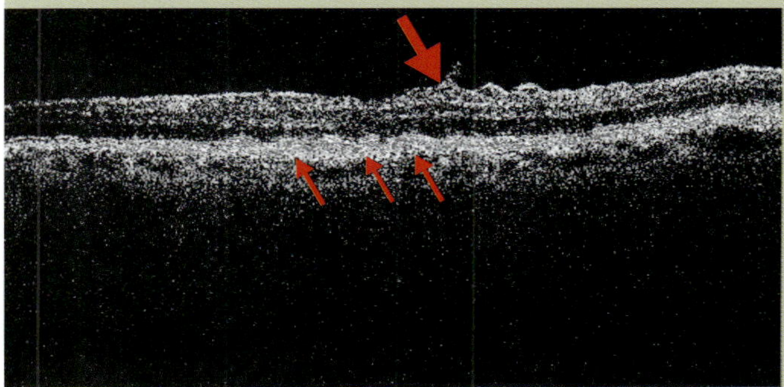

Patient with macular drusen. A There are multiple soft coalescent drusen in the posterior pole (the arrow shows the scan direction). B. Multiple nodular elevations of the retinal pigment epithelium-choriocapillaries layer with an underlying high reflective tissue are illustrated and correspond to macular drusen (small arrows). Notice the thin area of high reflectivity on the surface of the retina and its wrinkling due to an epiretinal membrane (big arrow).

DRY TYPE AGE-RELATED MACULAR DEGENERATION

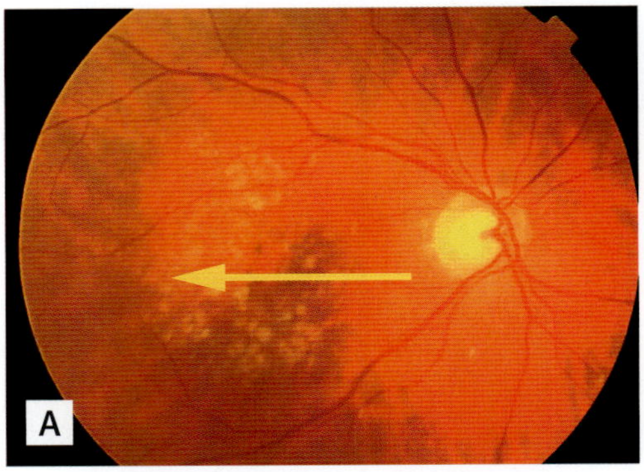

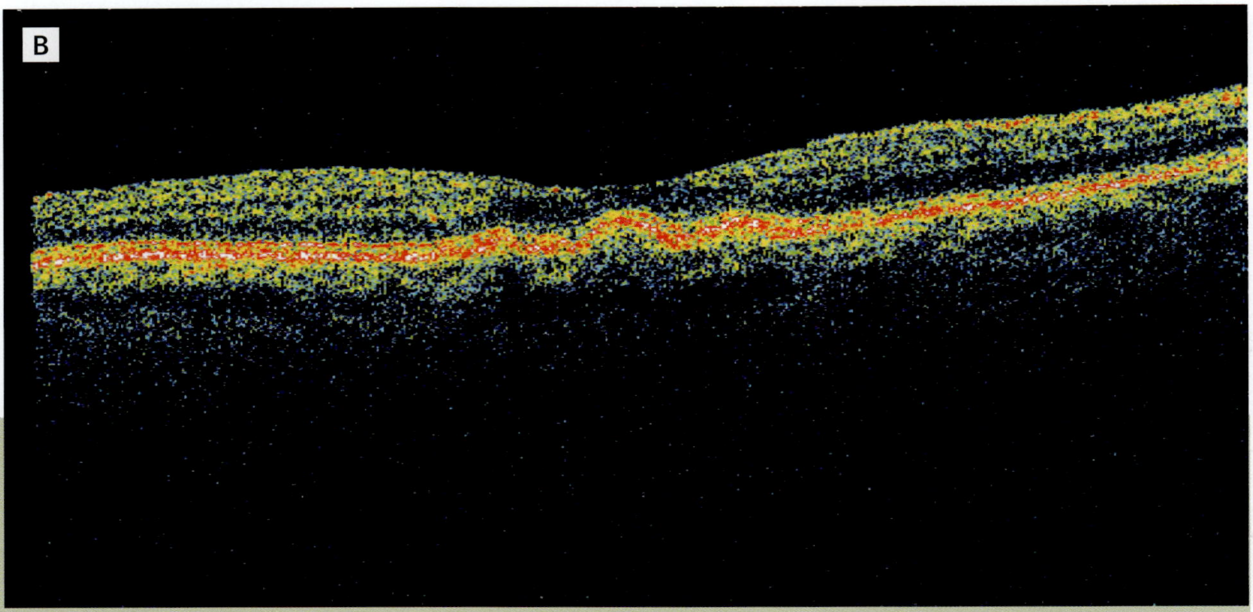

A patient with macular drusen. A. There are multiple soft coalescent drusen in the posterior pole (the arrow shows the scan direction). B. Optical Coherence Tomography depicts multiple nodular elevations of the retinal pigment epithelium-choriocapillaries complex with an underlying tissue of high reflectivity which correspond to macular drusen (arrows).

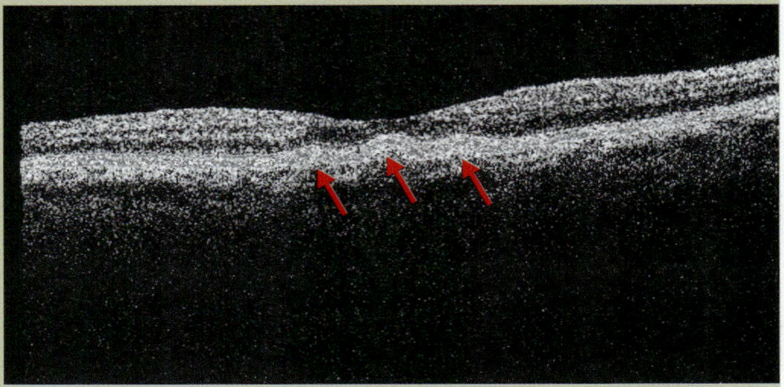

DRY TYPE AGE-RELATED MACULAR DEGENERATION

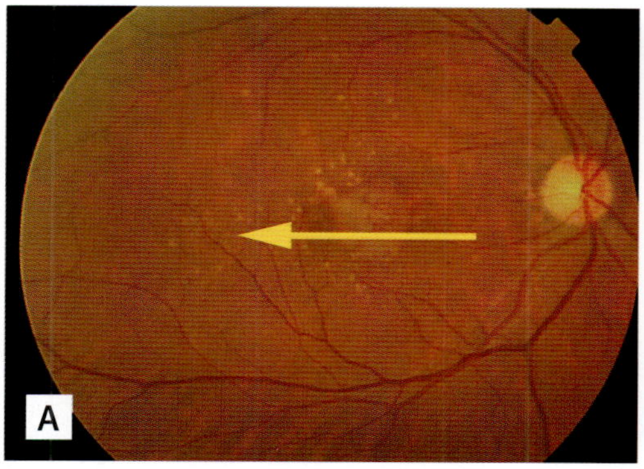

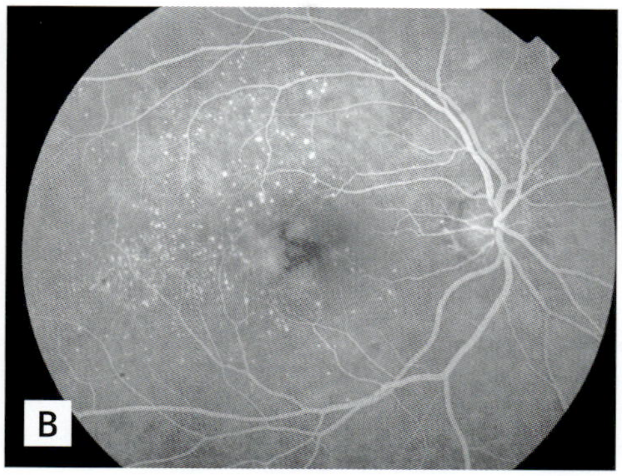

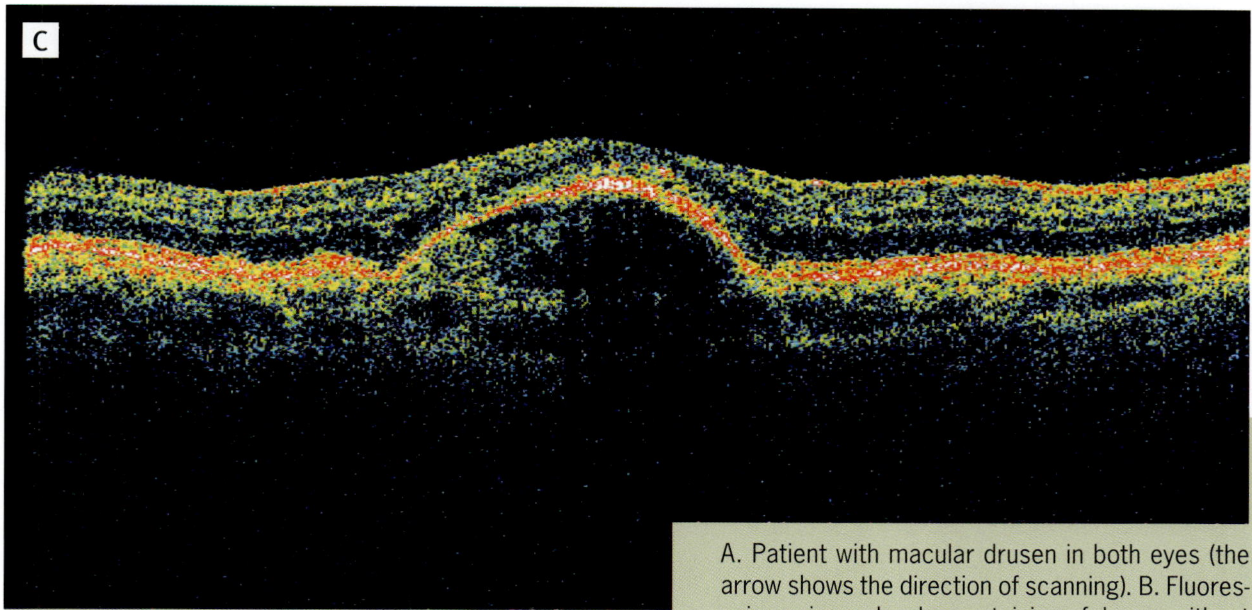

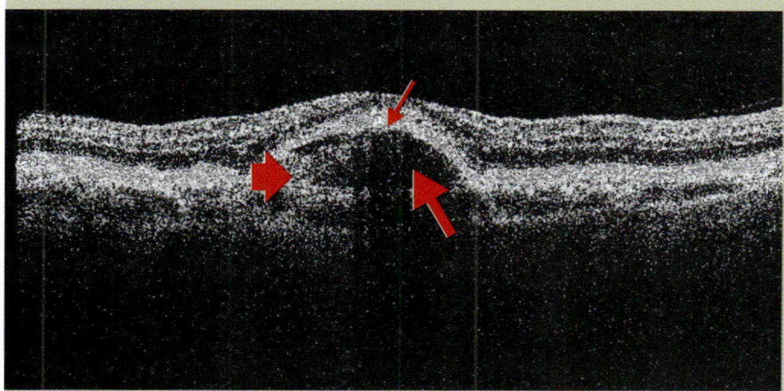

A. Patient with macular drusen in both eyes (the arrow shows the direction of scanning). B. Fluorescein angiography shows staining of drusen without leakage. C. Optical Coherence Tomography shows an elevation of retinal pigment epithelium in the fovea corresponding to a drusenoid retinal pigment epithelium detachment (small arrow). The underlying area is of mixed reflectivity, low because of the retinal pigment epithelium detachment (big arrow) and high because of its solid elements (thick arrow). This mixed condition differentiates the drusenoid retinal pigment epithelium detachment from the serous one, in which the underlying area is evenly optically free.

RETINAL PIGMENT EPITHELIUM RUPTURE

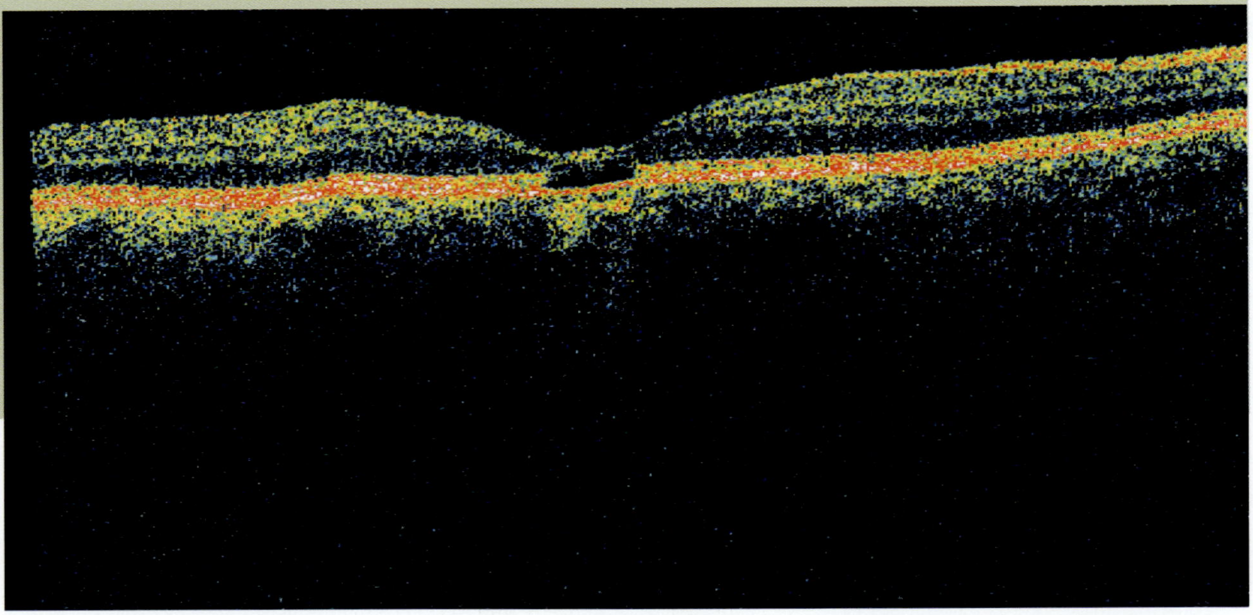

Patient with dry type age related macula degeneration. Notice the retinal pigment epithelium defect at the fovea (arrow). The overlying macula thickness is within normal limits.

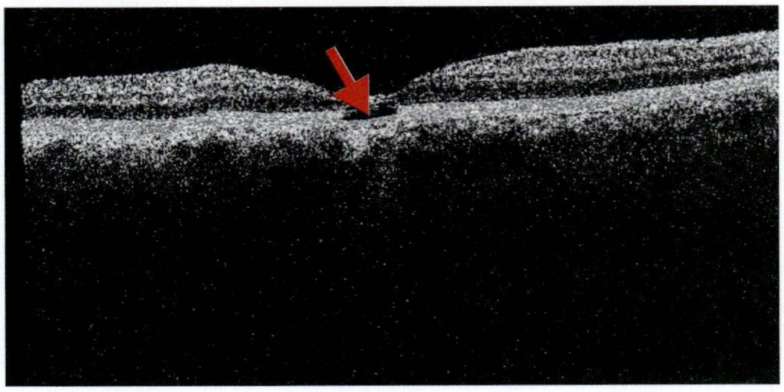

RETINAL PIGMENT EPITHELIUM INTERRUPTION

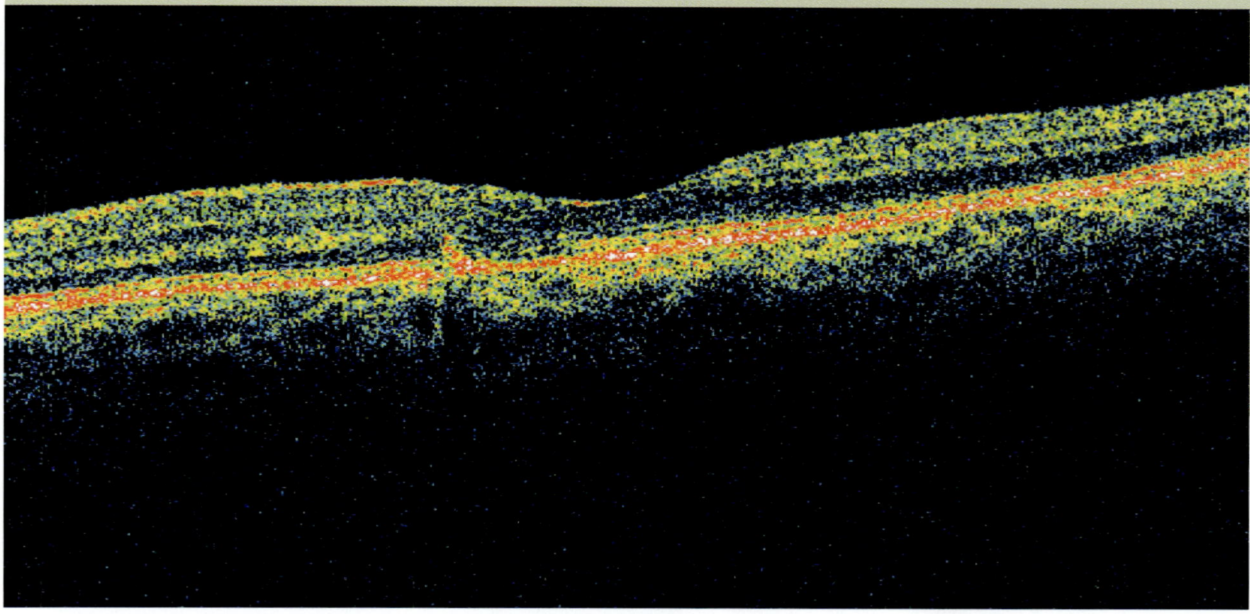

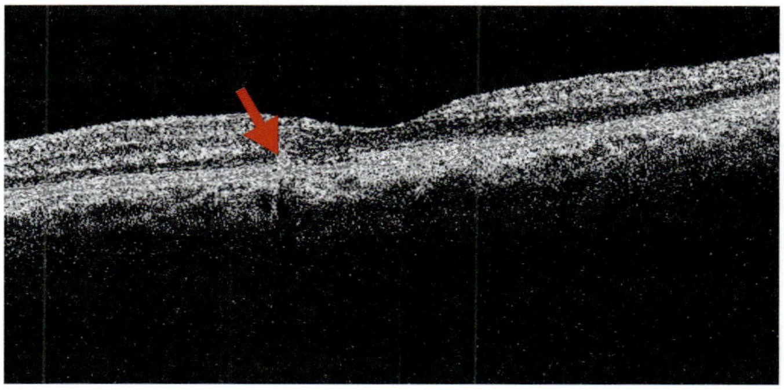

Asymptomatic patient with normal visual acuity. An interruption of the continuity of the retinal pigment epithelium-choriocapillaries complex due to a local break of that layer is illustrated in Optical Coherence Tomography (arrow). The retinal structure has not been disturbed.

RETINAL PIGMENT EPITHELIUM RUPTURE

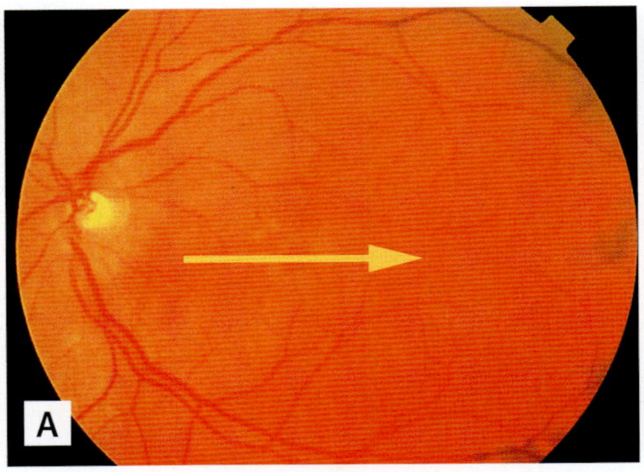

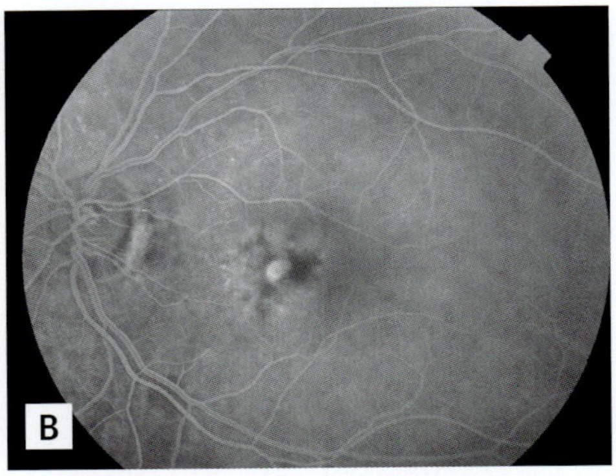

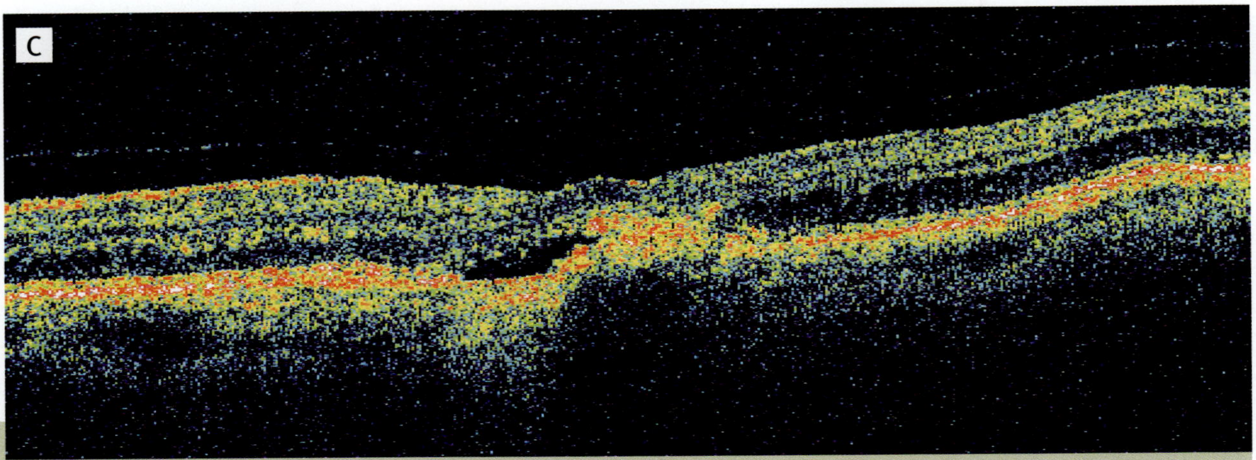

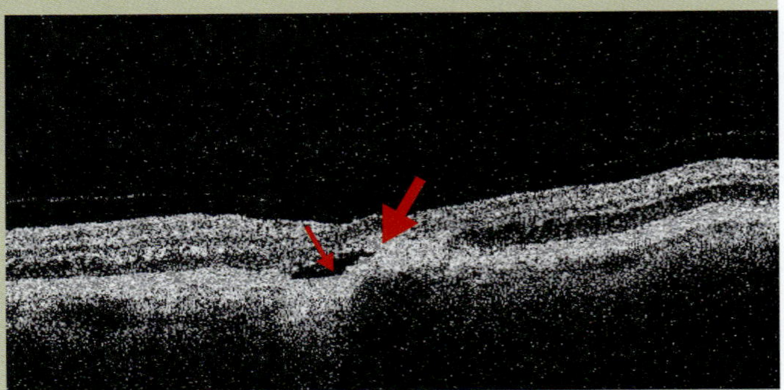

A. An 82 year old patient with low visual acuity in the left eye. Biomicroscopically there is an impression of lamellar macular hole (the arrow shows the scan direction). B. Fluorescein angiography shows hyperfluorescence of that lesion which is adjacent to an area of hypofluorescence temporally. These findings are compatible with a retinal pigment epithelium rip. C. Optical Coherence Tomography shows an area of low reflectivity at the retinal pigment epithelium layer that corresponds to a partial interruption of its integrity which is observed on biomicroscopy (small arrow). There is also an area of high reflectivity above the retinal pigment epithelium in the fovea that corresponds to the folded ripped retinal pigment epithelium (big arrow). In that case, where there is disagreement between biomicroscopy and fluorescein angiography, Optical Coherence Tomography confirms the diagnosis of a retinal pigment epithelium rip.

RETINAL PIGMENT EPITHELIUM RUPTURE

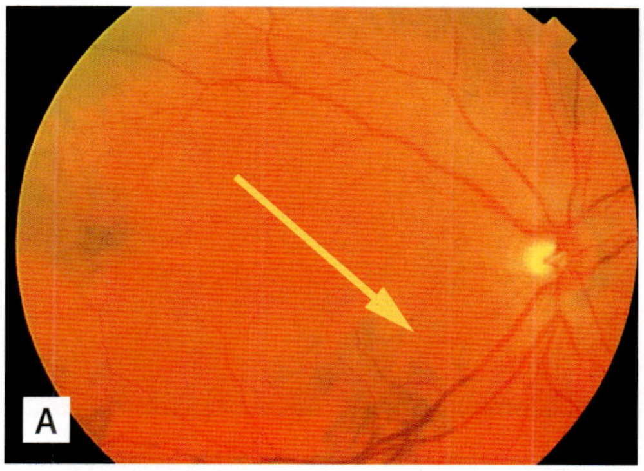

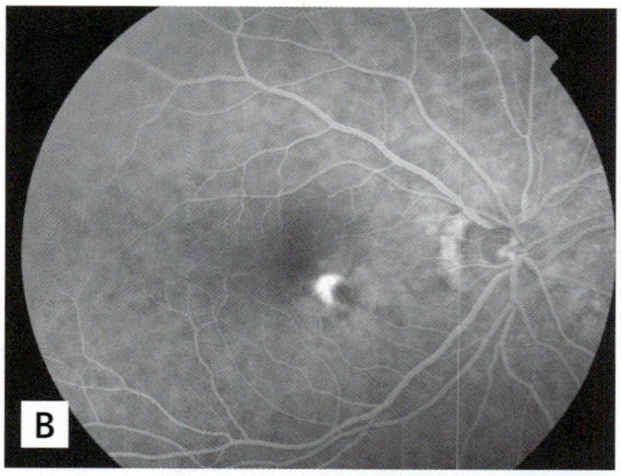

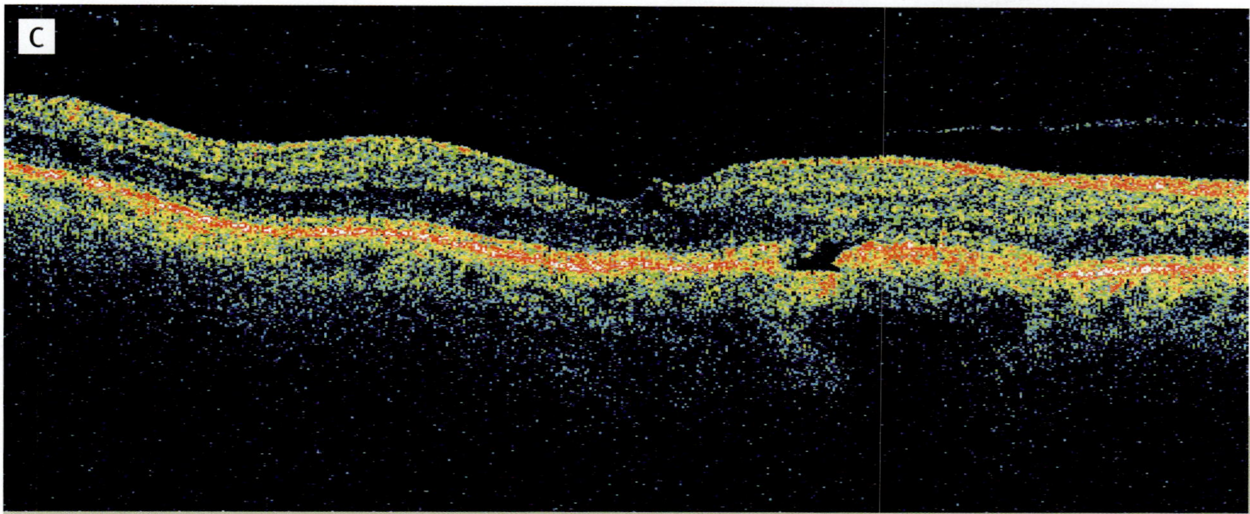

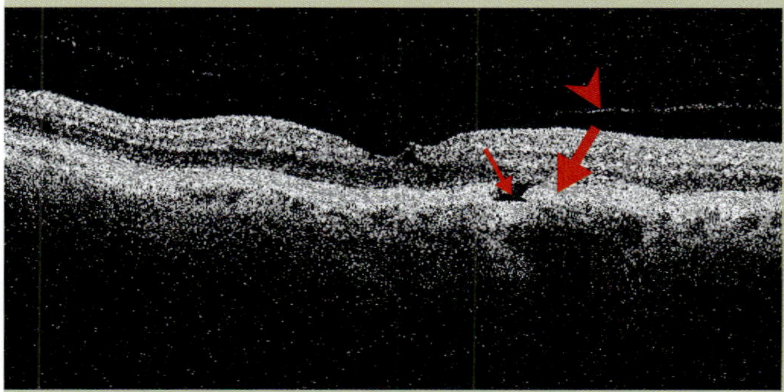

A. The other eye of the patient of page 34 has normal visual acuity, but there is a well delineated moon-shaped area, located inferonasally to the fovea, through which the choroid can be seen more clearly (the arrow shows the scan direction). B. Fluorescein angiography shows hyperfluorescence corresponding to the previous area which is adjacent to a hypofluorescence inferiorly and nasally to it. This finding is compatible with a rip of the retinal pigment epithelium. C. Optical Coherence Tomography shows a low reflectivity area at the retinal pigment epithelium layer that corresponds to a rupture of that layer, as biomicroscopy reveals (small arrow). There is also an area of high reflectivity above the retinal pigment epithelium that corresponds to the angiographic hypofluorescence and that represents the folded ripped part of the retinal pigment epithelium (big arrow). A partial vitreous detachment can also be seen (arrow head).

DRY TYPE AGE-RELATED MACULAR DEGENERATION

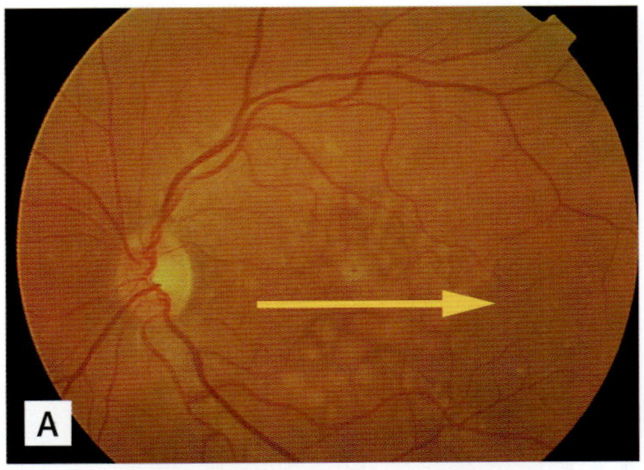

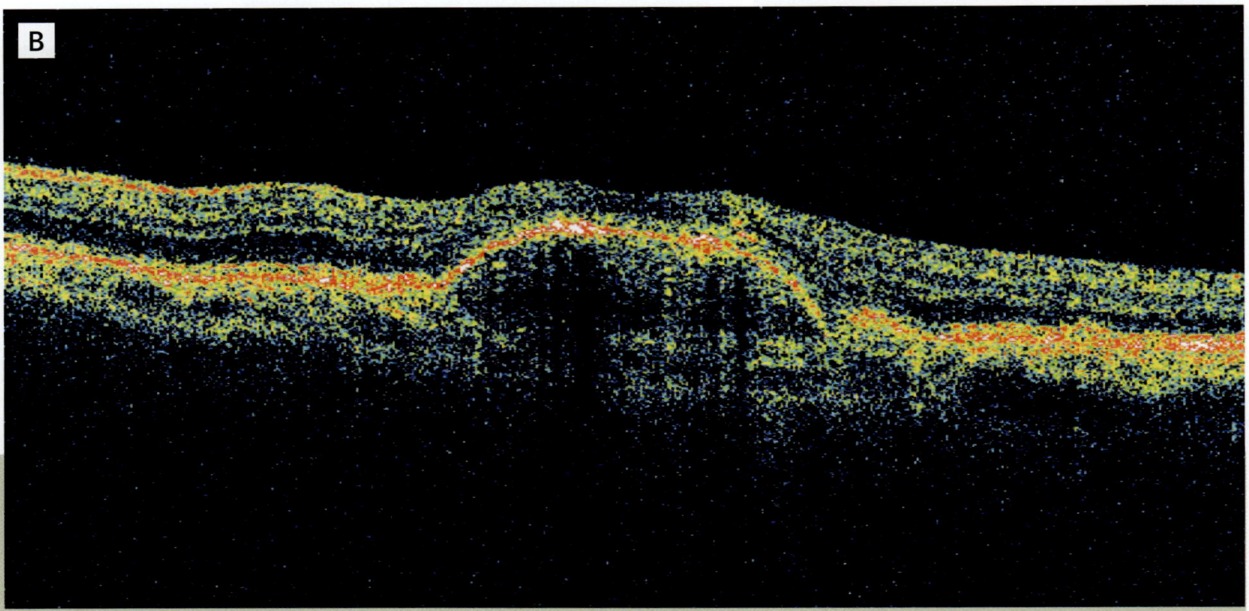

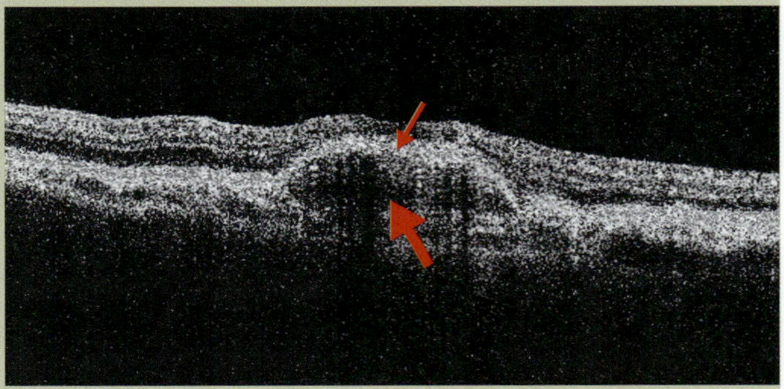

A. A 55 year old patient with reduction of visual acuity and metamorphopsia because of coalescent large soft drusen (the arrow shows the scan direction). A retinal elevation corresponding to the drusen can be seen in fundus biomicroscopy. Fluorescein angiography doesn't show any leakage. B. Optical Coherence Tomography shows a smooth elevation of the retinal pigment epithelium (small arrow). The cavity of the elevation is occupied by elements of low and high reflectivity (big arrow). Low reflectivity is due to the fluid presence and the comparatively higher reflectivity to the solid content of drusen.

DRY TYPE AGE-RELATED MACULAR DEGENERATION

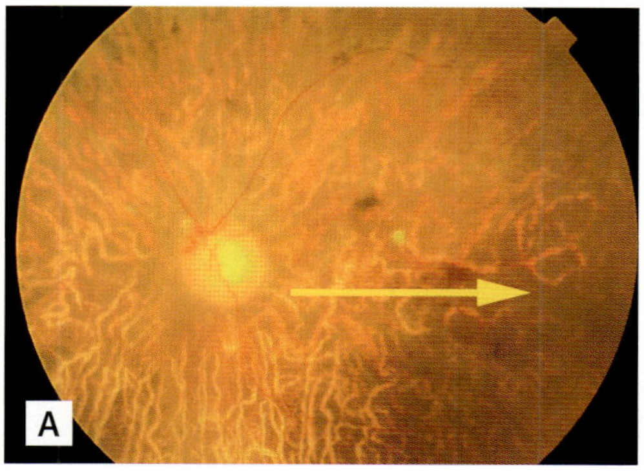

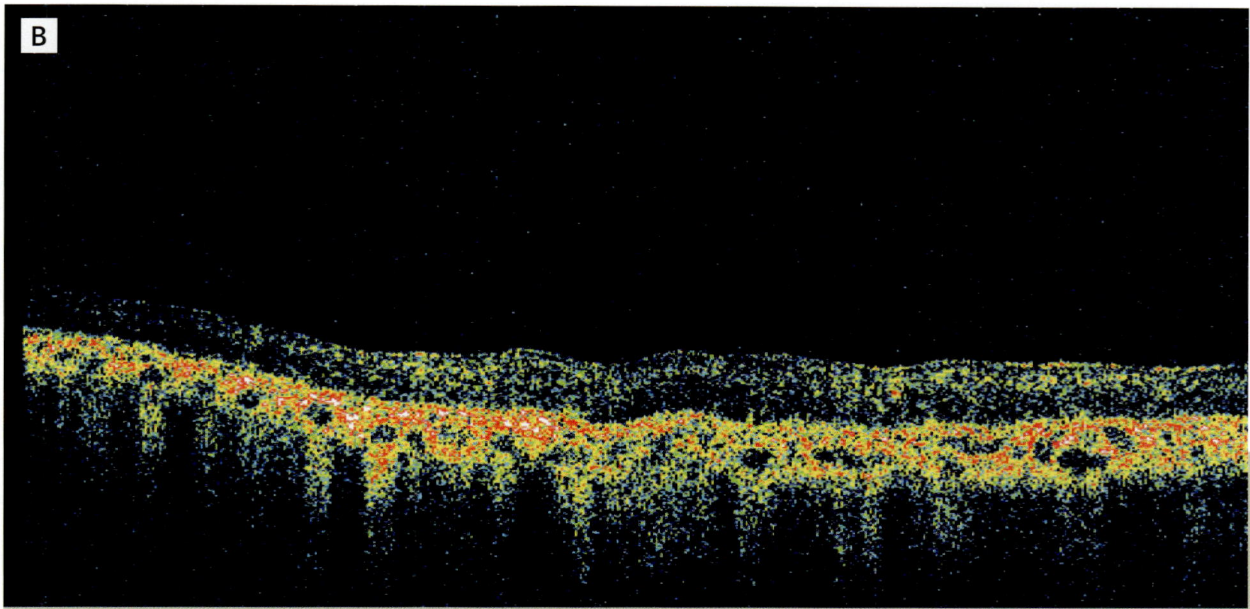

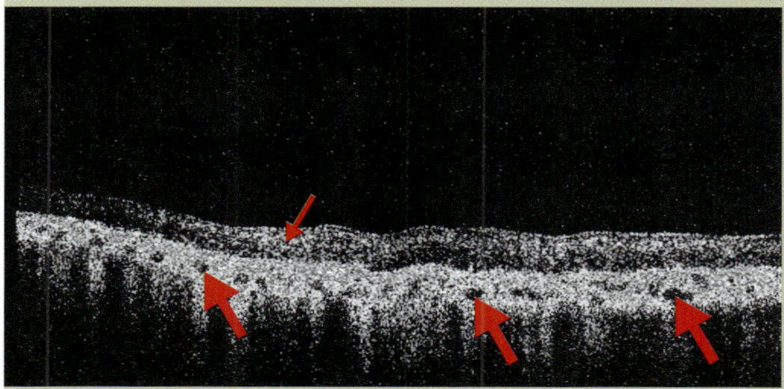

A. Patient with geographic macular atrophy (the arrow shows the scan direction) B. Optical Coherence Tomography shows a generalized retinal thinning (small arrow). The medium sized choroidal vessels appear as low reflectivity circular formations under the retinal pigment epithelium because of its atrophy (big arrows).

DRY TYPE AGE-RELATED MACULAR DEGENERATION

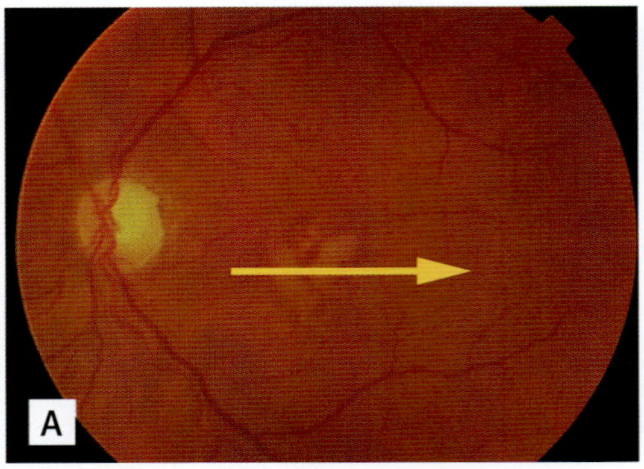

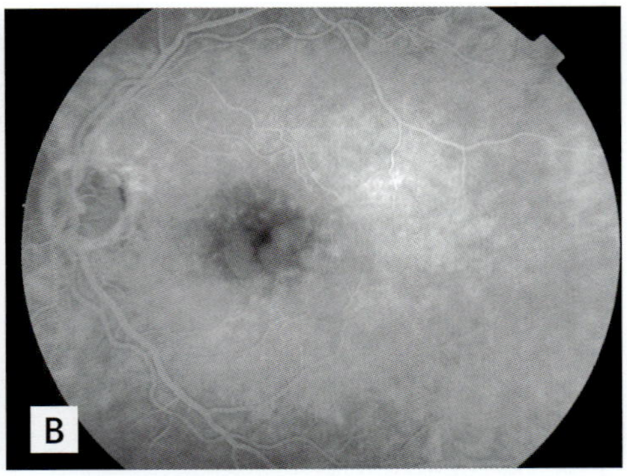

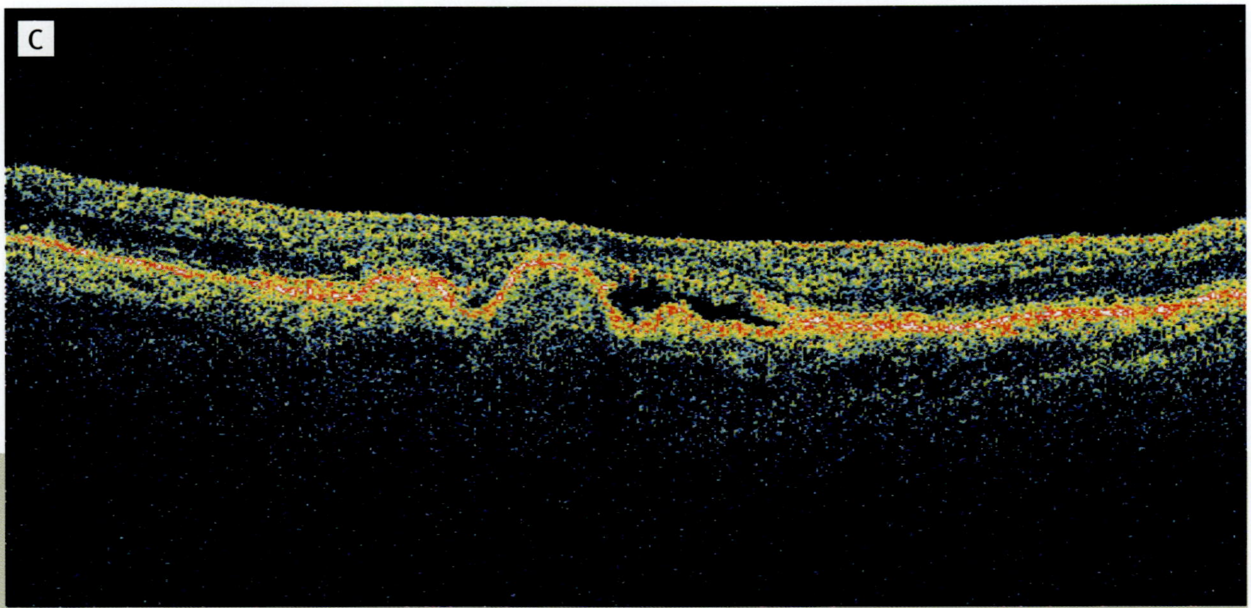

A. Patient with coalescent drusen of the posterior pole without any impression of subretinal fluid (the arrow shows the scan direction). B. Fluorescein angiography shows the drusen staining without any active leakage. C. Optical Coherence Tomography shows multiple elevated areas of high reflectivity under the retinal pigment epithelium corresponding to drusen (small arrows). There is also a low reflectivity area between the retina and the retinal pigment epithelium that corresponds to the presence of foveal subretinal fluid (big arrow). In this case indocyanine green angiography is mandatory in order to identify the presence or not of an occult choroidal neovascularization.

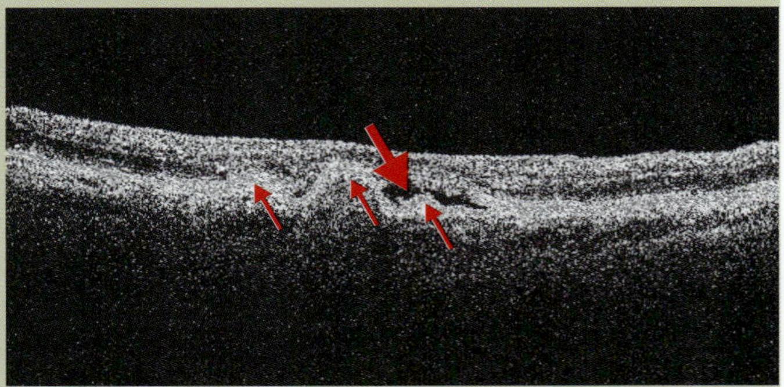

DRY TYPE AGE-RELATED MACULAR DEGENERATION

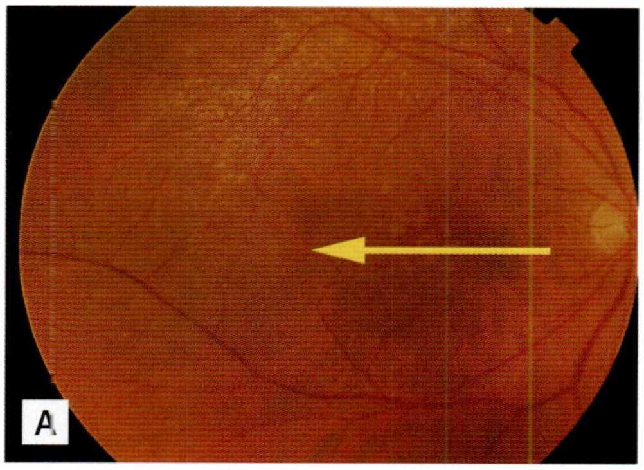

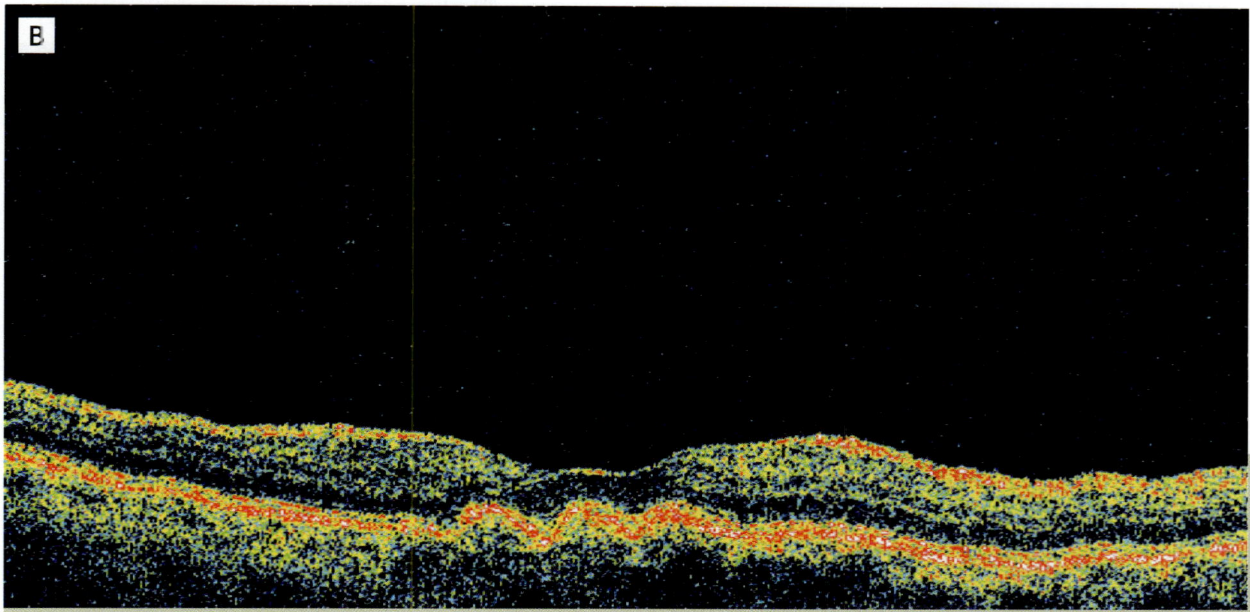

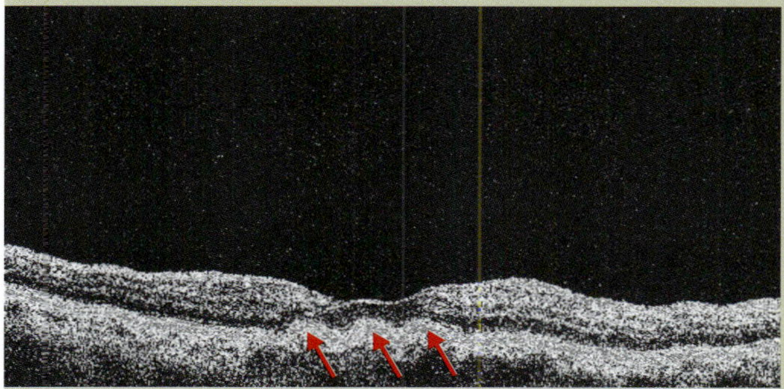

A. Patient with coalescent drusen of the posterior pole (the arrow shows the scan direction). B. Optical Coherence Tomography shows multiple elevated areas of high reflectivity under the retinal pigment epithelium corresponding to drusen (small arrows). The foveal morphology is maintained, but there is an enlargement of its depression.

DRY TYPE AGE-RELATED MACULAR DEGENERATION

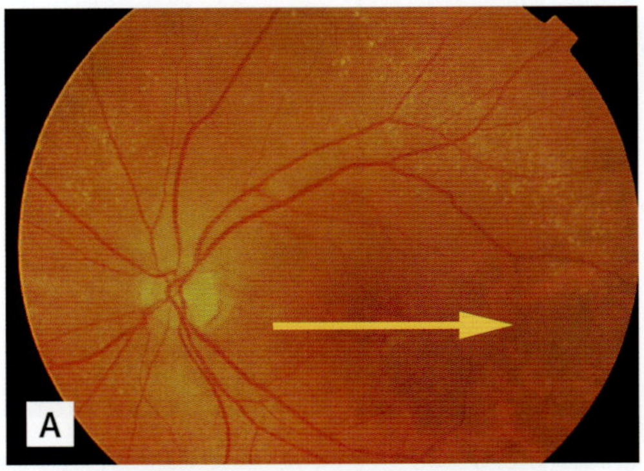

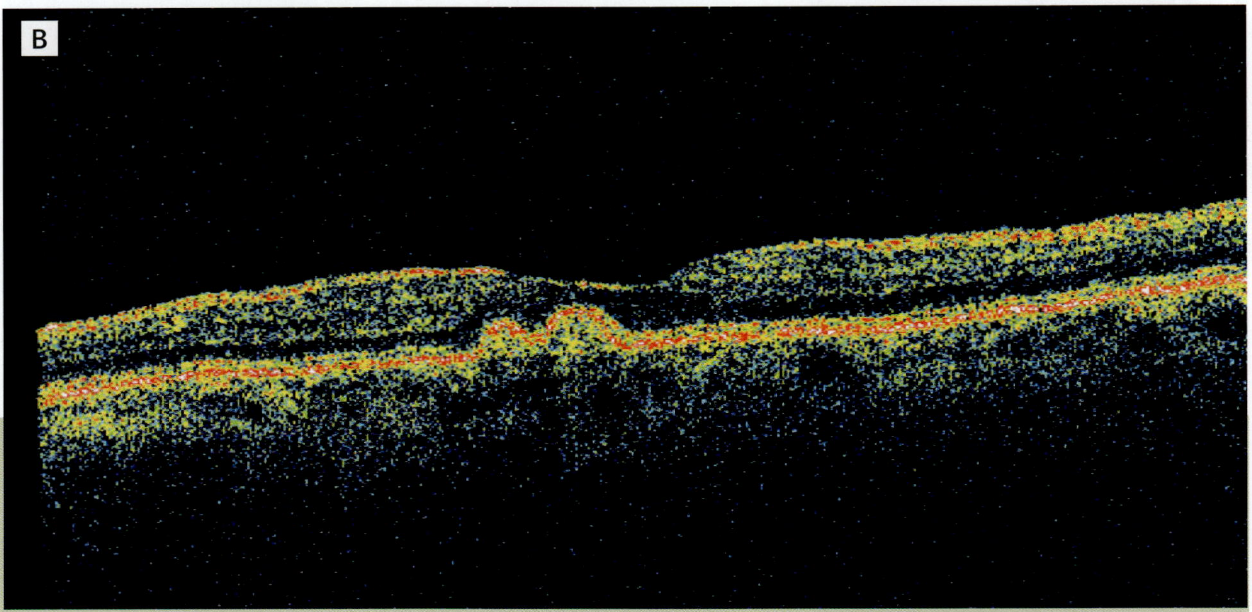

A. The other eye of the patient in page 39 where coalescent drusen are located at the posterior pole (the arrow shows the scan direction). B. Optical Coherence Tomography shows multiple elevated areas of high reflectivity under the retinal pigment epithelium corresponding to drusen (arrows). As in the fellow eye the foveal morphology is maintained, but there is an enlargement of the foveal depression.

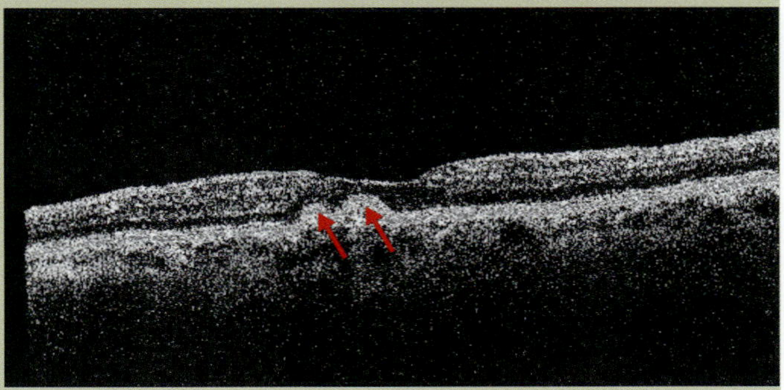

CLASSIC CHOROIDAL NEOVASCULAR MEMBRANE

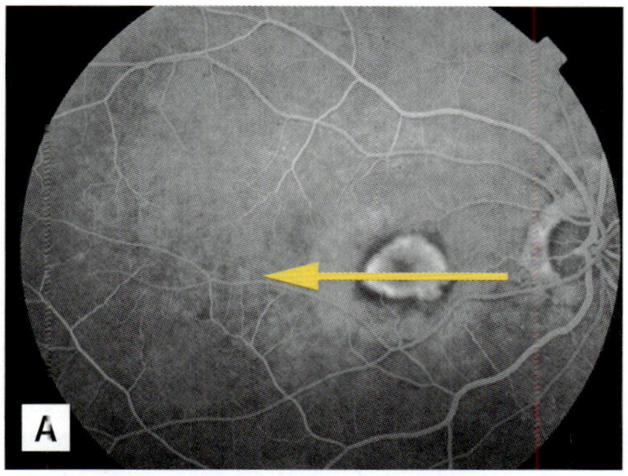

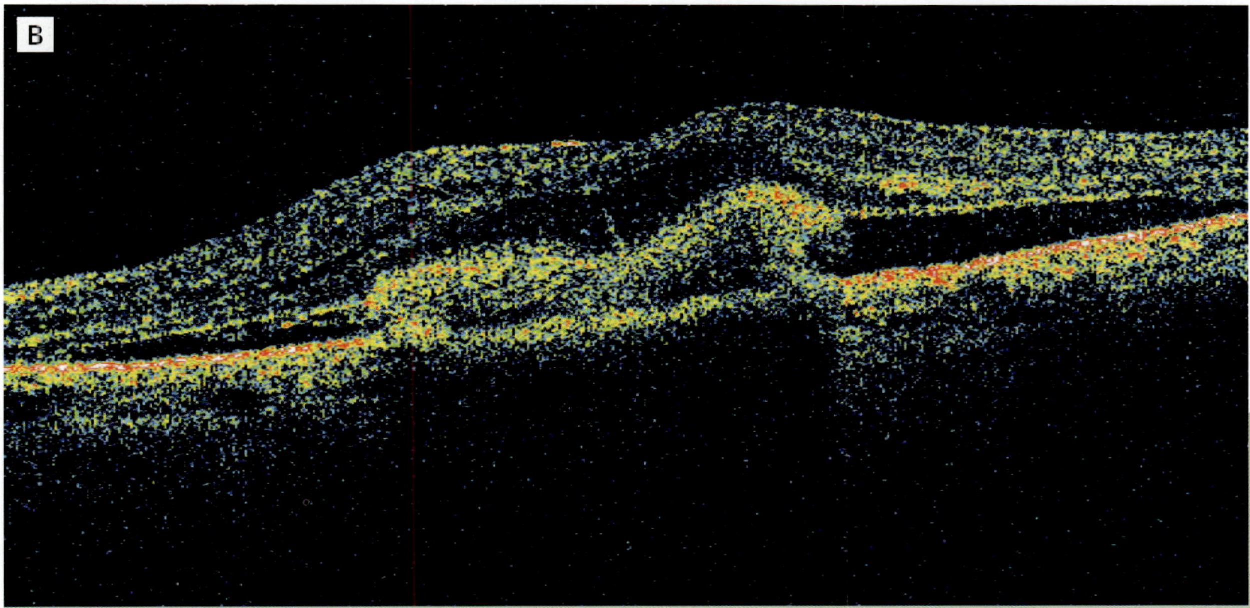

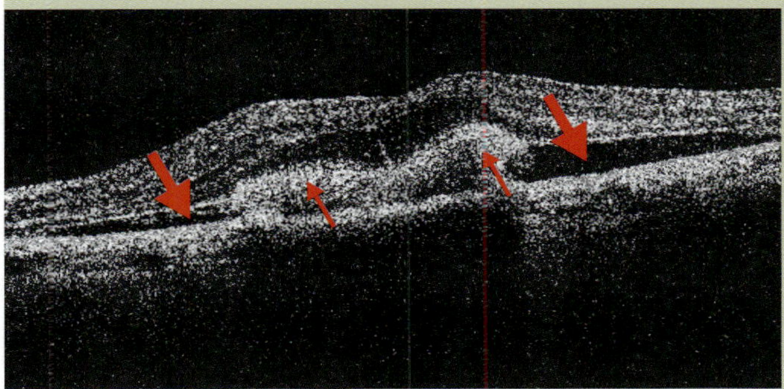

Patient with classic choroidal neovascularization secondary to age-related macular degeneration. A. Fluorescein angiography shows a subfoveal choroidal neovascularization (the arrow shows the scan direction). B. Optical Coherence Tomography shows a large area of adequate thickness and high reflectivity at the fovea due to the choroidal neovascularization (small arrows) that is surrounded by a low reflectivity area between the retina and the retinal pigment epithelium corresponding to subretinal fluid (big arrows). The retinal thickness is increased because of diffuse edema.

CLASSIC CHOROIDAL NEOVASCULAR MEMBRANE

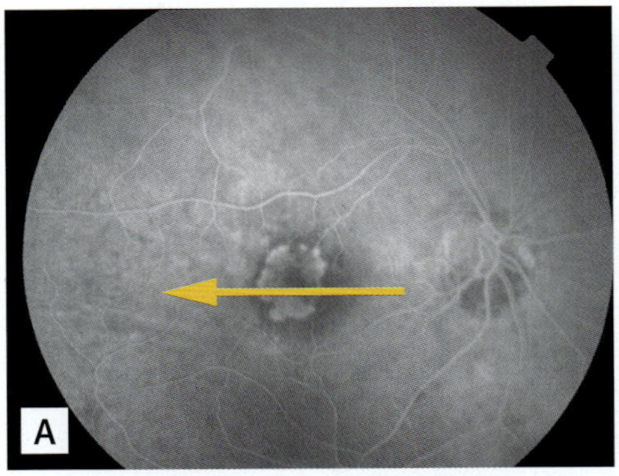

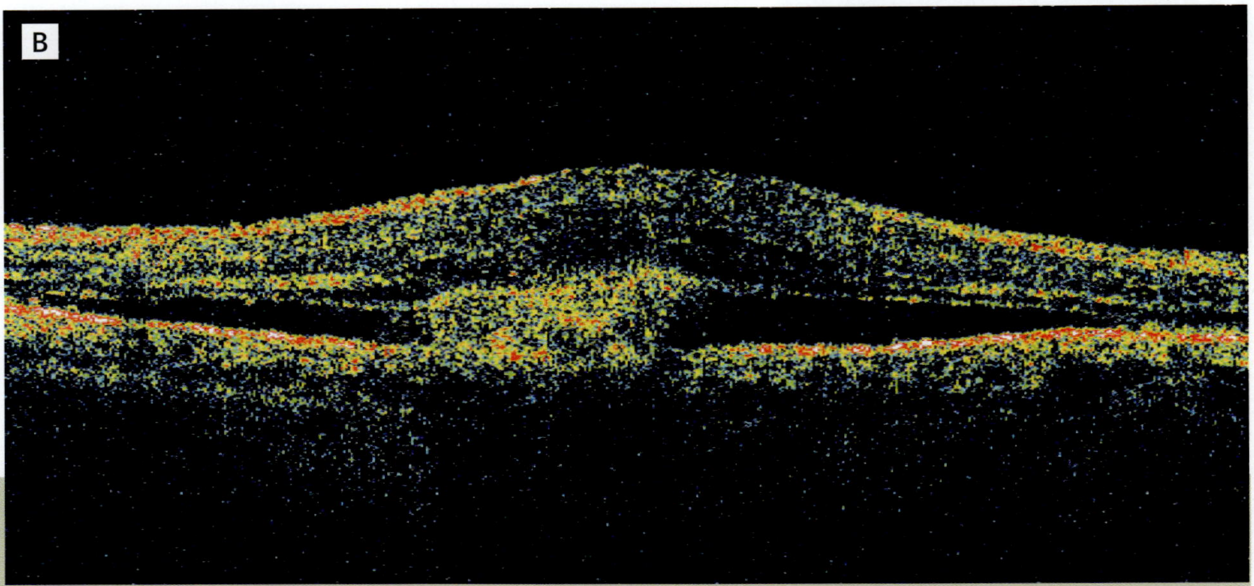

A. Patient with classic choroidal neovascularization secondary to age-related macular degeneration (the arrow shows the scan direction). B. Optical Coherence Tomography shows a large thick area of high reflectivity in the fovea due to the choroidal neovascularization (small arrow) that is surrounded by an area of low reflectivity between the retina and the retinal pigment epithelium corresponding to the subretinal fluid (big arrows). The retinal thickness is increased because of diffuse edema.

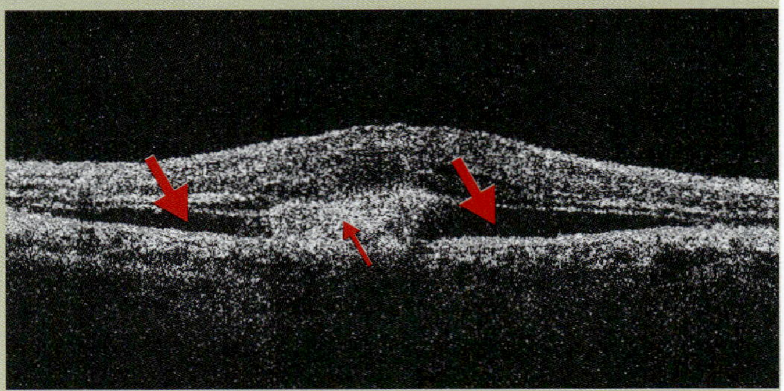

CLASSIC CHOROIDAL NEOVASCULAR MEMBRANE

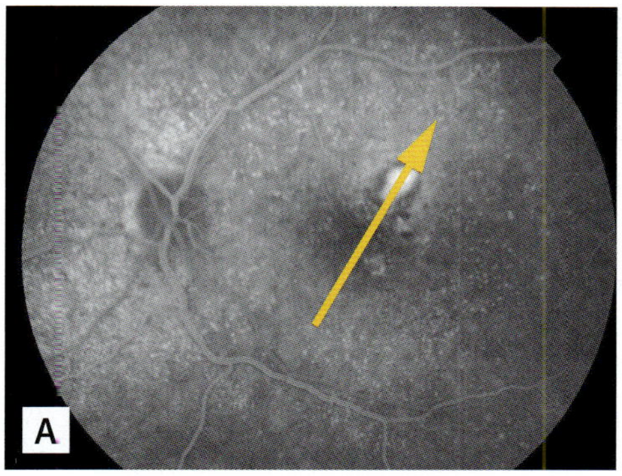

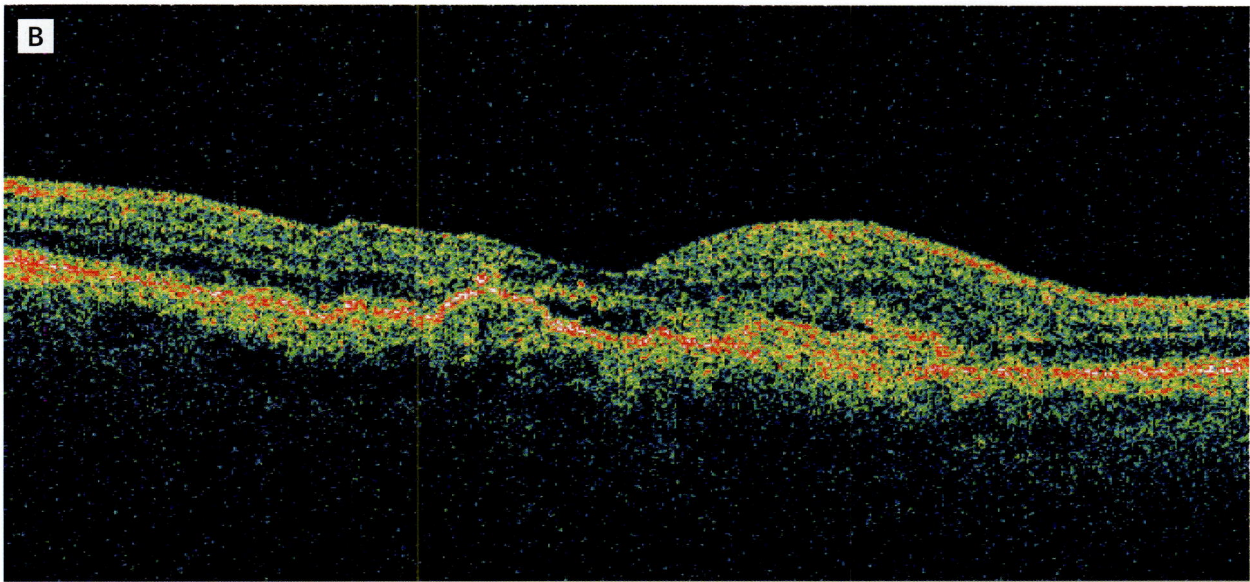

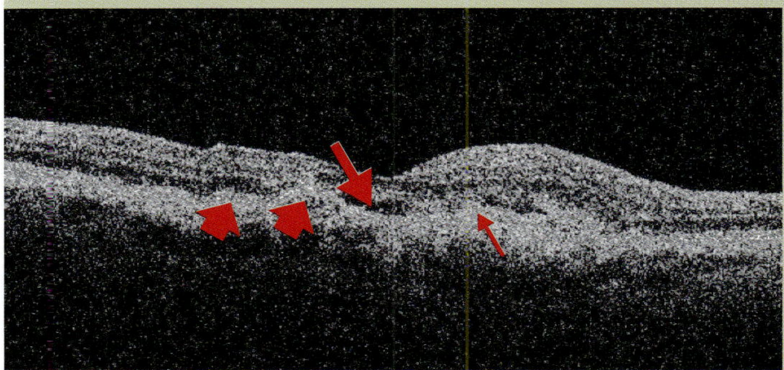

A. Patient with predominantly classic choroidal neovascularization secondary to age-related macular degeneration (the arrow shows the scan direction). B. Optical Coherence Tomography shows an area of high reflectivity (small arrow) located at the retinal pigment epithelium level, which extends superotemporally to the fovea, corresponding to the choroidal neovascularization. There is an area of low reflectivity between the retina and the retinal pigment epithelium corresponding to the subfoveal retinal detachment (big arrow). Areas of high reflectivity under the retinal pigment epithelium are also observed and correspond to the macular drusen (thick arrows).

OCCULT CHOROIDAL NEOVASCULAR MEMBRANE

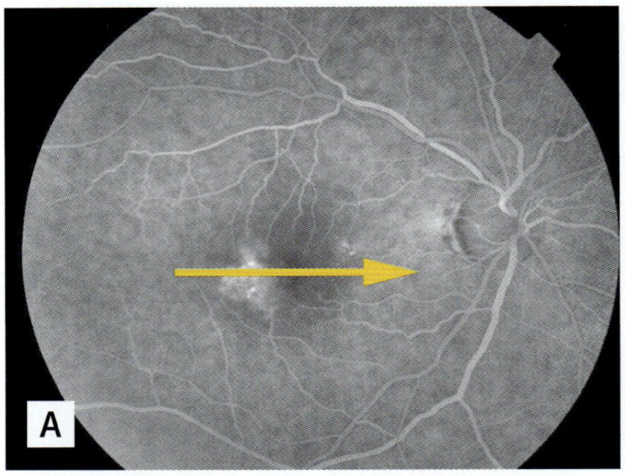

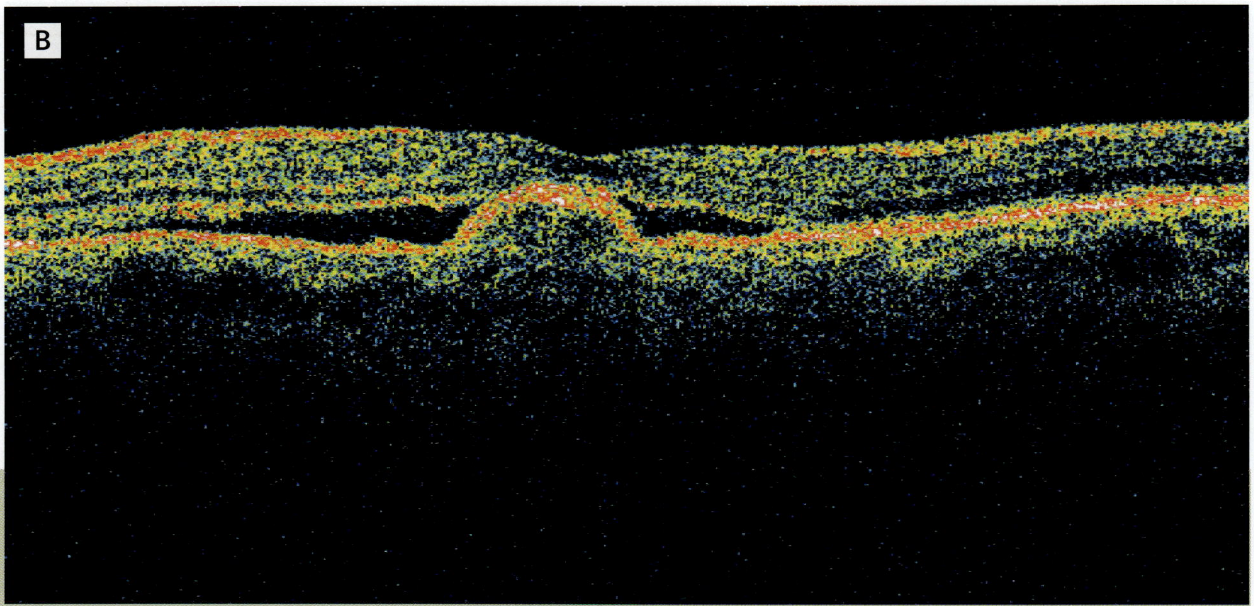

Patient with occult choroidal neovascularization due to age related macula degeneration. A. Fluorescein angiography shows the choroidal neovascularization at the fovea and temporally to it (the arrow shows the scan direction). B. Optical Coherence Tomography shows an area of high reflectivity under the retinal pigment epithelium in the fovea (small arrow) due to the choroidal neovascular membrane, that is surrounded by an area of low reflectivity between the retina and the retinal pigment epithelium corresponding to retinal detachment (big arrows).

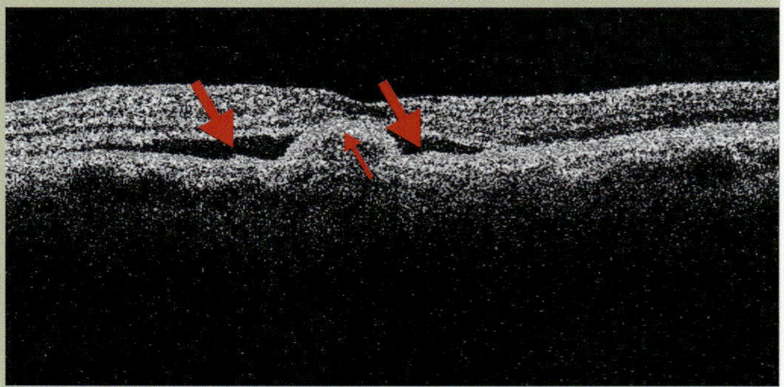

OCCULT CHOROIDAL NEOVASCULAR MEMBRANE

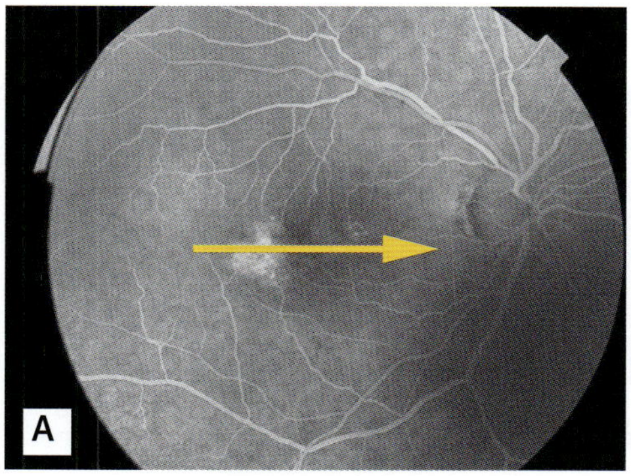

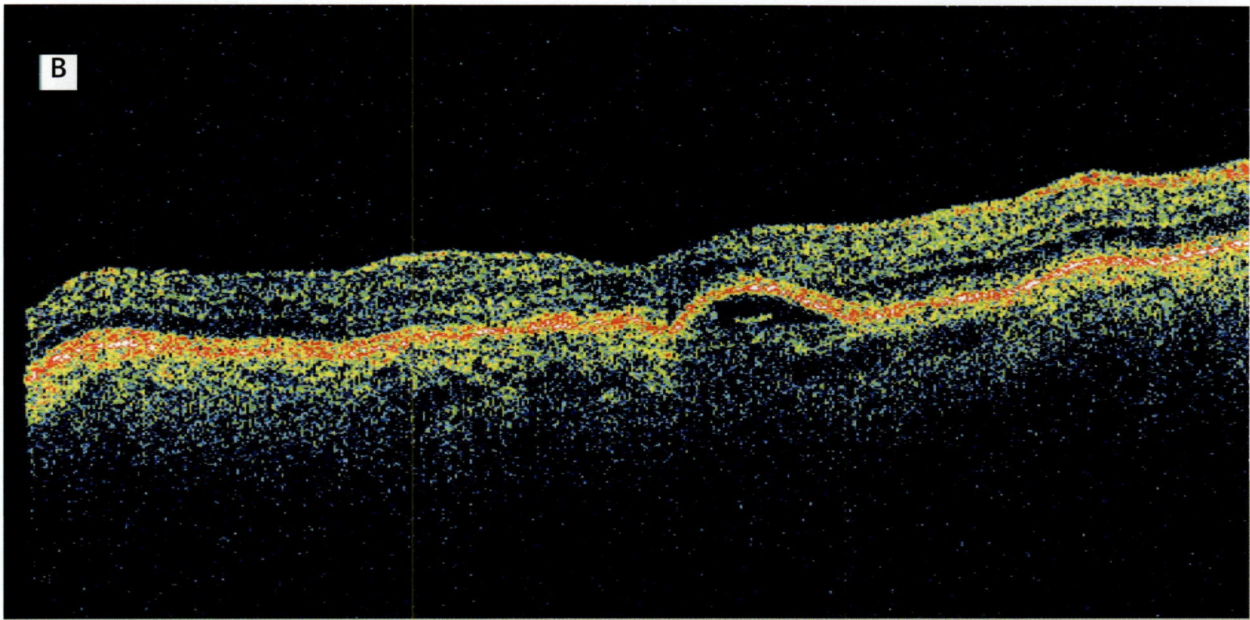

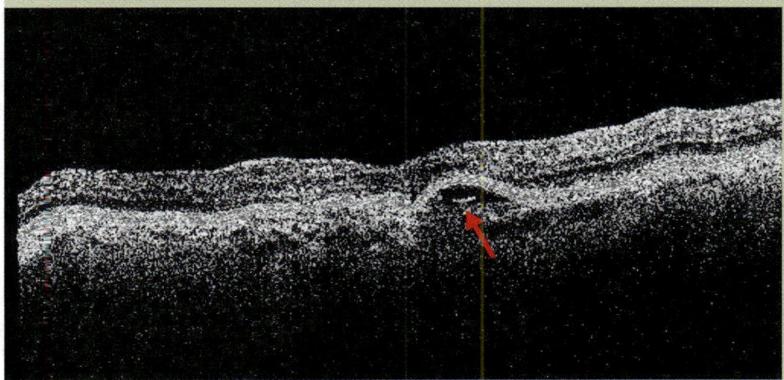

The patient of page 44, three months after photodynamic therapy. A. The angiographic findings are similar to these of the previous examination (the arrow shows the scan direction). B. Optical Coherence Tomography shows the retinal pigment epithelium detachment (arrow) with a complete absorption of the subretinal fluid.

CLASSIC CHOROIDAL NEOVASCULAR MEMBRANE

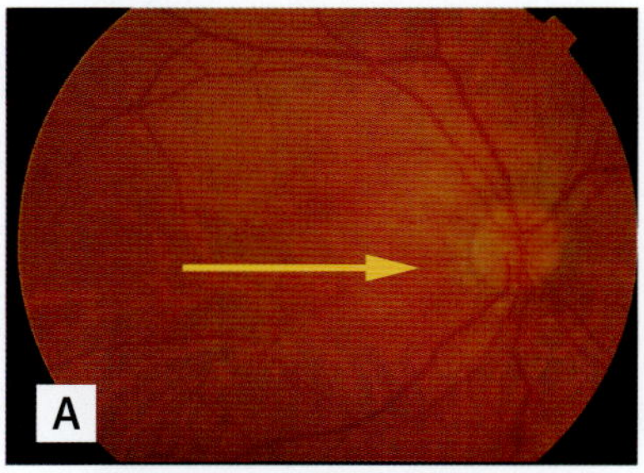

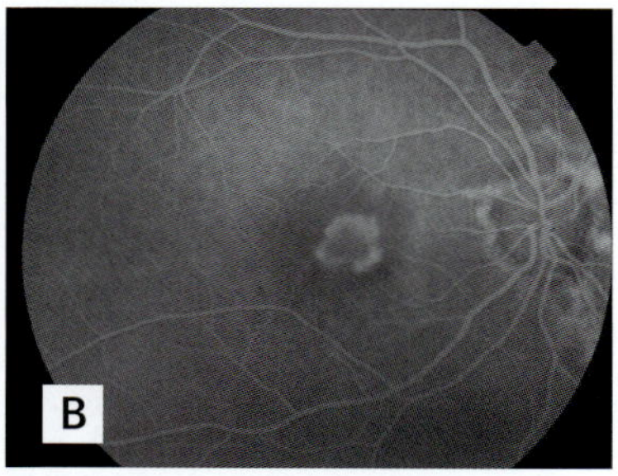

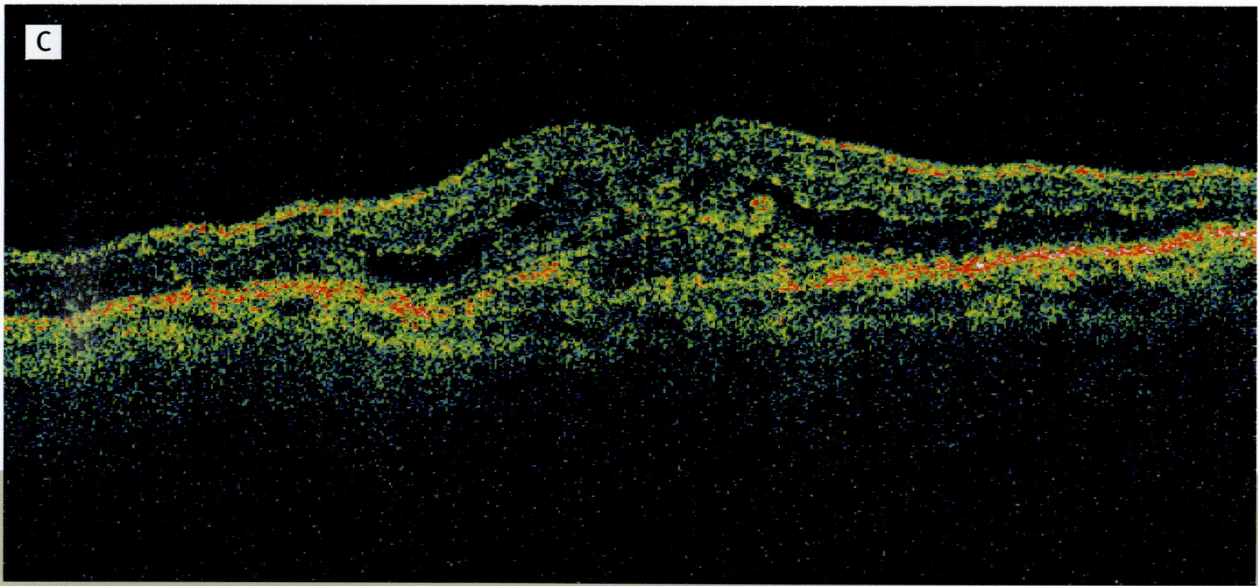

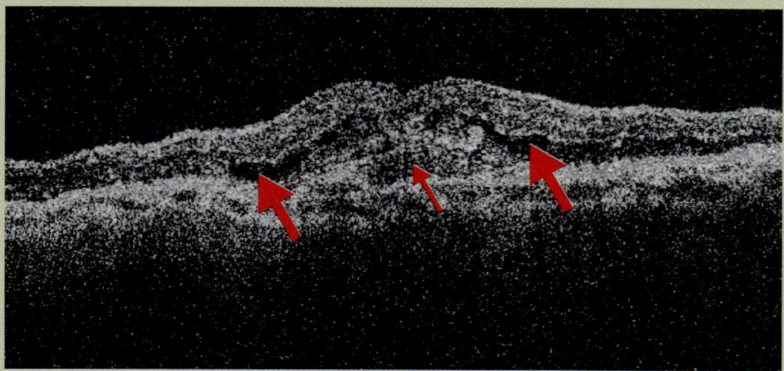

A, B. Patient with classic choroidal neovascular membrane (the arrow shows the scan direction). C. Optical Coherence Tomography shows a disruption of the retinal pigment epithelium layer by a mass of high reflectivity that represents the neovascular complex (small arrow). There are also areas of low reflectivity in the deeper retinal layers at both sides of the foveola corresponding to intraretinal oedema (thick arrows).

CLASSIC CHOROIDAL NEOVASCULAR MEMBRANE

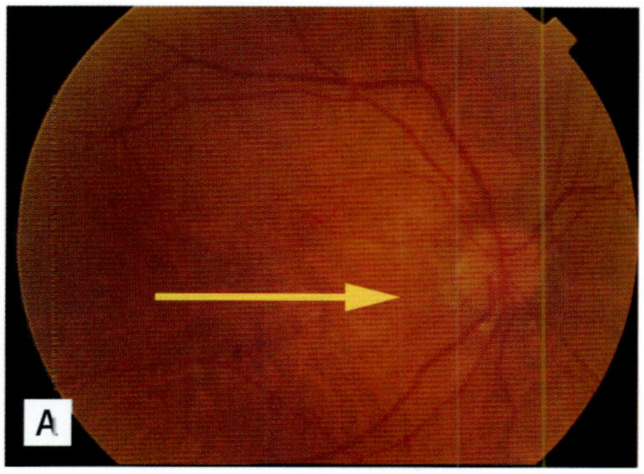

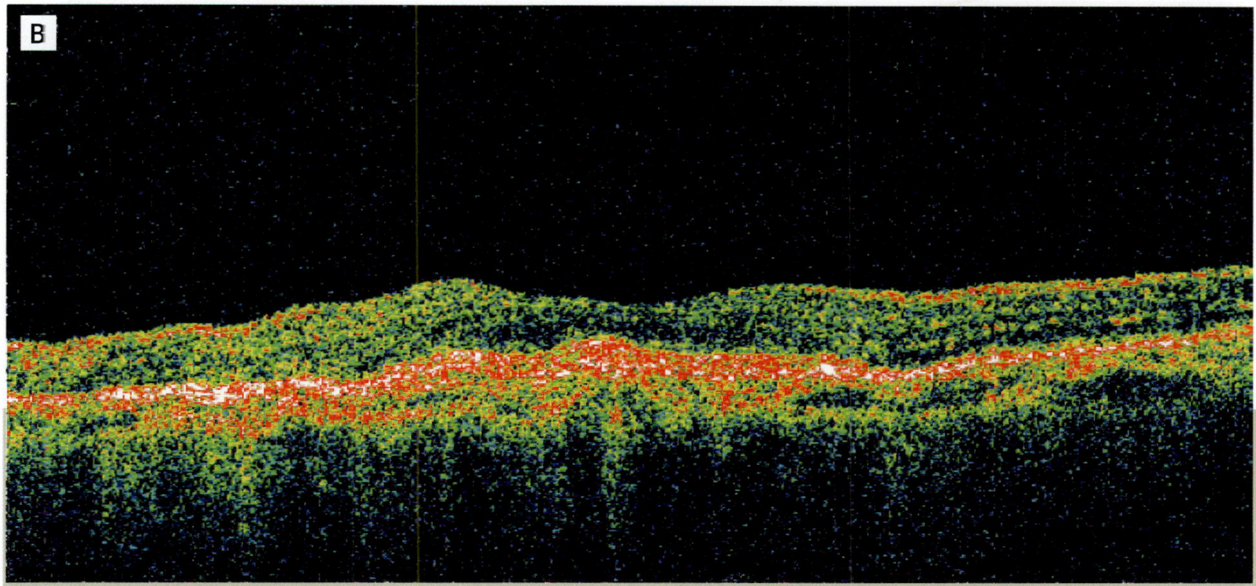

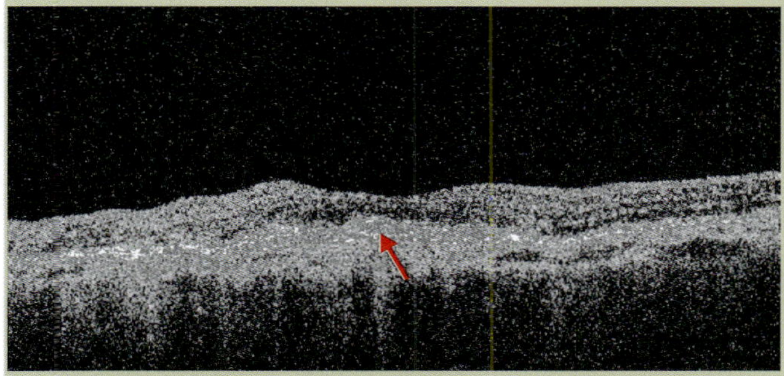

A. The same patient of page 46, one month after an intravitreal injection of anti-VEGF drug (the arrow shows the scan direction). B. Optical Coherence Tomography shows elimination of the intraretinal fluid. An area of high reflectivity below the retinal pigment epithelium layer represents the neovascular tissue (arrow).

OCCULT CHOROIDAL NEOVASCULAR MEMBRANE

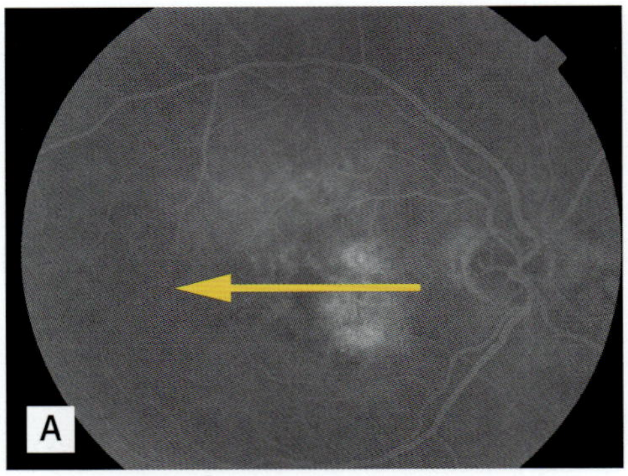

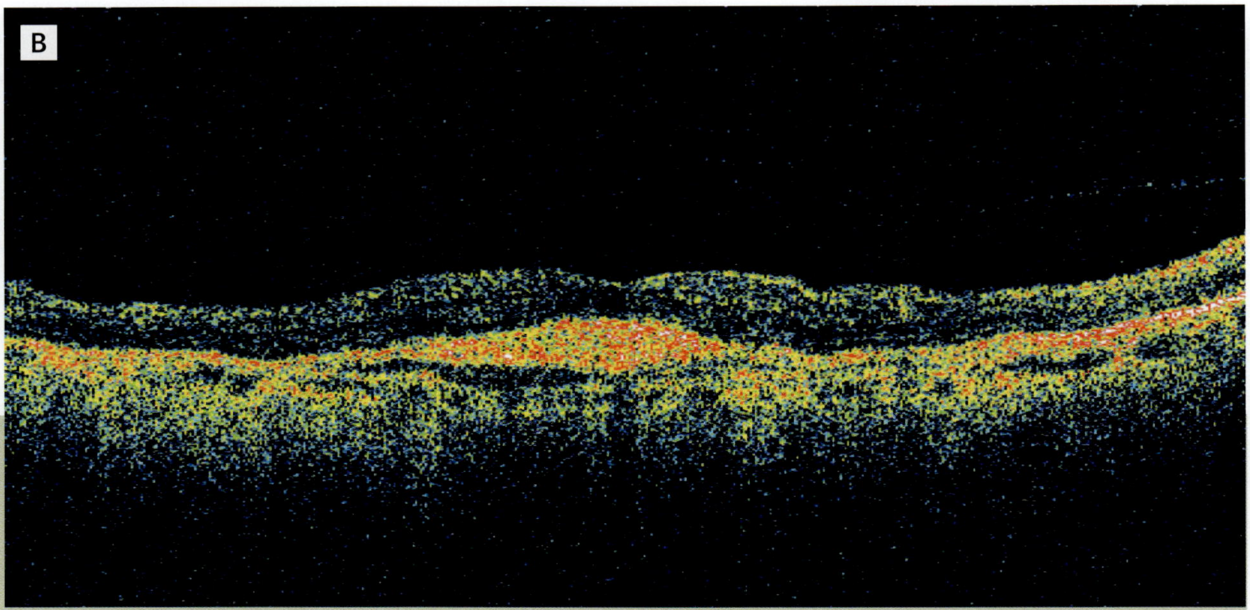

Patient with an occult choroidal neovascular membrane. A. Fluorescein angiography shows the choroidal neovascularization at the macula (the arrow shows the scan direction). B. Optical Coherence Tomography shows a thick area of high reflectivity under the retinal pigment epithelium, at the fovea (arrow) due to the choroidal neovascularization. There is no subretinal fluid.

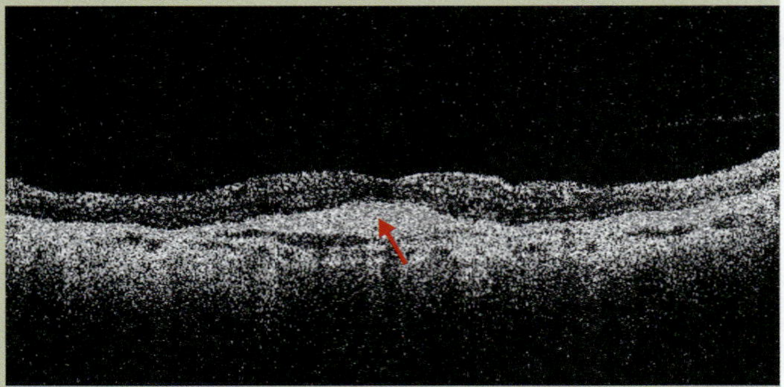

OCCULT CHOROIDAL NEOVASCULAR MEMBRANE

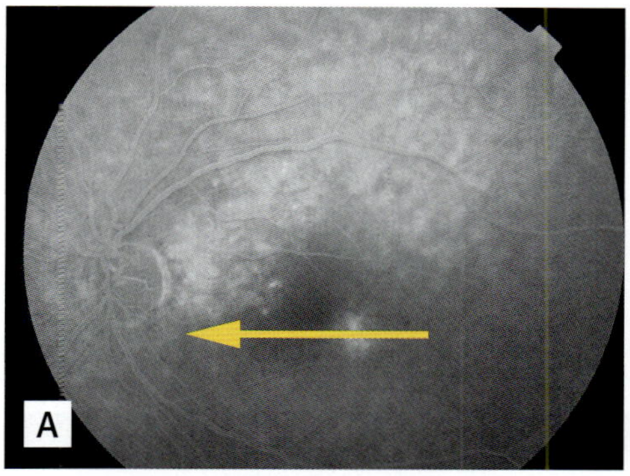

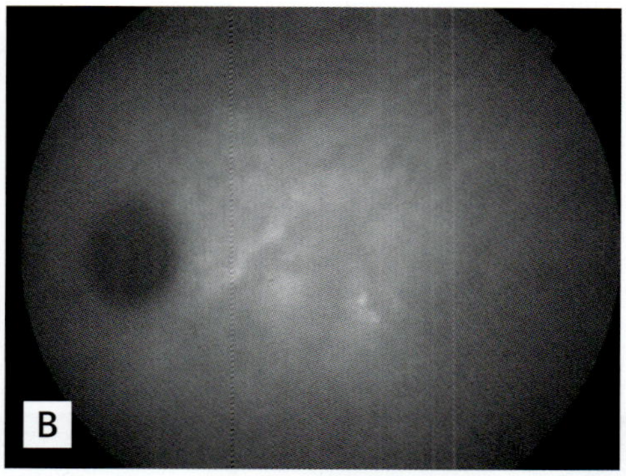

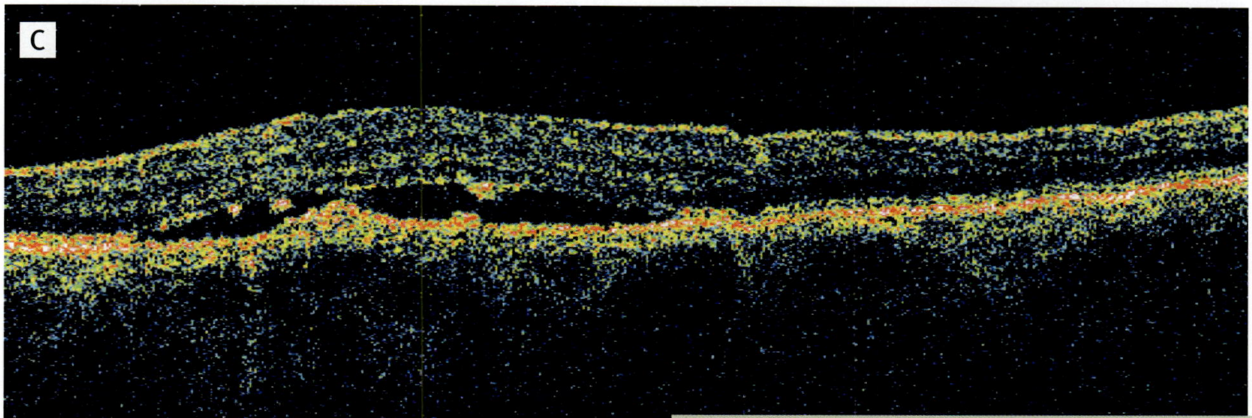

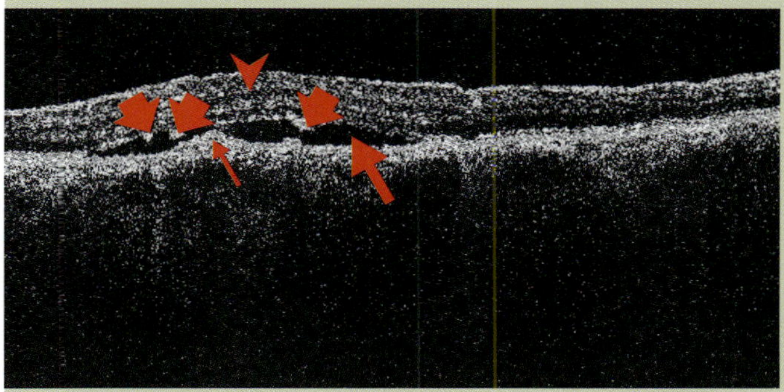

Patient with a choroidal neovascularization. A, B. Fluorescein angiography and especially indocyanine green angiography show an occult choroidal neovascularization (the arrow shows the scan direction). C. Optical Coherence Tomography shows a limited area of high reflectivity, located at the choriocapillaries layer which represents the active choroidal neovascularization (small arrow). There is also a low reflectivity area between the retina and the retinal pigment epithelium, corresponding to the retinal detachment (big arrow). Note the irregular inner surface of the retinal detachment due to the irregular separation of the photoreceptors from the retinal pigment epithelium (thick arrows). The presence of diffuse retinal edema is clearly noticeable (arrow head).

WET TYPE AGE-RELATED MACULAR DEGENERATION

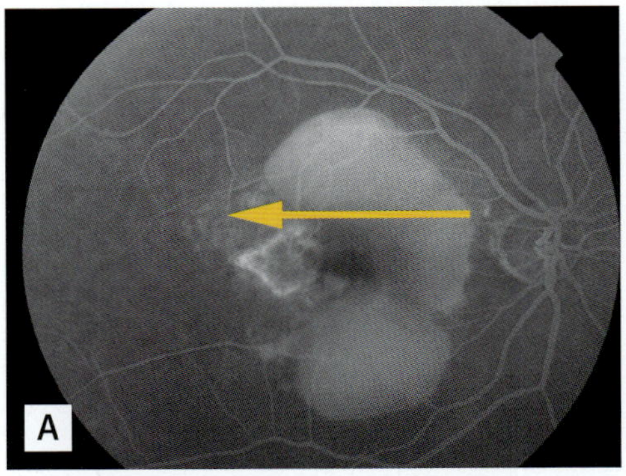

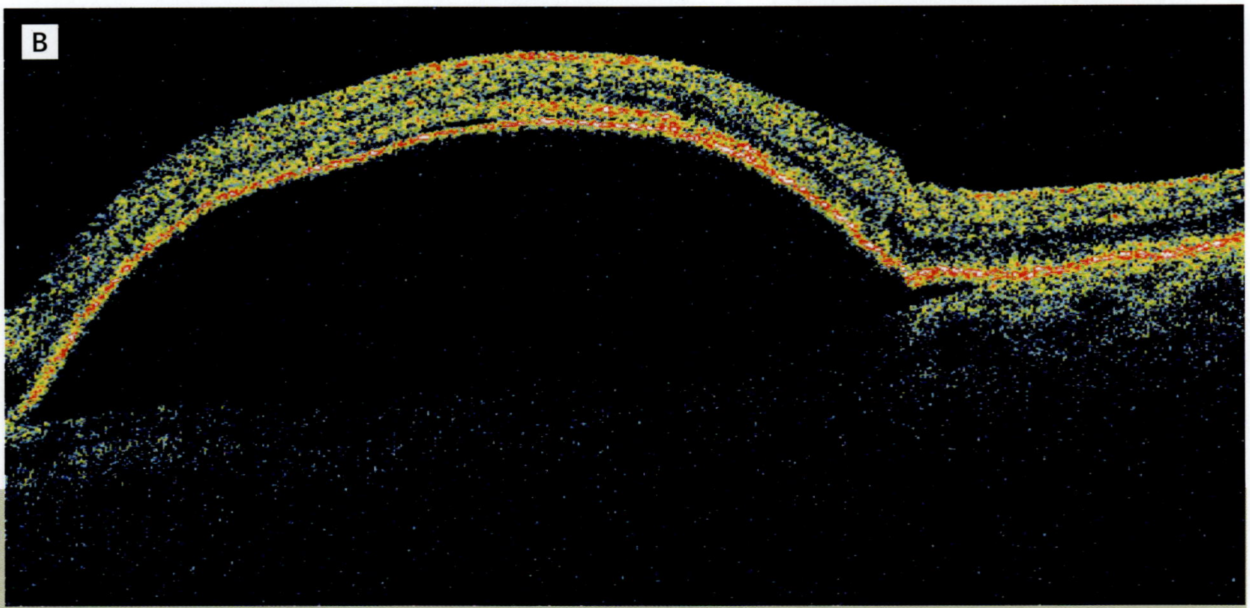

A. Fluorescein angiography image of a patient with a kidney-shaped retinal pigment epithelium detachment that surrounds the central area. There is also atrophy at the fovea. The patient presented with a retinal pigment epithelium detachment 48 hours after photodynamic therapy, which was performed because of occult choroidal neovascularization (the arrow shows the scan direction). B. Optical Coherence Tomography shows a large area of low reflectivity located under the retinal pigment epithelium that corresponds to a retinal pigment epithelium detachment (arrow), which accompanies the choroidal neovascularization.

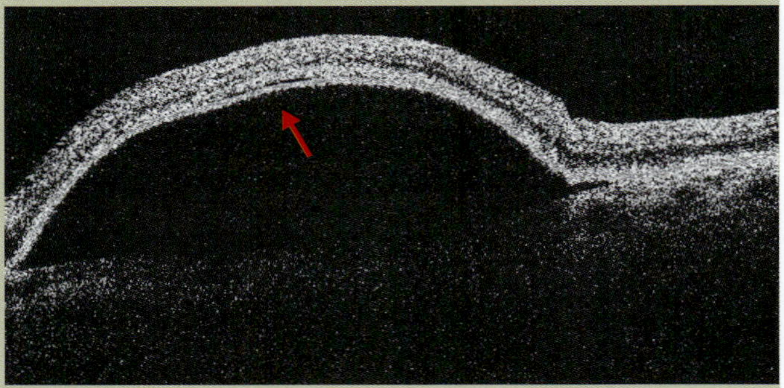

WET TYPE AGE-RELATED MACULAR DEGENERATION

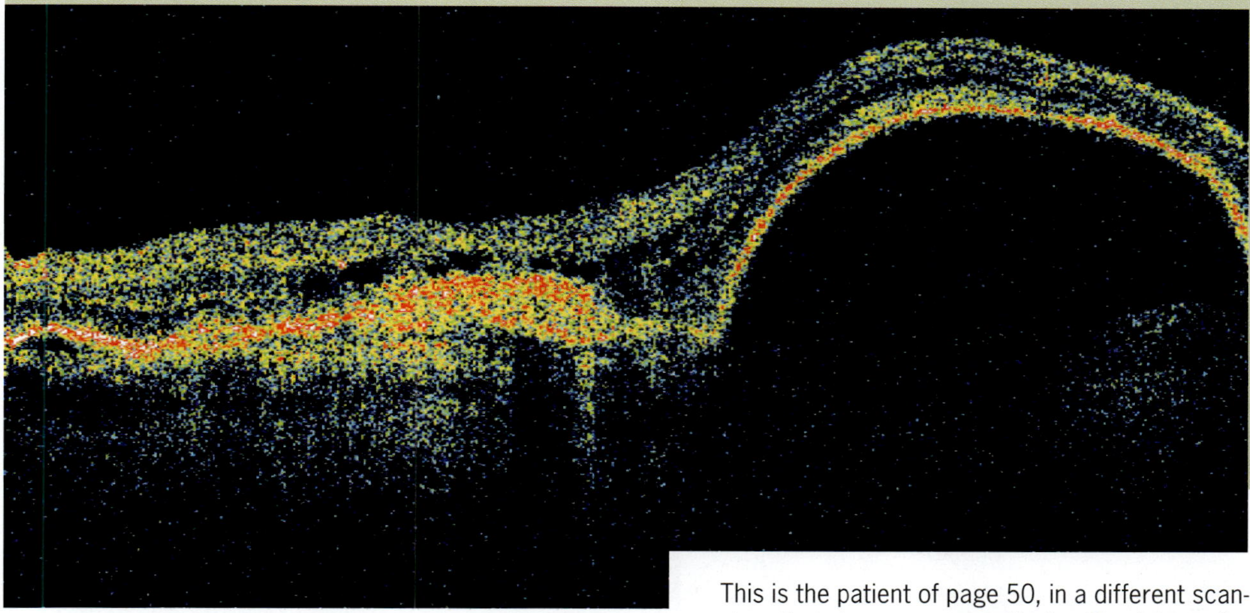

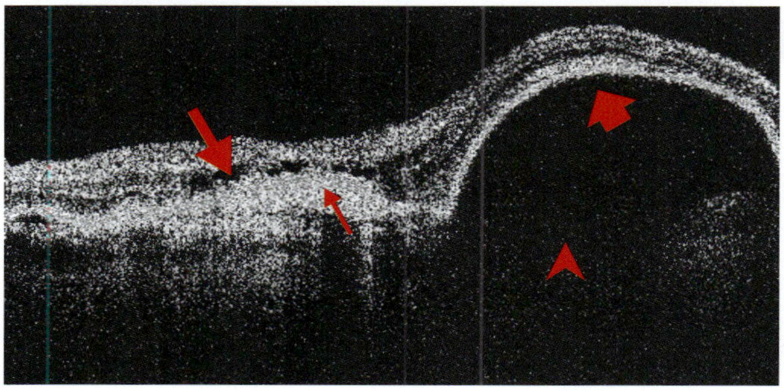

This is the patient of page 50, in a different scanning, that shows an area of high reflectivity under the retinal pigment epithelium, which corresponds to an active choroidal neovascularization (small arrow). Note the multiple areas of low reflectivity inside the retina, over the choroidal neovascularization that correspond to the cystic retinal edema (big arrow). There is a large area of low reflectivity, under the retinal pigment epithelium that corresponds to the retinal pigment epithelium detachment (thick arrow). Note the almost complete disappearance of the tissues under the detachment due to shadowing effect because of the increased reflectivity of the retinal pigment epithelium detachment (arrow head).

WET TYPE AGE-RELATED MACULAR DEGENERATION

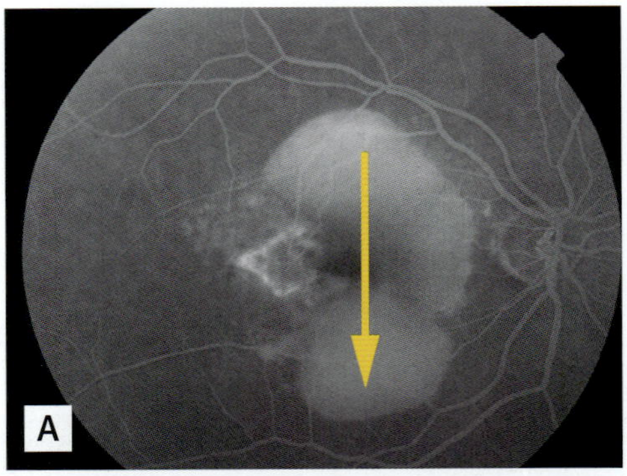

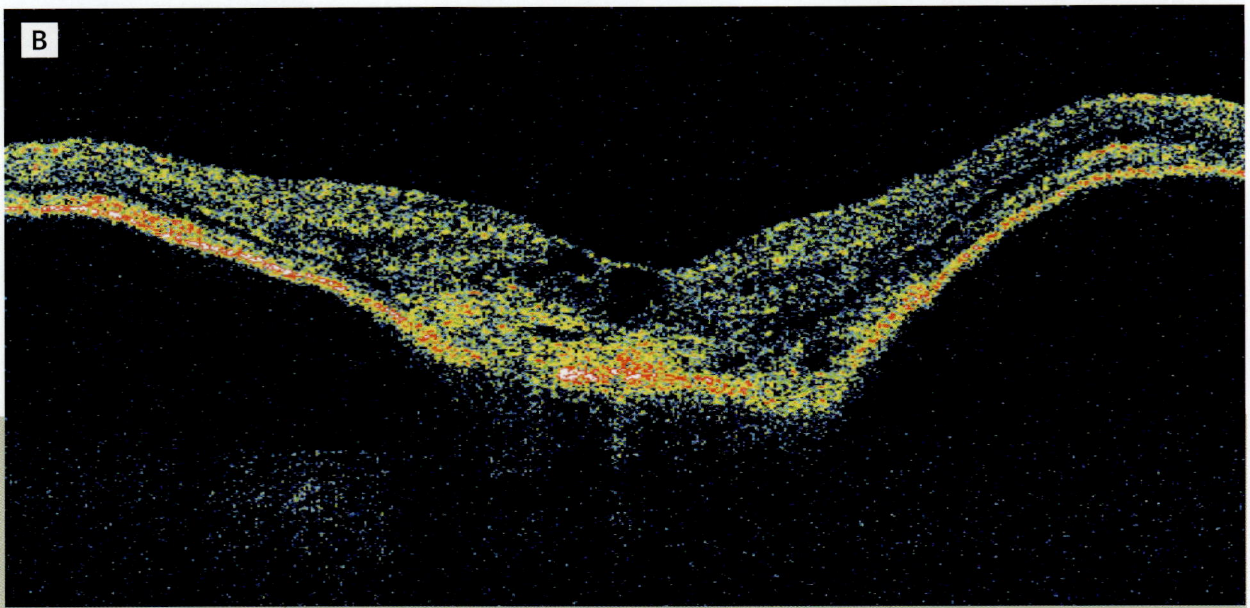

A. A different scanning of the patient of page 50 that shows the double (superior and inferior) kidney-shaped detachment of the retinal pigment epithelium (small arrows) B. Note the multiple areas of low reflectivity inside the retina which correspond to cystoid retinal edema (big arrow).

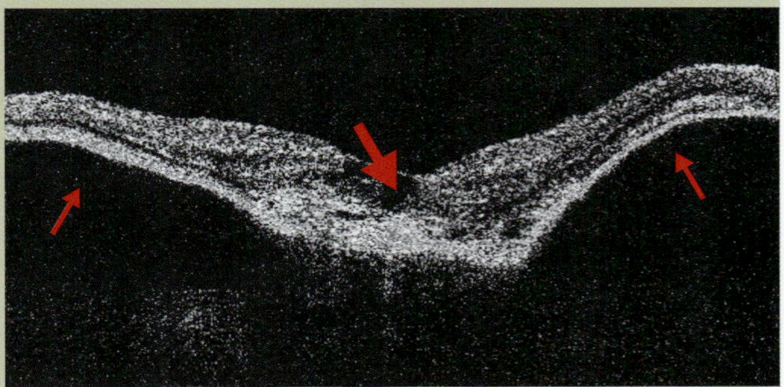

WET TYPE AGE-RELATED MACULAR DEGENERATION

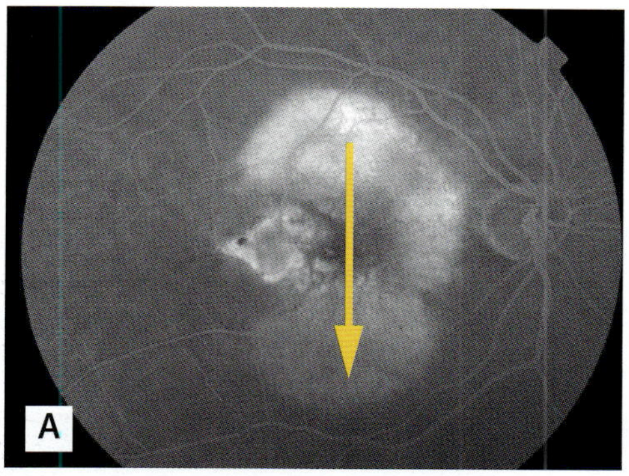

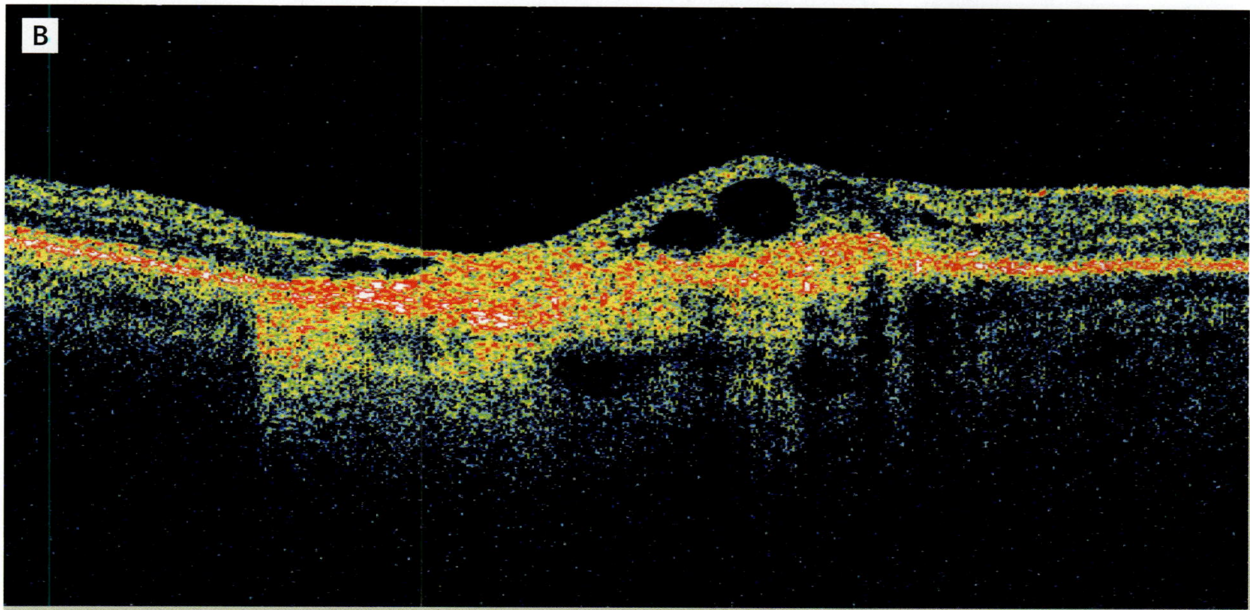

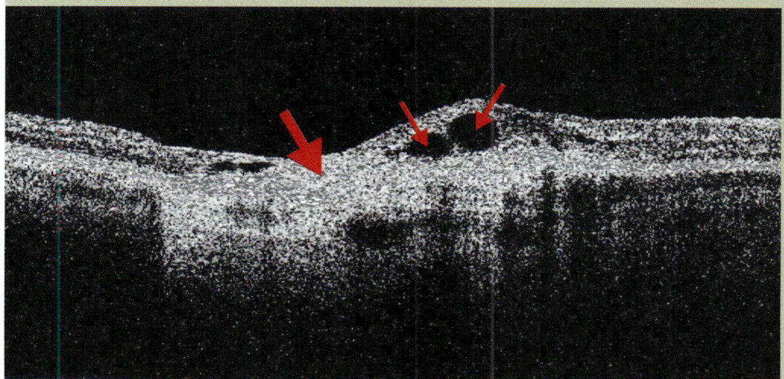

The patient of page 50, one year later. A. Fluorescein angiography shows the area of the retinal pigment epithelium detachment that remains the same, regarding the size of the hyperfluorescence, but with decreased intensity (the arrow shows the scan direction). B. Optical Coherence Tomography shows that the retinal pigment epithelium detachment has completely resolved. Intraretinal areas of low reflectivity, (small arrows) corresponding to cystoid retinal edema still exist. There are signs of membrane scarring (big arrow).

WET TYPE AGE-RELATED MACULAR DEGENERATION

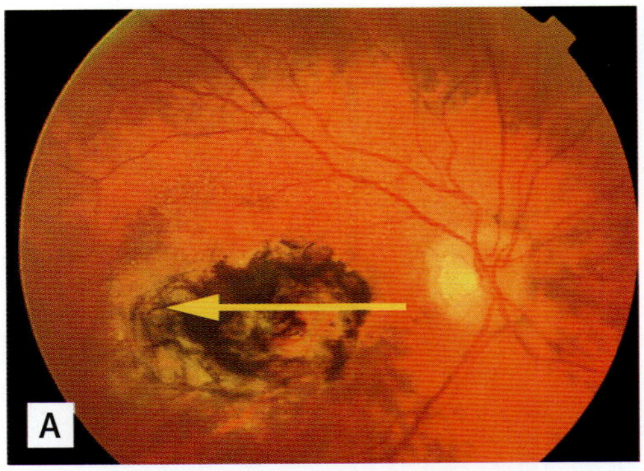

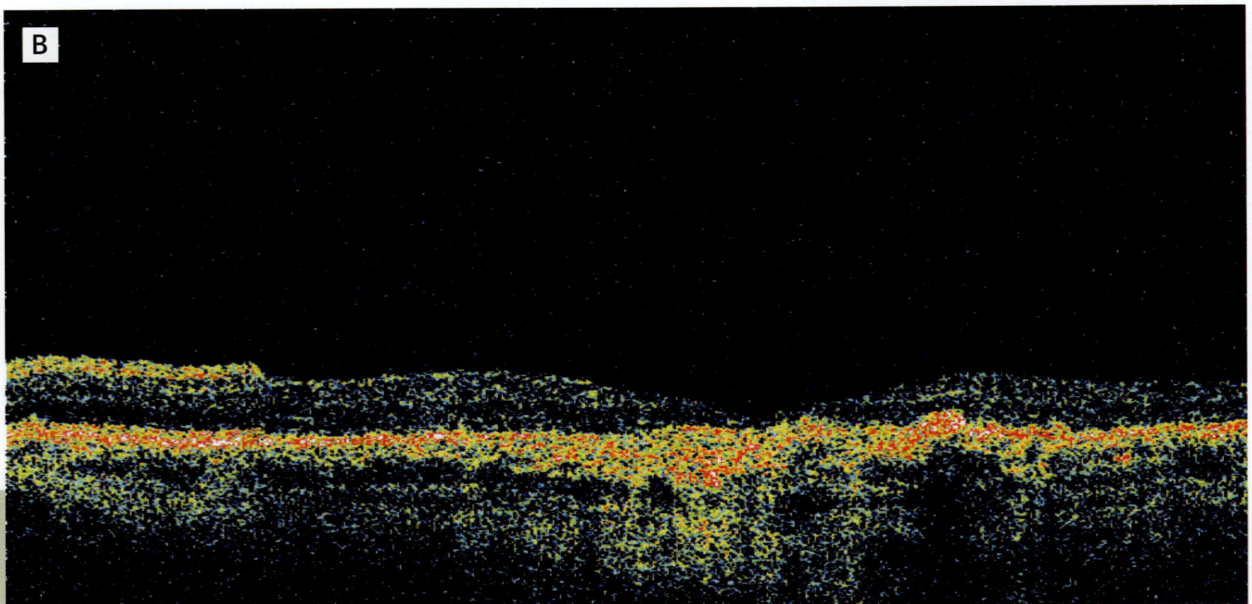

Patient after the third photodynamic therapy for choroidal neovascularization. A. Profound atrophy in the central fovea is observed (the arrow shows the scan direction). B. Optical Coherence Tomography shows an area of high reflectivity under the retinal pigment epithelium due to the scarring formation (small arrow). Subretinal fluid is not observed. The overlying retina appears thin due to its atrophy (big arrow).

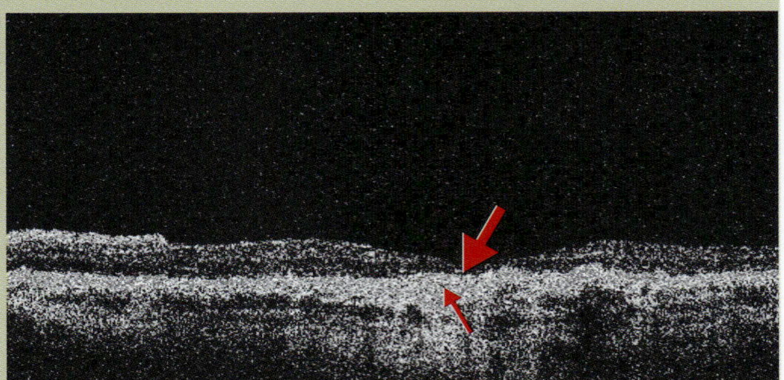

WET TYPE AGE-RELATED MACULAR DEGENERATION

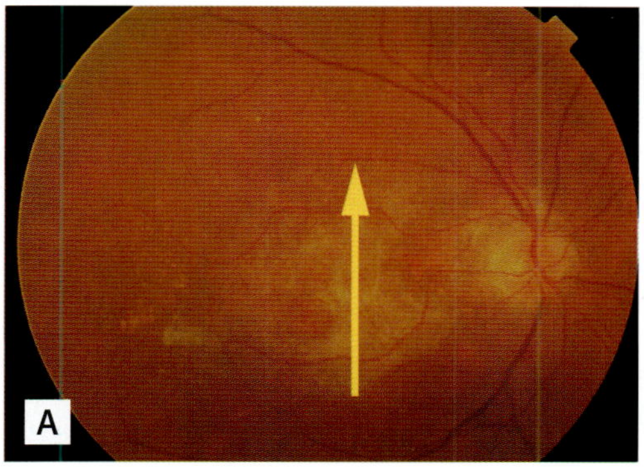

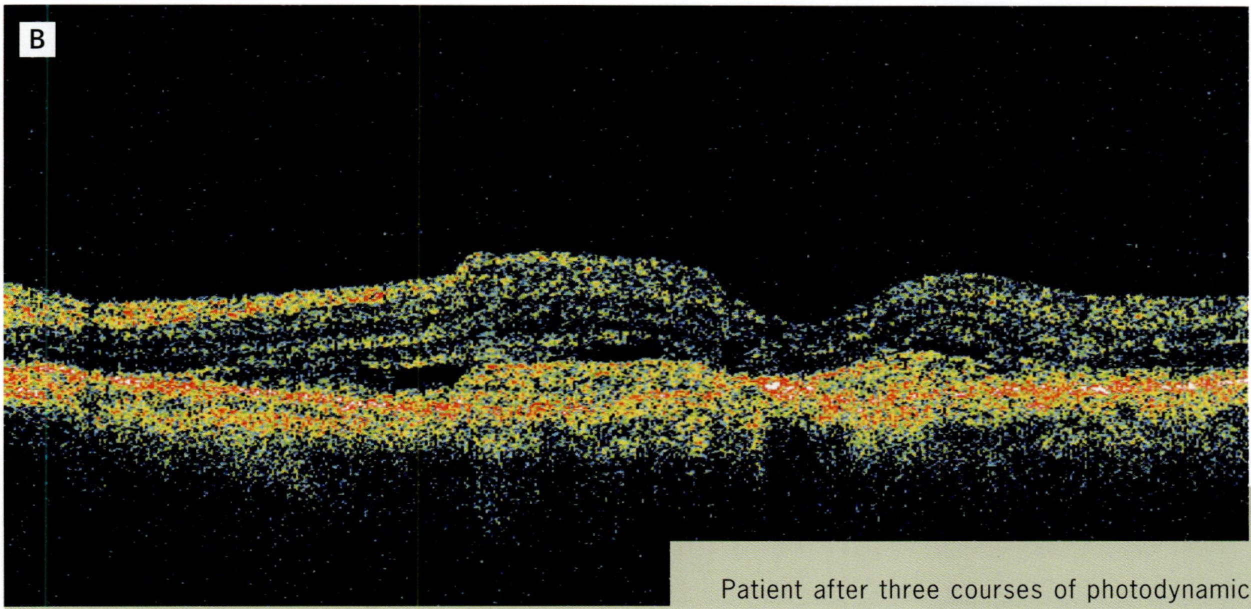

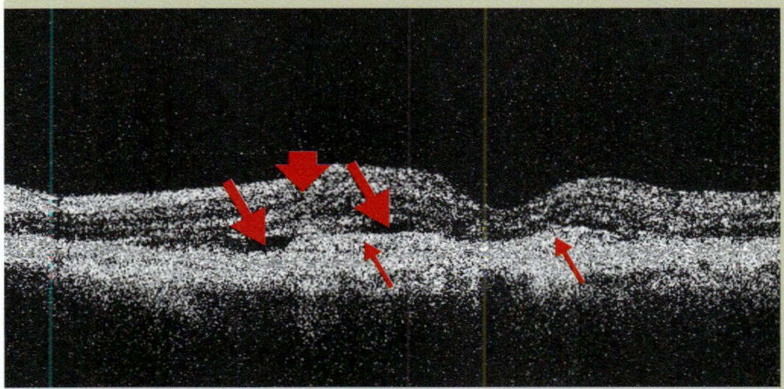

Patient after three courses of photodynamic therapy for choroidal neovascularization. A. Extensive macular scarring is observed (the arrow shows the scan direction). B. Optical Coherence Tomography shows a large area of high reflectivity at the retinal pigment epithelium due to the neovascular formation (small arrows). Note the small area of low reflectivity between the retina and the retinal pigment epithelium due to the presence of subretinal fluid (big arrows). An increase of retinal thickness because of the diffuse edema is also shown (thick arrow). In general, the persistence of subretinal fluid and retinal edema, combined with dubious fluorescein angiography findings, should direct the ophthalmologist towards continuation of treatment.

IDIOPATHIC CHOROIDAL NEOVASCULAR MEMBRANE

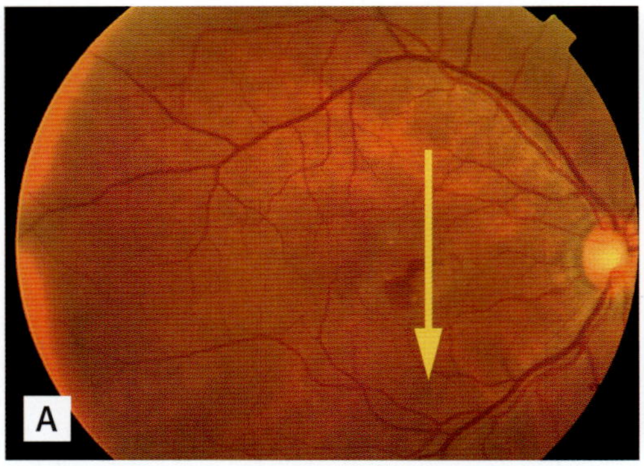

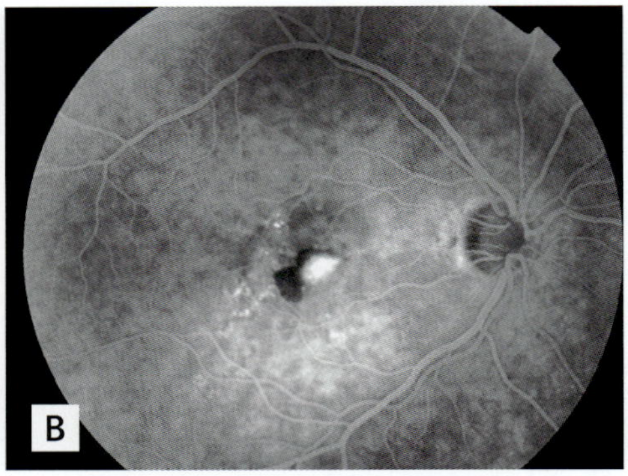

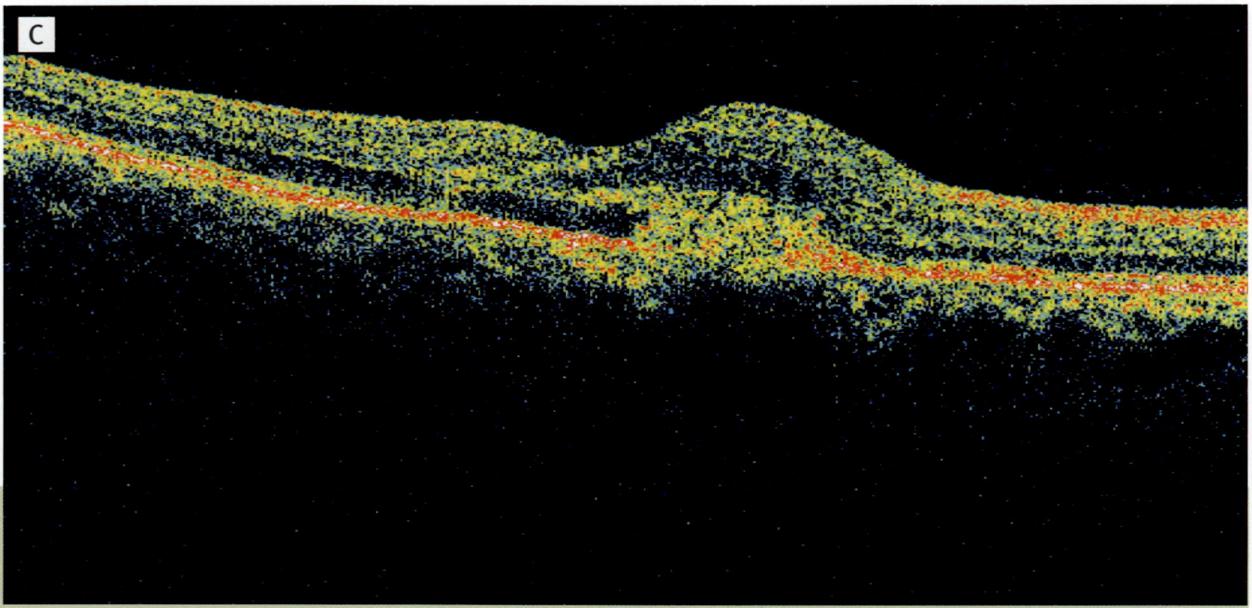

A 35 year old patient with idiopathic choroidal neovascular membrane. A. Notice the central foveal haemorrhage (the arrow shows the scan direction). B. Fluorescein angiography shows the subfoveal choroidal neovascularization that extends nasally to the fovea. C. Optical Coherence Tomography shows a thick area of high reflectivity above the retinal pigment epithelium inferonasally to the fovea (big arrow) due to the choroidal neovascularization. There is no presence of subretinal fluid but an increase of the retinal thickness due to edema is observed (small arrow).

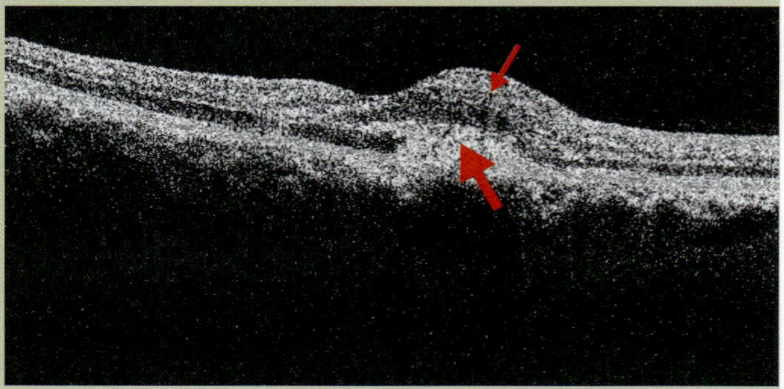

IDIOPATHIC CHOROIDAL NEOVASCULAR MEMBRANE

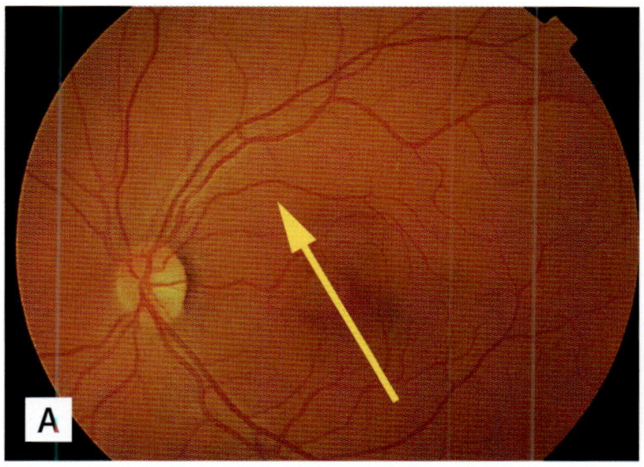

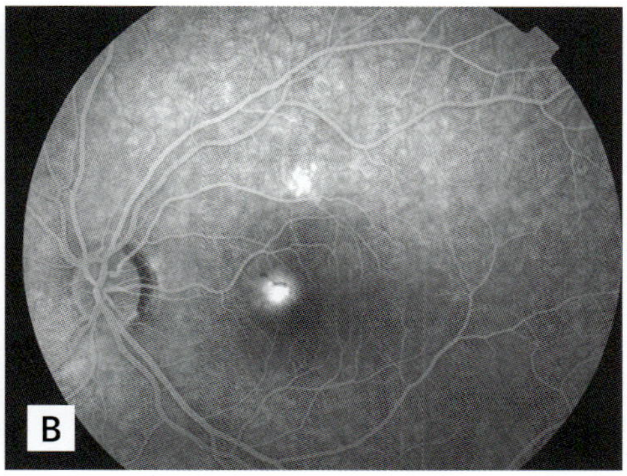

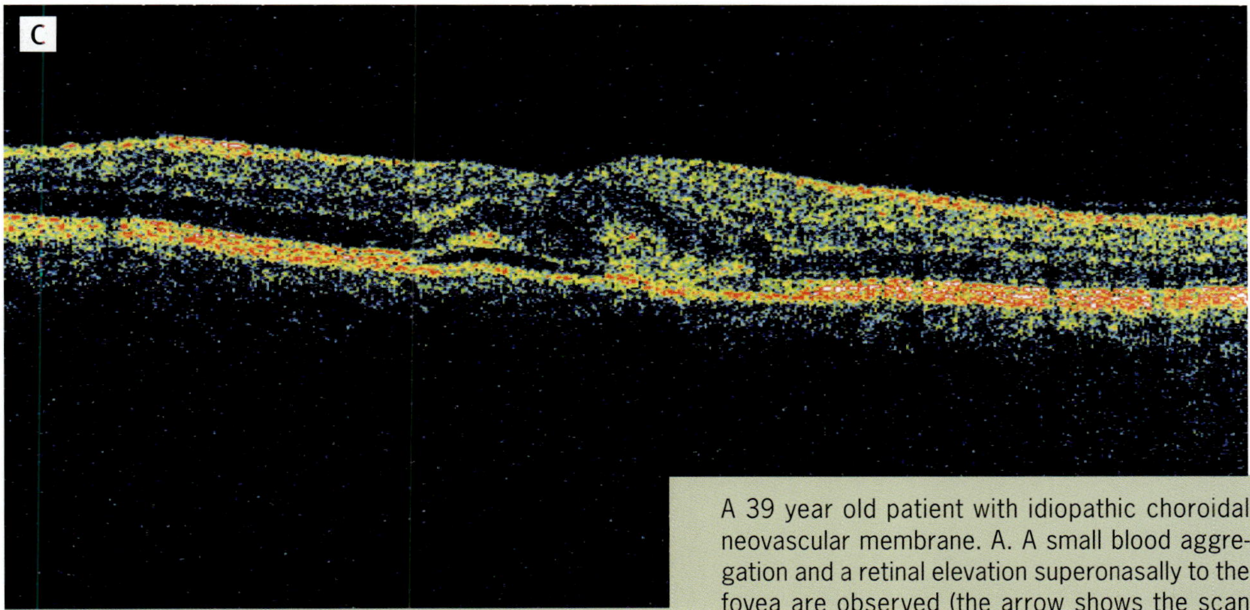

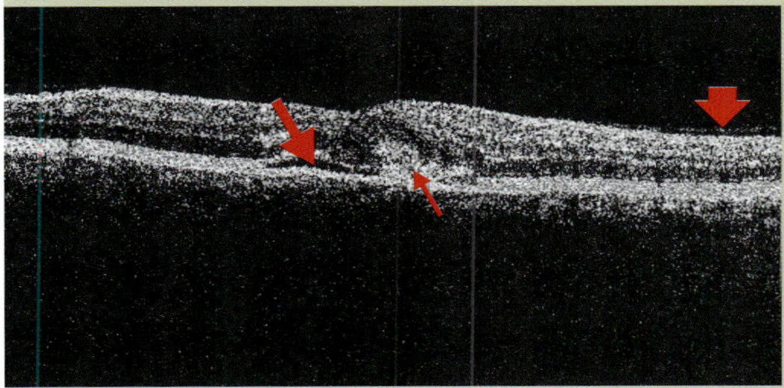

A 39 year old patient with idiopathic choroidal neovascular membrane. A. A small blood aggregation and a retinal elevation superonasally to the fovea are observed (the arrow shows the scan direction). B. In fluorescein angiography the dye leakage is obvious and corresponds to a classic choroidal neovascularization at the same area. C. Optical Coherence Tomography shows an area of high reflectivity located above the retinal pigment epithelium in the parafoveal area corresponding to a “type 2” choroidal neovascular membrane (small arrow). An area of low reflectivity, between the retina and the retinal pigment epithelium, that extends to the central fovea and is connected to the choroidal neovascularization is also observed corresponding to the subretinal fluid (big arrow). The vitreous seems to be attached to the retina in the macular area (thick arrow).

IDIOPATHIC POLYPOIDAL CHOROIDAL VASCULOPATHY

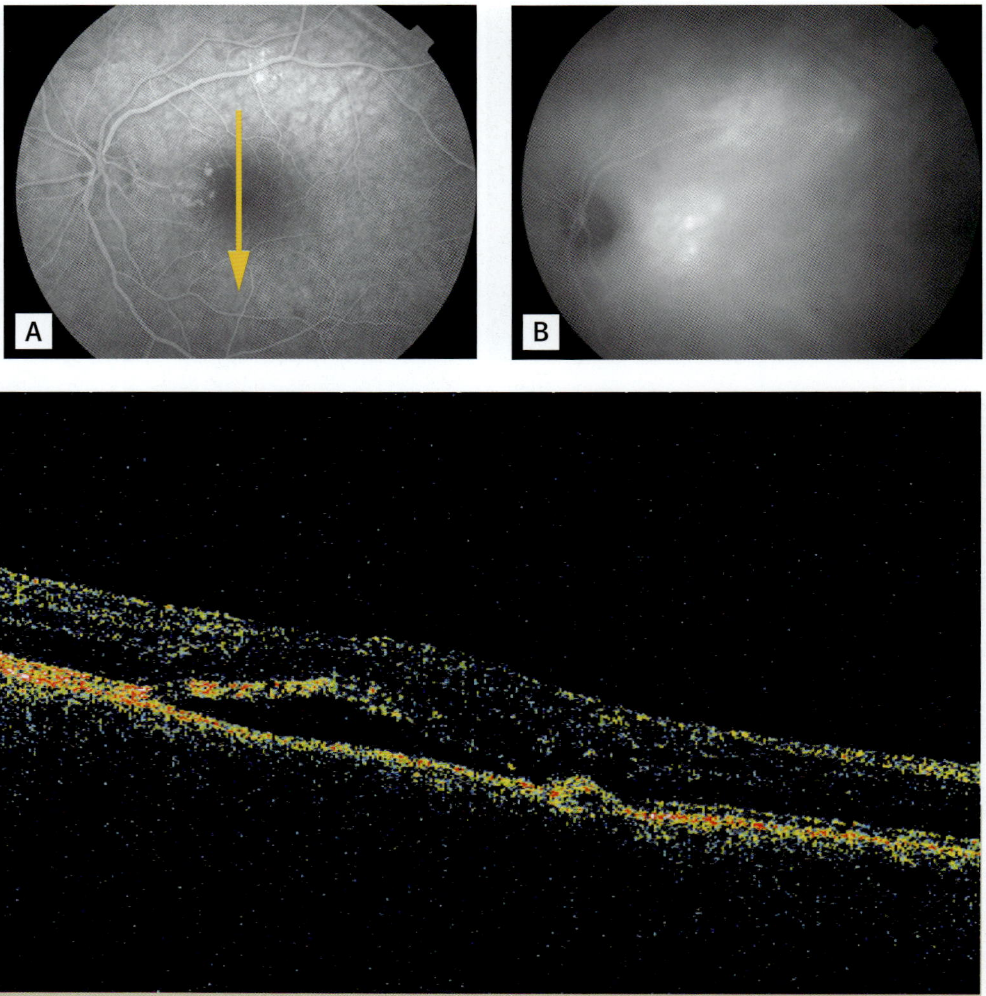

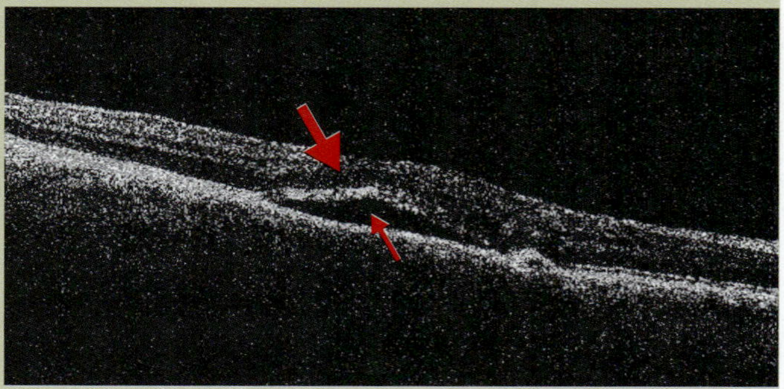

Patient with idiopathic polypoidal choroidal vasculopathy A. Fluorescein angiography shows multiple, small, subretinal areas of hyperfluorescence due to dye leakage, along the papillomacular bundle (the arrow shows the scan direction). B. Indocyanine green angiography shows polypoidal hyperfluorescent formations nasally to the macula. C. Notice the subfoveal area of low reflectivity located between the retina and the retinal pigment epithelium corresponding to the retinal detachment (small arrow). An increase of retinal thickness also coexists, corresponding to diffuse retinal edema (big arrow). Optical Coherence Tomography image is not typical in this disease.

IDIOPATHIC POLYPOIDAL CHOROIDAL VASCULOPATHY

A. Patient with idiopathic polypoidal choroidal vasculopathy (the arrow shows the scan direction). B. Fluorescein angiography shows a subretinal area

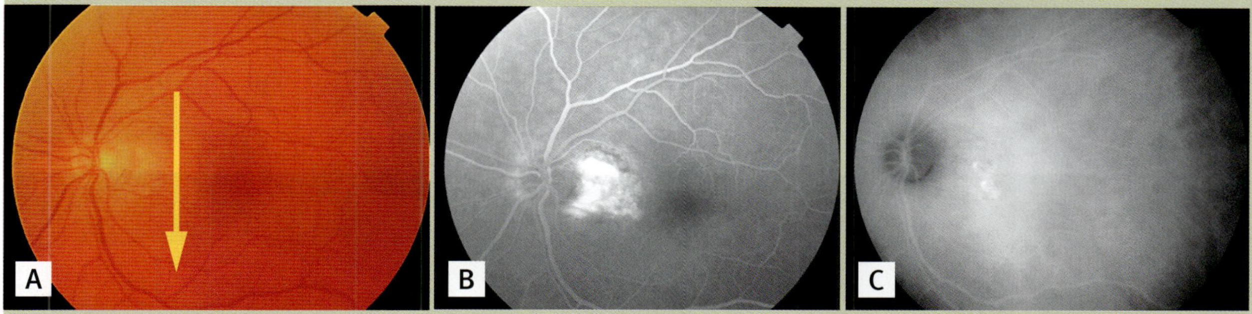

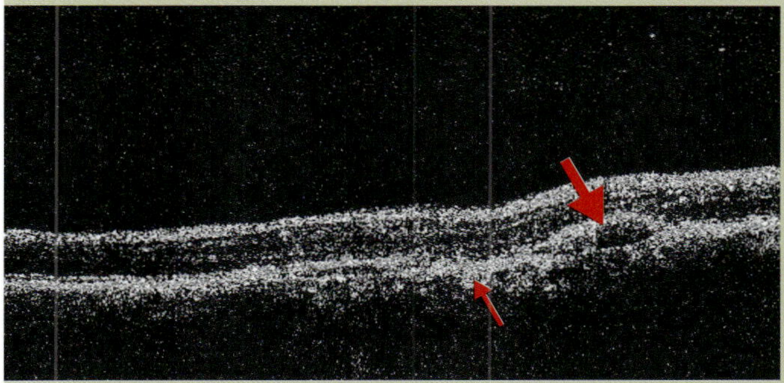

of hyperfluorescence due to dye leakage along the papillomacular bundle. C. Indocyanine green angiography shows the presence of polypoidal hyperfluorescent structures in the same area. D. Optical Coherence Tomography shows small areas of high reflectivity, located under the retinal pigment epithelium that correspond to the polypoidal formations (small arrow). A retinal pigment epithelium elevation of intermediate reflectivity is also observed (big arrow).

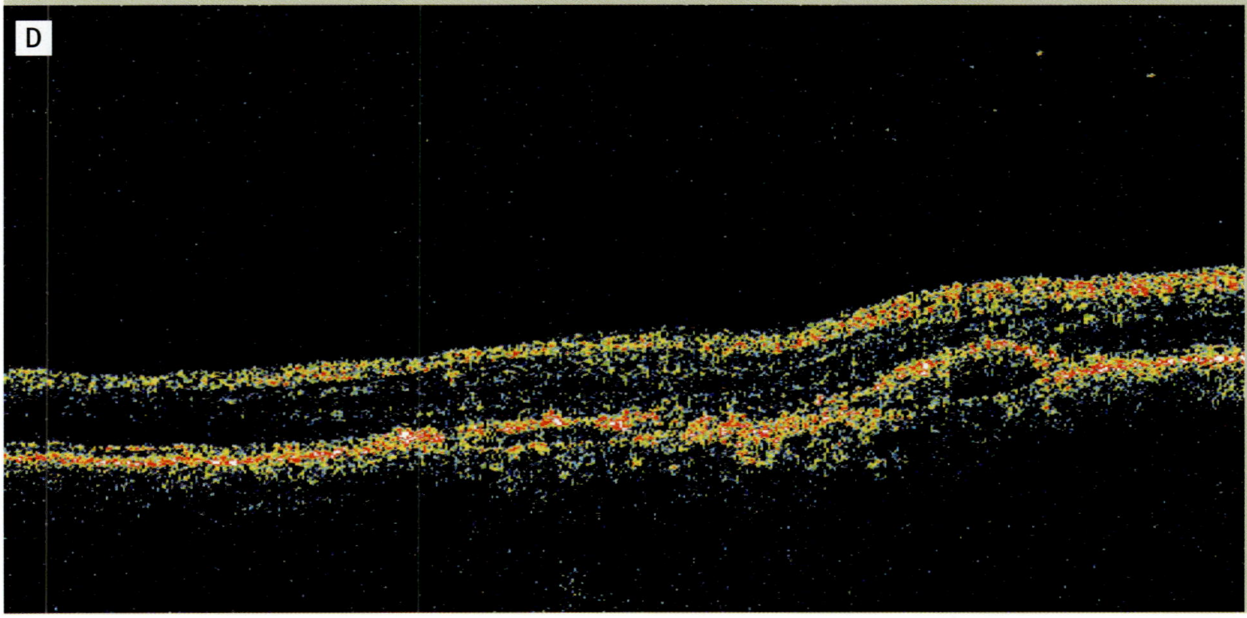

RETINAL PIGMENT EPITHELIUM DETACHMENT

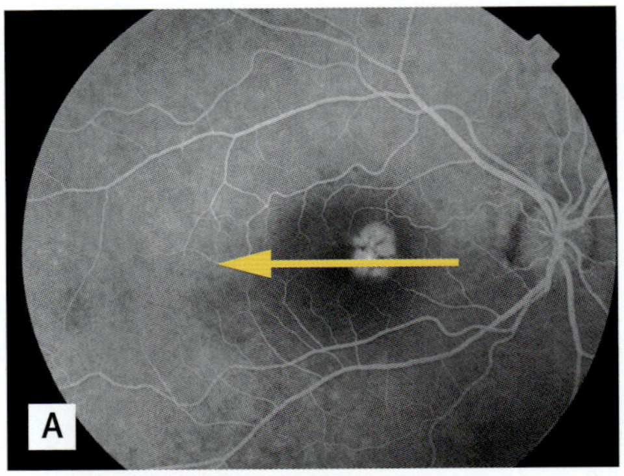

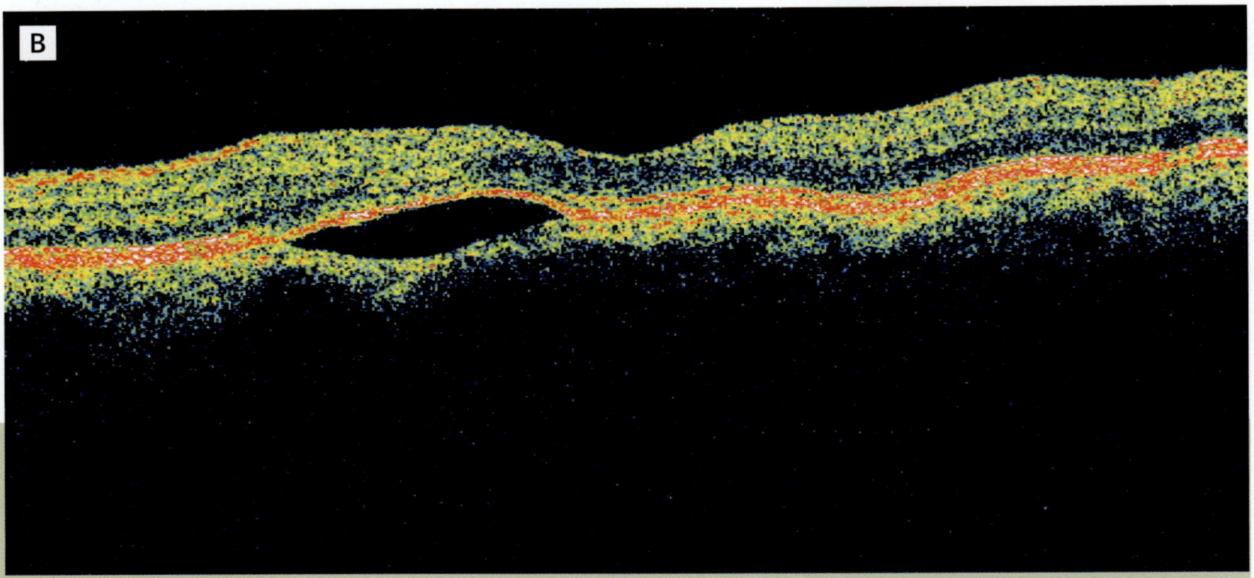

A 68 year old patient with normal visual acuity and a retinal pigment epithelium detachment that had already been observed by a colleague 5 years ago. A. Fluorescein angiography shows hyperfluorescence due to dye pooling that corresponds to the retinal pigment epithelium detachment with localized hypofluorescence due to pigment deposits (the arrow shows the scan direction). B. Optical Coherence Tomography shows an area of low reflectivity located under the retinal pigment epithelium near the central fovea, corresponding to a retinal pigment epithelium detachment (small arrow). There are no signs of choroidal neovascularization. Indocyanine green angiography is warranted in order to differentiate age-related macular degeneration from idiopathic central serous chorioretinopathy.

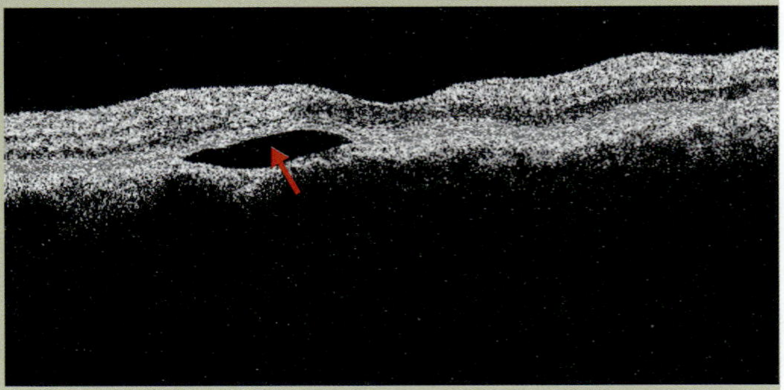

RETINAL ANGIOMATOUS PROLIFERATION

A. Patient with retinal angiomatous proliferation and the characteristic retinal haemorrhages (the arrow shows the scan direction). B. Fluorescein angiography shows the intraretinal anastomosis in the early phases. C. Indocyanine green angiography shows an area of hyperfluorescence (hot spot) corresponding to the angiomatous hyperplasia and an area of hypofluorescence corresponding to the retinal pig-

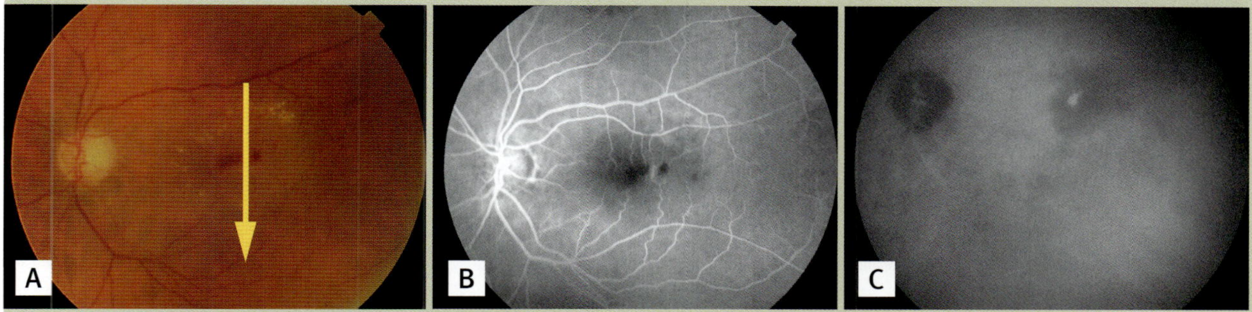

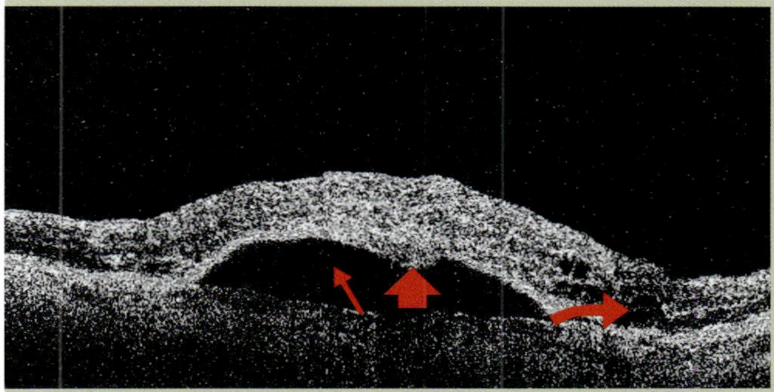

ment epithelium detachment. D. Optical Coherence Tomography depicts an area of low reflectivity under the retinal pigment epithelium due to its detachment (small arrow). An area of high reflectivity is illustrated at the intermediate retinal layers, corresponding to the angiomatous hyperplasia, which protrudes into the retinal pigment epithelium detachment cavity (thick arrow). Areas of low reflectivity inside the retinal layers are also observed, corresponding to cystoid retinal edema (convex arrow).

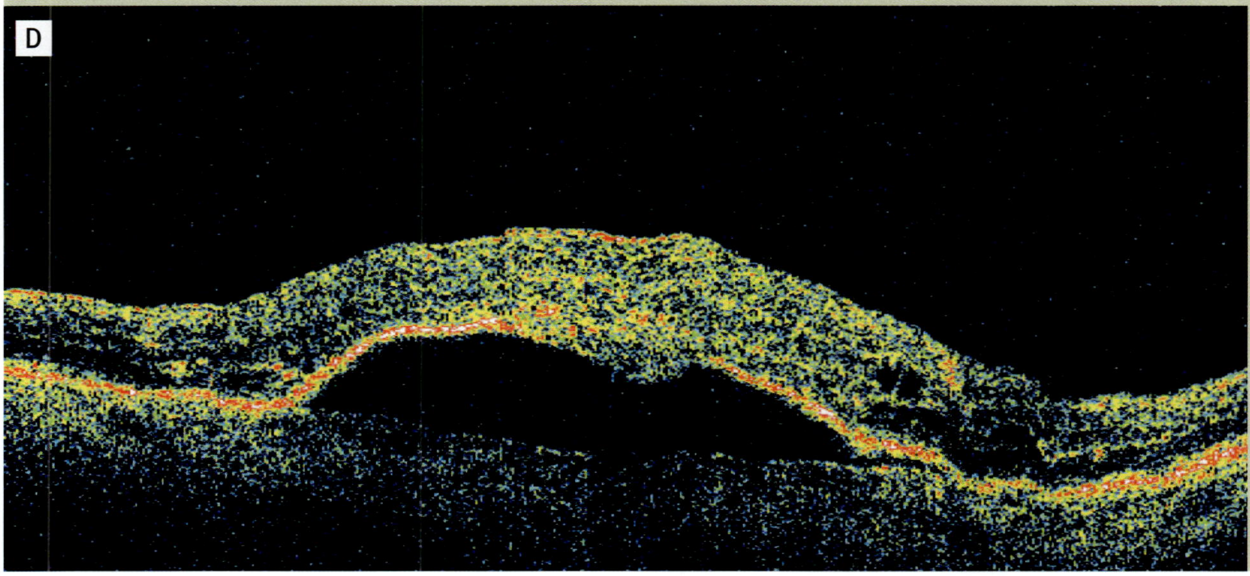

RETINAL ANGIOMATOUS PROLIFERATION

A. Patient with retinal angiomatous proliferation (the arrow shows the scan direction). B. Fluorescein angiography shows the intraretinal anastomosis in the early phases and the retinal pigment epithelium detachment in the middle and late phases. C. Indocyanine green angiography illustrates an area of hyperfluorescence (hot spot) corresponding to the angiomatous hyperplasia and an area of hypofluorescence corresponding to the retinal pigment epithelium detachment. D. Optical Coherence Tomography shows areas of low reflectivity under the retinal pigment epithelium, due to its detachment (small arrows). There is a high reflectivity area in the intermediate retinal layers, corresponding to the angiomatous hyperplasia (thick arrow). Multiple cystic spaces of low reflectivity, due to cystic edema, are observed in the retinal layers (convex arrows).

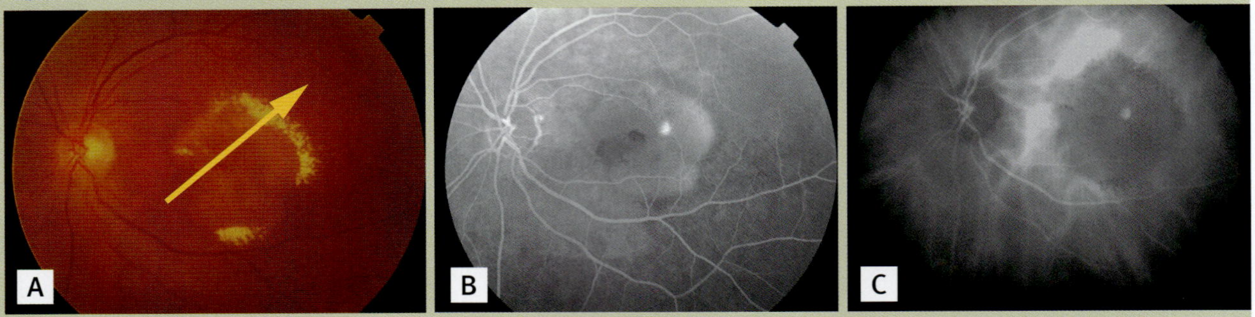

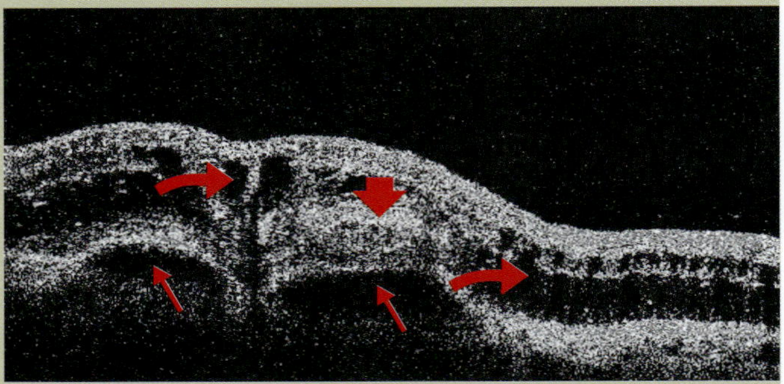

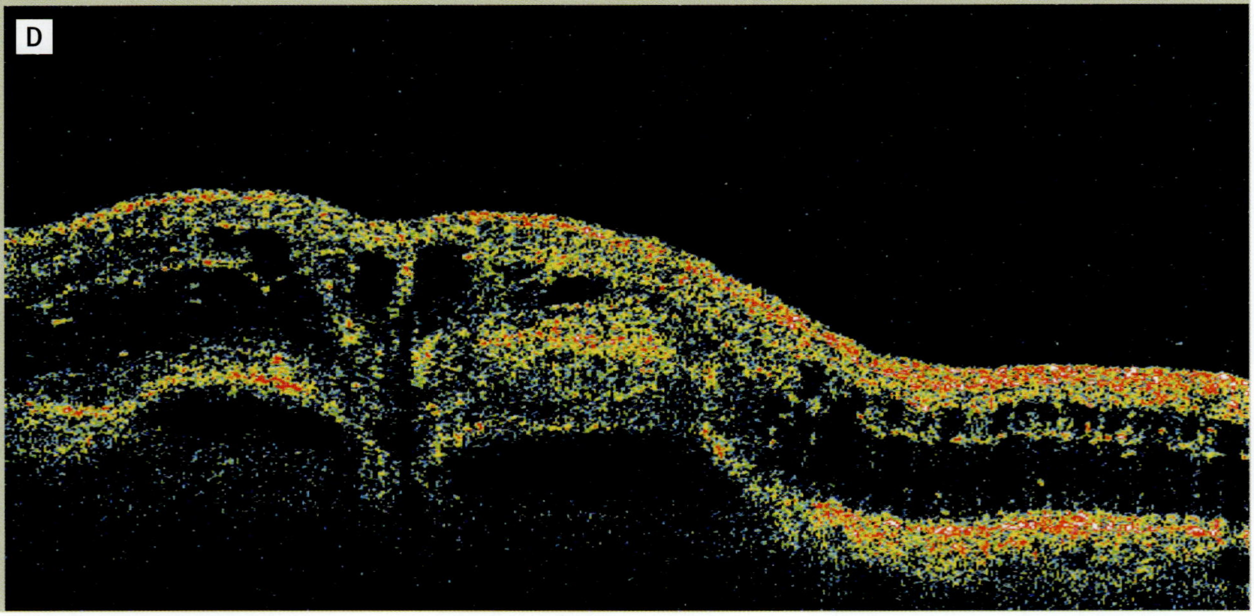

CHAPTER 3

EPIRETINAL MEMBRANE

Panagiotis Theodossiadis

Ivanoff (1865) first described the pathologic characteristics of the epiretinal membrane. However, real advances to this pathologic entity have been carried out the last 25 years. The epiretinal membrane that develops in the posterior pole of the eye can be idiopathic or can occur as a result of secondary conditions.

The disease is characterized by decrease in visual acuity, metamorphopsia and/or diplopia. Its evolution varies. In some cases it evolves rapidly and in other cases slowly. The epiretinal membrane can be distinguished clinically, according to its morphology, in stages as defined by Gass:

Grade (stage) 0: The membrane is transparent without changes of the retina.

Grade 1: The membrane causes distortion of the retinal surface.

Grade 2: The membrane appears white and causes retinal wrinkling obscuring the visibility of the underlying retinal vessels.

Pathogenesis: The cause of the epiretinal membrane has not been determined yet and most of the times it remains uncertain. In some cases it is due to inflammation, trauma, vascular disease, laser application, cryotherapy and vitrectomy.

An epiretinal membrane can be accompanied by vitreous detachment[11]. In that case one of the following situations is possible:

1. Epiretinal membrane with partial posterior vitreous detachment.
2. Epiretinal membrane with complete posterior vitreous detachment.
3. Epiretinal membrane with vitreous traction.

IDIOPATHIC EPIRETINAL MEMBRANE

Idiopathic epiretinal membrane occurs in approximately 20% of patients over the age of 75 years and its incidence increases with age.
The visual acuity decreases when the membrane is located at the center of the macula.
The decrease is mild and rarely reaches the level of 20/200[9].

When visual acuity is severely affected, there is usually displacement of the retinal vessels, occasionally microaneurysms and dye leakage in fluorescein angiography.
An epiretinal membrane can remain stable for a long time.
In other cases it evolves and affects the visual acuity.
In these cases vitrectomy is recommended.
Automatic separation from the retina surface has been observed in a few cases (1%).

OPTICAL COHERENCE TOMOGRAPHY AND IDIOPATHIC EPIRETINAL MEMBRANE

Optical Coherence Tomography is a very useful method of examination for the diagnosis of the epiretinal membrane[1,2,13]. With Optical Coherence Tomography the membrane appears like a thin area of high reflectivity which is located on the retinal surface. According to its extension and its retinal attachment, the membrane can be distinguished as continuous or interrupted (not continually adherent).

In cases where the membrane is partially adherent to the posterior pole, it must be differentiated from a posterior vitreous detachment[3,4,6]. In this case, apart from the physician's experience, the structure and the thickness of the membrane can help in the differential diagnosis.

Optical Coherence Tomography also helps in:

1. The calculation of the retinal thickness under the membrane in the macula[5]. An increase in retinal thickness is often accompanied by a decrease in visual acuity.
2. The diagnosis of pseudohole and its differentiation from a full thickness or a lamellar macular hole[7]. In this case the morphology and the thickness of the fovea will determine the nature of the hole.
3. The precise preoperative evaluation of the membrane and in particular the extent, the morphology and the adherence on the retinal surface[2,8].
4. The measurment and comparison of the preoperative and postoperative macular thickness[10,12,14].

EPIRETINAL MEMBRANE

1. Azzolini C, Patelli F, Codenotti M, Pierro L, Brancato R. Optical coherence tomography in idiopathic epiretinal macular membrane surgery. Eur J Ophthalmol 1999 ; 9 : 206-211.

2. Carpineto P, Ciancaglini M, Aharrh-Gnama A, Agnifili L, Mastropasqua L. Optical coherence tomography and retinal thickness analyzer features of spontaneous resolution of vitreomacular traction syndrome: a case report. Eur J Ophthalmol 2004; 14: 67-70.

3. Gallemore RP, Jumper JM, McCuen BW 2nd, Jaffe GJ, Postel EA, Toth CA. Diagnosis of vitreoretinal adhesions in macular diseases with optical coherence tomography. Retina 2000; 20: 115-120.

4. Hillenkamp J, Saikia P, Cora F, Sachs HG, Lohmann CP, Roider J, Baumler W, Gabel VP. Macular function and morphology after peeling of idiopathic epiretinal membrane with and without the assistance of indocyanine green. Br J Ophthalmol 2005; 89: 437-443.

5. Johnson MW. Tractional cystoid macular edema: a subtle variant of the vitreomacular traction syndrome. Am J Ophthalmolo 2005; 140: 184-192.

6. Meyer CH, Rodrigues EB, Mennel S, Schmidt JC. Spontaneous separation of epiretinal membrane in young subjects: personal observations and review of the literature. Graefes Arch Clin Exp Ophthalmol 2004; 242: 977-985.

7. Mizushima T, Uemure A, Sakamoto T. Prefoveolar membrane in macular hole opercula formation. Jpn J Ophthalmol 2004; 48: 478-485.

8. Niwa T, Terasaki H, Kondo M, Piao CH, Suzuki T. Miyake Y. Function and morphology of macula before and after removal of idiopathic epiretinal membrane. Invest Ophthalmol Vis Sci 2003; 44:1652-1656.

9. Sandberg MA, Brockhurst RJ, Gaudio AR, Berson EL. The association between visual acuity and central retinal thickness in retinitis pigmentosa. Invest Ophthalmol Vis Sci 2005; 46: 3349-3354.

10. Suzuki T, Terasaki H, Niwa T, Mori M, Kondo M, Miyake Y. Optical coherence tomography and focal macular electroretinogram in eyes with epiretinal membrane and macular pseudohole. Am J Ophthalmo 2003; 136: 62-67.

11. Thomas D, Bunce C, Moorman C, Laidlaw AH, Frequency and associations of a taut thickened posterior hyaloid, partial vitreomacular separation, and subretinal fluid in patients with diabetic macular edema. Retina 2005; 25: 883-888.

12. Uemoto R, Yamamoto S, Takeuchi S. Epimacular proliferative response following internal limiting membrane peeling for idiopathic macular holes. Graefes Arch Clin Exp Ophthalmol 2004; 242: 177-180.

13. Wilkins JR, Puliafito CA, Hee MR, Duker JS, Reichel E, Coker JG, Schuman JS, Swanson EA, Fujimoto JG. Characterization of epiretinal membranes using optical coherence tomography. Ophthalmology 1996; 103: 2142-2151.

14. Yamada N, Kishi S. Tomographic features and surgical outcomes of vitreomacular traction syndrome. Am J Ophthalmol 2005; 139: 112-117.

DIABETIC EPIRETINAL MEMBRANE

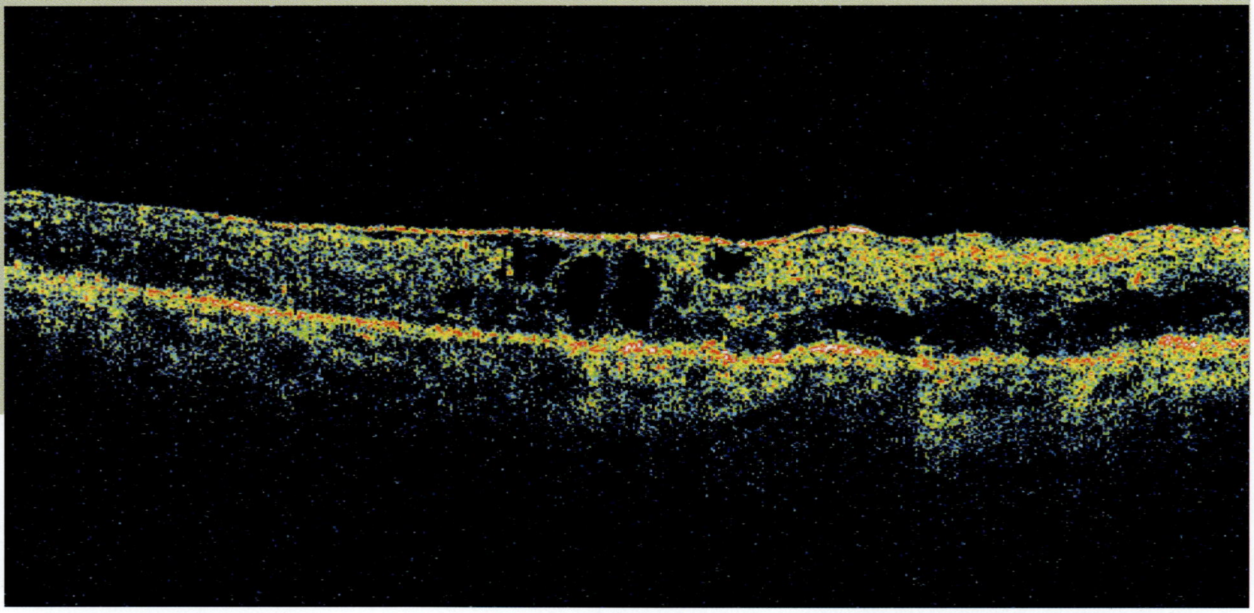

Patient with diabetic maculopathy. Note the multiple cystic formations of low intraretinal reflectivity corresponding to the diffuse cystoid retinal edema (small arrow). There is a thin area of high reflectivity on the retinal surface that corresponds to an epiretinal membrane in the macula (big arrow). Note the empty spaces between the membrane and the inner retinal surface (arrow head). The surgical excision of the membrane will be more beneficial than the laser treatment for this patient.

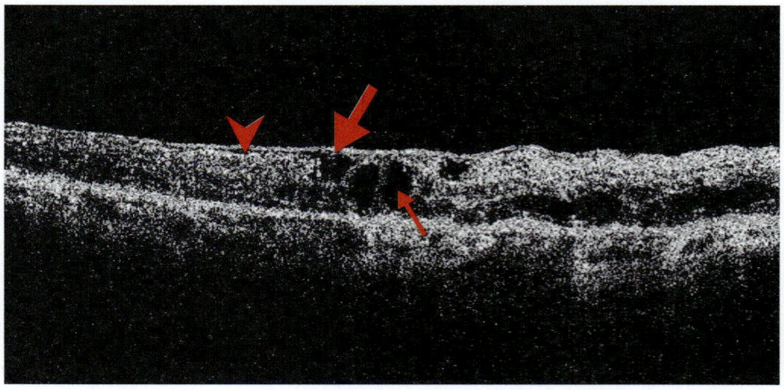

EPIRETINAL MEMBRANE

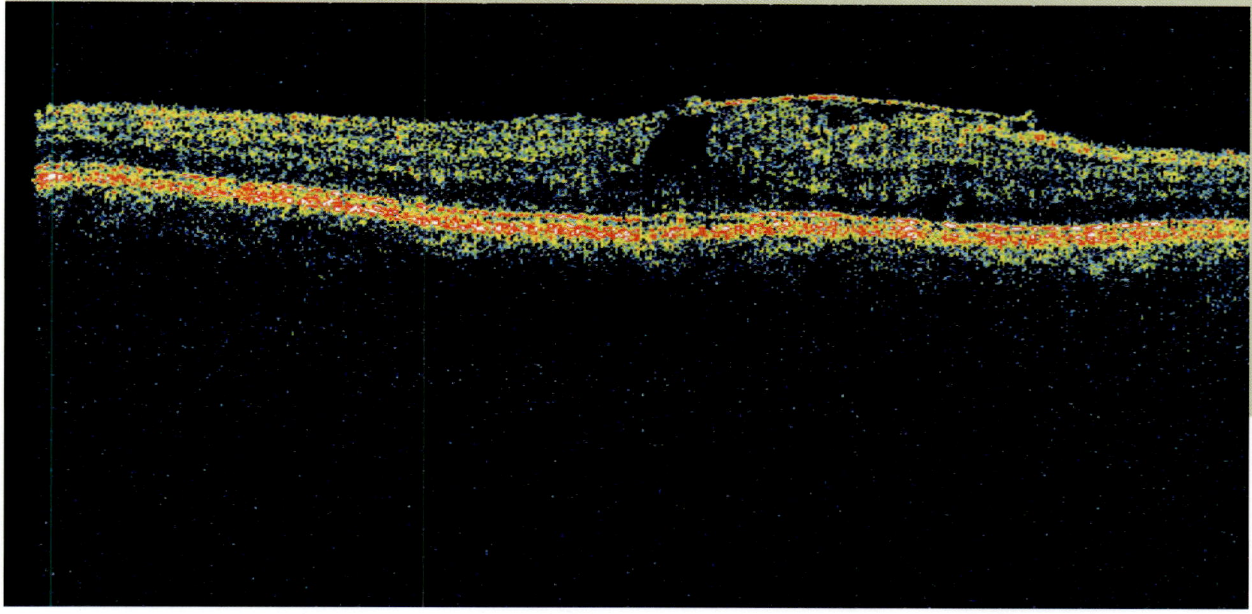

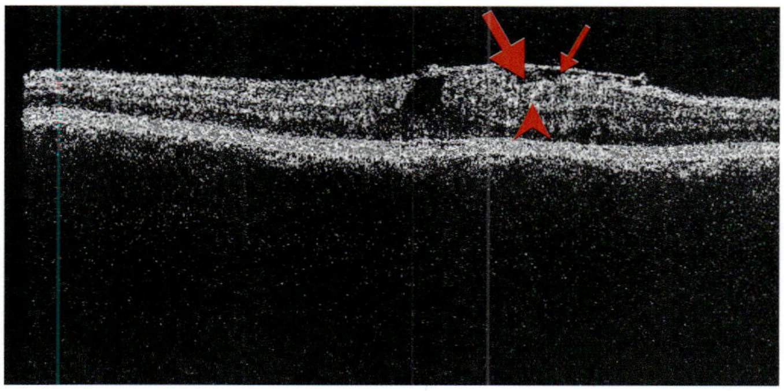

Patient with epiretinal membrane. Note the thin area of high reflectivity on the surface of the retina that corresponds to an epiretinal membrane in the fovea and to the right side of it (small arrow). The areas of low reflectivity located under the membrane consist of empty spaces between the membrane and the distorted retinal surface (big arrow). Note also the coexisting retinal edema (arrow head).

EPIRETINAL MEMBRANE

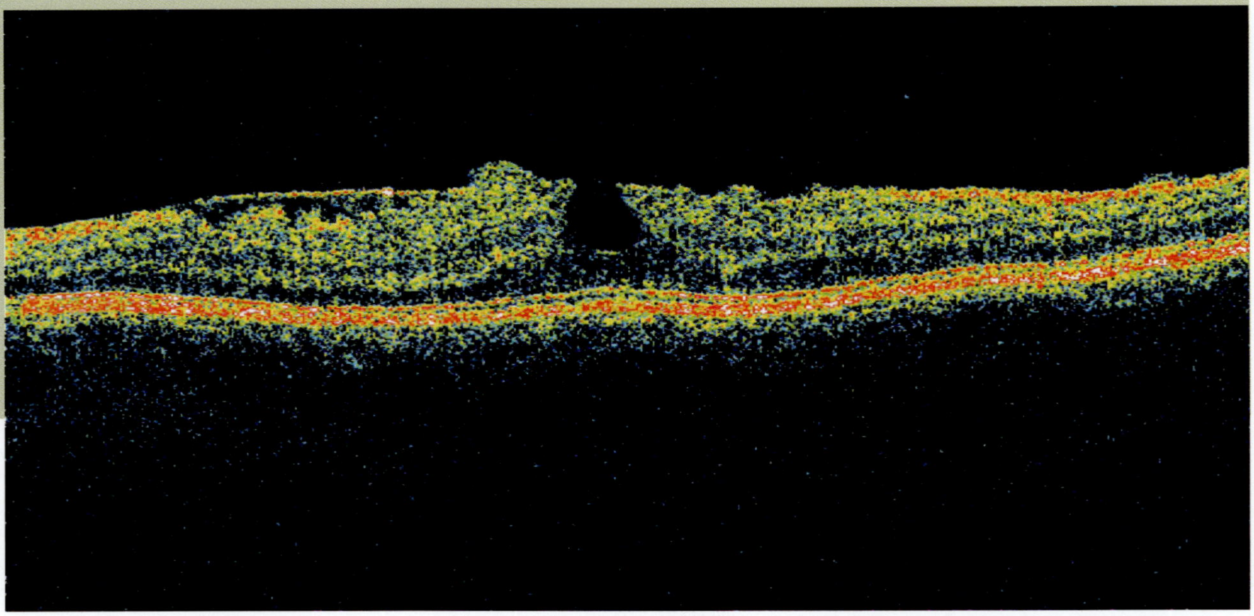

The patient of page 69, six months later. The membrane continues to be detected as a thin area of high reflectivity located at the left of the fovea (small arrow). A retinal defect is clearly visible at the fovea and corresponds to a macular pseudohole that has been created by the traction of the membrane (big arrow). The borders of the hole appear regular and vertical to its bed (arrow head). The retinal thickness around the hole has increased. This represents a complication of the epiretinal membrane.

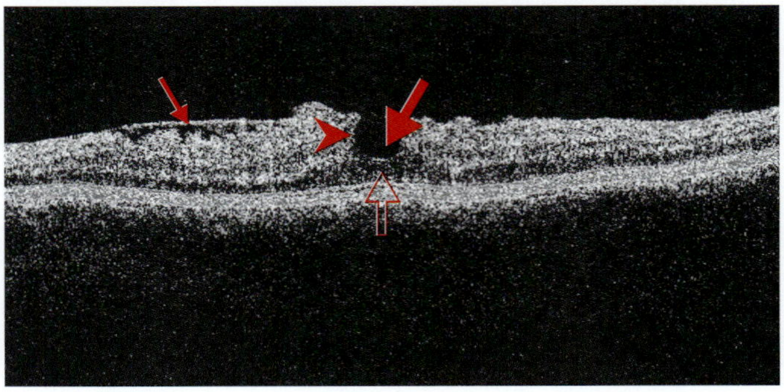

EPIRETINAL MEMBRANE

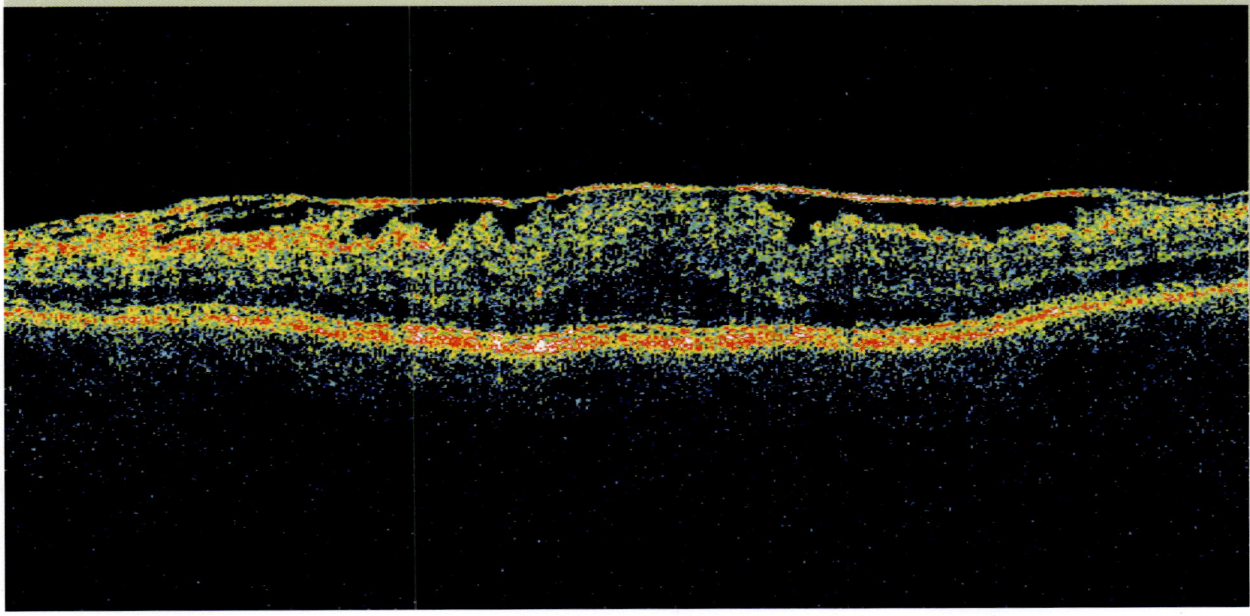

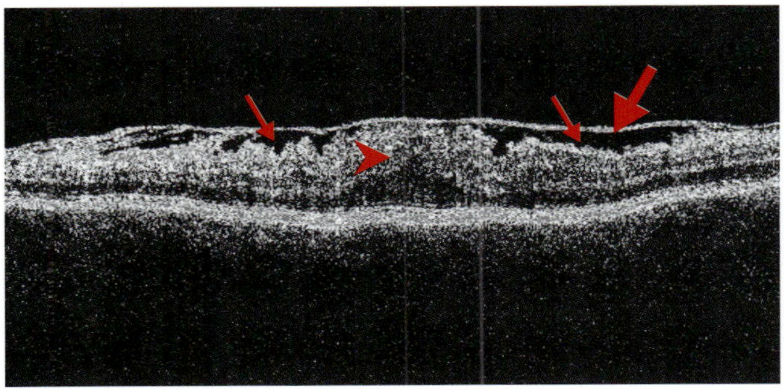

Patient with epiretinal membrane. A thin area of high reflectivity is detected on the retinal surface and corresponds to an epiretinal membrane in the macula (big arrow). Note the empty space detected between the membrane and the irregular inner retinal surface (small arrows).The retina appears thicker due to edema, mainly in the outer layers (arrow head).

EPIRETINAL MEMBRANE

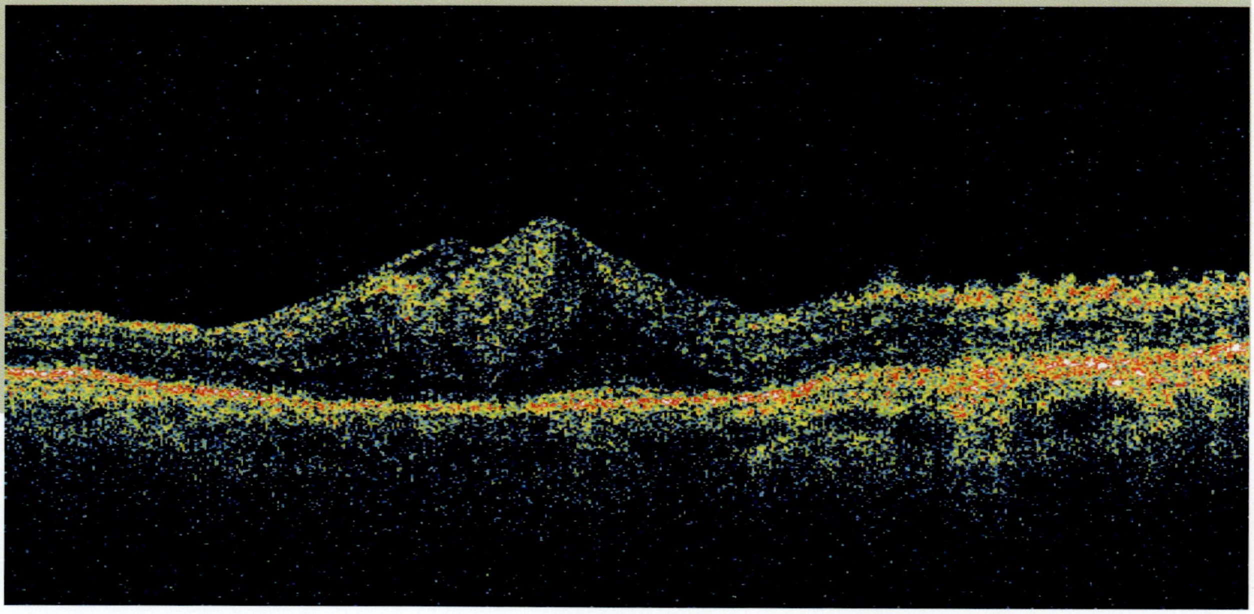

Patient with epiretinal membrane. Note the thin area of high reflectivity located on the retinal surface corresponding to an epiretinal membrane in the fovea (small arrow). The retinal surface appears considerably distorted to the right of the fovea (big arrow). The fovea appears considerably thick because of the diffuse edema (arrow head).

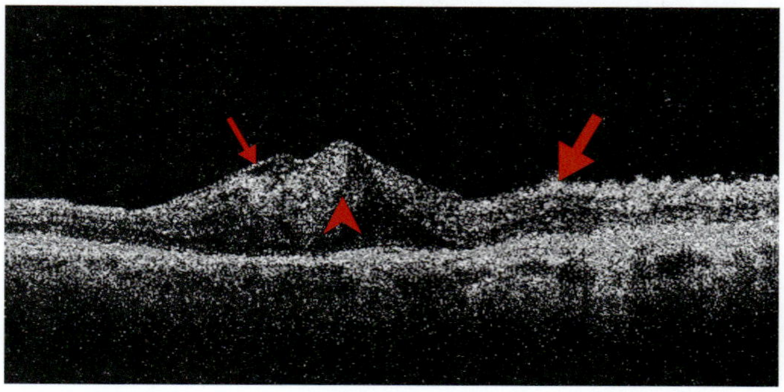

EPIRETINAL MEMBRANE

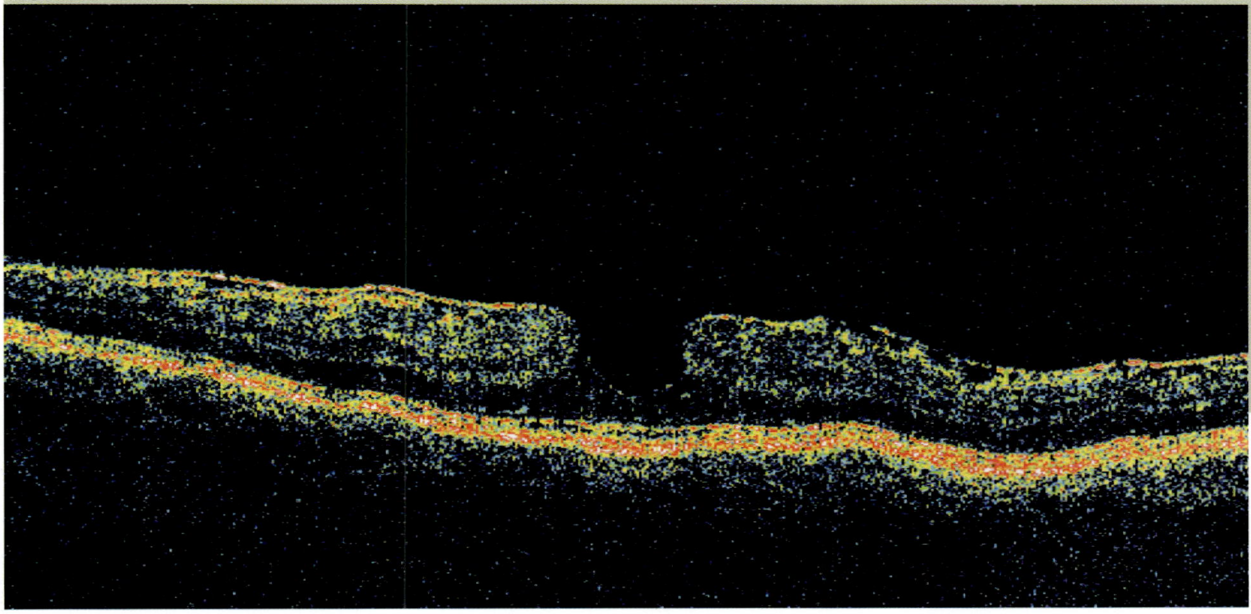

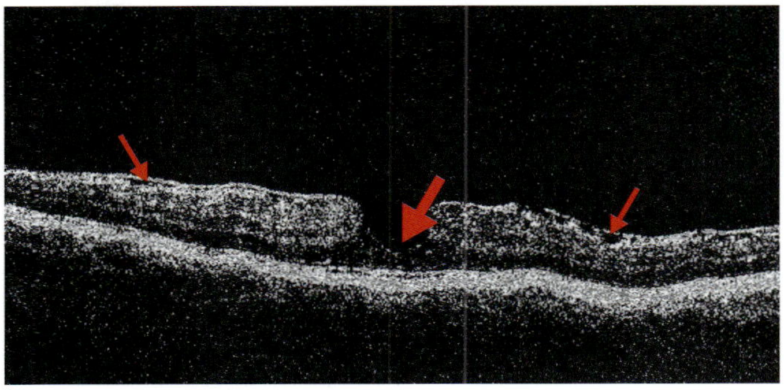

Patient with epiretinal membrane. Note the thin area of high reflectivity located on the retinal surface that corresponds to an epiretinal membrane in the fovea and around it (small arrows). There is a retinal defect corresponding to a lamellar hole in the fovea (big arrow).

EPIRETINAL MEMBRANE

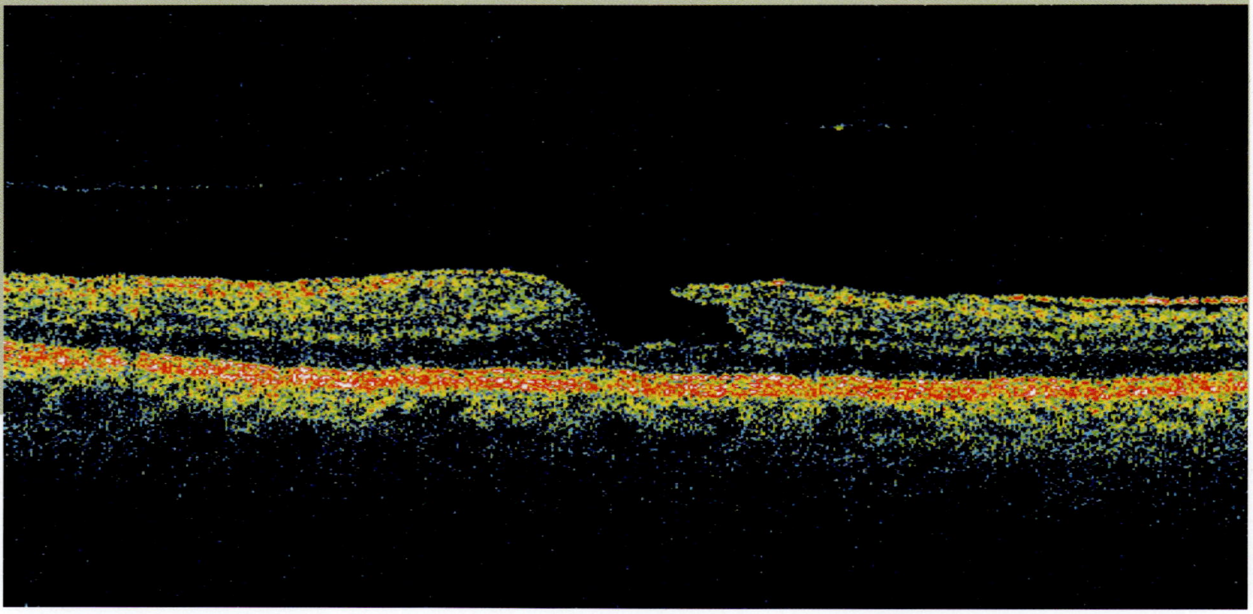

Patient with epiretinal membrane. Note the thin area of high reflectivity located on the retinal surface that corresponds to an epiretinal membrane in the fovea and around it (small arrows). There is a retinal defect corresponding to a lamellar hole in the fovea (big arrow). The vitreous appears detached from the retina and is represented as a thin horizontal line inside the vitreous cavity (arrow head).

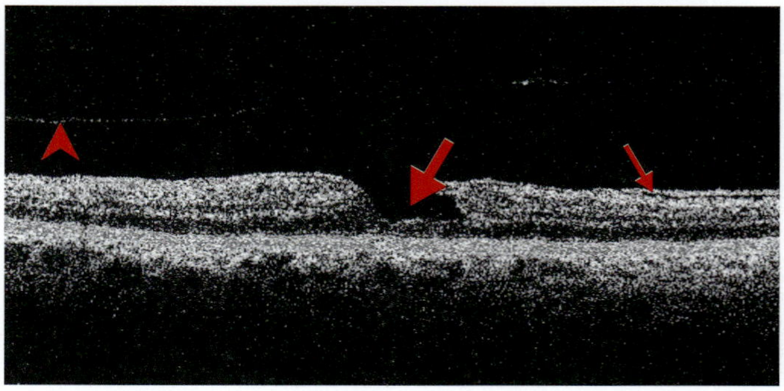

EPIRETINAL MEMBRANE

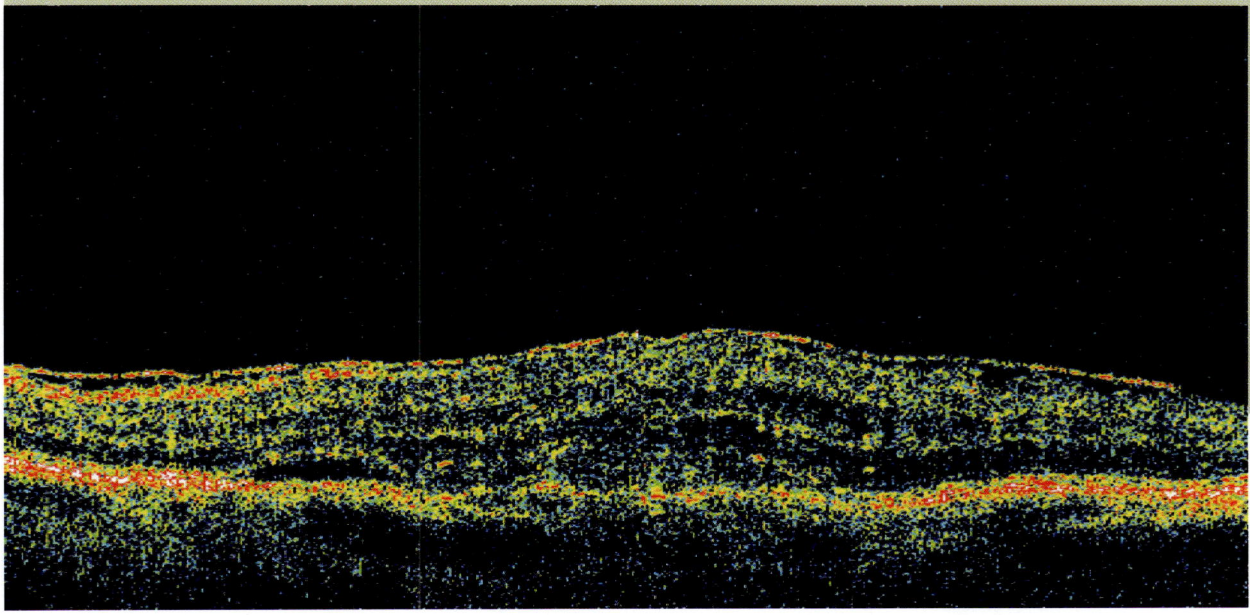

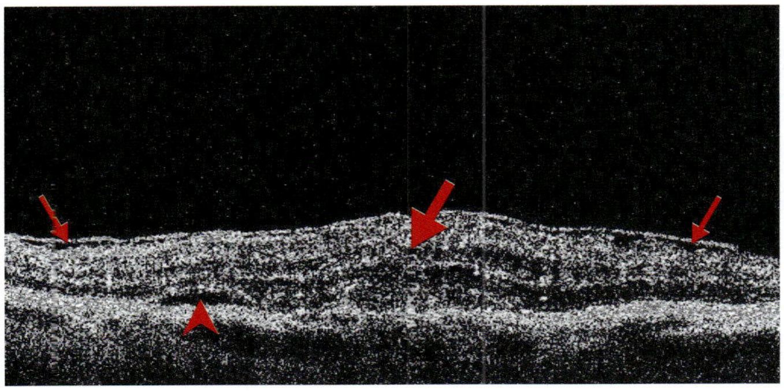

The thin area of high reflectivity on the retinal surface corresponds to an epiretinal membrane in the macula with global adherence to the retina (small arrows). Note the increased thickness in the central area due to edema (big arrow) and the limited retinal detachment (thick arrow).

DIABETIC EPIRETINAL MEMBRANE

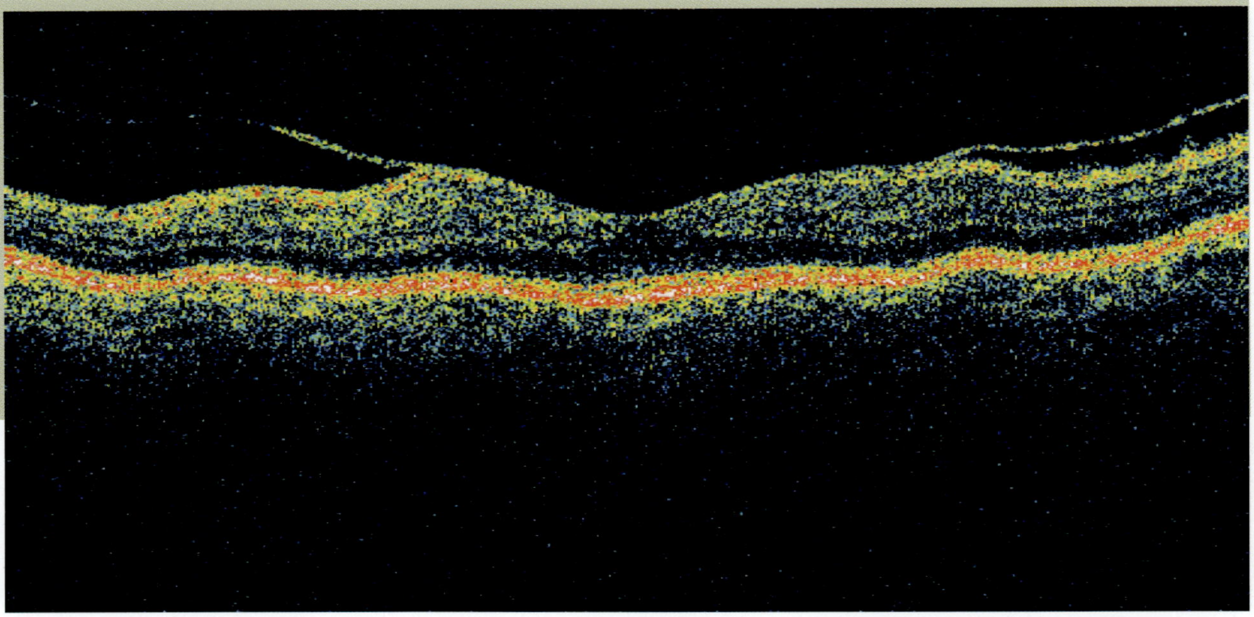

Diabetic patient with recent reduction in visual acuity. The posterior cortical vitreous is detected like a thick line of high reflectivity strongly attached to the fovea (big arrows). There is a very thin area of high reflectivity to the right of the fovea, located on the retina surface that corresponds to an epiretinal membrane (small arrow).

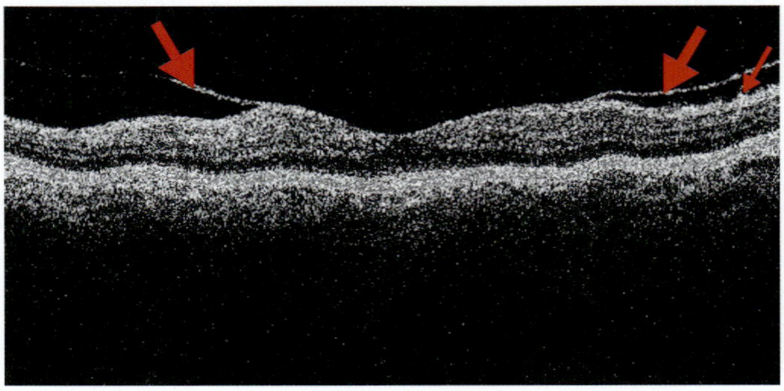

EPIRETINAL MEMBRANE

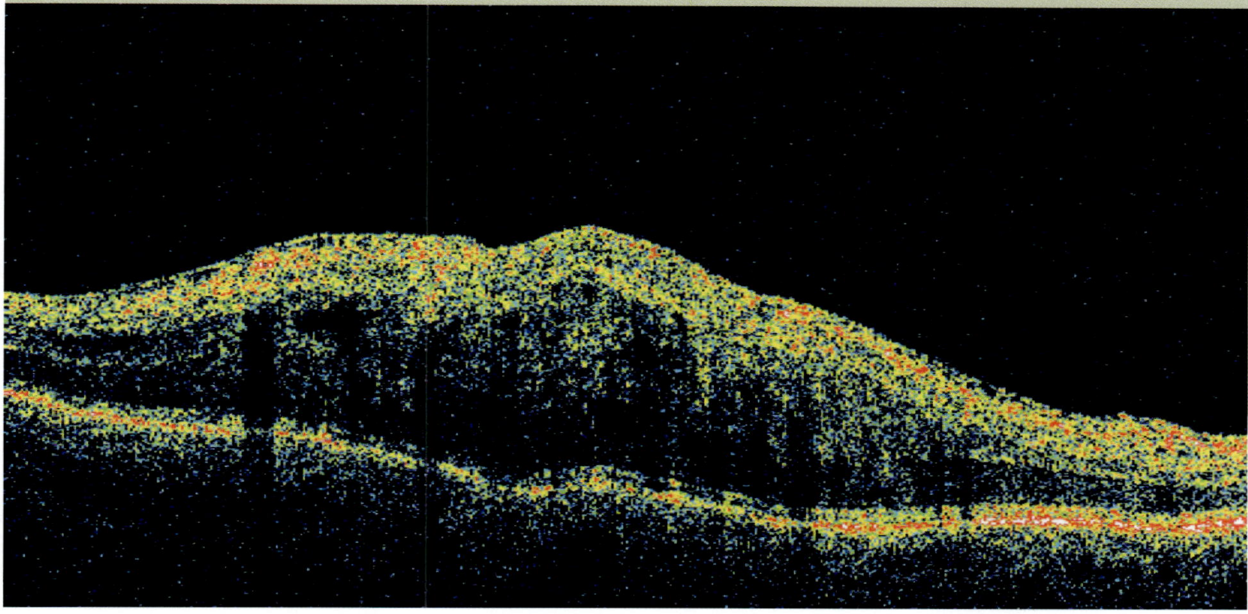

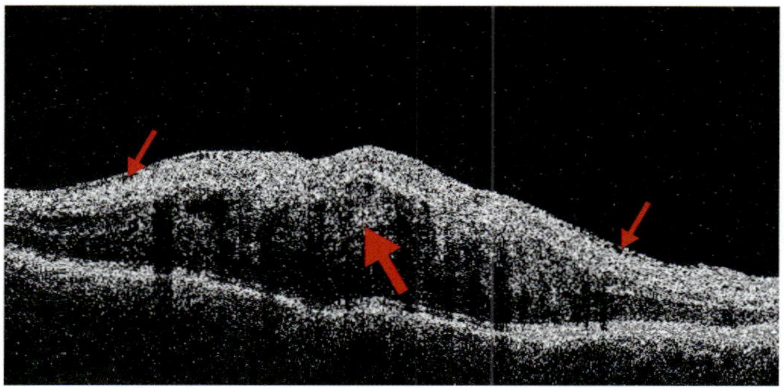

Patient with epiretinal membrane. Note the thin area of high reflectivity located on the retinal surface that corresponds to an epiretinal membrane in the fovea and around it (small arrows). The retina appears considerably thick with an area of low reflectivity in the outer layers corresponding to diffuse edema (big arrow).

MYOPIC EPIRETINAL MEMBRANE

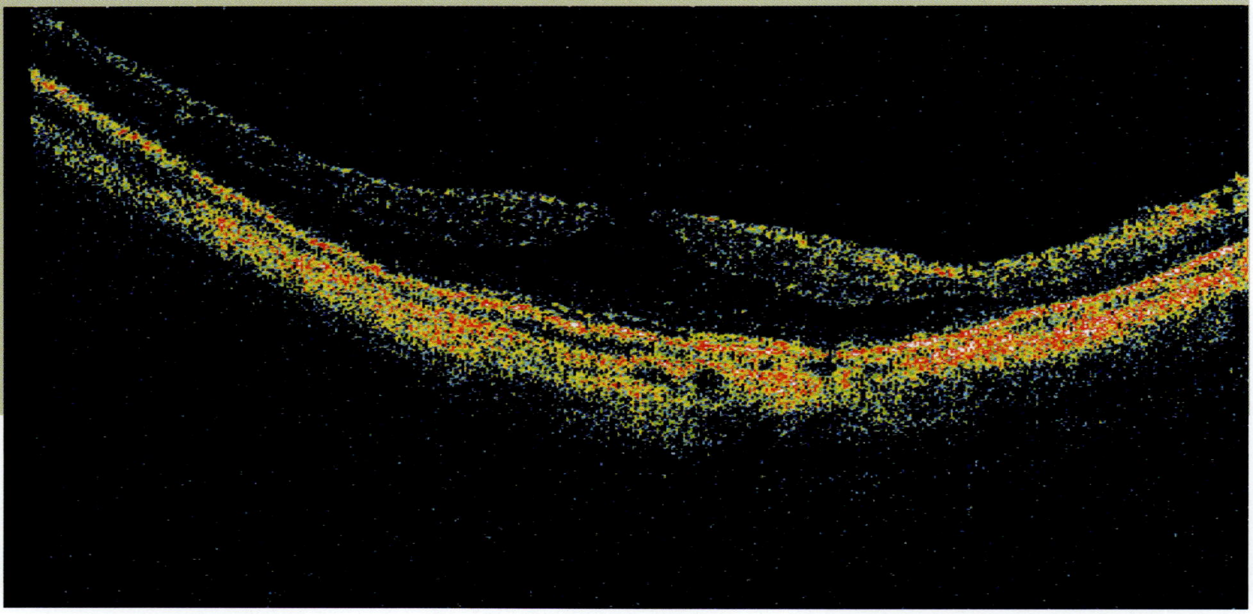

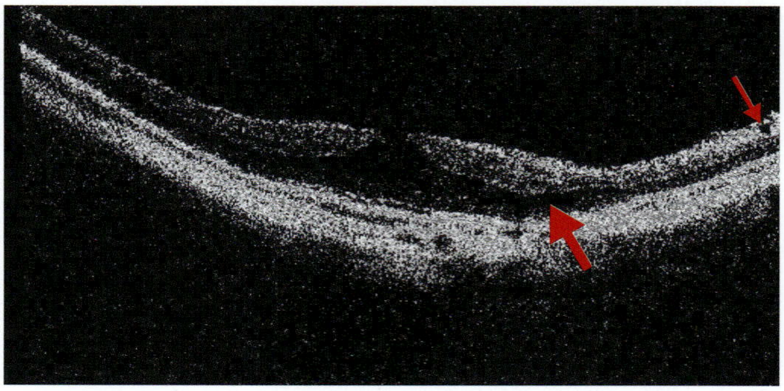

Patient with high myopia (-20D) and a recent decrease of visual acuity. There is a diffuse area of low reflectivity located in the outer retinal layers in the fovea that corresponds to a retinoschisis (big arrow). There is also an area of high reflectivity to the right of the macula, located on the retinal surface corresponding to an epiretinal membrane (small arrow). The retinal layers are not clearly distinguished because of the high myopia.

MYOPIC EPIRETINAL MEMBRANE

The patient of page 78 six months after the surgical excision of the epiretinal membrane. The retinoschisis has extended further (big arrow). Moreover, a retinal defect appears in the fovea that corresponds to a lamellar macular hole (small arrow). Multiple cystic formations of low reflectivity are located in the inner retinal layers and correspond

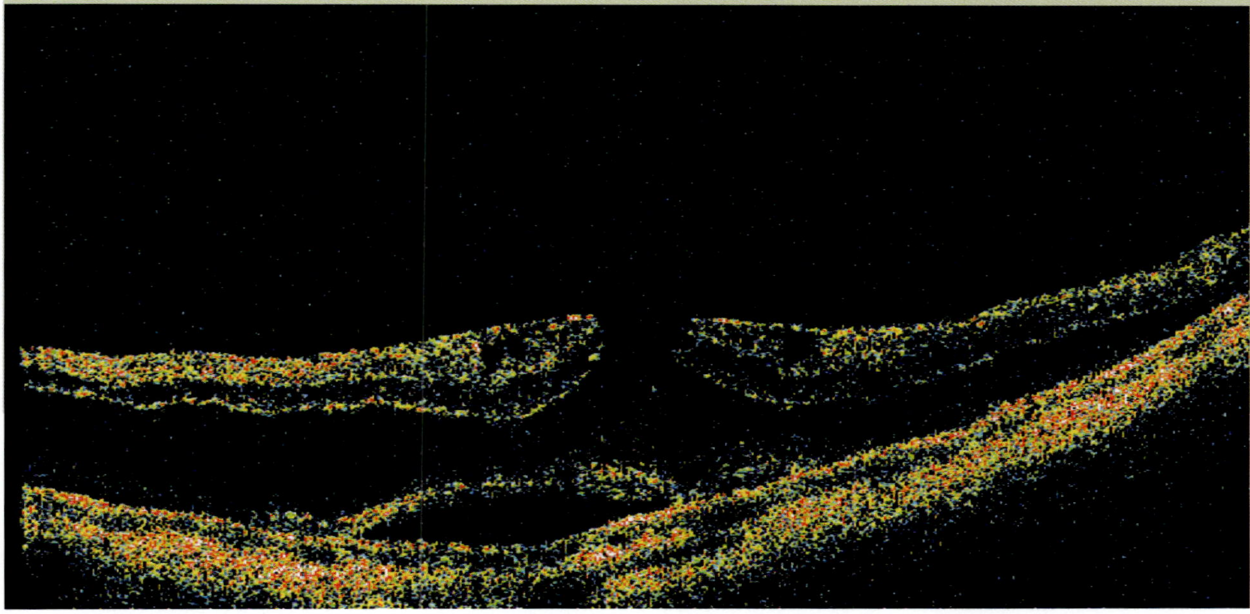

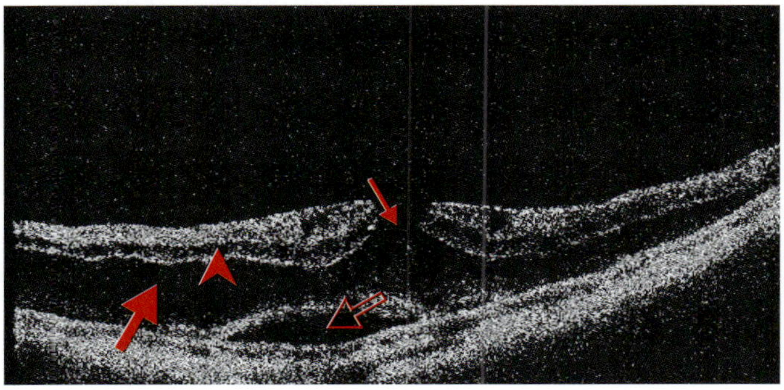

to macular cystic edema (arrow head). The area of low reflectivity located between the retina and the retinal pigment epithelium corresponds to a retinal detachment (empty arrow). The patient developed a total retinal detachment of the posterior pole due to a full thickness macular hole two months later.

EPIRETINAL MEMBRANE

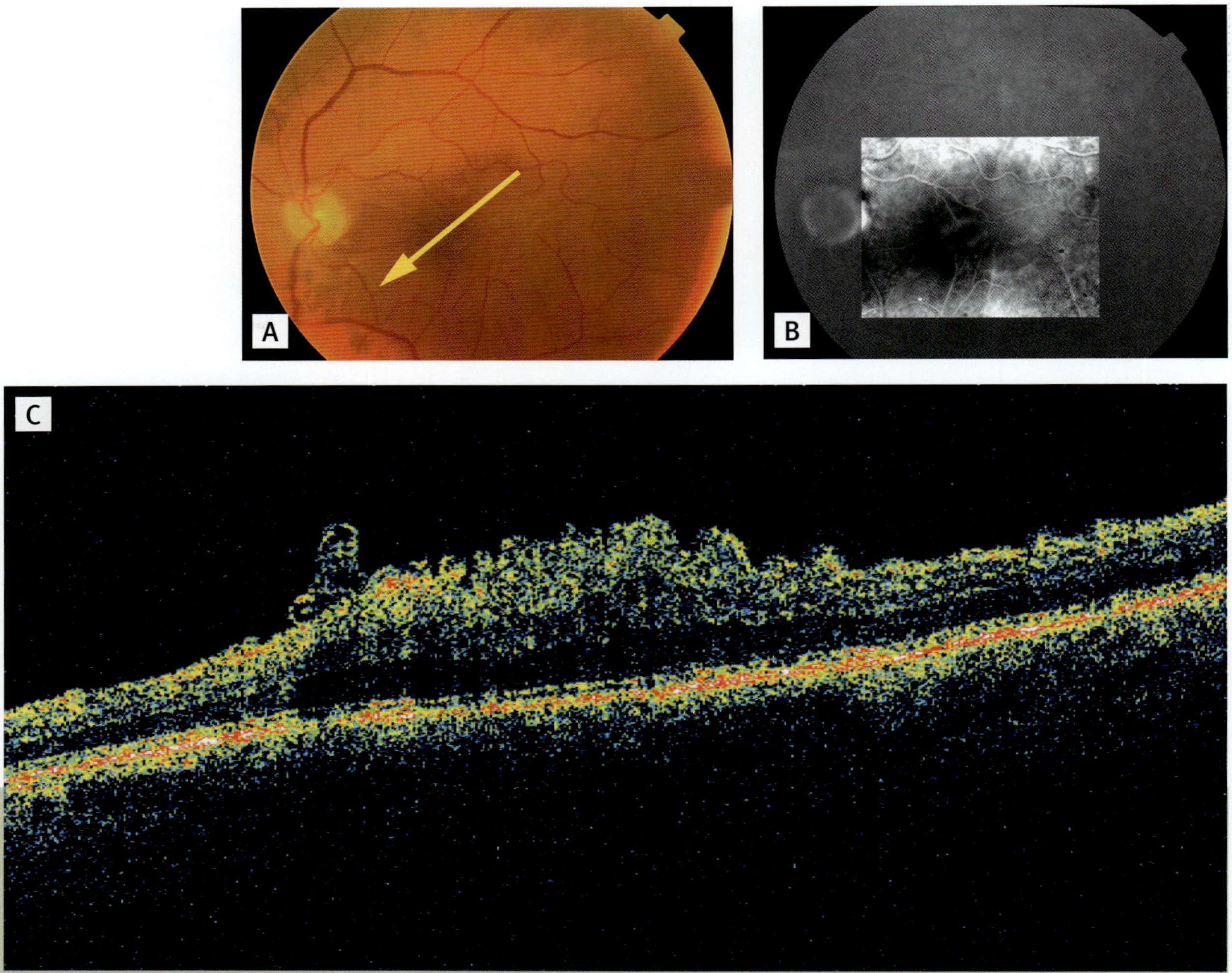

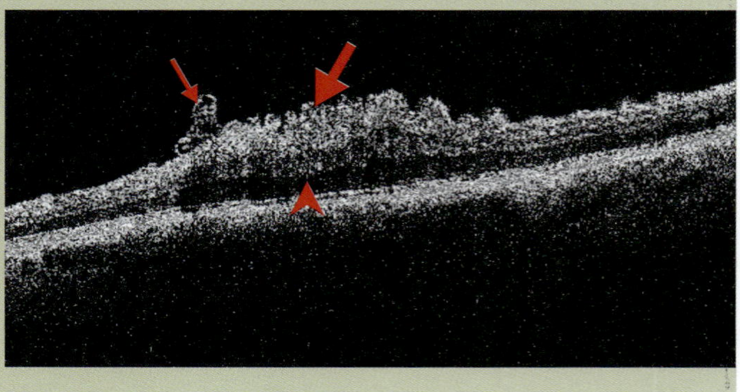

A. Patient with an epiretinal membrane (the arrow shows the scan direction). B. Fluorescein angiography shows leakage of dye in the fovea. C. Optical Coherence Tomography shows a diffuse distortion of the retinal surface due to the epiretinal membrane (big arrow). There is an area of high reflectivity on the retina surface that protrudes into the vitreous cavity and corresponds to the epiretinal membrane in the fovea and around it (small arrow). The retina appears thick with areas of low reflectivity in the outer layers corresponding to diffuse retina edema (arrow head).

DIABETIC EPIRETINAL MEMBRANE

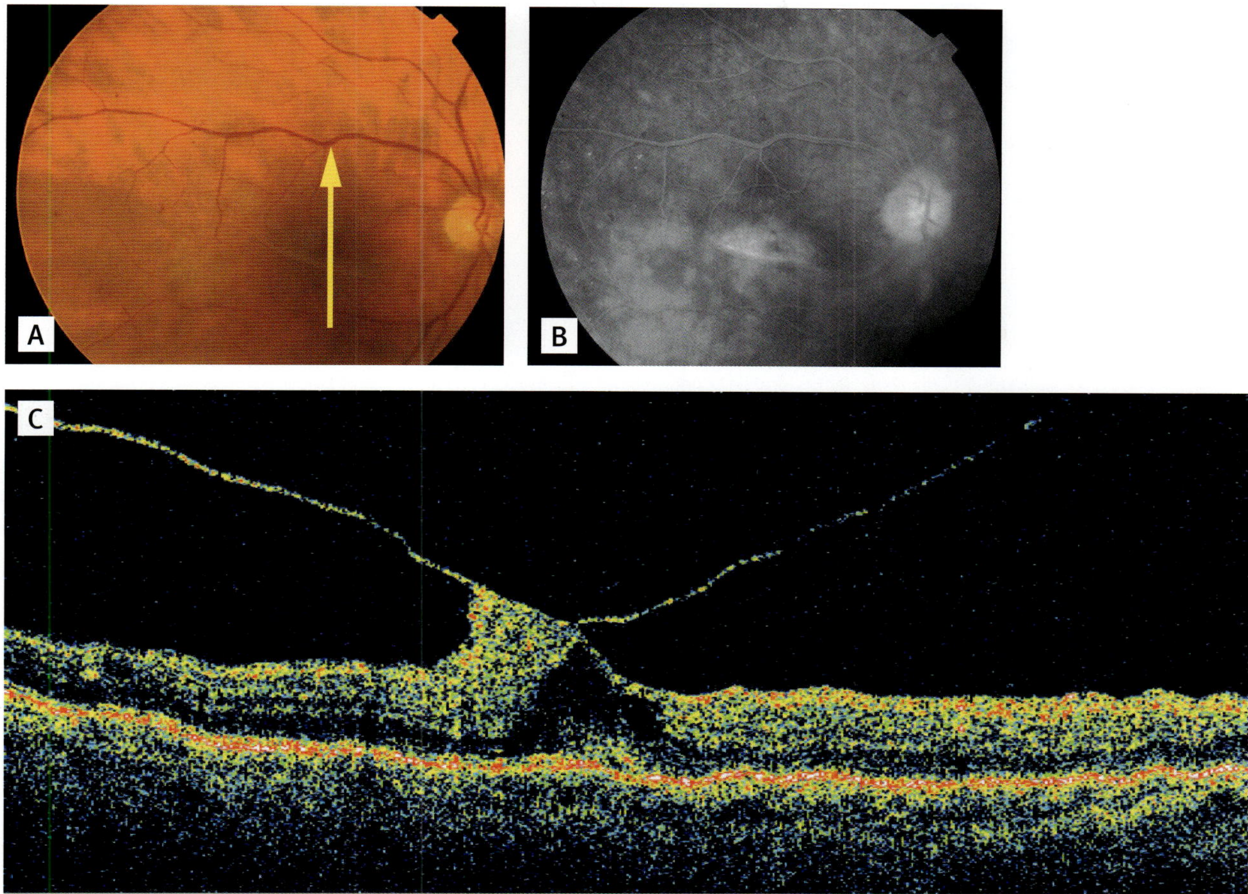

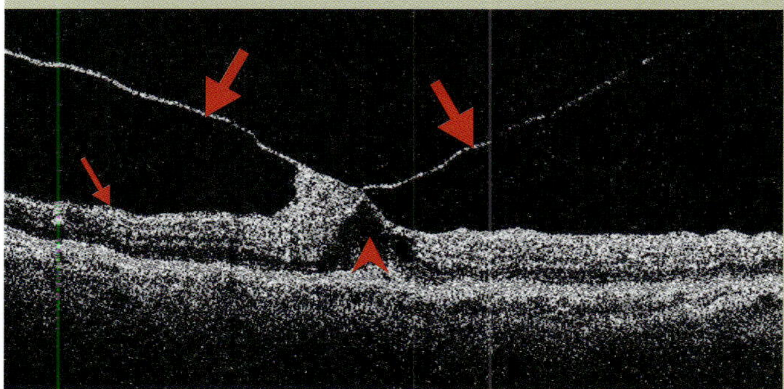

Diabetic patient with diabetic retinopathy and an epiretinal membrane. A. There is a thick epiretinal membrane that forms a fold in the macula (the arrow shows the scan direction). B. The folded area shows dye leakage in fluorescein angiography. There are also leaking points by microaneurysms due to diabetic maculopathy. C. The posterior cortical vitreous is detected as a thick area of high reflectivity strongly adherent to the fovea (big arrows). There is also a very thin area of high reflectivity to the left of the fovea, located on the retinal surface that corresponds to an epiretinal membrane (small arrow). The cystic intraretinal formations of low reflectivity correspond to cystic edema in the fovea (arrow head).

EPIRETINAL MEMBRANE

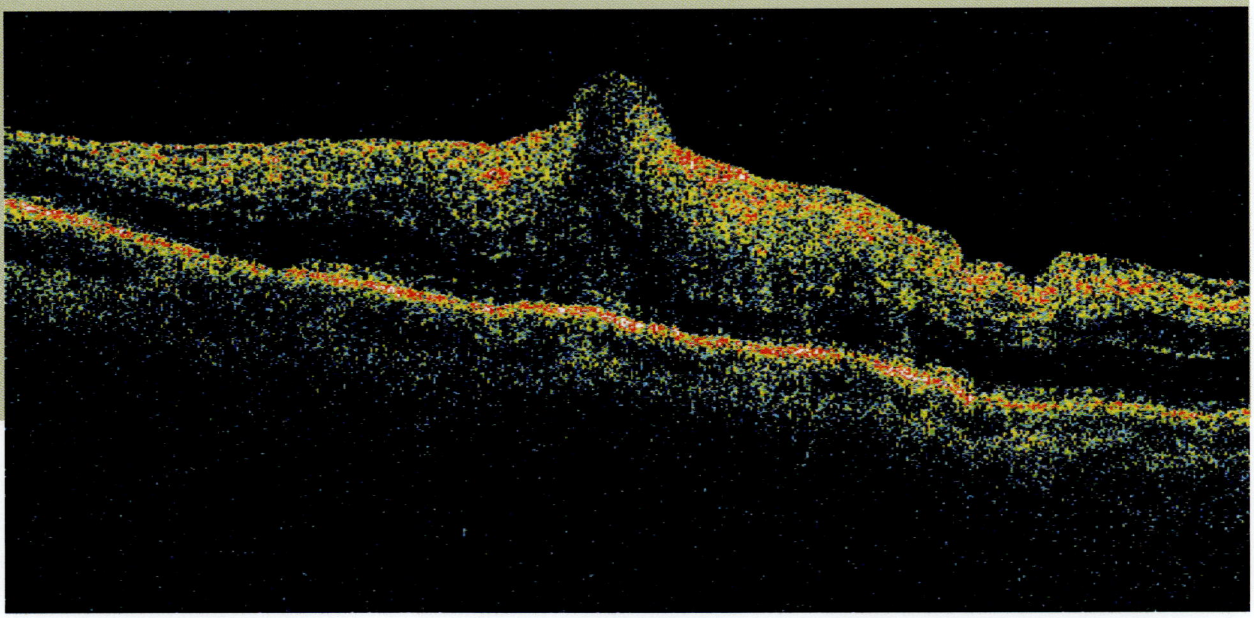

Patient with epiretinal membrane. There is an area of high reflectivity on the retinal surface that protrudes in the vitreous cavity and corresponds to the epiretinal membrane in the fovea and around it (small arrow). The retina appears increased in thickness with areas of low reflectivity in the outer layers that correspond to diffuse edema (arrow head). The retinal surface appears irregular due to the epiretinal membrane (big arrow).

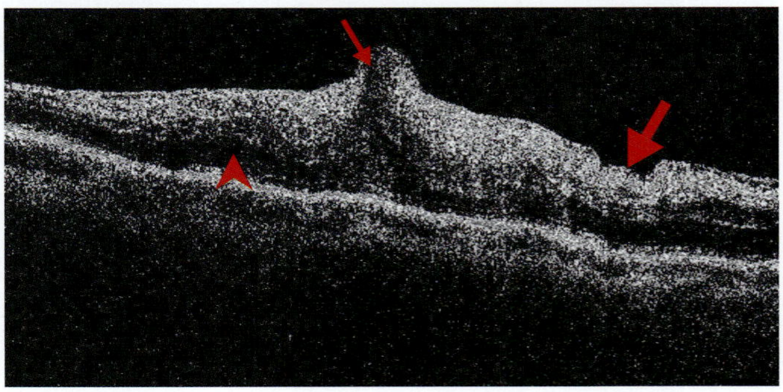

EPIRETINAL MEMBRANE

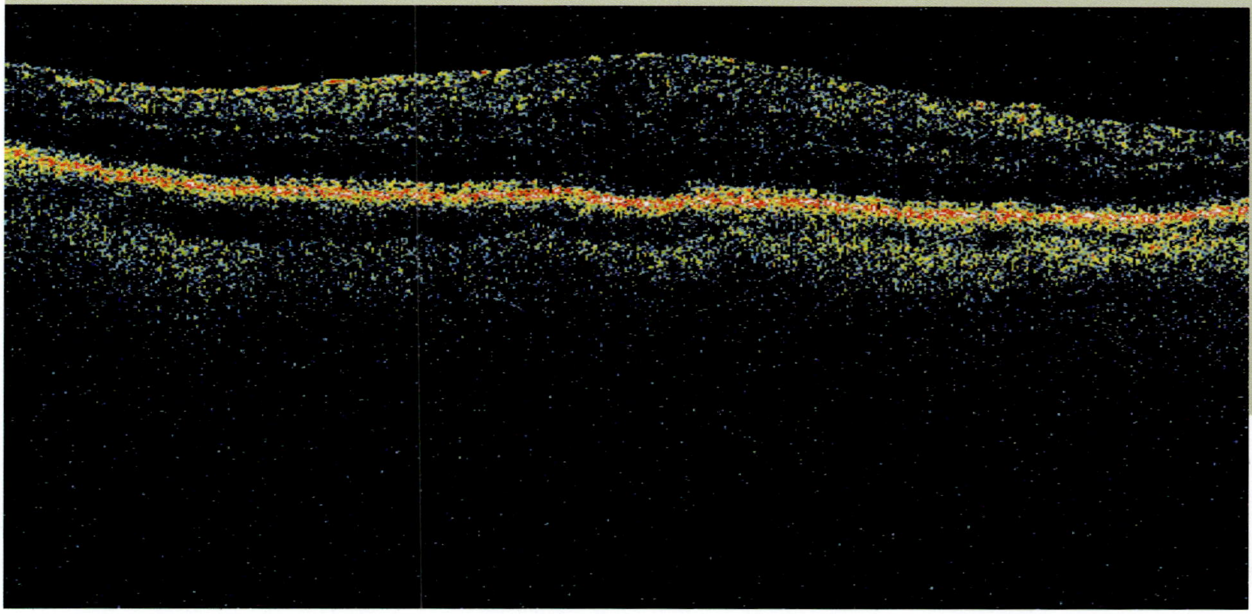

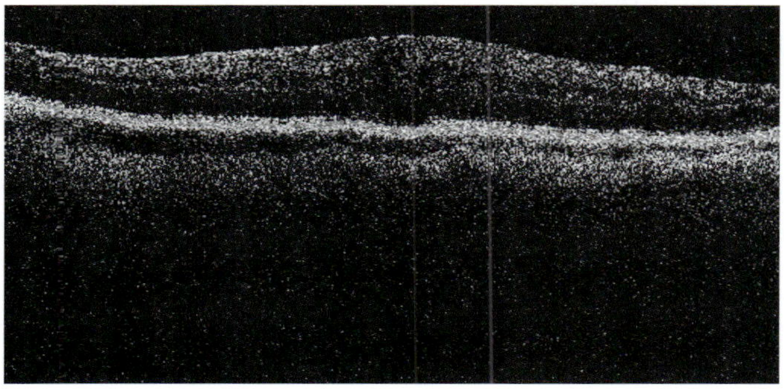

The patient of page 82, one month after the surgical excision of the membrane. Note the significant decrease of the macular edema, although the macular anatomy was not fully restored.

EPIRETINAL MEMBRANE

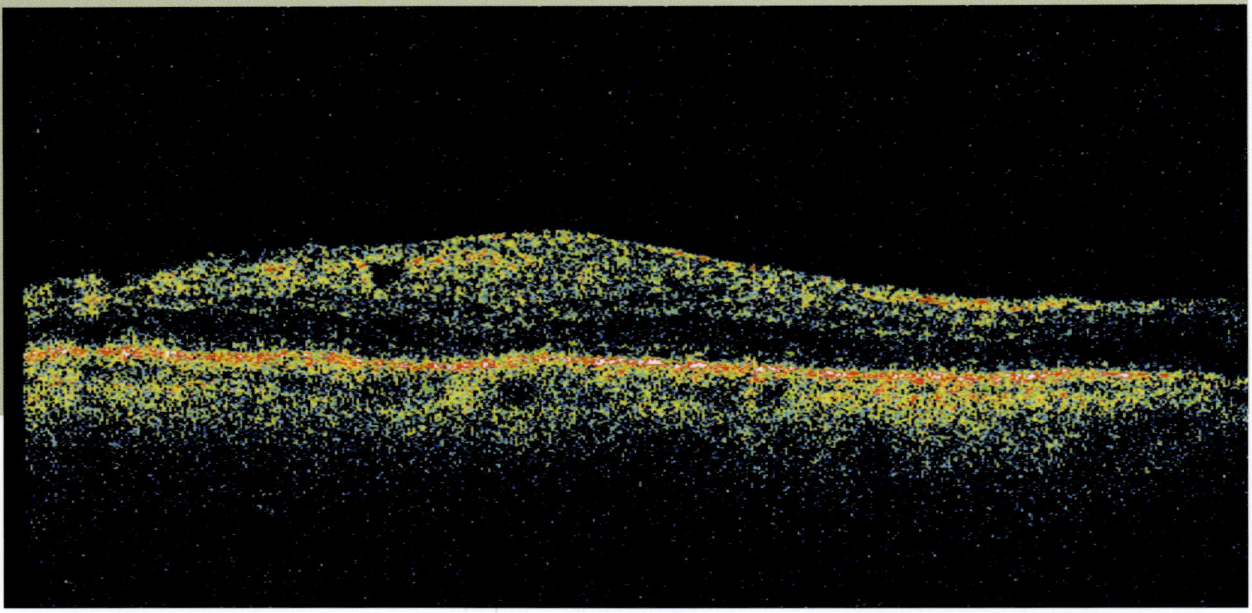

Patient who has been surgically treated two months earlier for a macula-off retinal detachment. The retinal thickness in the macula appears increased due to diffuse edema. A cystic intraretinal formation of low reflectivity corresponding to retinal cystic edema is also detected (big arrow). There is an area of high reflectivity on the retinal surface that corresponds to an epiretinal membrane (small arrow).

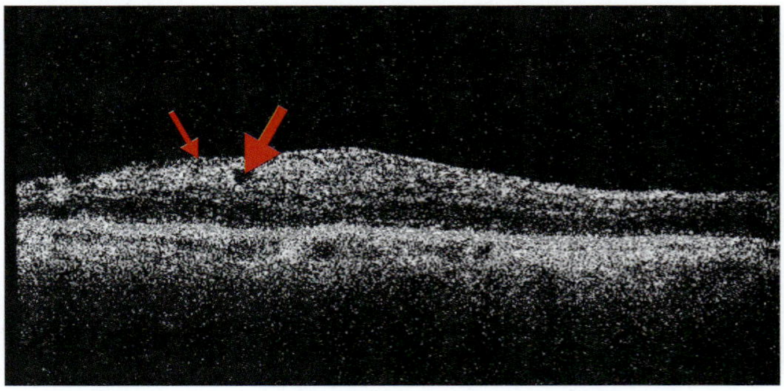

EPIRETINAL MEMBRANE

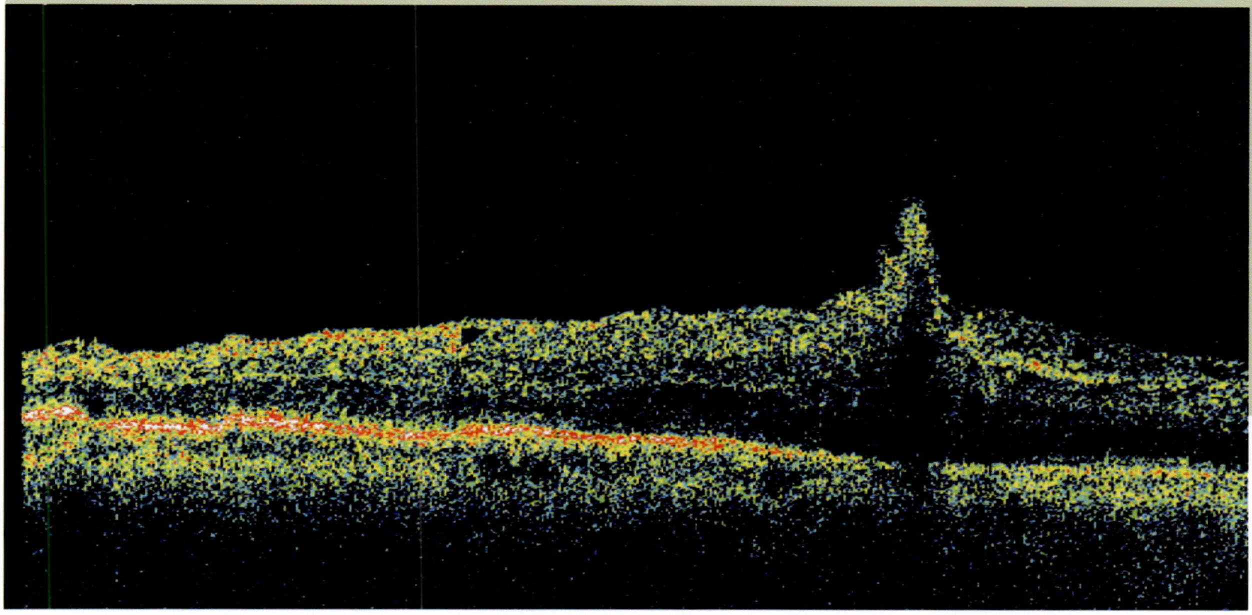

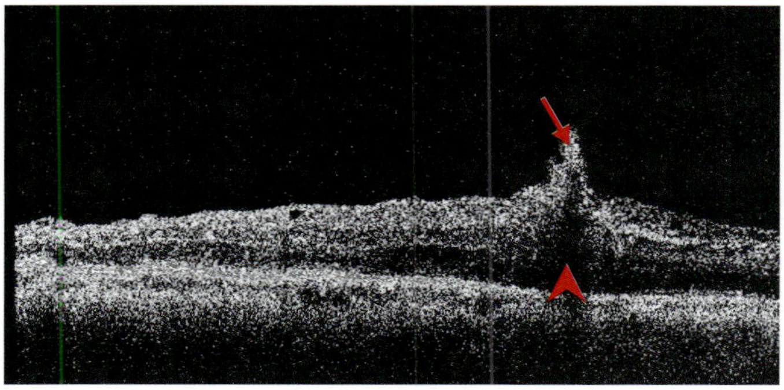

The patient of page 84 two months later developed an epiretinal membrane. The visual acuity is 20/200. There is an area of high reflectivity on the retinal surface protruding into the vitreous cavity and corresponding to the epiretinal membrane in the fovea and around it (small arrow). The retina appears thick with areas of low reflectivity in the outer layers that correspond to extensive diffuse edema (arrow head).

EPIRETINAL MEMBRANE

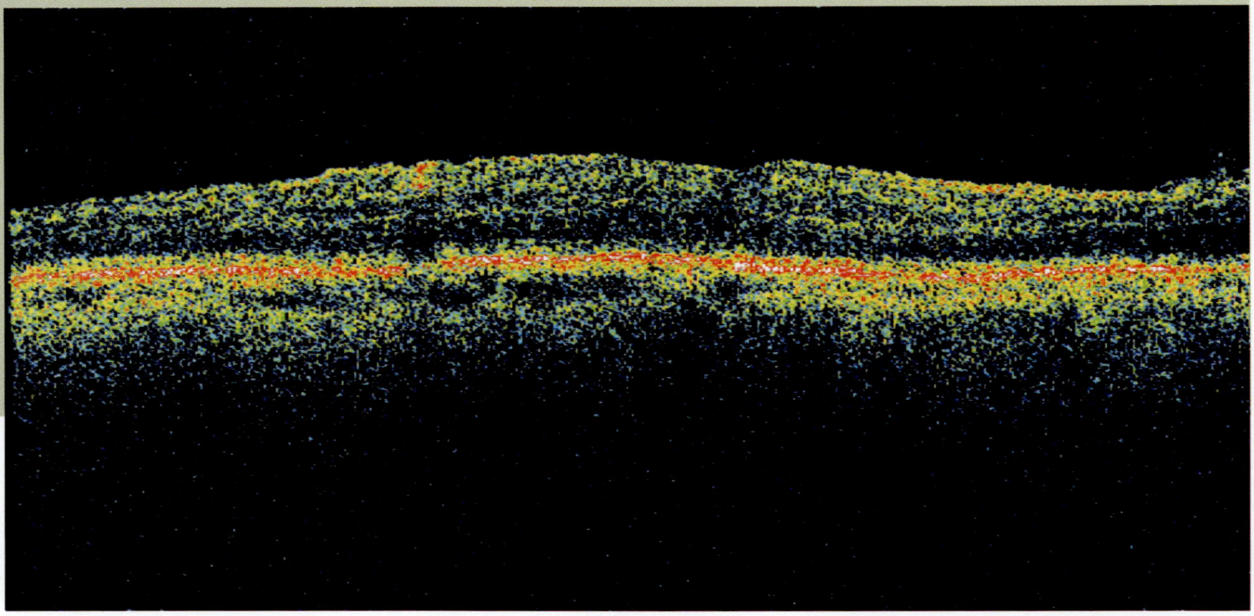

The patient of page 85, two months after surgical excision of the membrane. The visual acuity has improved to 20/30. Note the significant reduction of the edema, even though there is still not a complete recovery of the macular anatomy. There are elements of high reflectivity on the retina surface, to the right of the image that correspond to a residual membrane (small arrow).

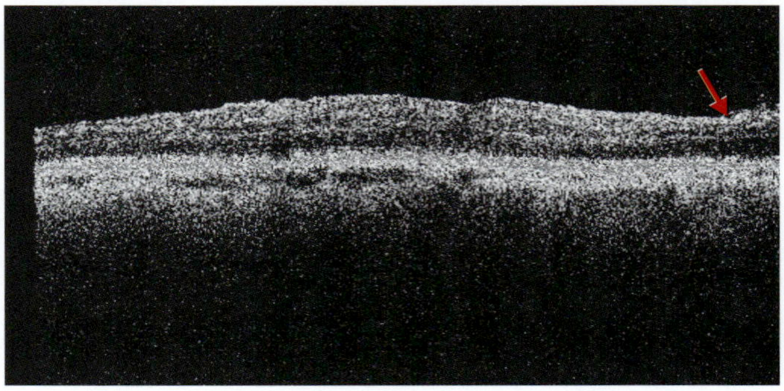

EPIRETINAL MEMBRANE

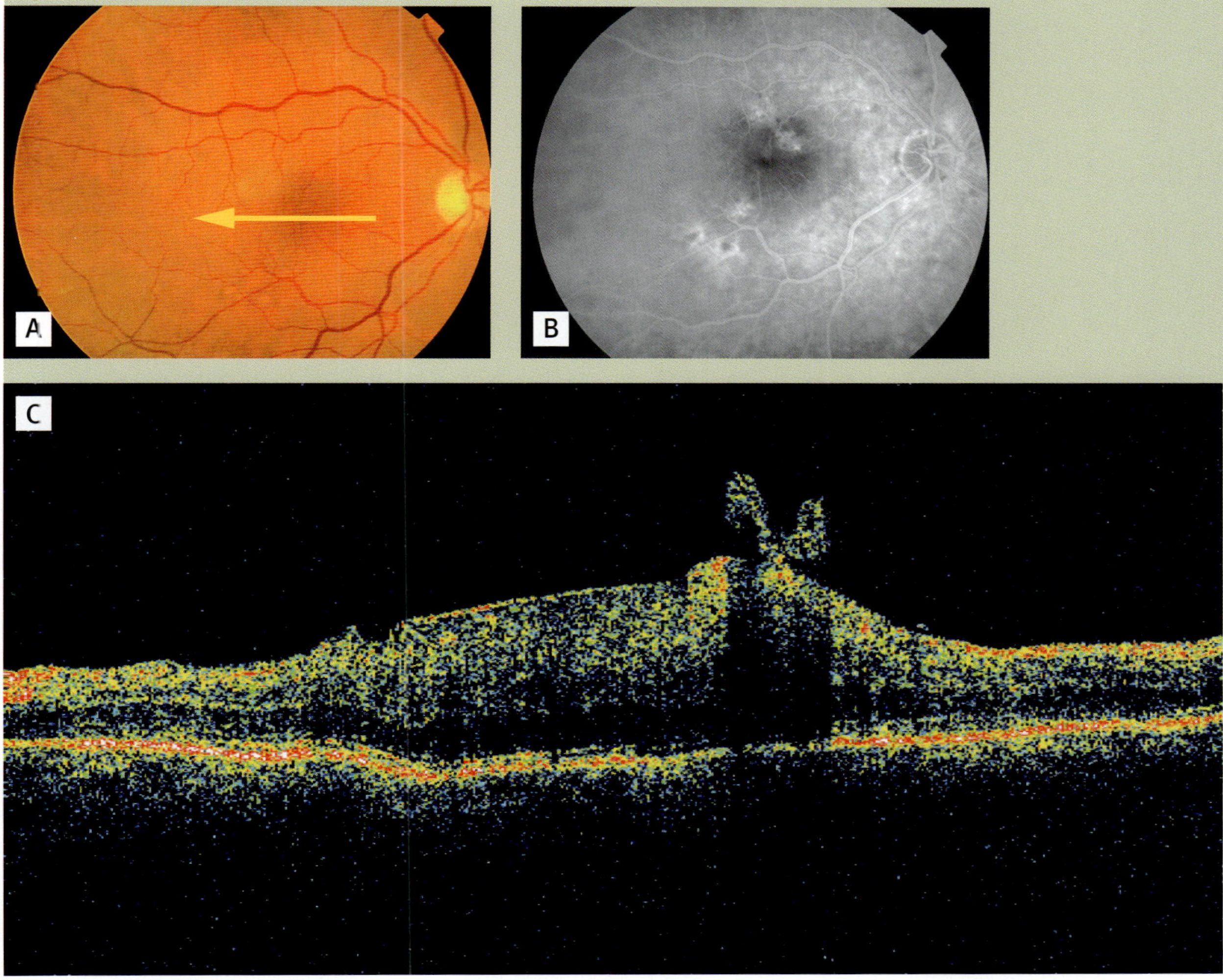

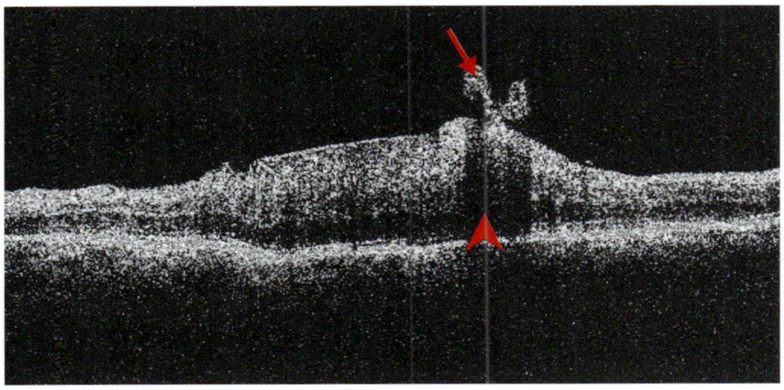

A. Patient with an epiretinal membrane. The visual acuity is 20/200 (the arrow shows the scan direction). B. Fluorescein angiography shows dye leakage in the macula. C. There is an area of high reflectivity on the retina surface protruding into the vitreous cavity and corresponding to an epiretinal membrane in the fovea and around it (small arrow).The retina appears thicker with areas of low reflectivity in the outer layers due to diffuse edema (arrow head).

EPIRETINAL MEMBRANE

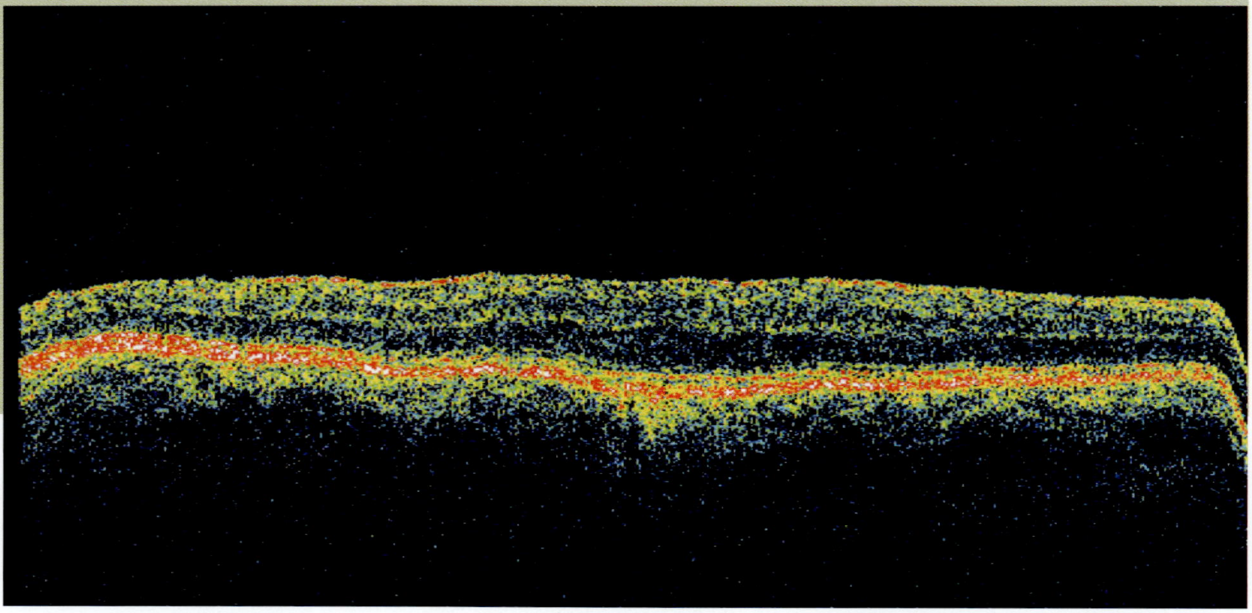

The patient of page 87, two years after surgical excision of the membrane. The visual acuity has improved to 20/30. Note the substantial reduction of the edema, even though there is still not a complete recovery of the macular anatomy.

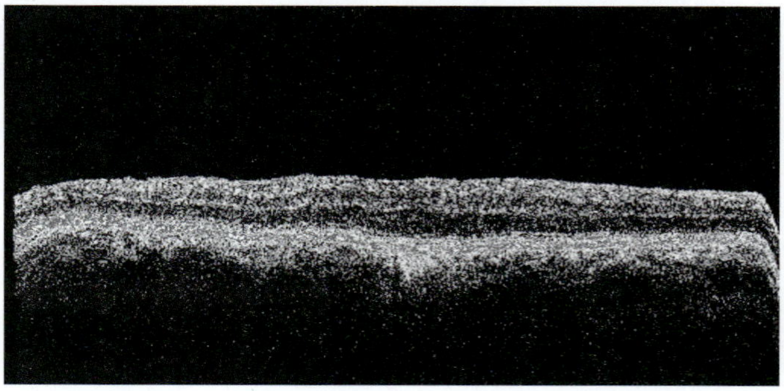

FULL THICKNESS MACULAR HOLE STAGE II WITH EPIRETINAL MEMBRANE

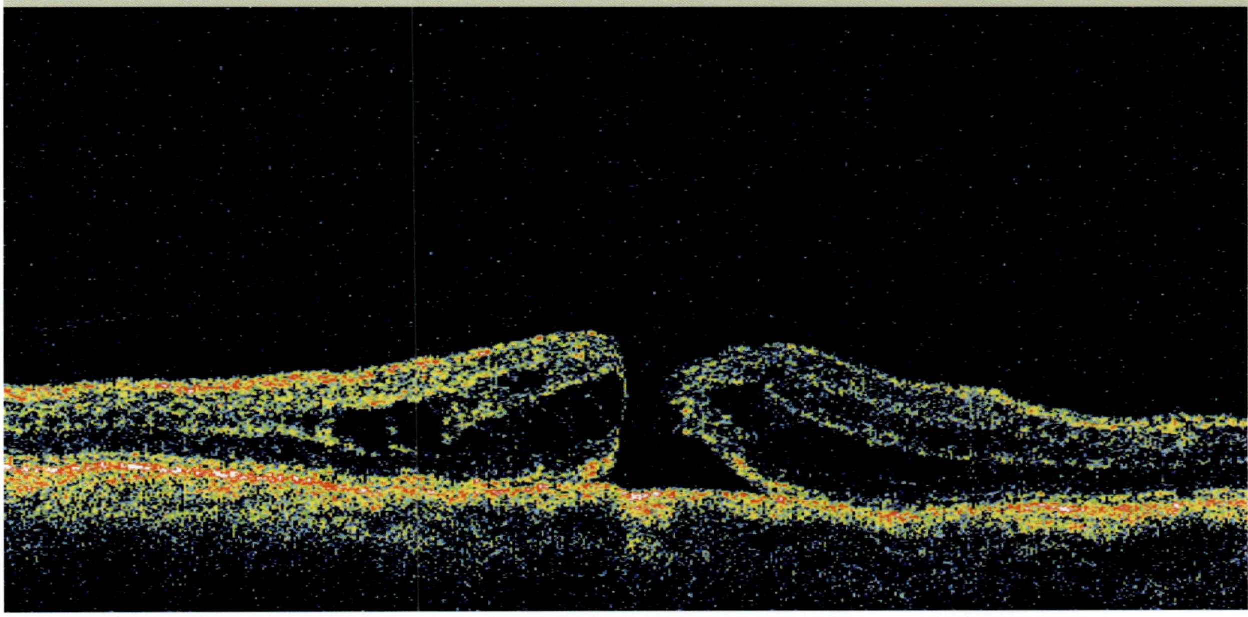

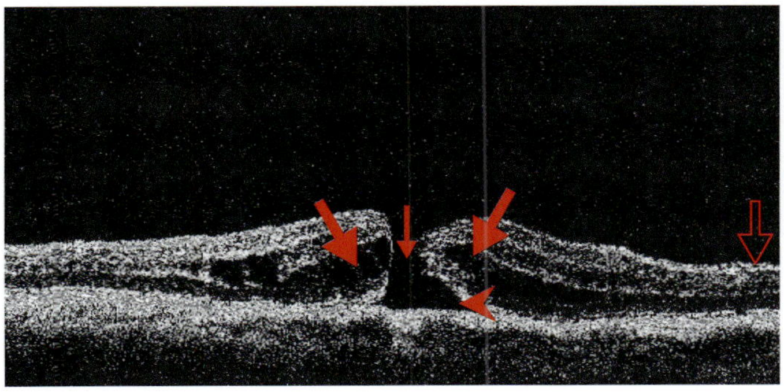

Stage II full thickness macular hole with central opening (small arrow), a cuff of subretinal fluid (arrow head) and cystic intraretinal formations of low reflectivity corresponding to cystic retinal edema at both sides (big arrows). There is a thin area of high reflectivity on the retinal surface corresponding to an epiretinal membrane (empty arrow).

EPIRETINAL MEMBRANE

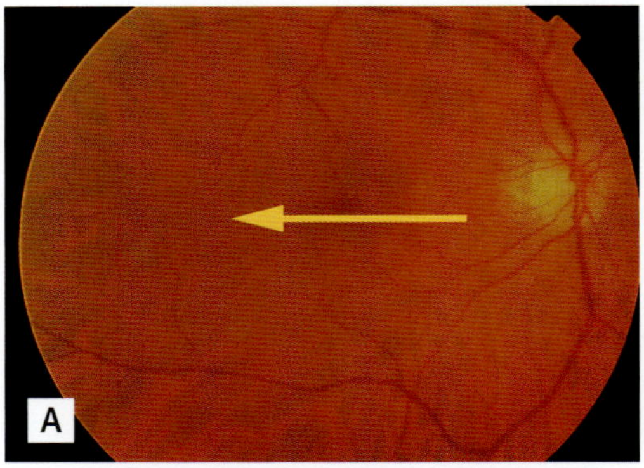

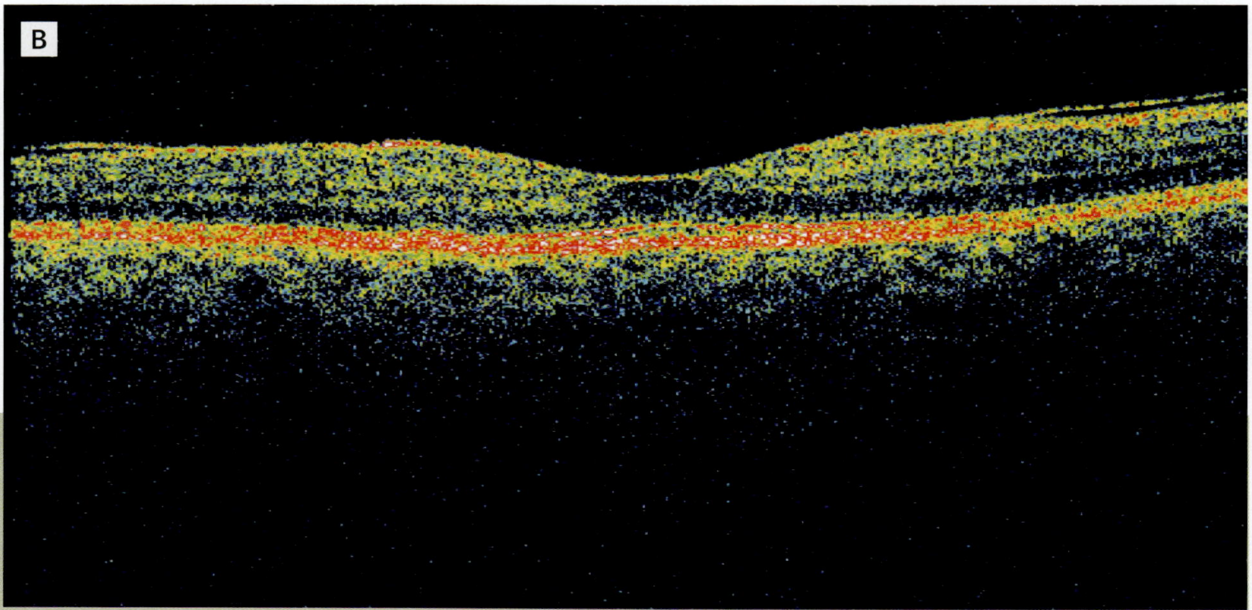

A. Patient with an epiretinal membrane (the arrow shows the scan direction). B. Optical Coherence Tomography shows a thin area of high reflectivity on the retinal surface that corresponds to an epiretinal membrane (arrows) at both sides of the fovea without retinal edema.

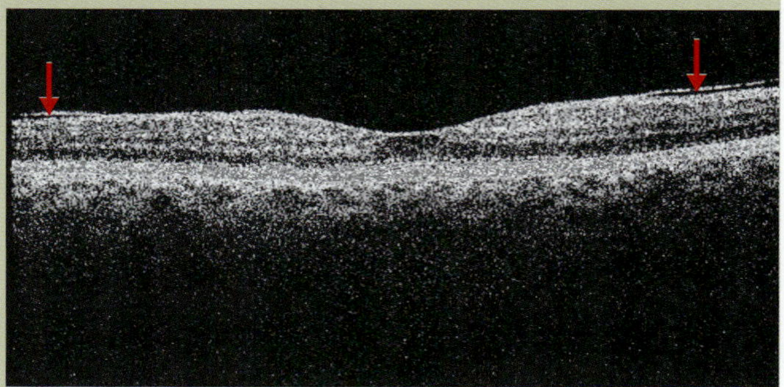

EPIRETINAL MEMBRANE

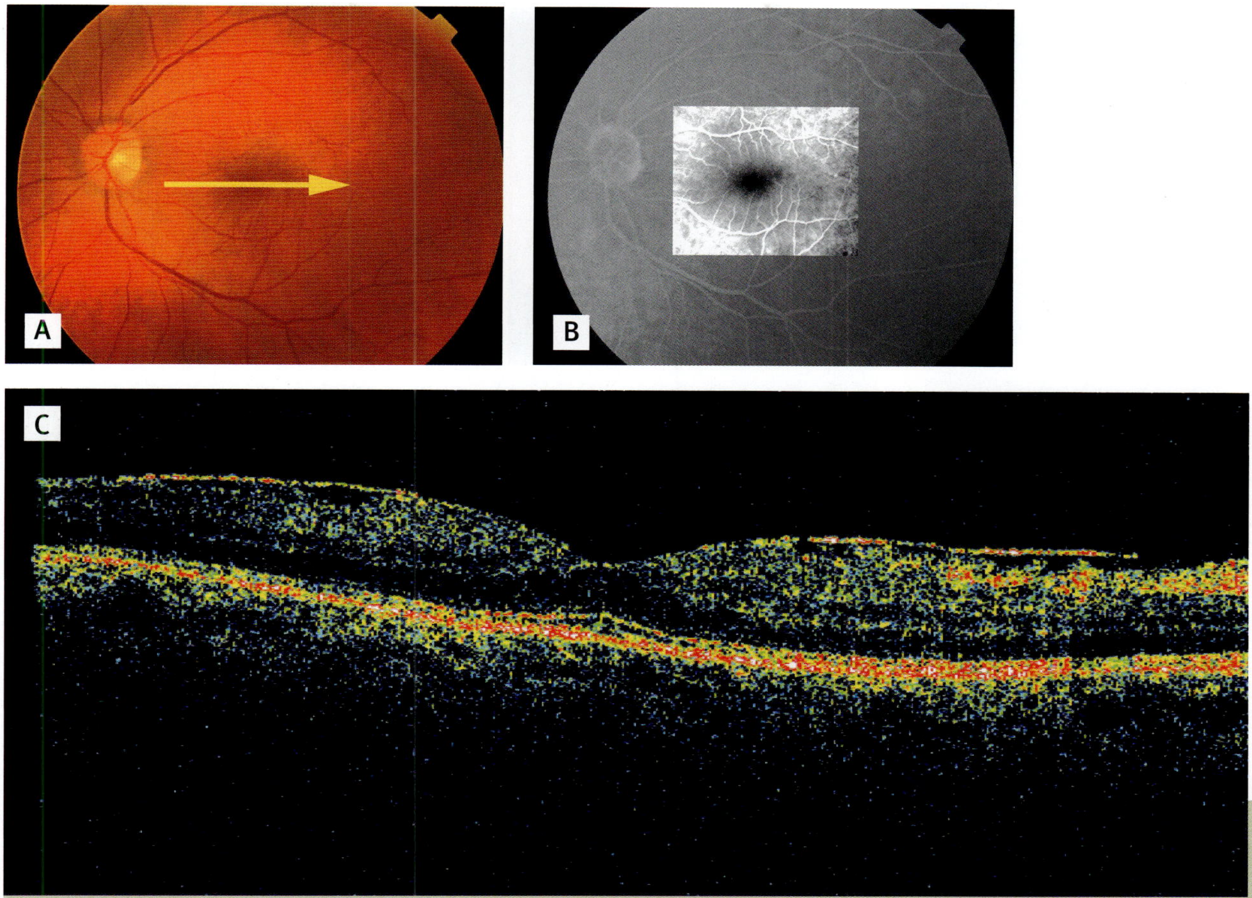

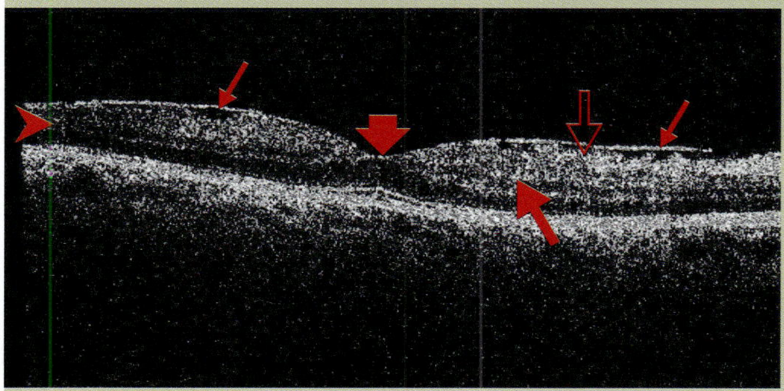

The other eye of the patient of page 90. A. The epiretinal membrane is evident and causes stretching of the vessels above the fovea (the arrow shows the scan arrow). B. Fluorescein angiography doesn't reveal dye leakage in the macula. C. Optical Coherence Tomography depicts a thin area of high reflectivity located on the retinal surface that corresponds to the epiretinal membrane (small arrows) in both sides of the fovea with subtle diffuse retinal edema (big arrow). There is also retinal distortion (empty arrow). The morphology of the fovea is within normal limits (thick arrow). The weak chromatic appearance of the retinal layers is due to the presence of a mild cataract (arrow head).

EPIRETINAL MEMBRANE WITH BRANCH RETINAL ARTERY OCCLUSION

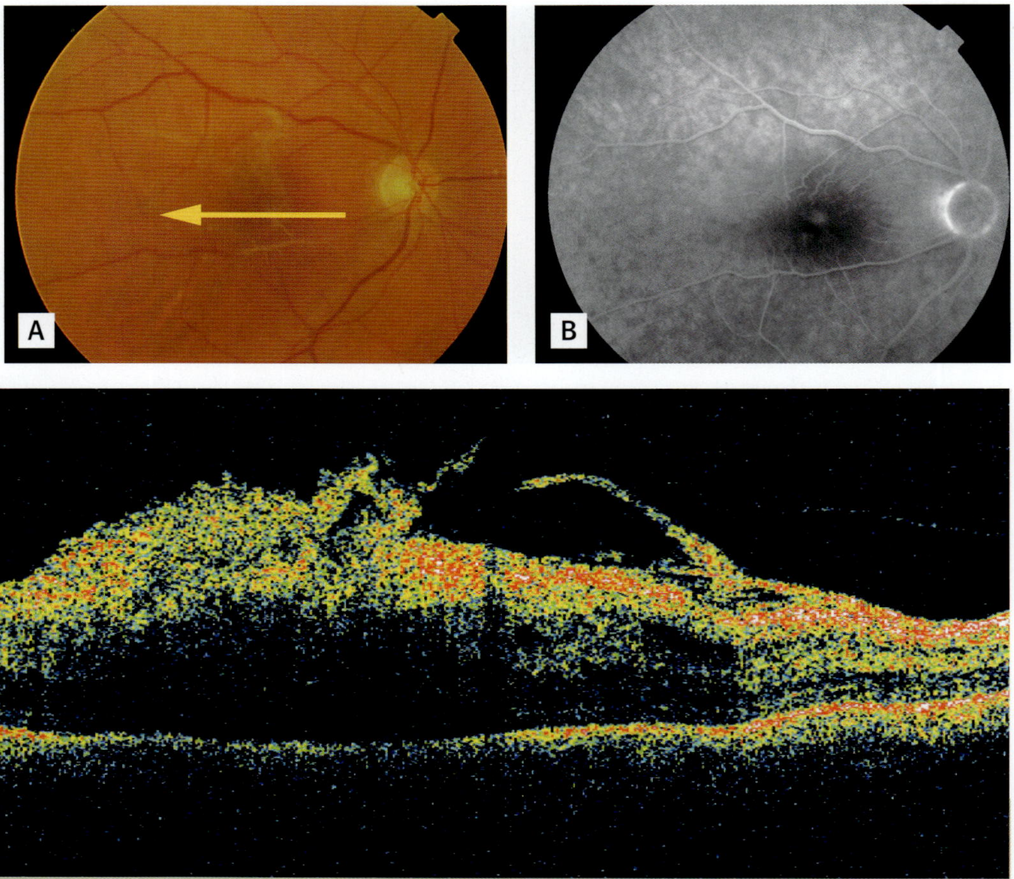

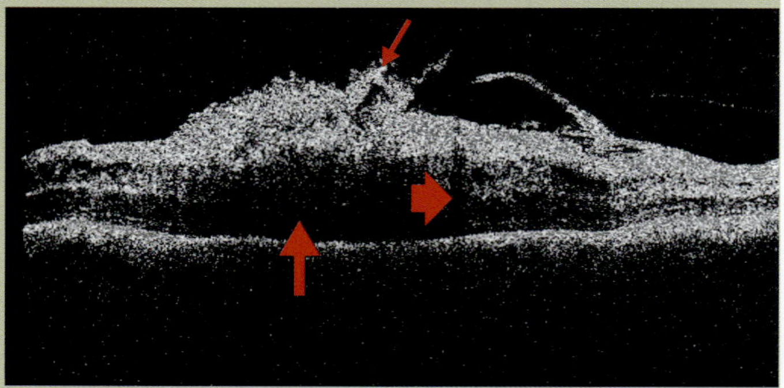

A. Patient with an epiretinal membrane and an inferotemporal branch retinal artery occlusion (the arrow shows the scan direction). B. Fluorescein angiography shows dye leakage in the macula. C. Optical Coherence Tomography shows an area of high reflectivity on the inner retinal surface that corresponds to a thick epiretinal membrane (small arrow). There is also low reflectivity of the outer retinal layers due to diffuse macular edema (big arrow). The presence of isolated and scattered retinal elements in the edematous retina (thick arrow) differentiates the edema from the serous retinal detachment. The diffuse shadowing of the outer retinal layers is due to the increased reflectivity of the thick epiretinal membrane.

EPIRETINAL MEMBRANE WITH BRANCH RETINAL ARTERY OCCLUSION

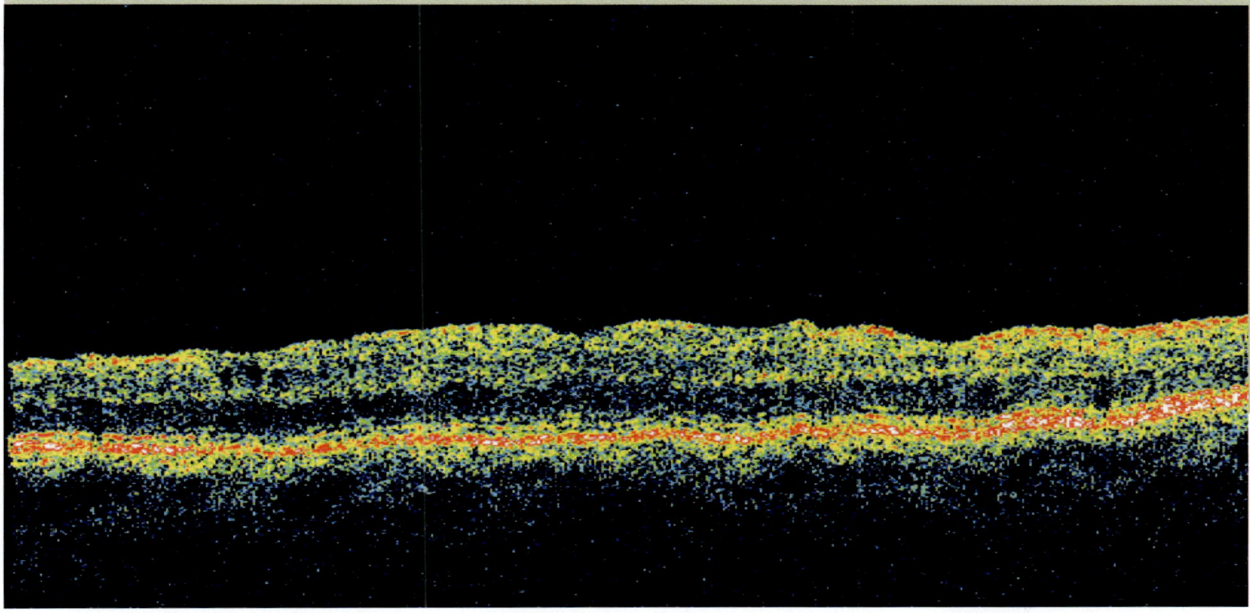

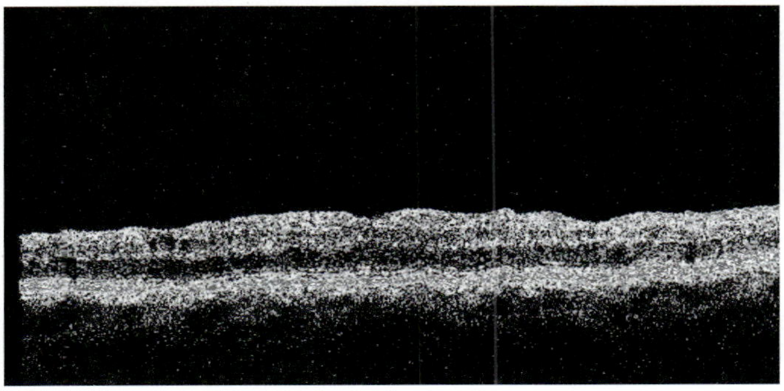

Postoperative image of the patient of page 92, twelve months later. Note the significant decrease of the macular edema, even though there is still not a complete recovery of the macular anatomy.

EPIRETINAL MEMBRANE

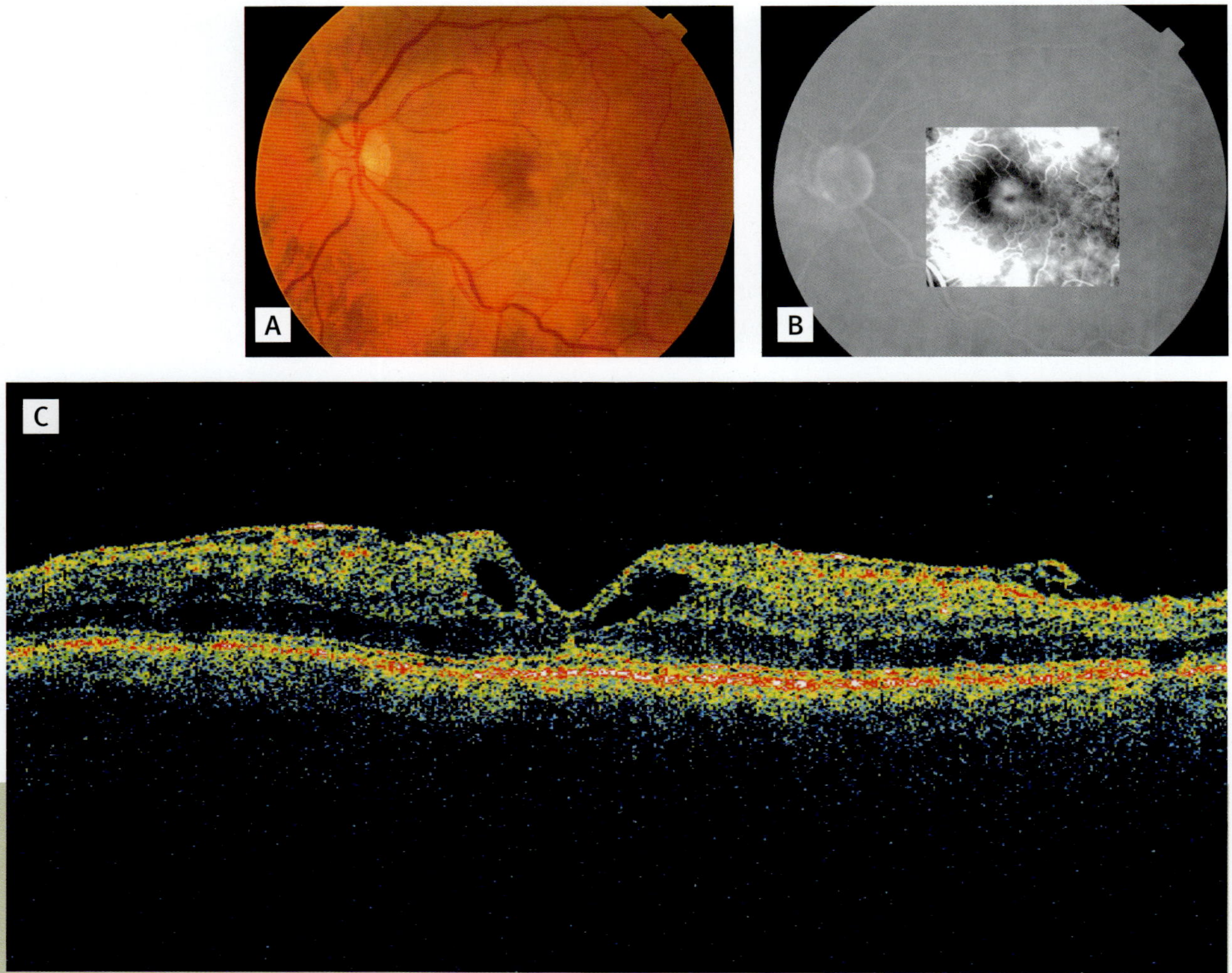

A. Patient with an epiretinal membrane (the arrow shows the scan direction). B. Fluorescein angiography shows mild leakage of dye around the fovea in the late phases. C. Optical Coherence Tomography shows a linear area of high reflectivity on the inner surface of the retina that corresponds to an epiretinal membrane (small arrows). The retinal thickness is increased due to edema. There are also cystic areas of low intraretinal reflectivity on either side of the fovea indicating cystoid edema (big arrows).

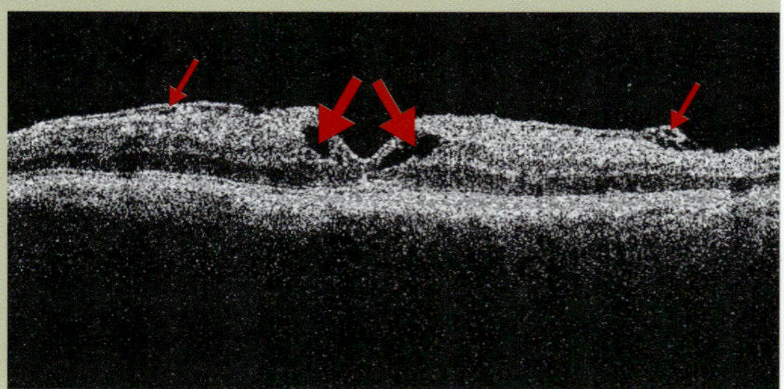

EPIRETINAL MEMBRANE

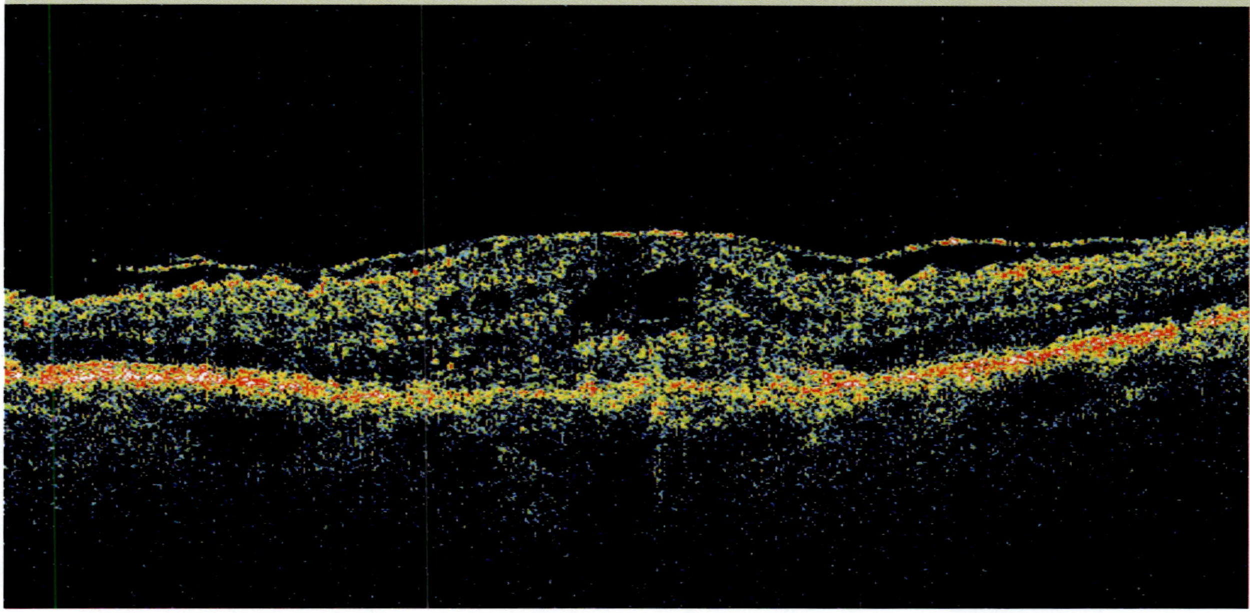

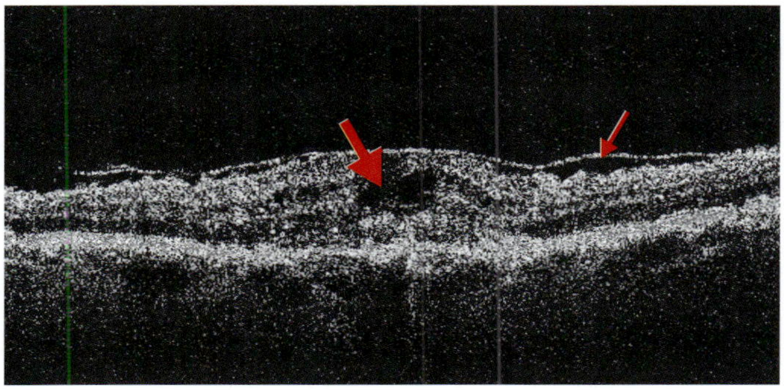

Epiretinal membrane of the macula. There is a linear area of high retinal reflectivity corresponding to the epiretinal membrane in the macula (small arrow) and there are also cystic formations of low reflectivity and thickening of the retina corresponding to diffuse and cystoid retinal edema (big arrow).

EPIRETINAL MEMBRANE

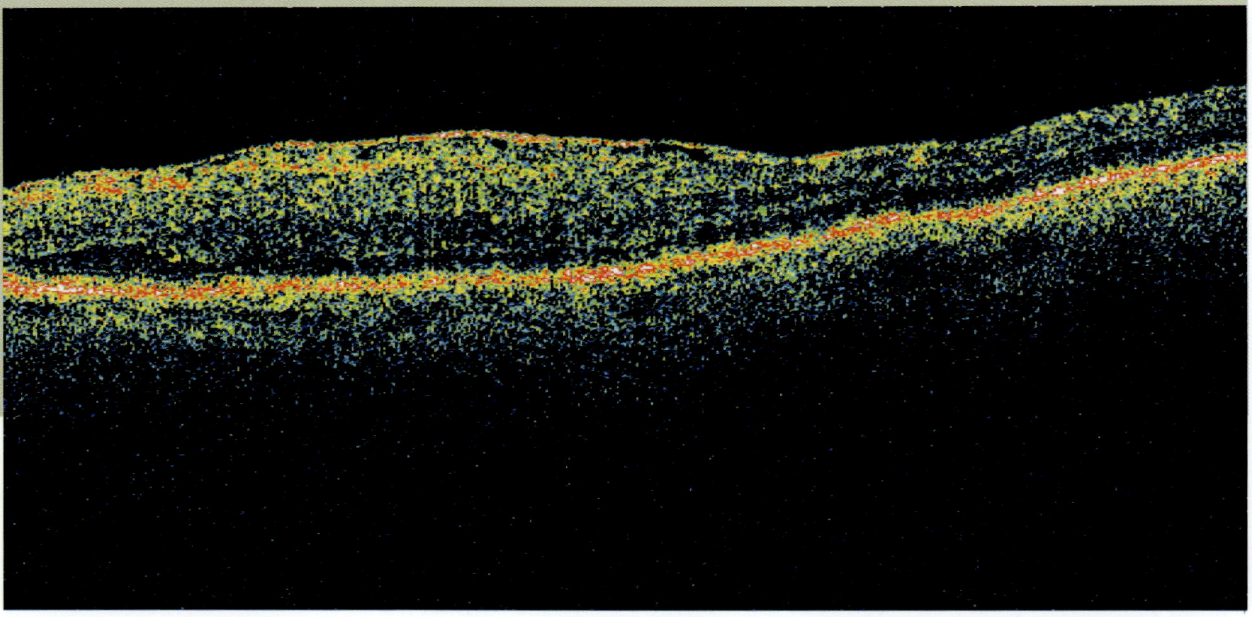

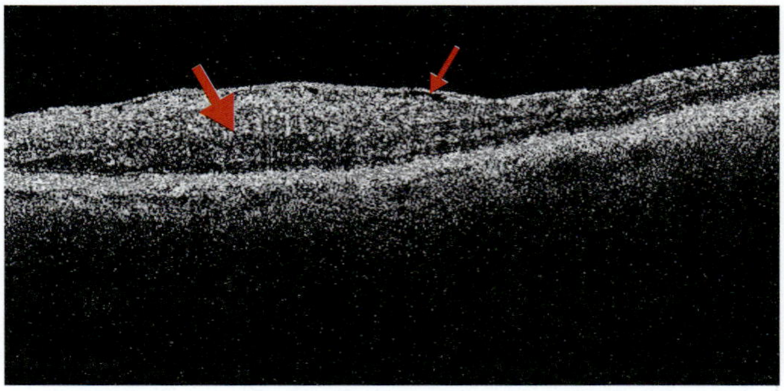

Epiretinal membrane of the macula. There is a linear area of high reflectivity on the retinal surface that corresponds to a macular epiretinal membrane (small arrow) with associated retinal thickening corresponding to diffuse edema (big arrow).

CHAPTER 4

VITREORETINAL TRACTION

VLASSIS GRIGOROPOULOS

IDIOPATHIC FULL THICKNESS MACULAR HOLE

Alterations to the vitreous attachment to the retina can cause many macular diseases. Optical Coherence Tomography is able to detect many of them in a more complete way than biomicroscopy, ultrasonography, fluorescein angiography or other examination modalities. It can also evaluate very small alterations of the retinal surface and perform quantitative calculations that may be useful to the diagnosis and follow-up of the patient as well as to the assessment of the applied treatment.

Idiopathic full thickness macular hole occurs mainly in women of 60-70 years of age. The most common symptoms are decreased visual acuity, metamorphopsia and central scotoma. In 15-20% of cases the macular hole may be bilateral. The disease should be differentiated from epiretinal membrane with lamellar macular hole, retinal cysts or cystoid macular edema and macular detachment. Optical Coherence Tomography shows an alteration of the normal anatomy and a full thickness retinal deficit of the fovea. In contrast, in cases of epiretinal membrane with lamellar hole of the macula there is a small deficit of retinal tissue with preservation of the outer retinal layers at the bottom of the hole[3]. In cases of macular cysts there are optically empty areas within the retinal layers, while in macular detachment there is an optically empty area between the neurosensory retina and the pigment epithelium[6].

Gass described in detail the macular hole stages by biomicroscopy. Stage I or impending hole is characterized by a macular detachment that appears on biomicroscopy like a yellow spot (Ia) or a yellow ring (Ib). Almost half of these patients will develop a complete macular hole, while the rest will spontaneously resolve when the vitreous is completely detached. Stage II macular hole is characterized by a full thickness retinal defect with diameter under 400μm. In stage III there is an enlargement of the diameter of the hole above 400μm with the vitreous attached to the hole and detached around it. In stage IV there is further enlargement of the hole with a complete vitreous detachment.

Optical Coherence Tomography confirmed the role of vitreous traction in macular hole pathology. Vitreous traction on the fovea with vitreous detachment around it has been detected[2]. It is possible that continuous macular traction may lead to the formation of a stage I macular hole. Patients who had full thickness macular hole in one eye had the fellow eye studied by Optical Coherence Tomography. The results showed that if the vitreous was attached to the fovea and detached around it, they were more likely to develop a macular hole in the fellow eye. For these patients, the term stage 0 has been proposed because of the special vitreous attachment to the retina[1]. These patients have increased chances to develop a macular hole.
Other studies have showed that a pseudocyst may be the initial stage of formation of a macular hole. It appears on Optical Coherence Tomography as an area of low reflectivity into the retina corresponding to the area of vitreous traction. The enlargement of the cyst may lead to a defect of the inner retinal layers and to their rupture with the development of a stage II macular hole. Sometimes, an operculum is observed, attached to one side of the hole or in front of the hole into the vitreous cavity. In stage III a hole enlargement is observed and around it a cuff of subretinal fluid is detected located between the neurosensory retina and the retinal pigment epithelium[4]. Also, intraretinal edema and cystic changes may be observed. Frequently, the operculum is clearly detached from the retina and remains in a small distance from the hole inside the vitreous cavity and attached to the posterior hyaloid. In stage IV a large hole is observed without visible vitreous because of its complete detachment and withdrawal into the vitreous cavity. Optical Coherence Tomography produces quantitative information related to the diameter of the hole, the diameter of the base of the hole as well as the retinal thickness around the hole. Various studies have shown that these measurements may have a prognostic value regarding the anatomical and functional results of macular hole repair.

Nowadays, vitrectomy is the treatment of choice for a full thickness macular hole. Optical Coherence Tomography offers the possibility to observe the development and anatomical results after the surgical repair of a macular hole[7]. Postoperatively, the hole can appear open[5], closed but with a thin retina (retinal thickness under 100μm), closed with a normal retinal anatomy and thickness or with a small foveolar detachment that is absorbed within a few weeks or months[8]. Improvement in Optical Coherence Tomography often corresponds to an increase in visual acuity.

IDIOPATHIC FULL THICKNESS MACULAR HOLE

1. Chan A, Duker JS, Schuman JS, Fujimoto JG. Stage 0 macular holes: observations by optical coherence tomography. Ophthalmology 2004;111:2027-32

2. Gross JG. Late reopening and spontaneous closure of previously repaired macular holes. Am J Ophthalmol 2005;140:556-558.

3. Haouchine B, Massin P, Tadayoni R, Erginay A, Gaudric A. Diagnosis of macular pseudoholes and lamellar macular holes by optical coherence tomography. Am J Ophthalmol 2004;138:732-739.

4. Kitchens JW, Flynn HW Jr, Moshfeghi AA, Puliafito CA. Idiopathic macular hole with extensive subretinal fluid: clinical and optical coherence tomography features before and after surgery. Am J Ophthalmol 2005;139:383-386.

5. Moshfeghi AA, Flynn HW Jr, Elner SG, Puliafito CA, Gass JD. Persistent outer retinal defect after successful macular hole repair. Am J Ophthalmol 2005;139:183-184.

6. Ratoglia R, Osnaghi S, Bindella A, Pirondini C. Posterior traction retinal detachment in highly myopic eyes: clinical features and surgical outcome as evaluated by optical coherence tomography. Retina 2005;25:473-478.

7. Sato H, Kawasaki R, Yamashita H. Observation of idiopathic full-thickness macular hole closure in early postoperative period as evaluated by optical coherence tomography. Am J Ophthalmol 2003;136:185-187.

8. Uemoto R, Yamamoto S, Aoki T, Tsikahara I, Yamamote T, Yakeuchi S. Macular configuration determined by optical coherence tomography after idiopathic macular hole surgery with or without internal limiting membrane peeling. Br J Ophthalmol 2002;86:1240-1242.

VITREOMACULAR TRACTION SYNDROME

Vitreomacular traction is becoming one of the most frequent causes of visual acuity decrease due to chronic or non responding to therapy macular edema. The edema can be idiopathic or secondary to other ophthalmic diseases like diabetic retinopathy. In this syndrome there is a partial vitreous detachment, while the posterior vitreous remains attached to the macula and the optic disc. The attachment can be focal, linear or diffuse and can cause anteroposterior as well as tangential traction to the macula. This appears clinically by a decrease in visual acuity and an apparently normal looking macula. However, a careful examination of the macula will reveal the presence of macular edema in most cases[3].

The presence of folds and elevation of the retina, distortion of blood vessels, retinal elevation nasally to the optic disc or vitreous condensation above the optic disc are all indications of vitreomacular traction. Epiretinal membrane may coexist. Macular edema can be detected by fluorescein angiography, while the vitreous traction can also be observed by B-scan ultrasonography.

Optical Coherence Tomography is the most appropriate method to observe the vitreoretinal interface at the fovea[2]. The vitreomacular traction syndrome is characterized by the presence of highly reflective linear areas located inside the vitreous cavity connected to the retinal surface at the macula area, that correspond to focal vitreomacular attachments.
They are usually accompanied by retinal elevation due to a tractional detachment. Another usual finding is the increased retinal thickness and the cystic macular appearance that are due to cystic or diffuse retinal edema because of the strong vitreous traction on the macula. The usually coexisting epiretinal membrane can augment the exerted macular traction, thus accelerating the formation of a lamellar or full thickness macular hole.

In some cases, spontaneous posterior vitreous detachment can lead to the alleviation of symptoms without any treatment[1,4,7]. However, vitrectomy is often necessary to remove the vitreous traction[6]. Optical Coherence Tomography can be helpful in the preoperative assessment of the patient, in estimating the intraoperative risk of lamellar or full thickness macular hole[8] formation and in the postoperative follow-up[5].

VITREOMACULAR TRACTION SYNDROME

1. Carpineto P, Ciancaglini M, Aharrh-Gnama A, Agnifili L, Mastropasqua L. Optical coherence tomography and retinal thickness analyzer features of spontaneous resolution of vitreomacular traction syndrome: a case report. Eur J Ophthalmol 2004;14;67-70.
2. Gallemore RP, Jumper JM, McCuen BW 2nd, Jaffe GJ, Postel EA, Toth CA. Diagnosis of vitreoretinal adhesions in macular disease with Optical coherence tomography. Retina 2000;20;115-120.
3. Johnson MW. Tractional cystoid macular edema: a subtle variant of the vitreomacular traction syndrome. Am J Ophthalmol 2005;140;184-192.
4. Kusaka S, Saito Y, Okada AA, Sasamoto M, Hayashi A, Ohji M, Tano Y. Optical coherence tomography in spontaneously resolving vitreomacular traction syndrome. Ophthalmologica 2001;215(2):139-41.
5. Munuera JM, Garcia-Layana A, Maldonado MJ, Aliseda D, Moreno-Montanes J. Optical coherence tomography in successful surgery of vitreomacular traction syndrome. Arch Ophthalmol 1998;116(10):1388-9.
6. Smiddy WE, Michels RG, Glaser BM, deBustros S. Vitrectomy for macular traction caused by incomplete vitreous separation. Arch Ophthalmol 1988;106(5):624-8.
7. Sulkes DJ, Ip MS, Baumal CR, Wu HK, Puliafito CA. Spontaneous resolution of vitreomacular traction documented by optical coherence tomography. Arch Ophthalmol 2000;118(2):286-7.
8. Uchino E, Uemura A, Doi N, Ohba N. Postsurgical evaluation of idiopathic vitreomacular traction syndrome by optical coherence tomography. Am J Ophthalmol 2001;132(1):122-3.

IDIOPATHIC FULL THICKNESS MACULAR HOLE STAGE IA

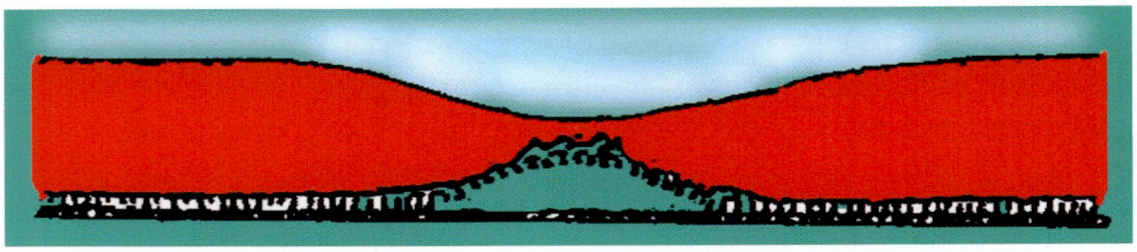

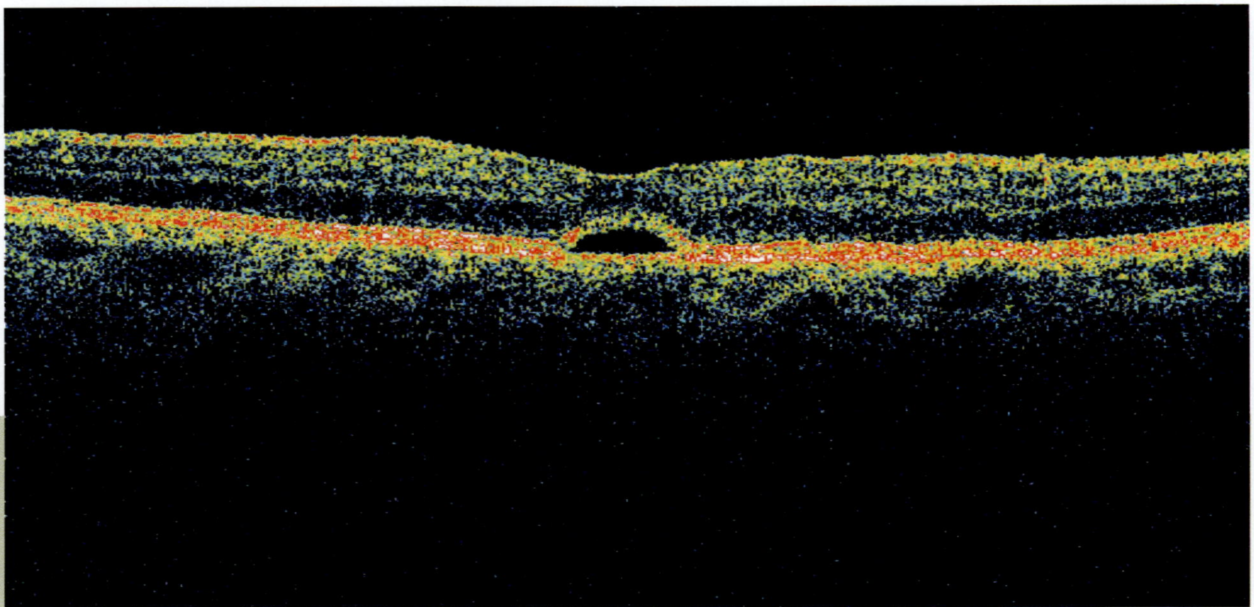

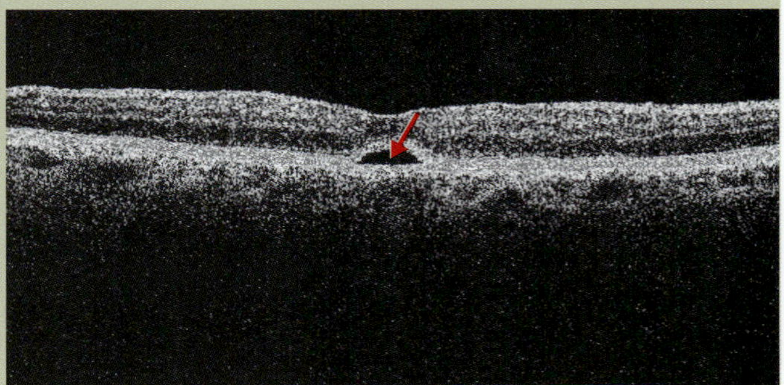

Stage Ia macular hole. Note the area of low reflectivity between the retina and the retinal pigment epithelium that corresponds to a partial retinal detachment in the fovea (arrow).

IDIOPATHIC FULL THICKNESS MACULAR HOLE STAGE IA

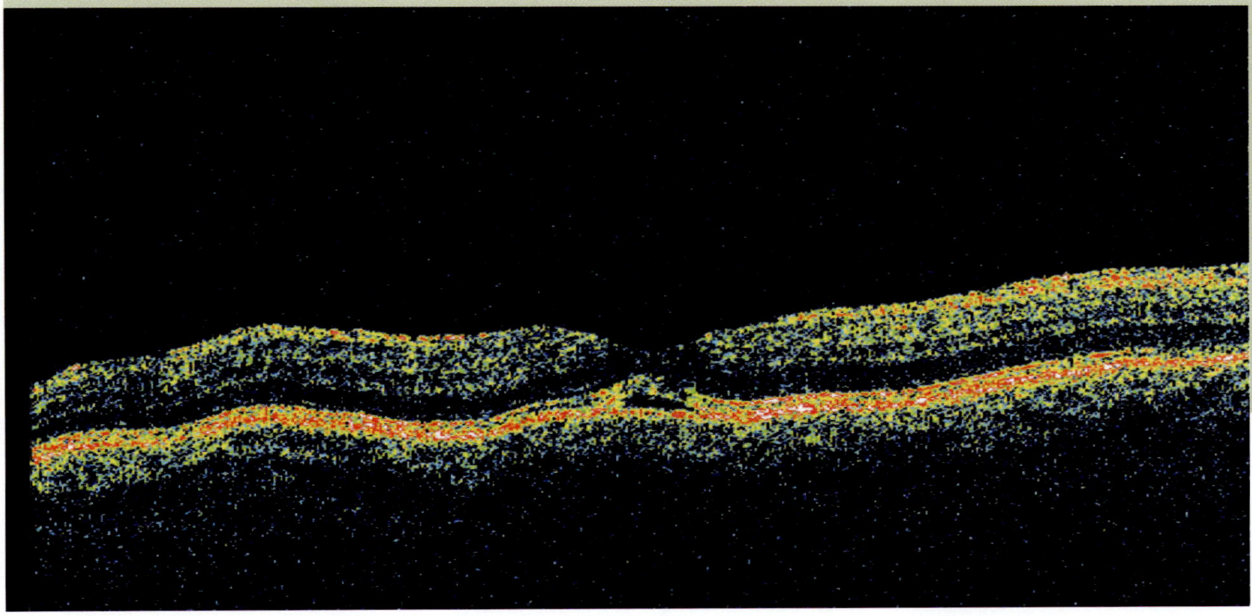

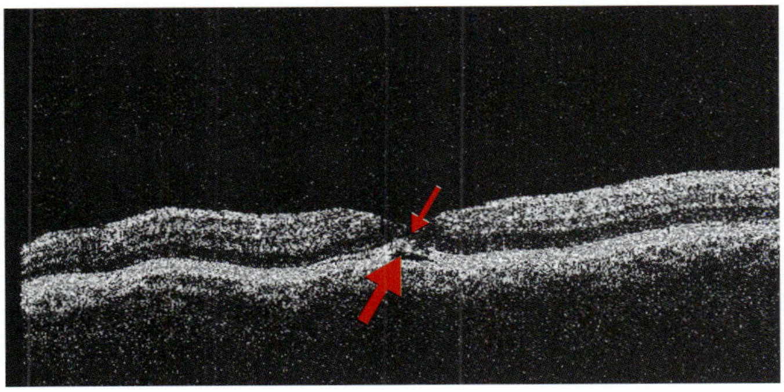

Stage Ia macular hole (impending hole). The retinal detachment appears as a low reflectivity area between the retina and the retinal pigment epithelium (big arrow), accompanied by thinning of the overlying retina (small arrow). The image looks like a retinal cyst in the fovea ready to rupture and convert to a full thickness macular hole.

IDIOPATHIC FULL THICKNESS MACULAR HOLE STAGE IB

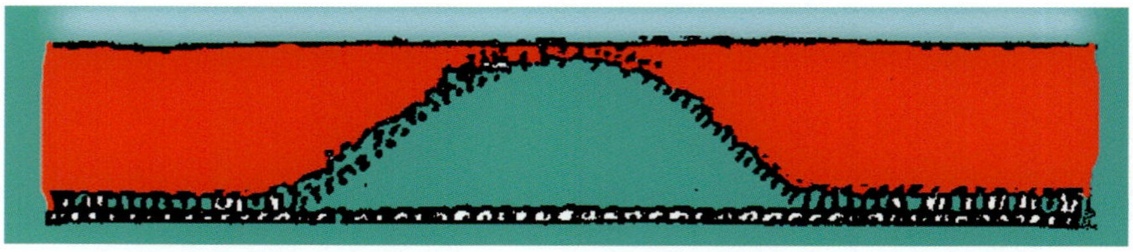

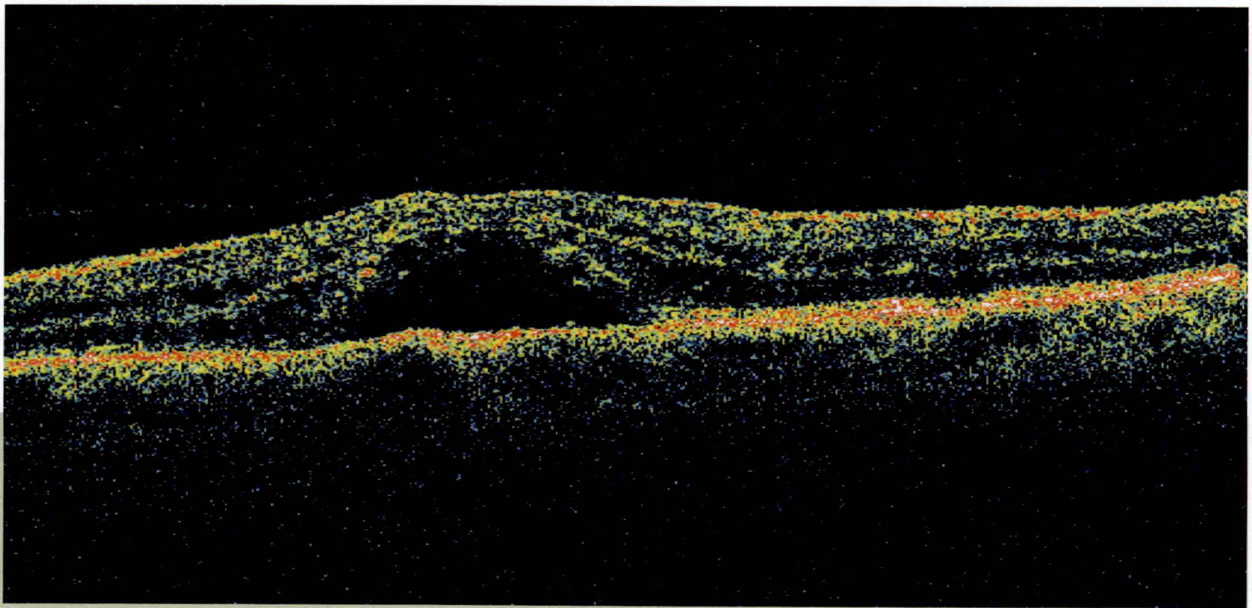

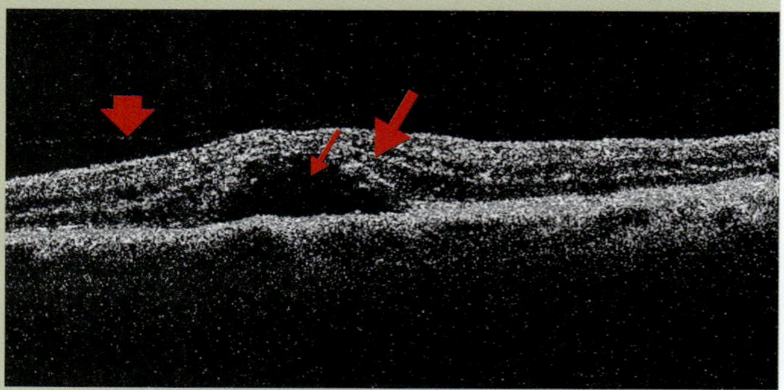

Stage Ib macular hole. In this stage the retinal detachment that is displayed like a low reflectivity area between the retina and the retinal pigment epithelium is larger and higher than in stage Ia (small arrow). There is also diffuse retinal edema in the central area around the detachment (big arrow). The vitreous is detected like a thin faint line of high reflectivity attached to the fovea (thick arrow).

IDIOPATHIC FULL THICKNESS MACULAR HOLE STAGE I

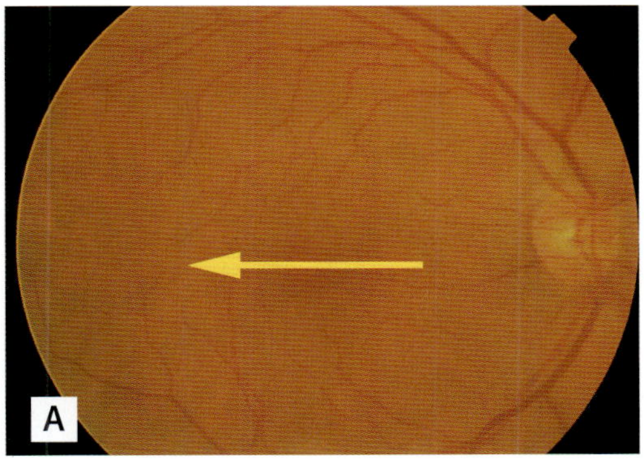

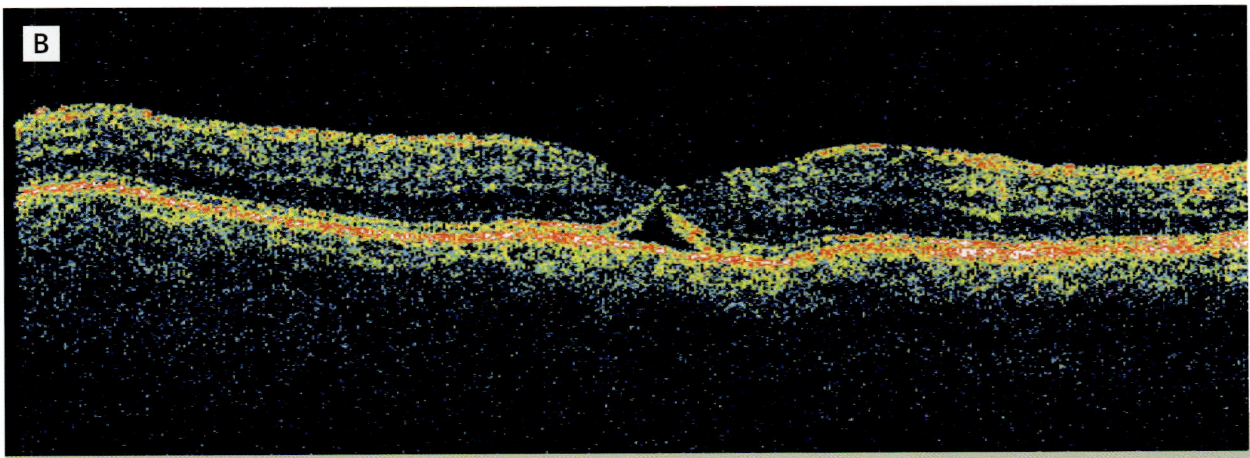

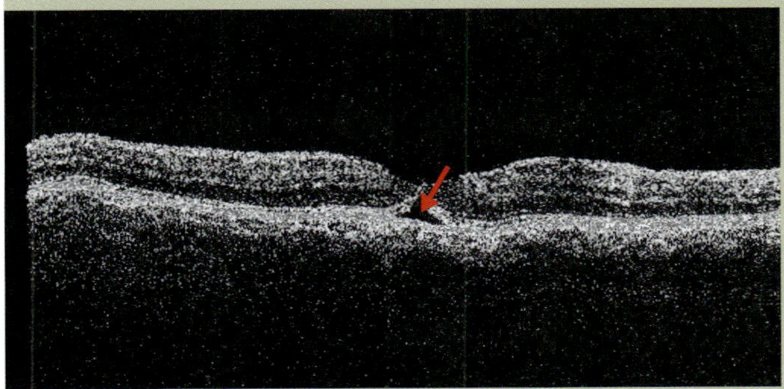

Patient with recent decrease of visual acuity. A. On biomicroscopy there is a foveal lesion with a small yellow ring around it (the arrow shows the scan direction). B. Optical Coherence Tomography shows a small low reflectivity area located between the retina and the retinal pigment epithelium that corresponds to subretinal fluid accumulation (small arrow). The vitreous is not detected. The subretinal fluid at the fovea is an indication of a stage I macular hole (impending). The fact that the vitreous is detached, as biomicroscopy shows, increases the likelihood of spontaneous regression of the development of a full thickness macular hole.

IDIOPATHIC FULL THICKNESS MACULAR HOLE STAGE II

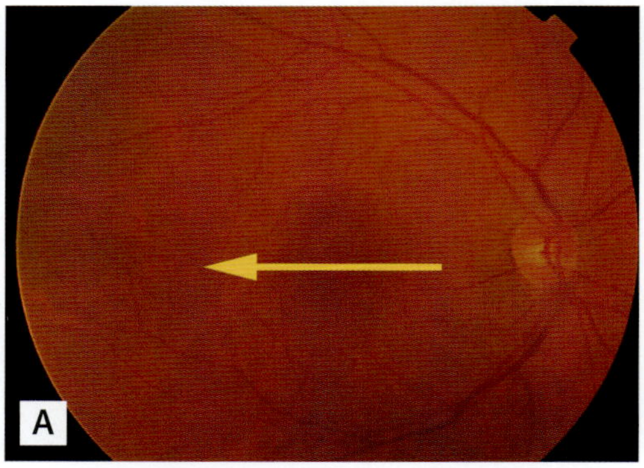

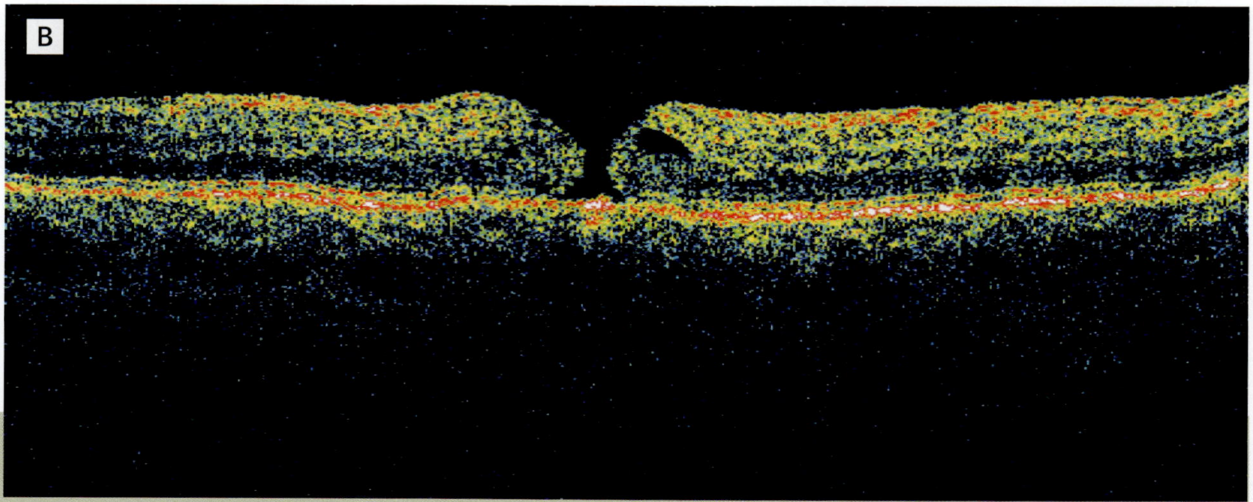

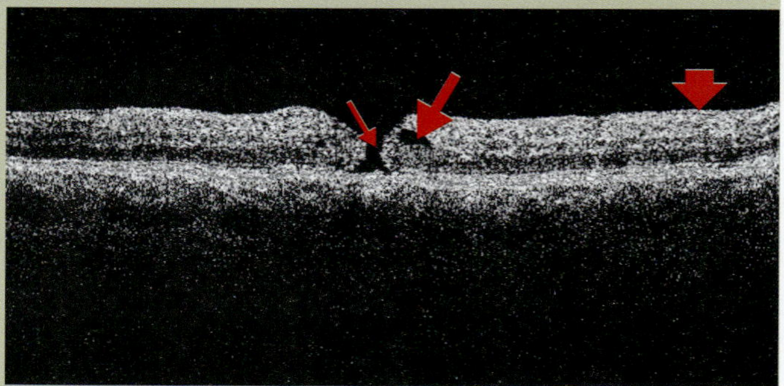

The patient of page 105, four months later. A. The macular hole is clearly visible on biomicroscopy (the arrow shows the scan direction). B. Optical Coherence Tomography shows a full thickness macular defect in the fovea corresponding to a stage II macular hole (small arrow). Note also the cystic intraretinal formations at both sides of the hole corresponding to cystic retinal edema (big arrow). There is a thin line of high reflectivity on the retinal surface that corresponds to an epiretinal membrane (thick arrow). It is possible that, despite the clinically obvious vitreous detachment, there is a vitreous schisis in the posterior pole with maintenance of cortical vitreous attachment on the retinal surface, thus justifying the progression of the impending hole to a full thickness macular hole.

IDIOPATHIC FULL THICKNESS MACULAR HOLE
STAGE II

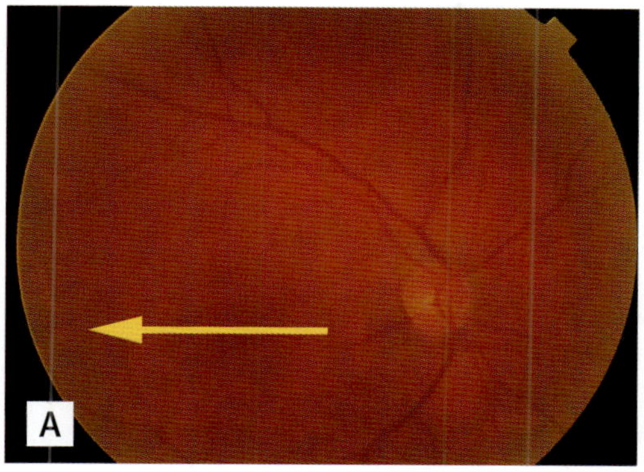

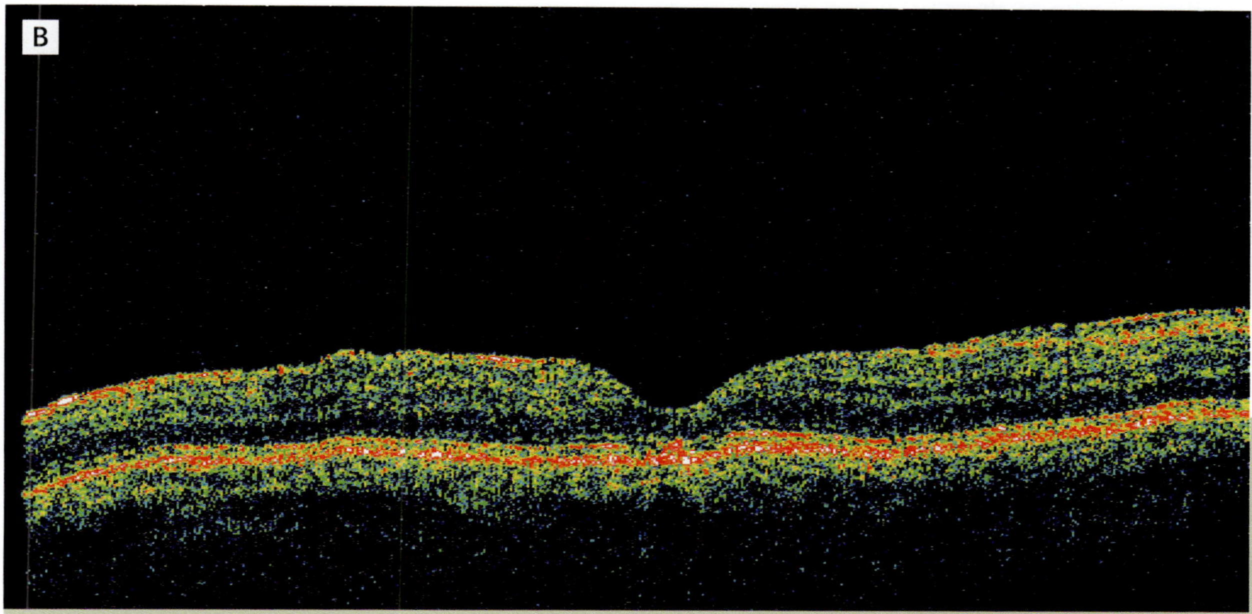

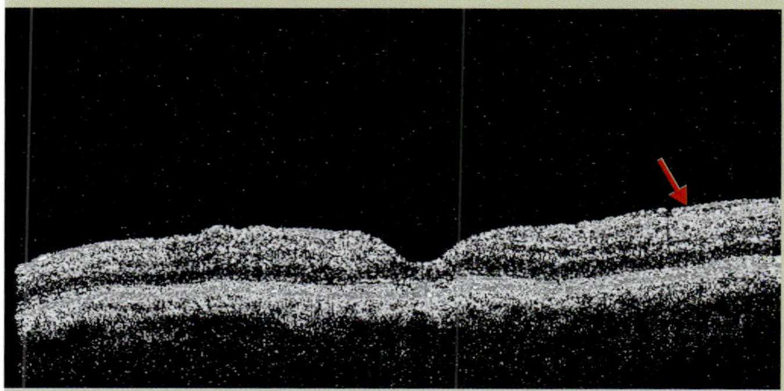

The patient of page 106, three months after surgical treatment. A. Biomicroscopically there is disappearance of the macular hole (the arrow shows the scan direction). B. Optical Coherence Tomography shows a reestablishment of the normal foveal anatomy with closure of the hole. Note the remnants of the epiretinal membrane around the fovea (small arrow).

IDIOPATHIC FULL THICKNESS MACULAR HOLE STAGE II

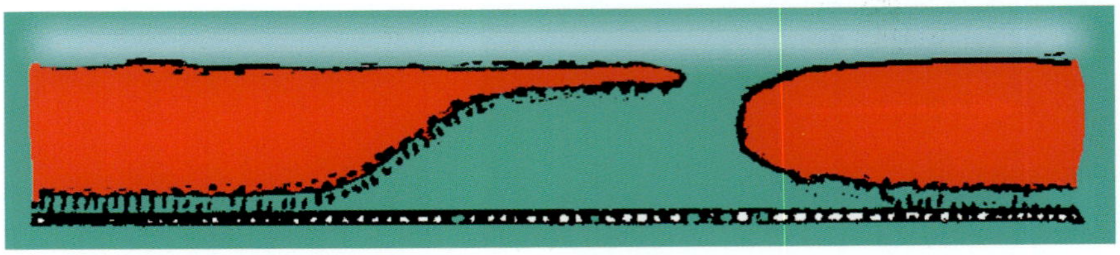

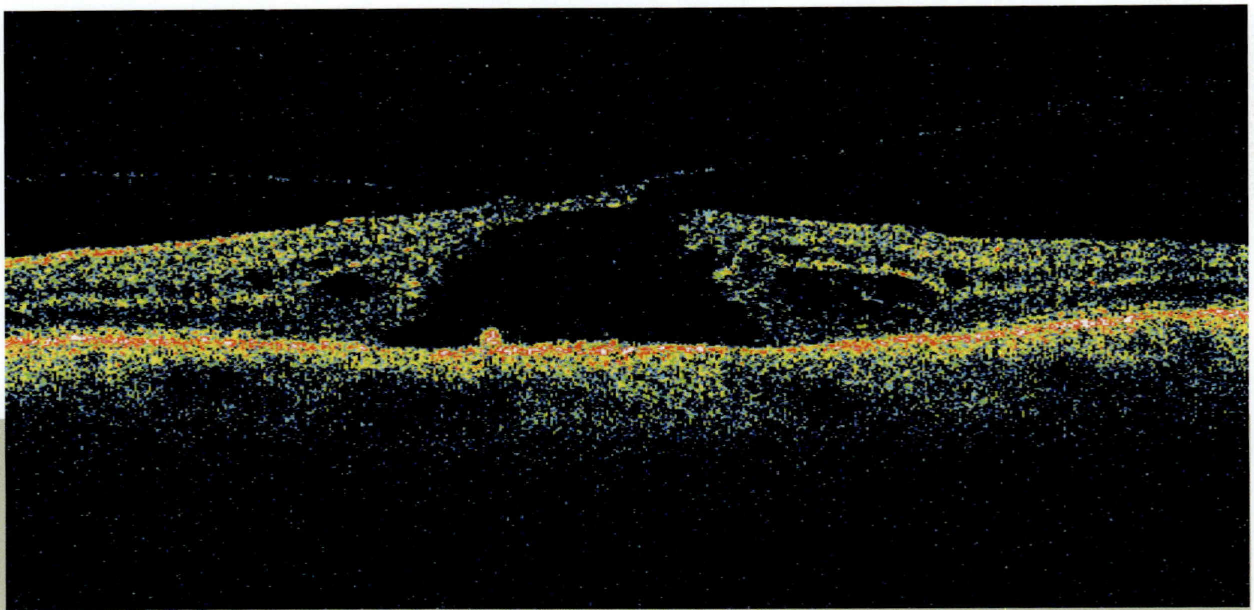

Stage II macular hole. A full-thickness hole with an eccentric opening and a coexisting vitreous attachment that appears like a high reflectivity line in the vitreous cavity (small arrow). Subretinal fluid collection is clearly detected (cuff), at both sides of the hole (big arrow). There is also a small elevated area of high reflectivity at the crater hole that corresponds to a thickening of the retinal pigment epithelium - choriocapillaries layer (thick arrow).

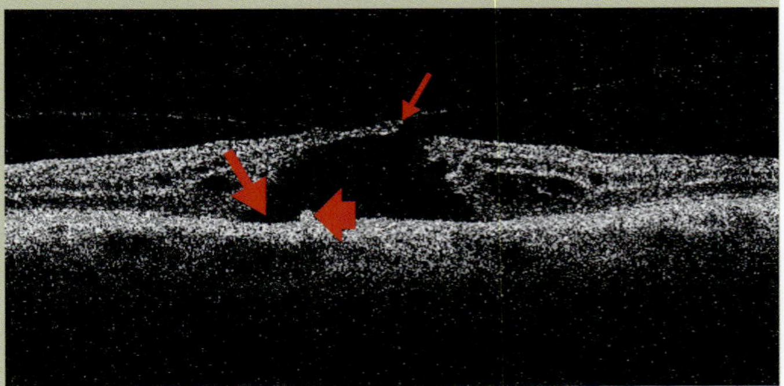

IDIOPATHIC FULL THICKNESS MACULAR HOLE STAGE II

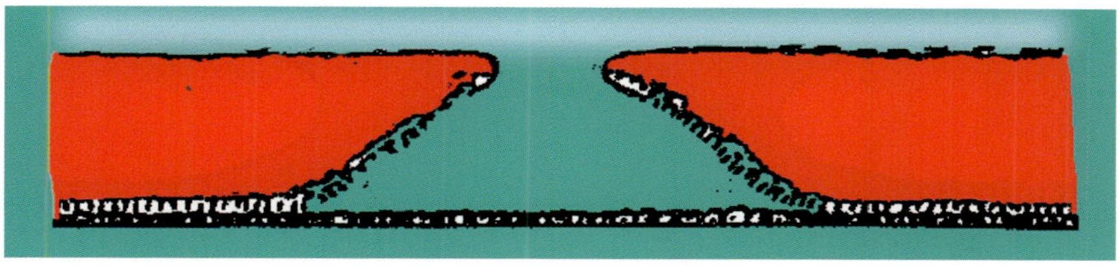

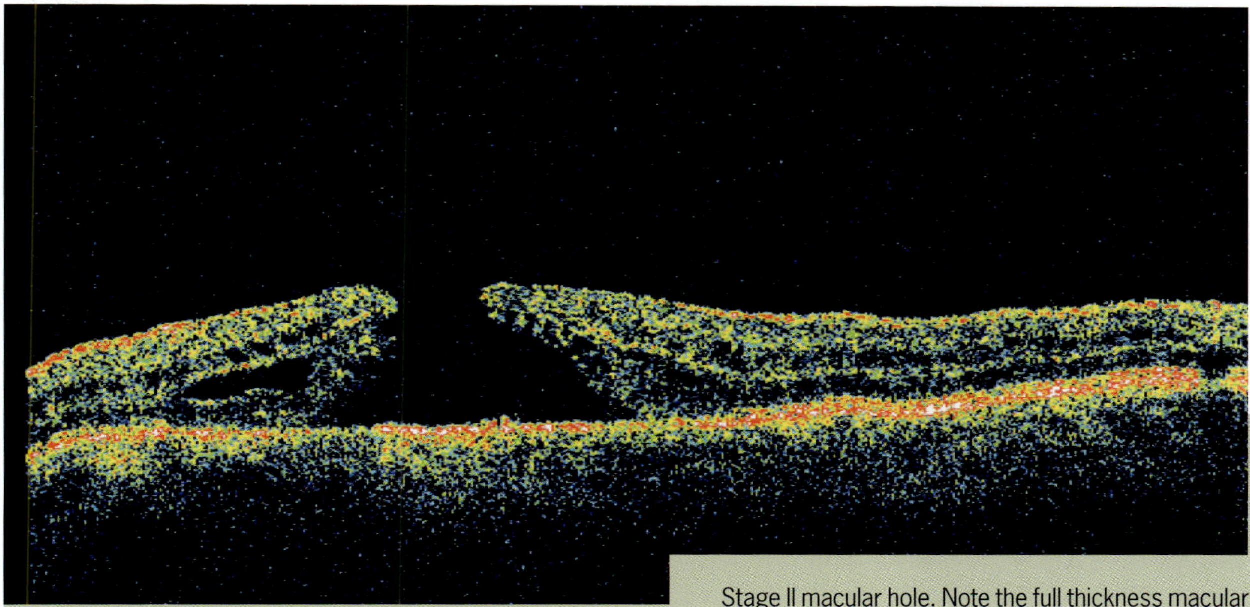

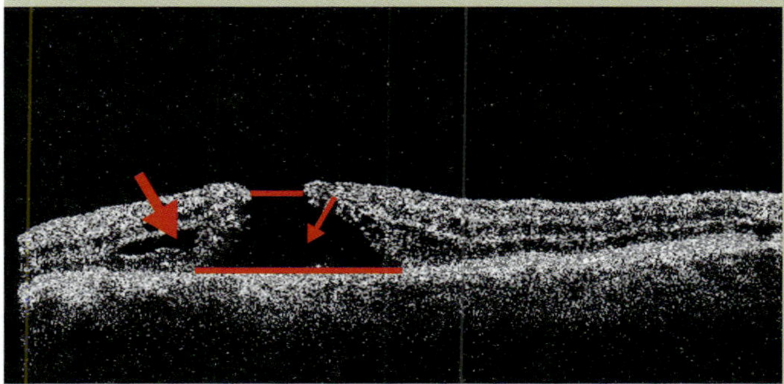

Stage II macular hole. Note the full thickness macular hole with a central opening (small arrow), the subretinal fluid collection (cuff) around the hole as well as the cystic intraretinal formations of low reflectivity corresponding to cystic edema at both sides of the hole (big arrow). Also Note the difference of the hole diameter at the level of the retina (343μm) and at the level of the retinal pigment epithelium (1260μm) (small and big line). The estimation of the hole diameter at the retinal pigment epithelium level and the correlation with its smaller diameter consists in a prognostic factor for the anatomical and functional results after surgical intervention.

IDIOPATHIC FULL THICKNESS MACULAR HOLE STAGE III

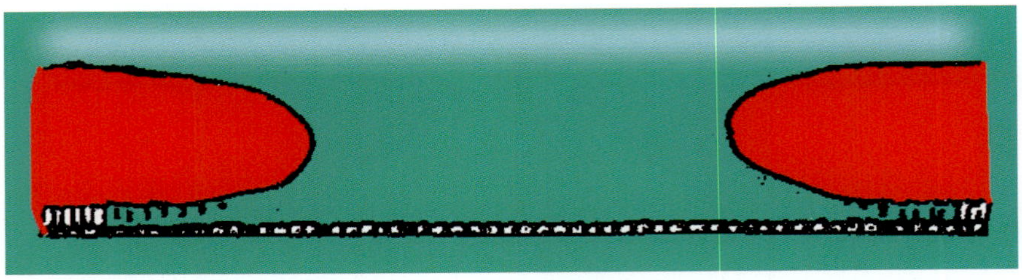

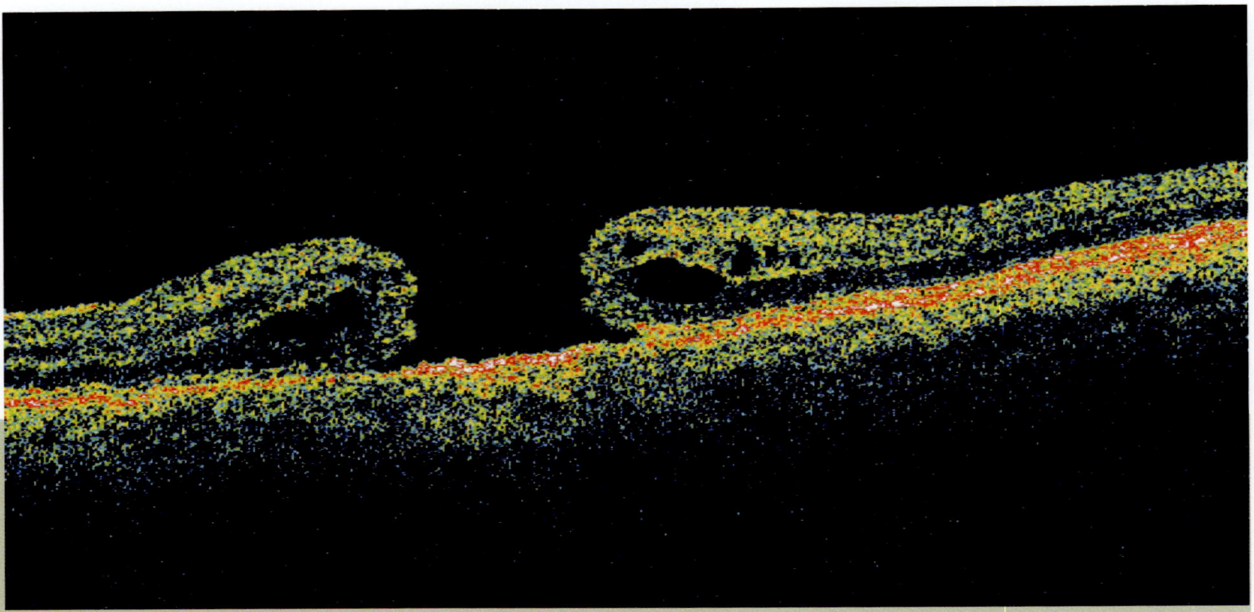

Stage III macular hole with a preoperative bottom diameter of 1480μm and top diameter 845μm. At both sides of the hole there are intraretinal cystic formations of low reflectivity corresponding to retinal cystic edema (arrows). There is also diffuse retinal edema.

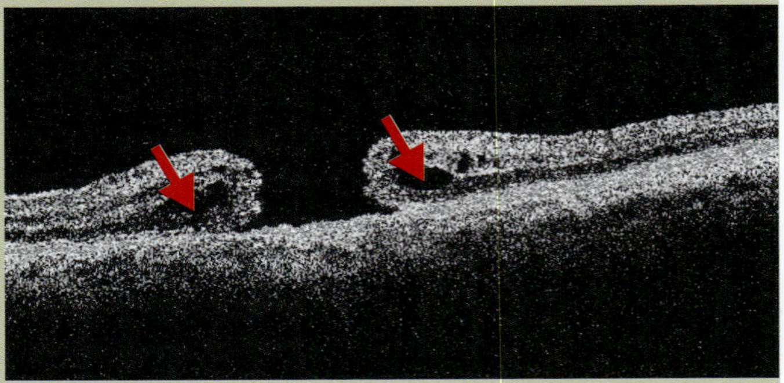

IDIOPATHIC FULL THICKNESS MACULAR HOLE STAGE III

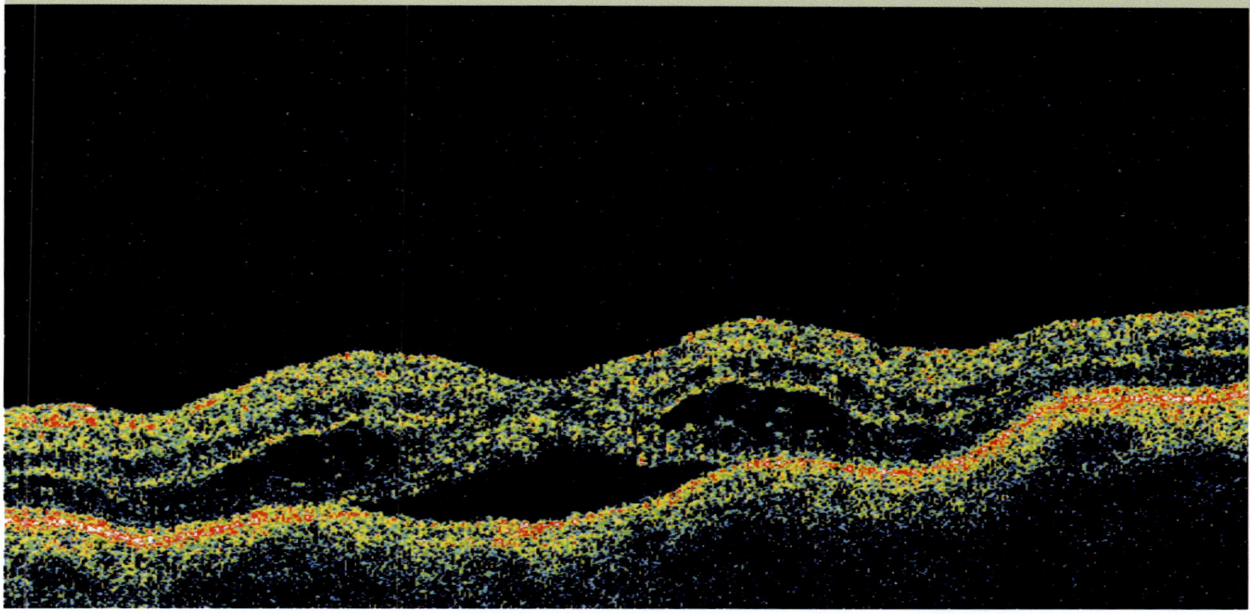

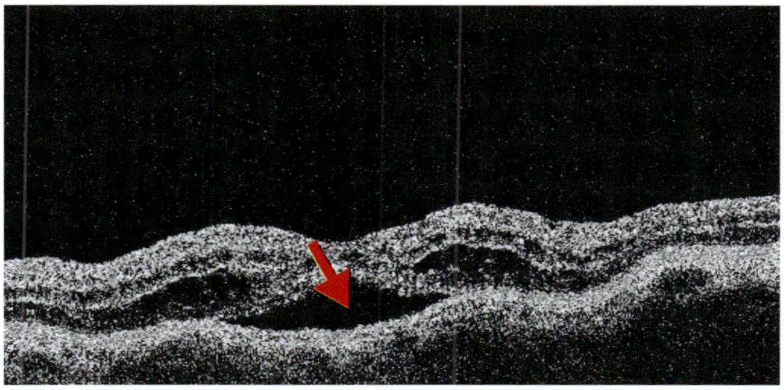

The patient of page 110 during the same examination. The scan area has been moved a few μm with respect to the previous image, resulting in failure to demonstrate the macular hole and giving the impression of a retinal detachment (arrow). The physician must be experienced and familiar with the instrument in order to be able to perform careful scanning of the entire area, to identify lesions and to correctly assess the images and the calculations performed by Optical Coherence Tomography.

IDIOPATHIC FULL THICKNESS MACULAR HOLE STAGE III

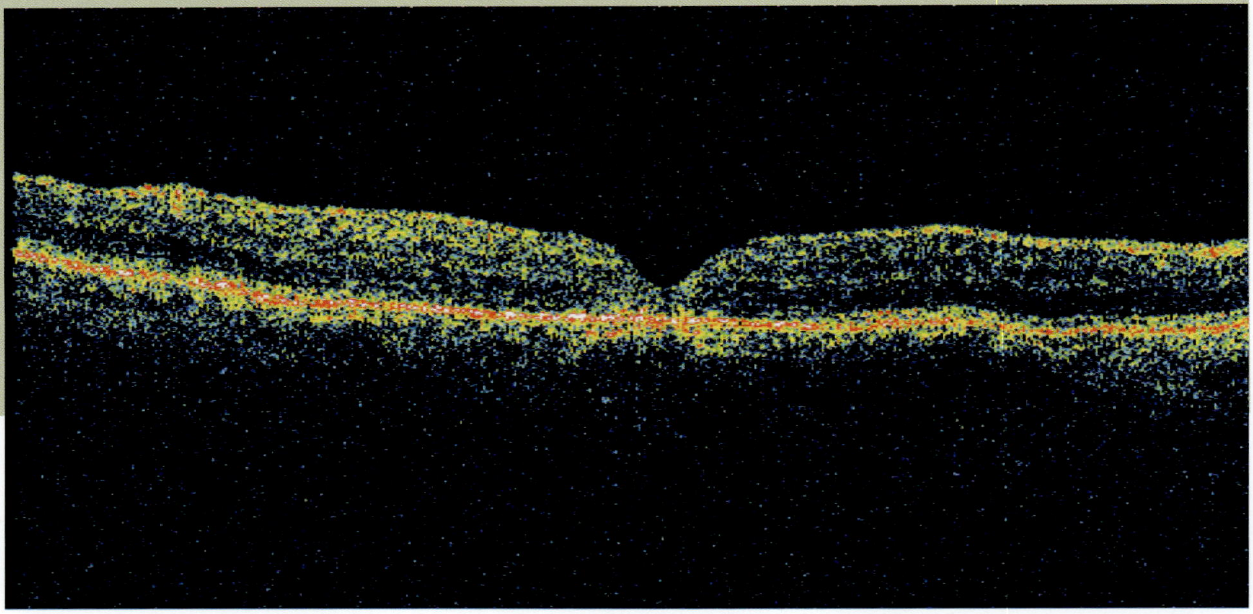

The patient of page 110, twelve months after surgery. The hole is completely closed and the retinal thickness in the fovea is 110μm.

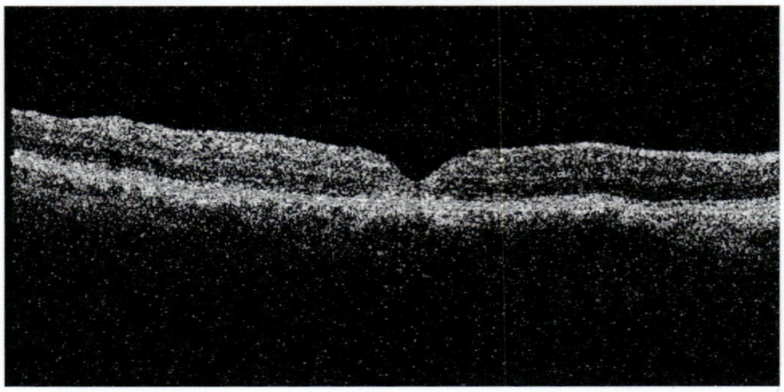

IDIOPATHIC FULL THICKNESS MACULAR HOLE STAGE III

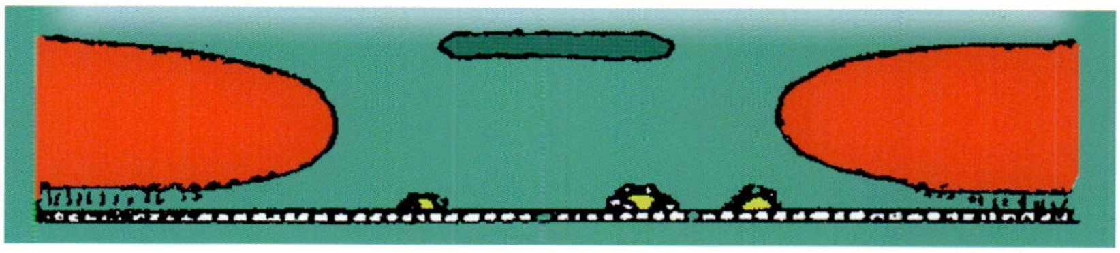

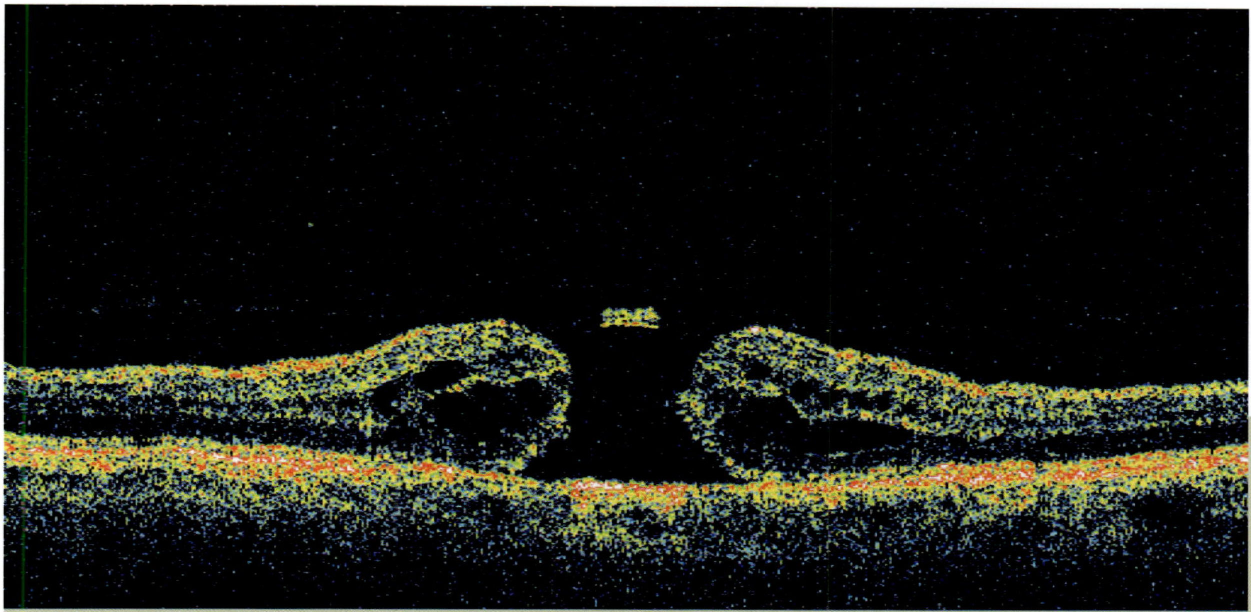

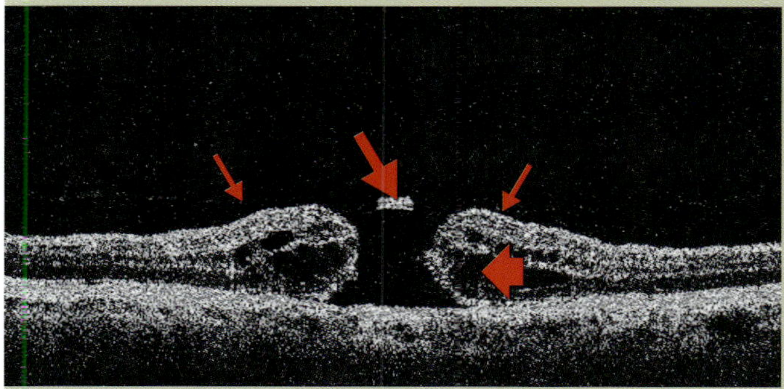

Stage III macular hole with a central pseudo-operculum, represented as a small area of high reflectivity in the vitreous cavity (big arrow). The vitreous is attached only to the edge of the hole and represented as a thin line of high reflectivity in the vitreous cavity (small arrows). The presence of cystic retinal edema at both sides of the hole shown as cystic formations of low intraretinal reflectivity is characteristic (thick arrow).

IDIOPATHIC FULL THICKNESS MACULAR HOLE STAGE III

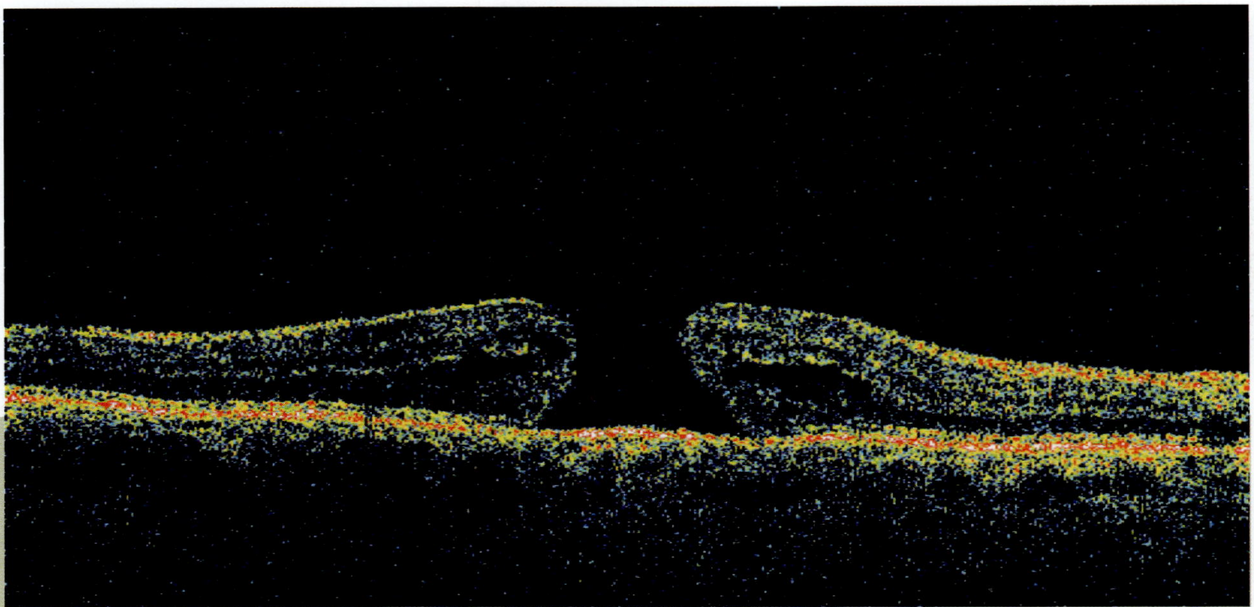

Stage III macular hole without a pseudo-operculum. The retina at both sides of the hole has cystic formations of low intraretinal reflectivity that correspond to cystic edema (arrow).

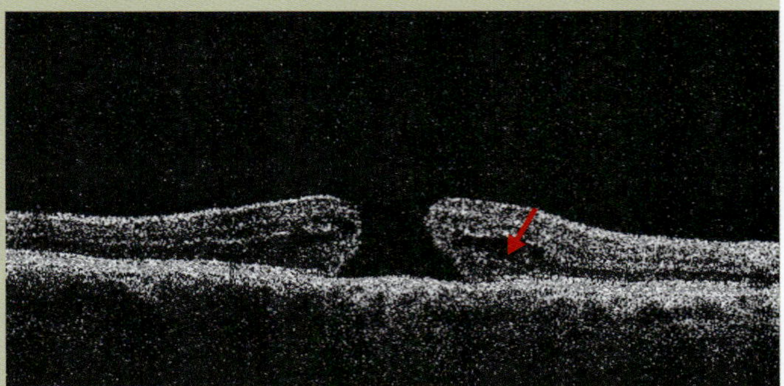

IDIOPATHIC FULL THICKNESS MACULAR HOLE STAGE IV

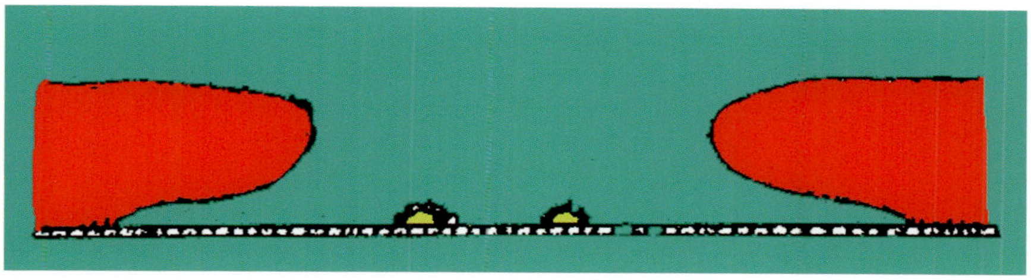

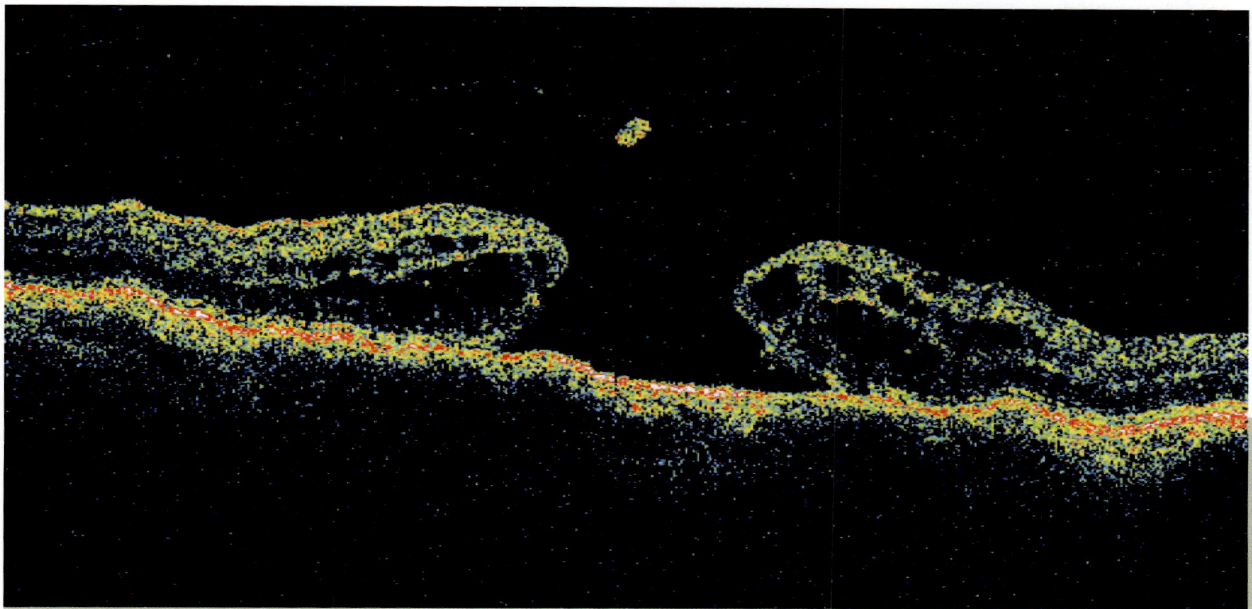

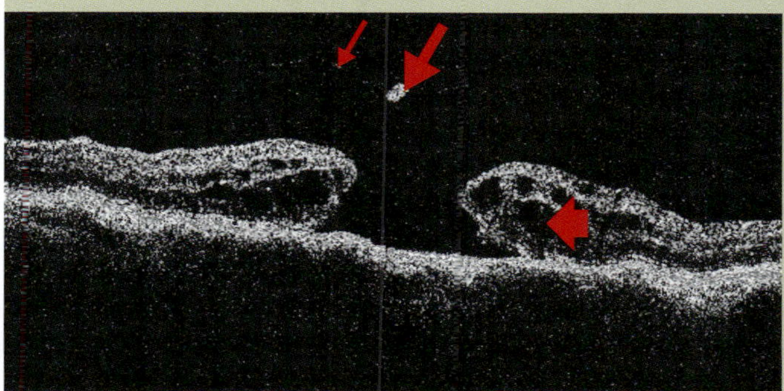

Stage IV macular hole with completely detached vitreous (the thin line of high reflectivity inside the vitreous cavity [small arrow]) and a pseudo-operculum (the small area of high reflectivity) in the vitreous cavity (big arrow). The presence of cystic formations of low intraretinal reflectivity is clearly detected corresponding to cystic retinal edema at both sides of the hole (thick arrow).

IDIOPATHIC FULL THICKNESS MACULAR HOLE STAGE IV

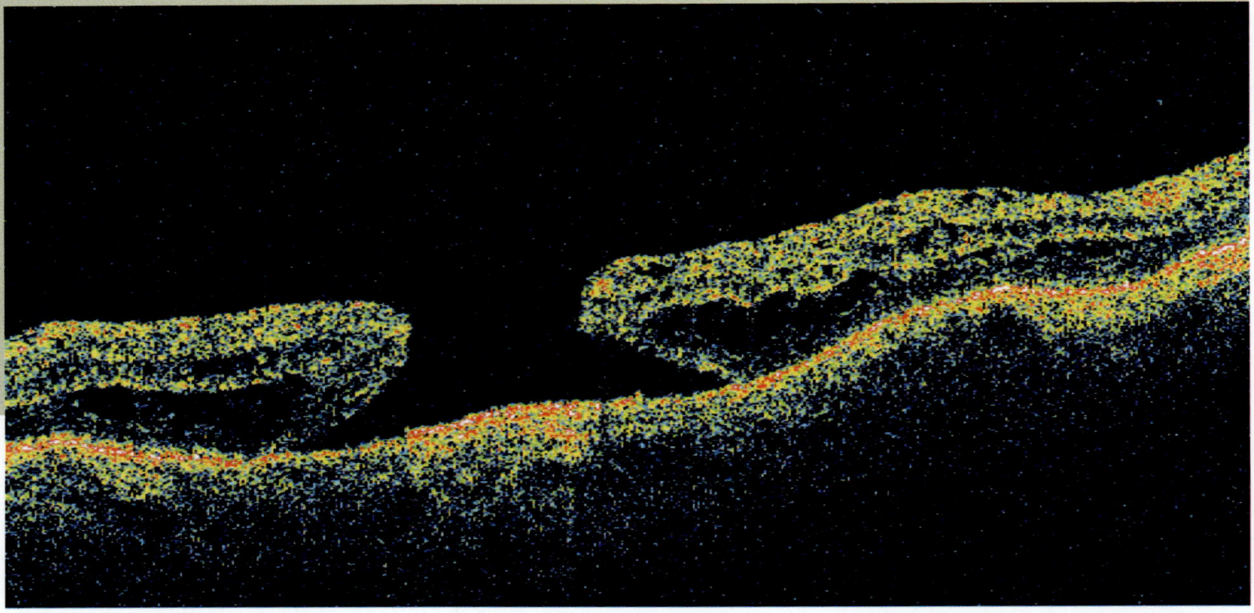

Stage IV macular hole. Cystic formations of low intraretinal reflectivity are clearly detected and correspond to cystic retinal edema at both sides of the hole (big arrow). Subretinal fluid collection (cuff) appears at both sides of the hole (small arrow). There is a thin area of high reflectivity on the retinal surface that corresponds to an epiretinal membrane (empty arrow).

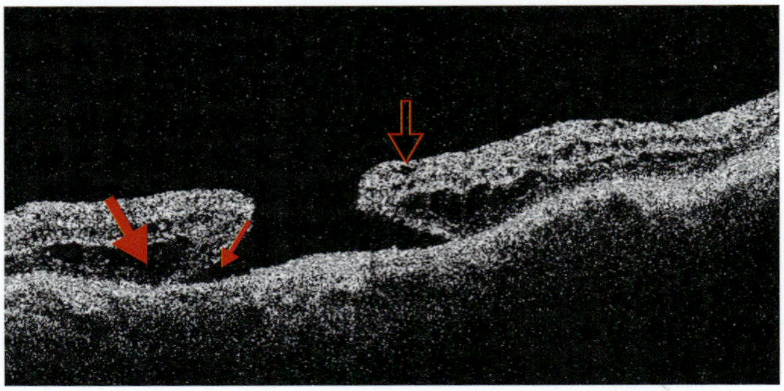

IDIOPATHIC FULL THICKNESS MACULAR HOLE STAGE IV

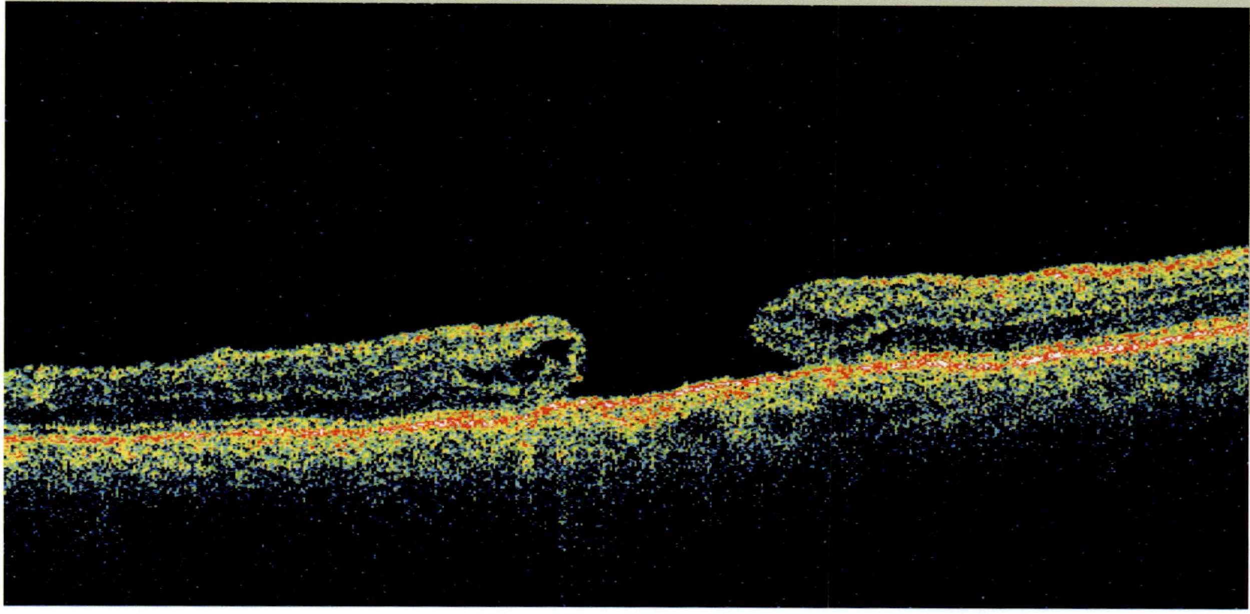

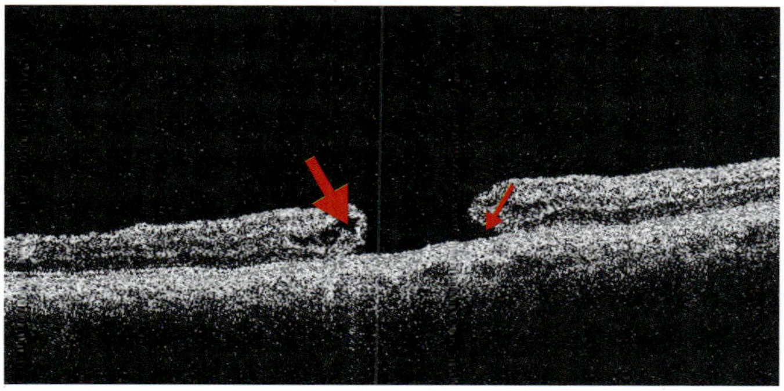

Stage IV macular hole of 8 years duration. There is a mild presence of cystic formations of low intraretinal reflectivity corresponding to cystic retinal edema at both sides of the hole (big arrow). There is a small quantity of subretinal fluid (cuff) at both sides of the hole (small arrow). Because of the chronicity the retina appears thinner around the hole.

MYOPIC FULL THICKNESS MACULAR HOLE

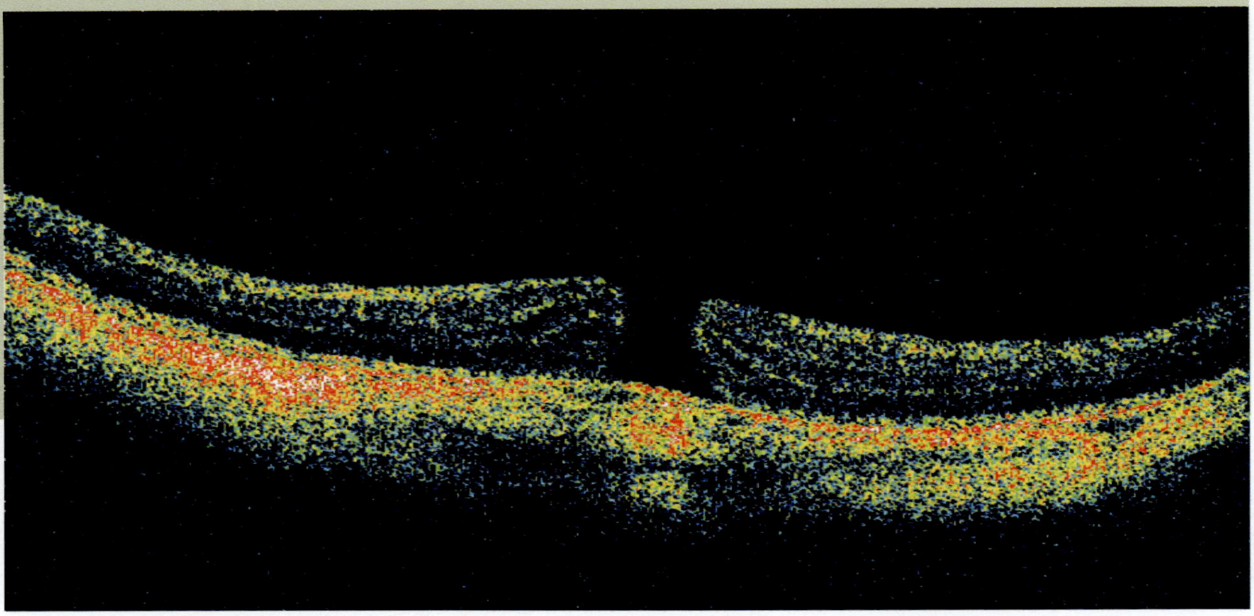

Patient with high myopia (-24D), visual acuity 20/200 and stage III full thickness macular hole. Around the opening of the hole (arrow) there is not any significant edema or subretinal fluid.

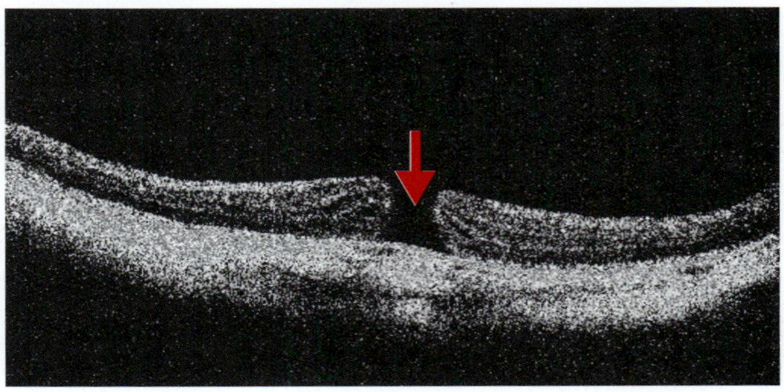

MYOPIC FULL THICKNESS MACULAR HOLE

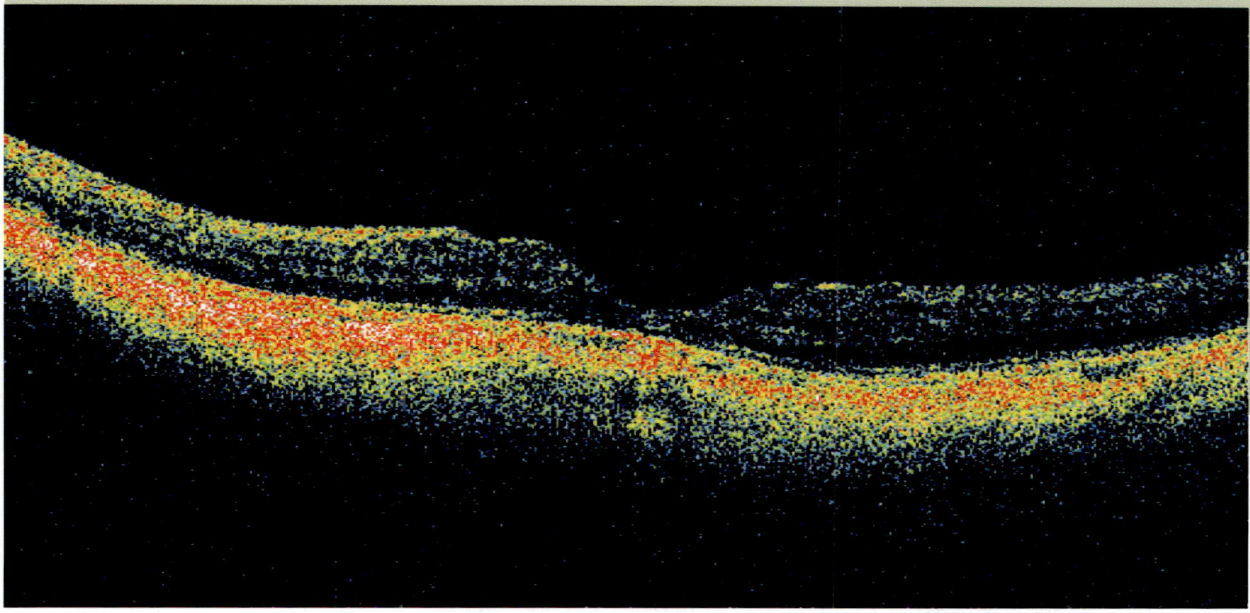

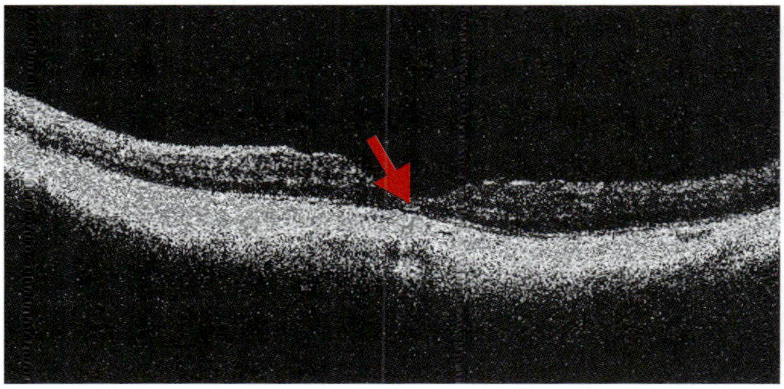

The patient of page 118, 4 months after surgical treatment. The visual acuity is 20/70. Note the closure of the hole and the relative retinal thinning in the foveola (arrow).

TRAUMATIC FULL THICKNESS MACULAR HOLE

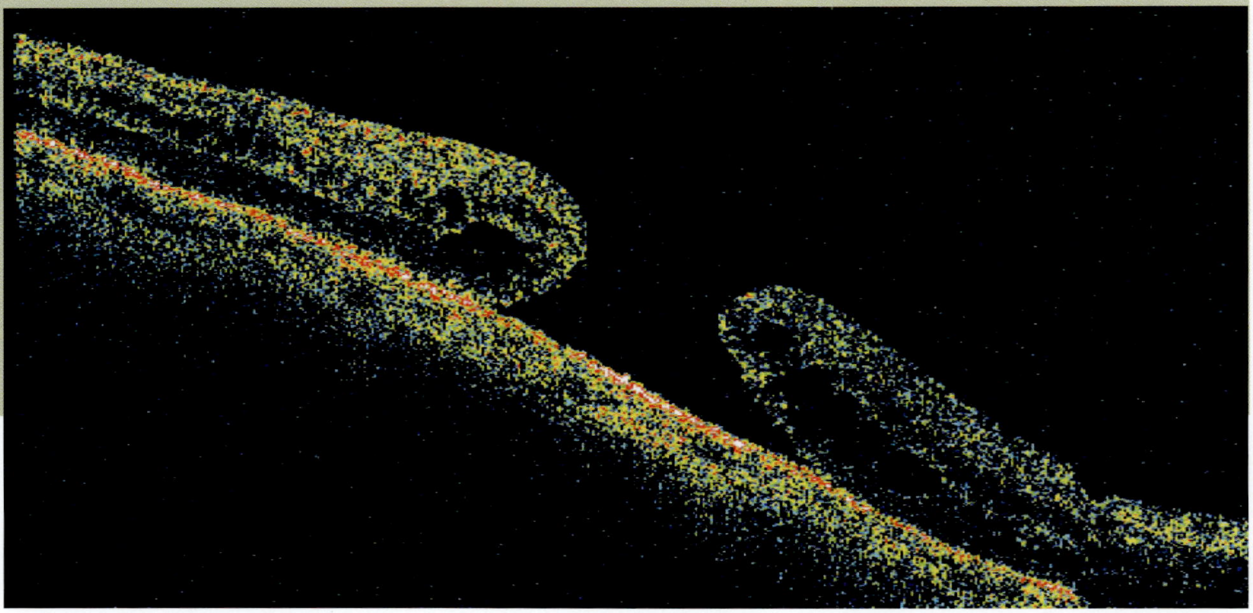

Stage IV traumatic macular hole of 30 years duration. The presence of cystic intraretinal formations of low reflectivity is clear and corresponds to cystic retinal edema at both sides of the hole (big arrow). There is also subretinal fluid collection (cuff) at both sides of the hole (small arrow). A thin area of high reflectivity is detected on the retinal surface and corresponds to an epiretinal membrane (empty arrow).

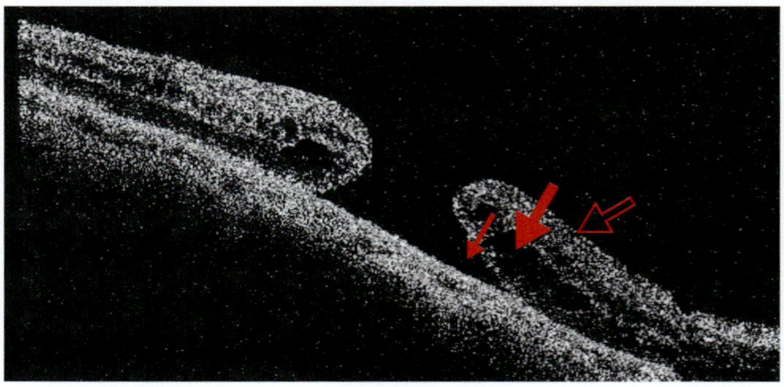

LAMELLAR MACULAR HOLE

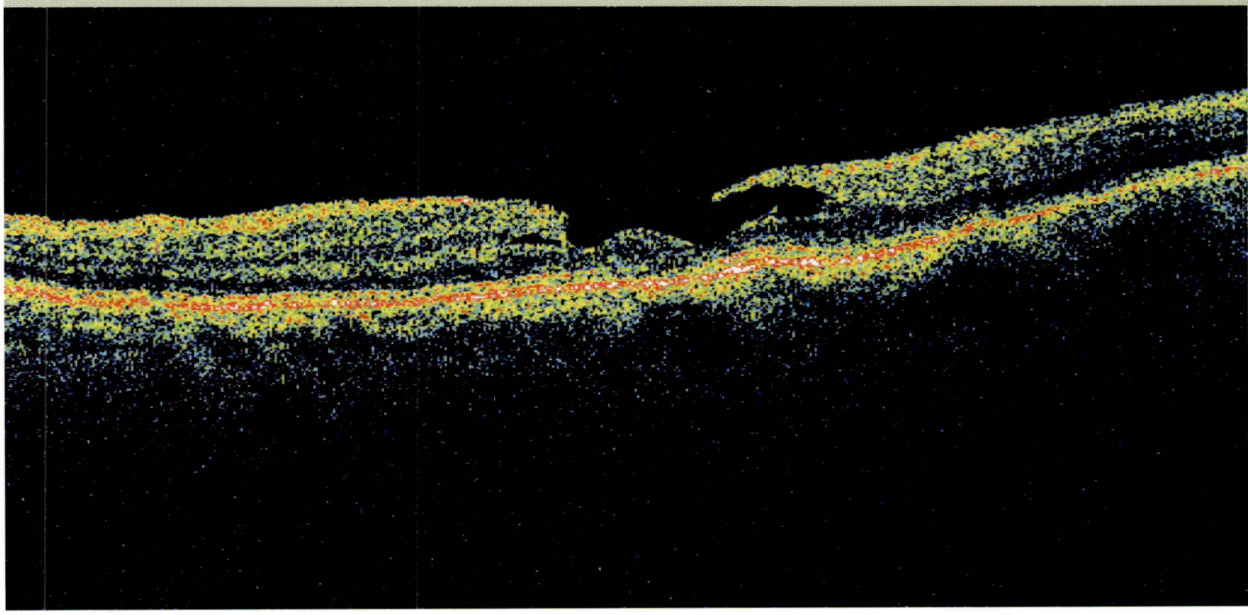

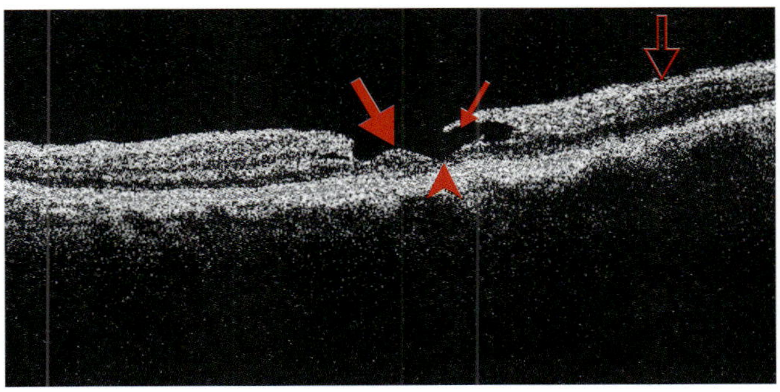

Patient with lamellar macular hole. There is a partial retinal defect in the fovea corresponding to a lamellar macular hole (big arrow). The edge of the hole appears irregular and away from the retina (small arrow), while the remaining retinal tissue at the bed of the hole is thin (arrow head). The retinal thickness around the hole is within normal limits. To the right of the fovea a thin area of high reflectivity is detected on the retinal surface and corresponds to an epiretinal membrane (empty arrow).

LAMELLAR MACULAR HOLE

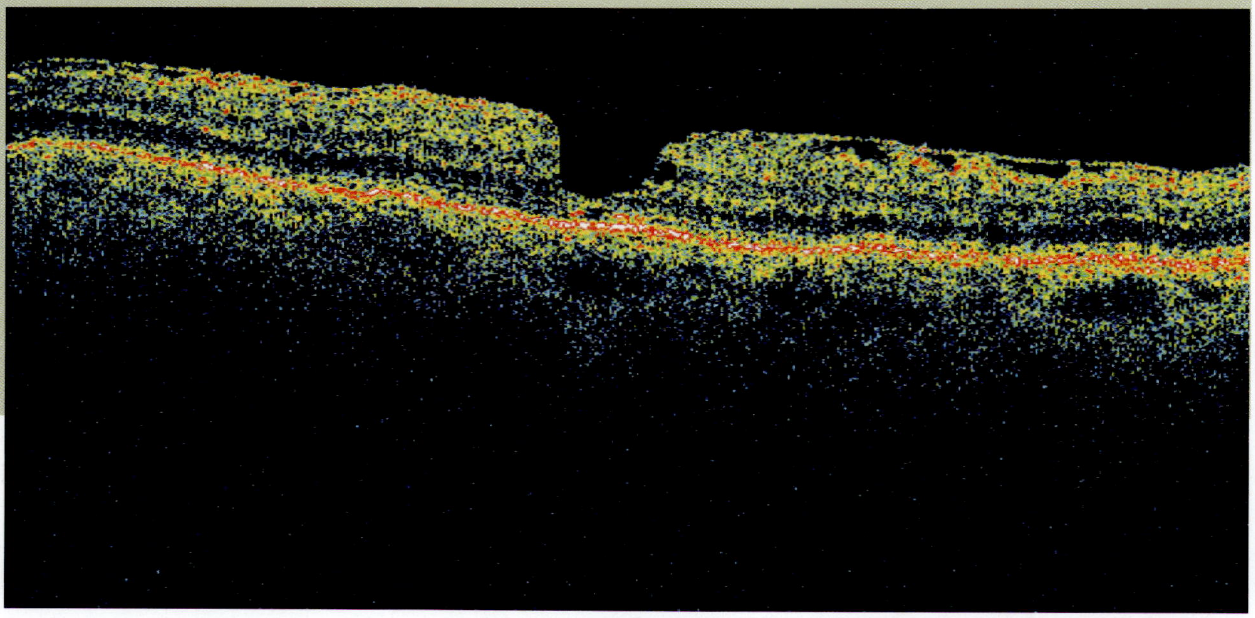

Patient with lamellar macular hole. There is a partial retinal defect in the fovea that corresponds to a lamellar macular hole (big arrow). A thin area of high reflectivity is detected around the fovea on the retinal surface and corresponds to an epiretinal membrane (empty arrow).

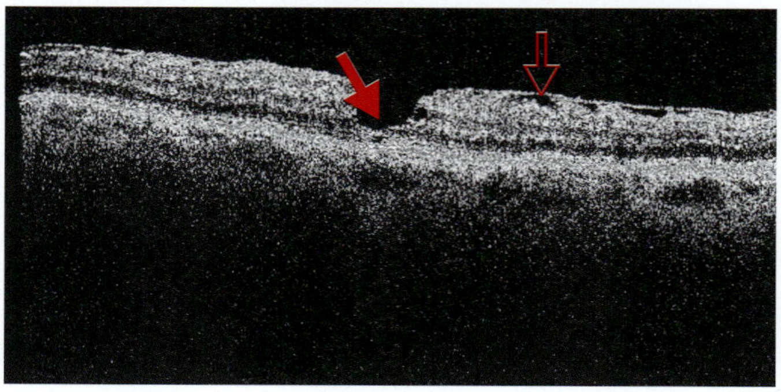

EPIRETINAL MEMBRANE WITH LAMELLAR MACULAR HOLE

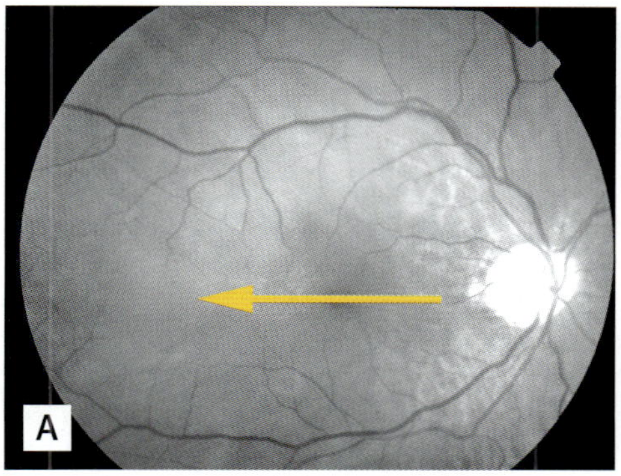

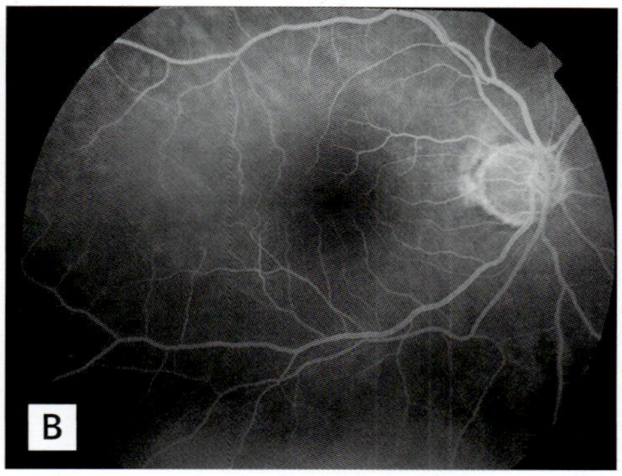

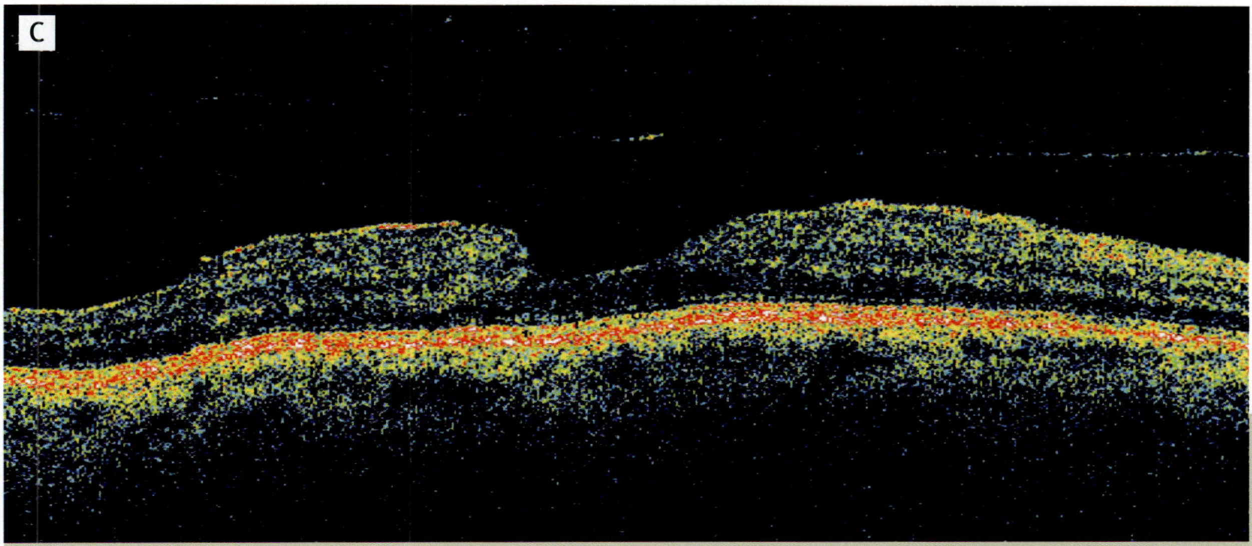

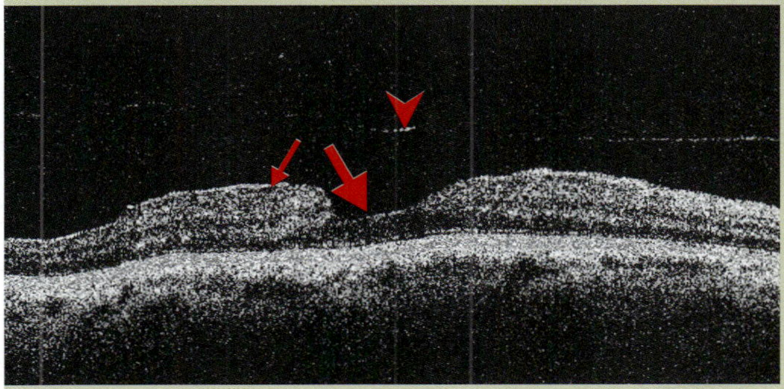

A. Patient with an epiretinal membrane and an obvious lamellar macular hole (the arrow shows the scan arrow). B. Fluorescein angiography doesn't detect any dye leakage. C. Note the thin area of high reflectivity located on the retinal surface that corresponds to the epiretinal membrane in the fovea and around it (small arrow). There is a partial retinal defect in the fovea that corresponds to a lamellar macular hole (big arrow). The vitreous appears detached from the retina and is displayed like a thin horizontal line inside the vitreous cavity (arrow head).

LAMELLAR MACULAR HOLE

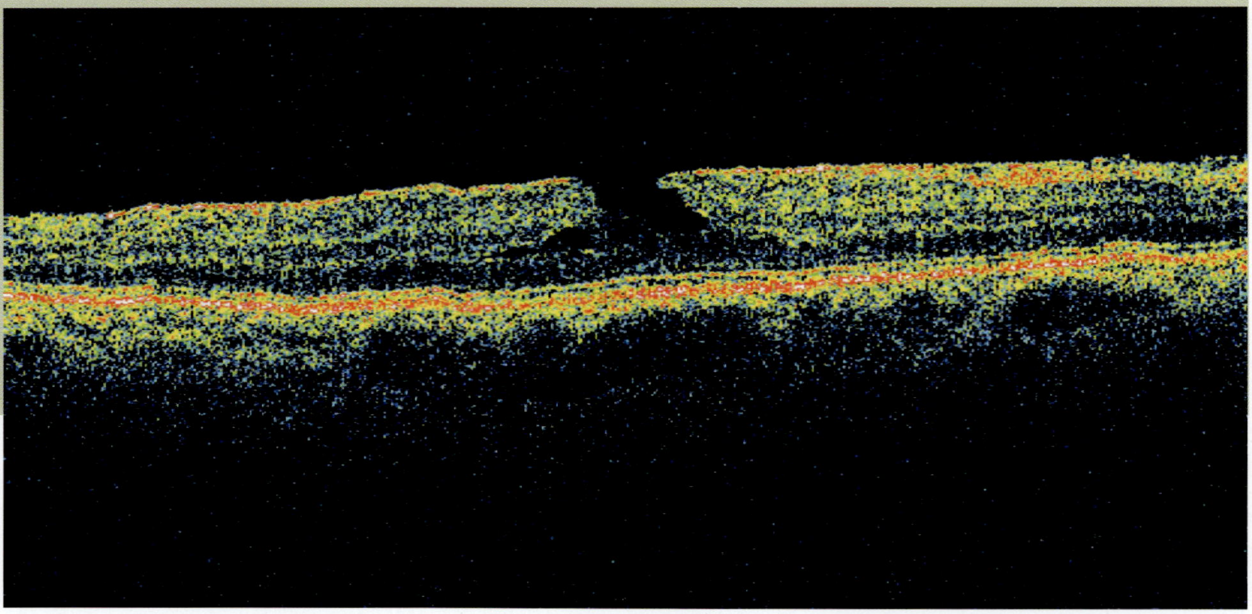

Patient with lamellar macular hole. A partial retinal defect is detected in the fovea corresponding to the lamellar macular hole (big arrow). There is a thin area of high reflectivity around the fovea on the retinal surface that corresponds to an epiretinal membrane (empty arrow).

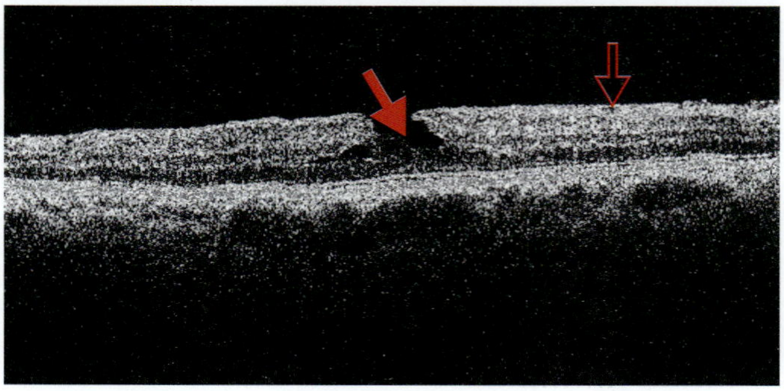

LAMELLAR MACULAR HOLE

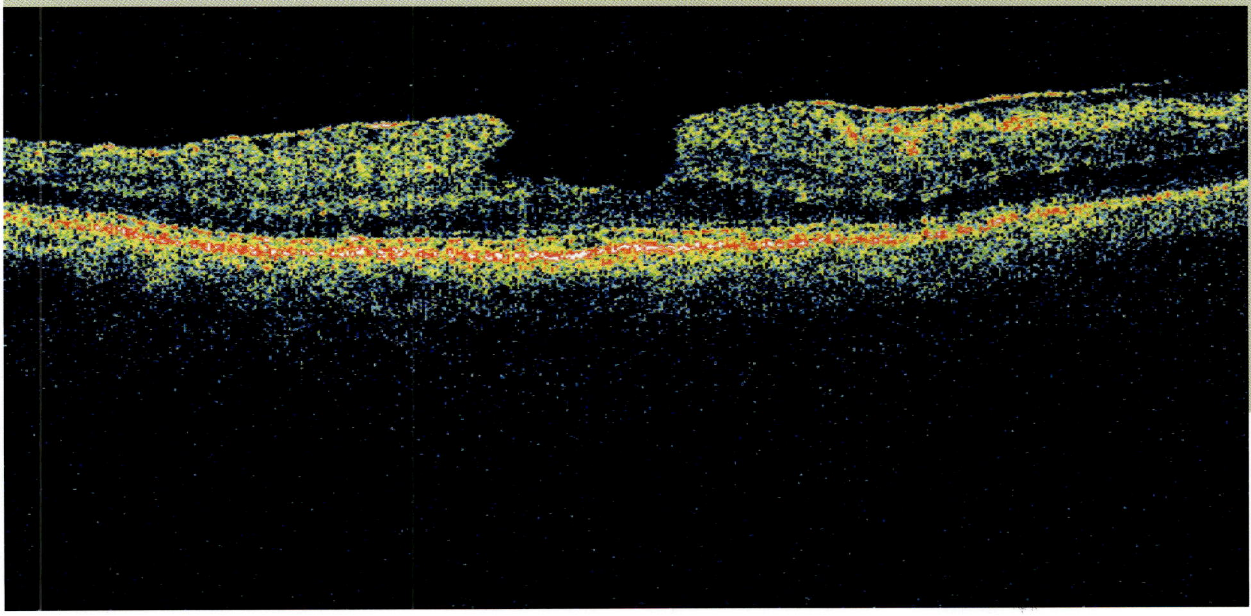

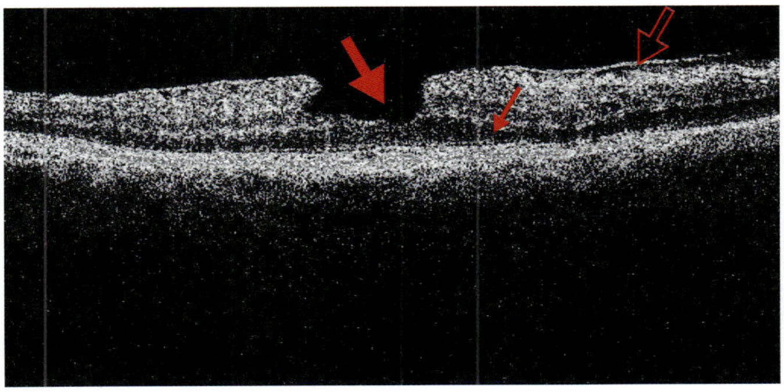

Patient with lamellar macular hole. A partial retinal defect is detected in the fovea and corresponds to the lamellar macular hole (big arrow). There is a thin area of high reflectivity around the fovea on the retinal surface corresponding to an epiretinal membrane (empty arrow). There is also an area of low reflectivity in the outer retinal layers that corresponds to diffuse edema (small arrow).

LAMELLAR MACULAR HOLE

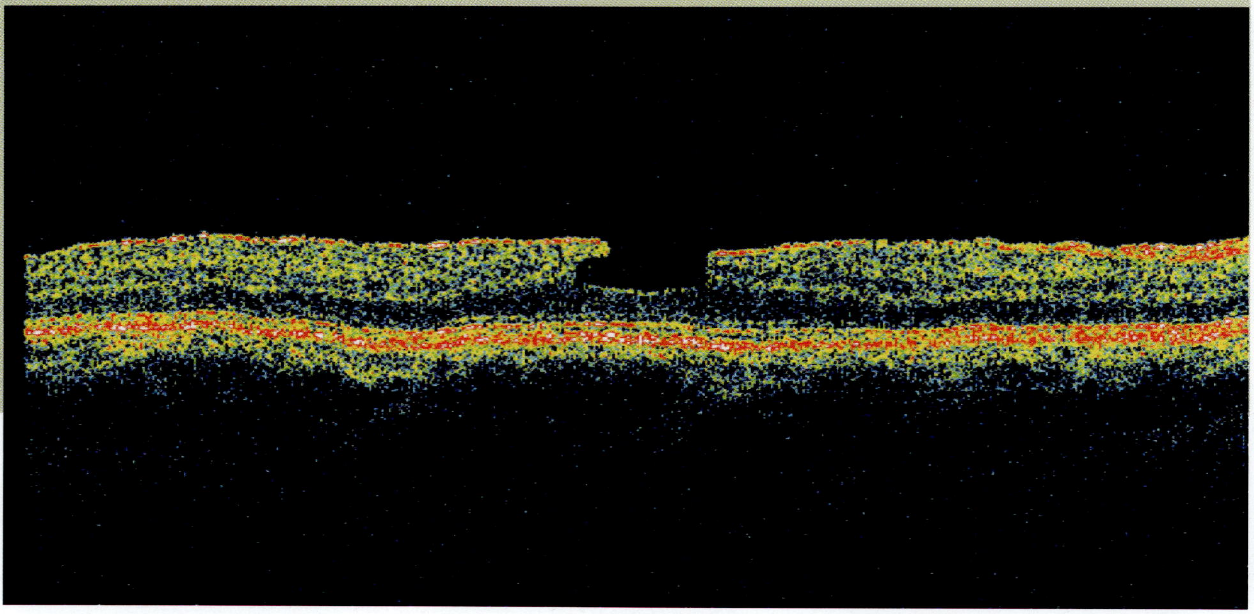

Patient with lamellar macular hole. A partial retinal defect is detected in the fovea corresponding to the lamellar macular hole (big arrow). The retinal thickness around the hole appears slightly increased.

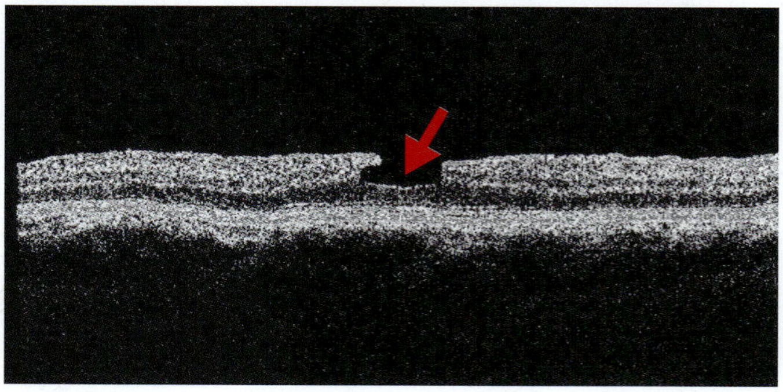

LAMELLAR MACULAR HOLE

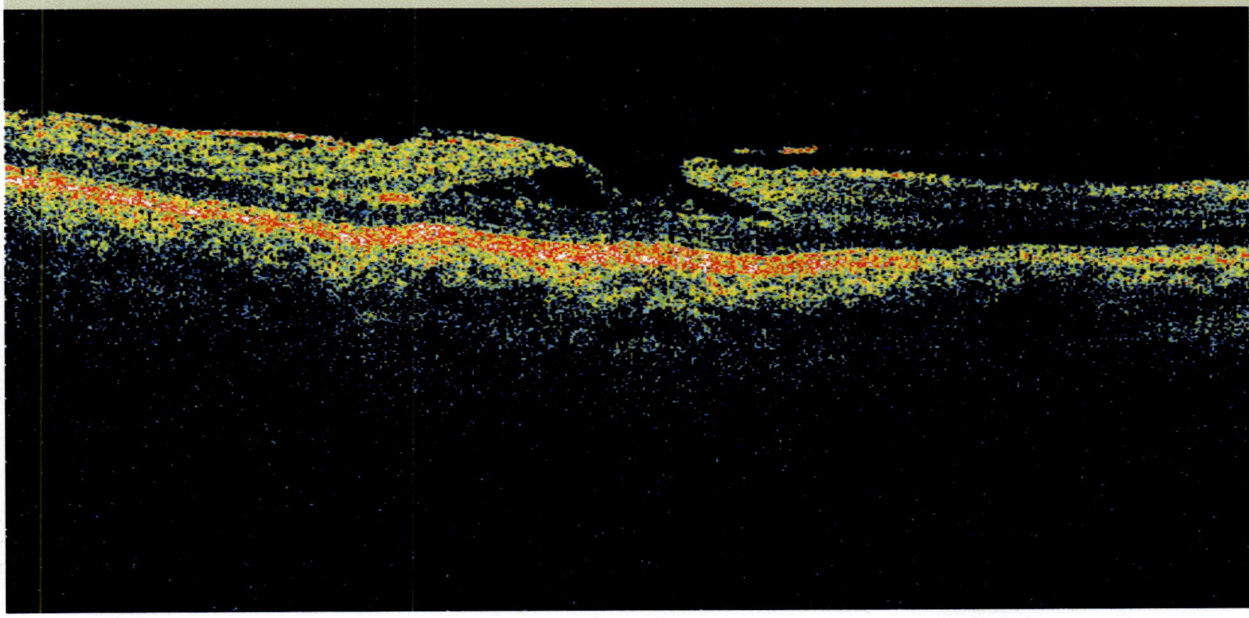

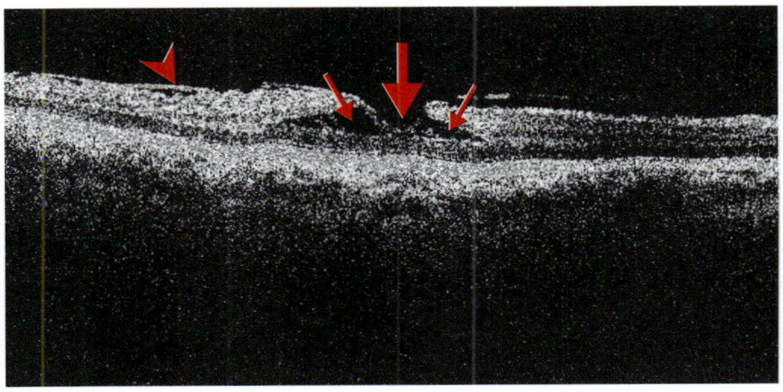

Patient with lamellar macular hole. A partial retinal defect is detected in the fovea and corresponds to the lamellar macular hole (big arrow). There is a thin area of high reflectivity around the fovea on the retinal surface that corresponds to an epiretinal membrane (arrow head). The cystic formations of low reflectivity in the inner retinal layers at the hole area correspond to cystic edema (small arrows).

EPIRETINAL MEMBRANE WITH LAMELLAR MACULAR HOLE

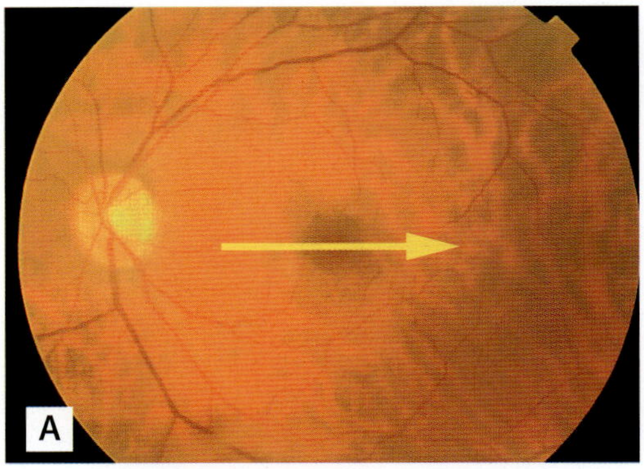

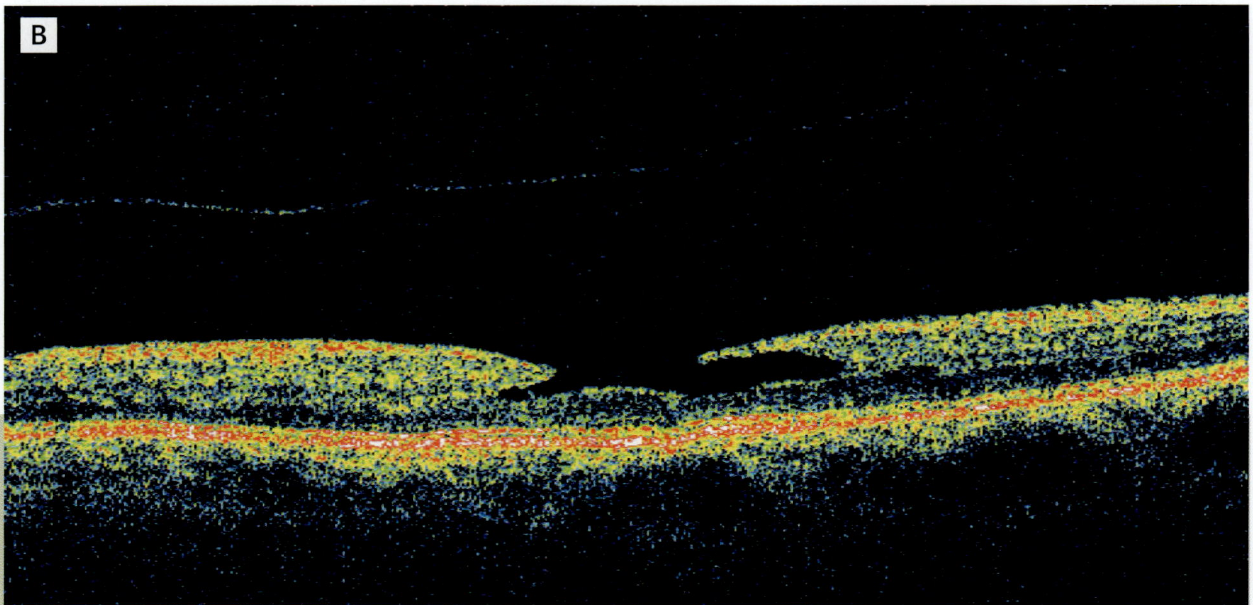

A. Patient with an epiretinal membrane and a lamellar macular hole (incomplete) (the arrow shows the scan direction). B. Optical Coherence Tomography shows the presence of retinal tissue in the outer layers (small arrow). The epiretinal membrane is detected as a local interruption of the continuity of the retinal surface (big arrow). The vitreous appears clearly detached from the retina (thick arrow).

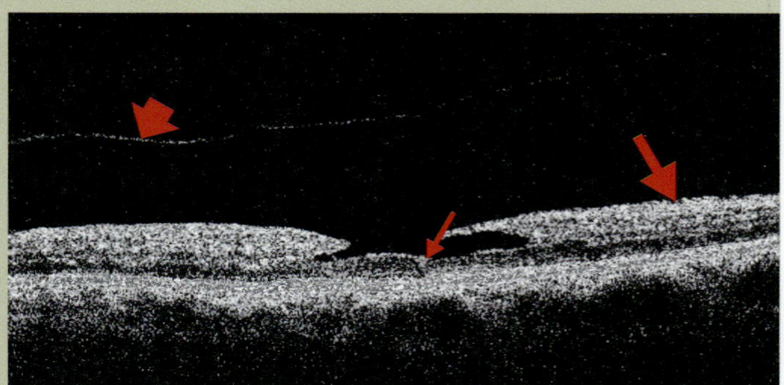

EPIRETINAL MEMBRANE WITH LAMELLAR MACULAR HOLE

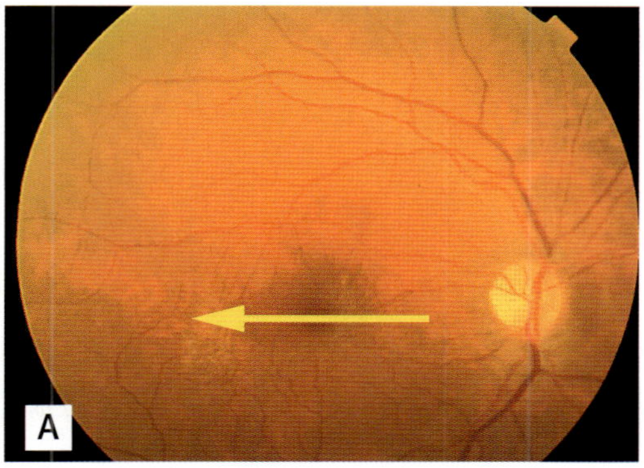

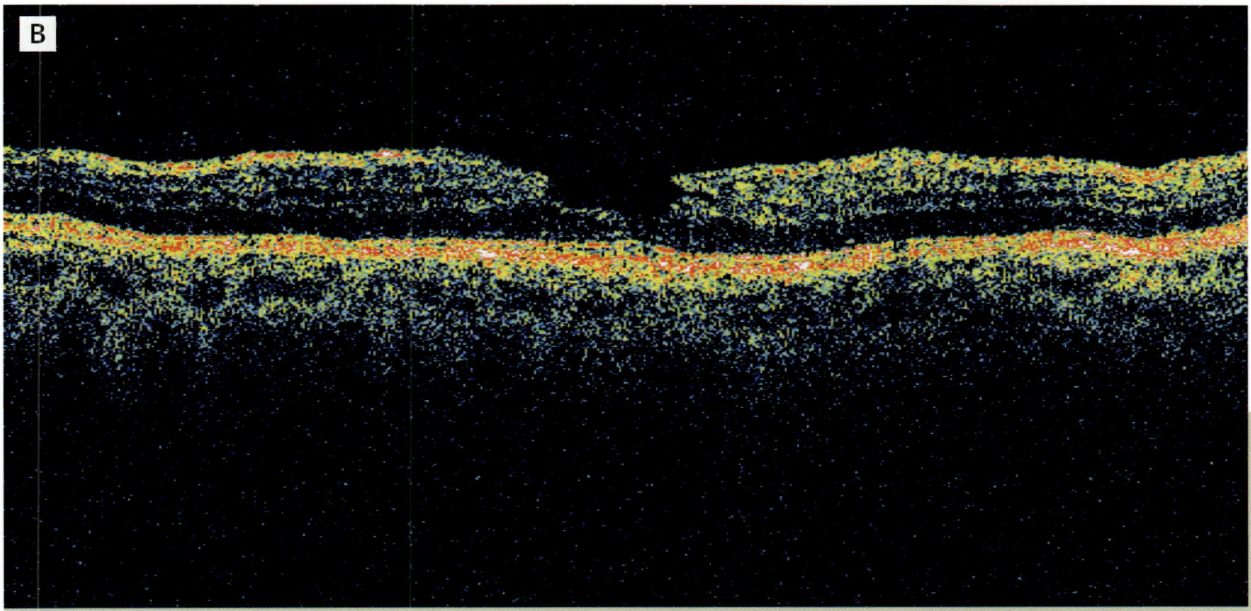

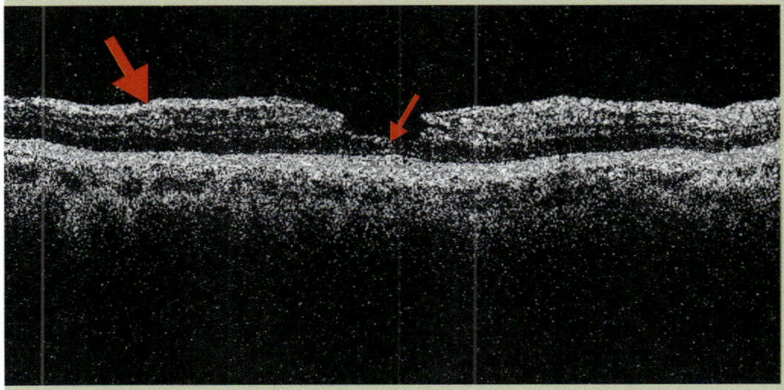

A. Patient with an epiretinal membrane and a lamellar macular hole (incomplete) (the arrow shows the scan direction). B. Optical Coherence Tomography shows the presence of retinal tissue only in the outer layers (small arrow). The epiretinal membrane is displayed as an increased reflectivity of the inner retinal layers (big arrow).

VITREOMACULAR TRACTION SYNDROME

Vitreomacular traction syndrome. A linear area of high reflectivity is detected inside the vitreous cavity, connected to the fovea and corresponding to the posterior cortical vitreous that exerts strong vitreoretinal traction on the macula (small

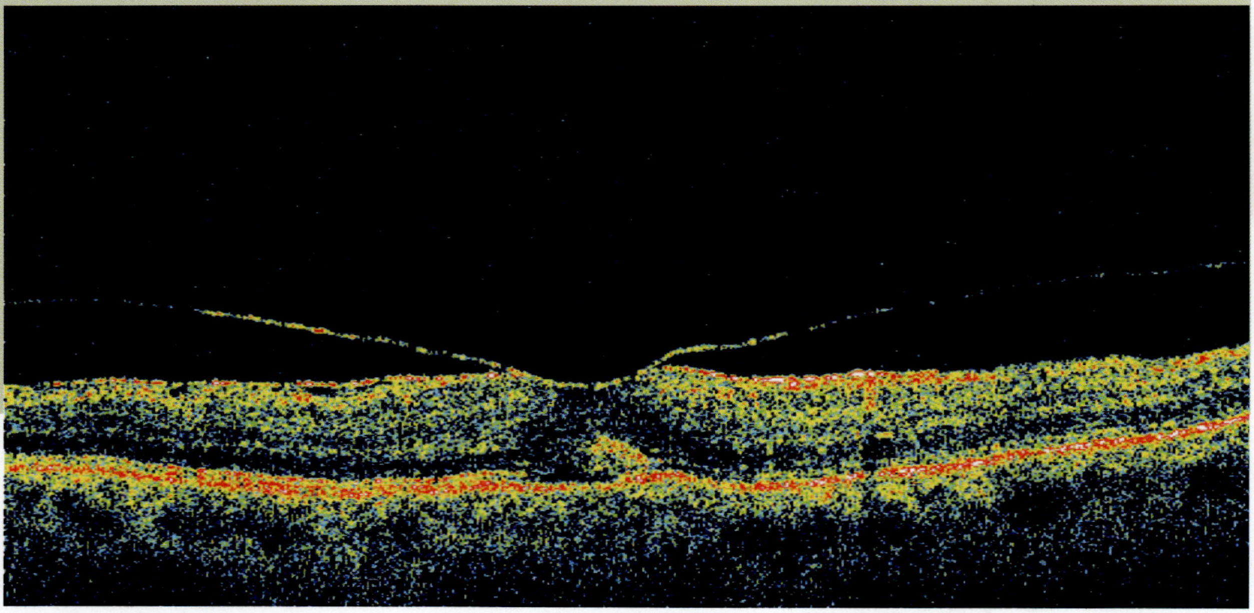

arrows). There is also an increase of retinal thickness with low reflectivity areas in the outer layers and diffuse edema in the fovea (big arrow). A high reflectivity area is detected on the retinal surface and corresponds to an epiretinal membrane around the fovea (arrow head). Note the absence of the normal photoreceptors' architecture in the foveola appearing like an elimination of the normal line that separates the inner from the outer parts of photoreceptors (empty arrow).

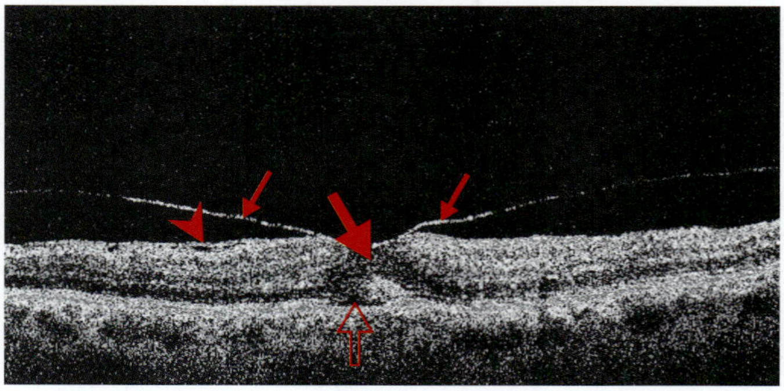

VITREOMACULAR TRACTION SYNDROME

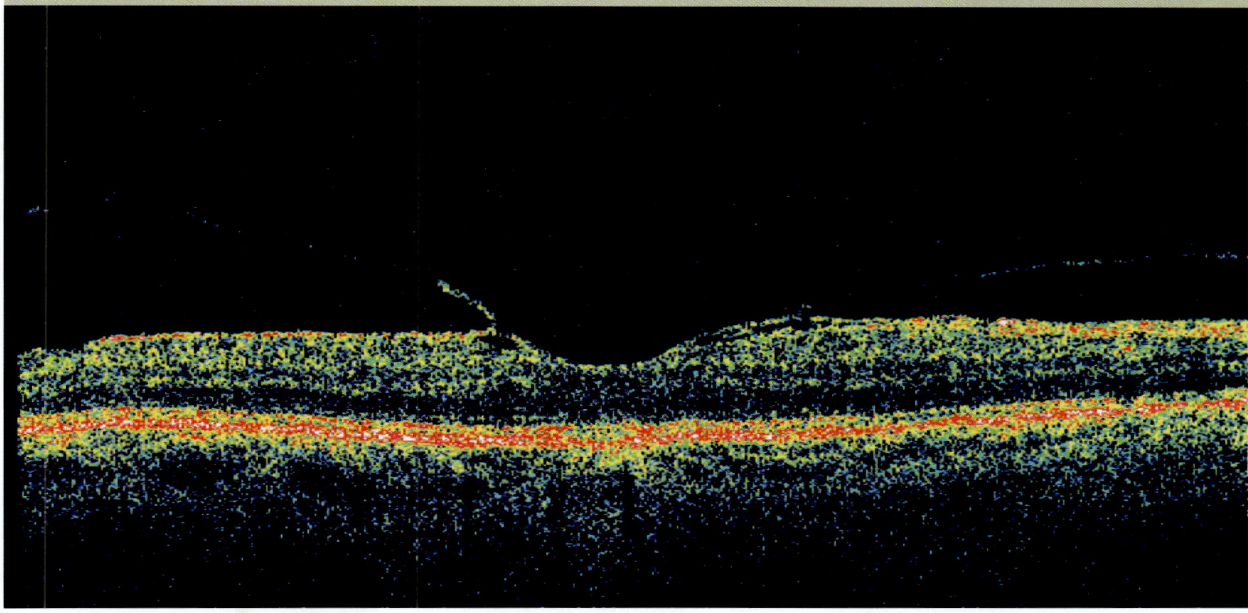

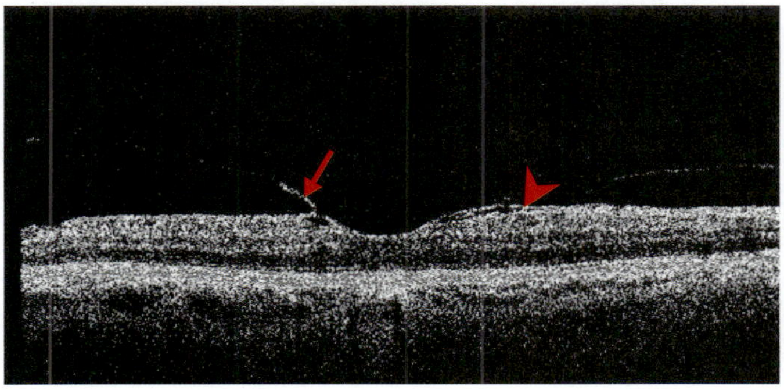

Vitreomacular traction syndrome. A linear area of high reflectivity is detected inside the vitreous cavity, connected to the fovea and corresponding to the posterior cortical vitreous that exerts strong vitreoretinal traction on the macula (small arrow). There is also a high reflectivity area on the retinal surface that corresponds to an epiretinal membrane around the fovea (arrow head). The macular morphology is not altered.

VITREOMACULAR TRACTION SYNDROME

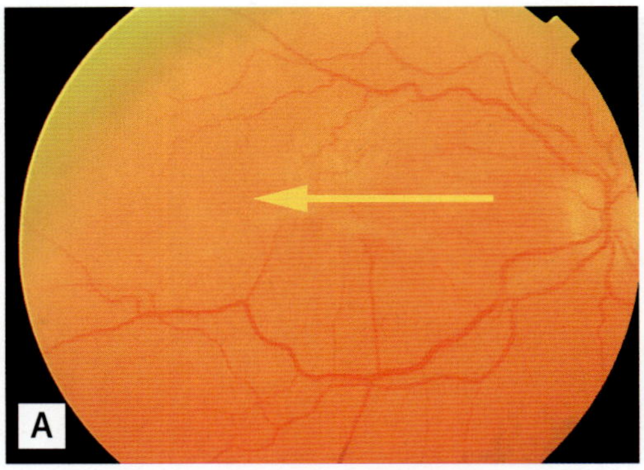

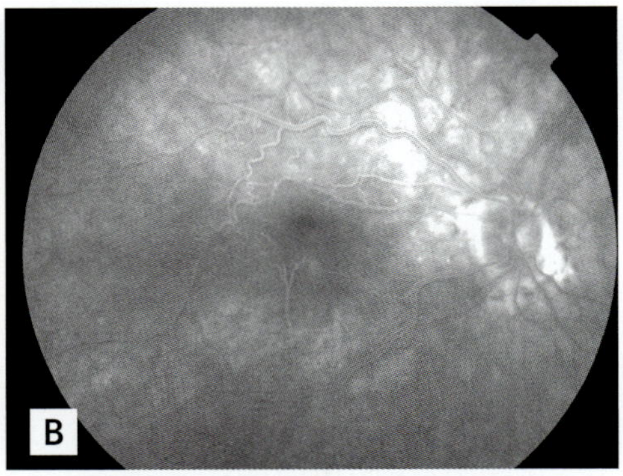

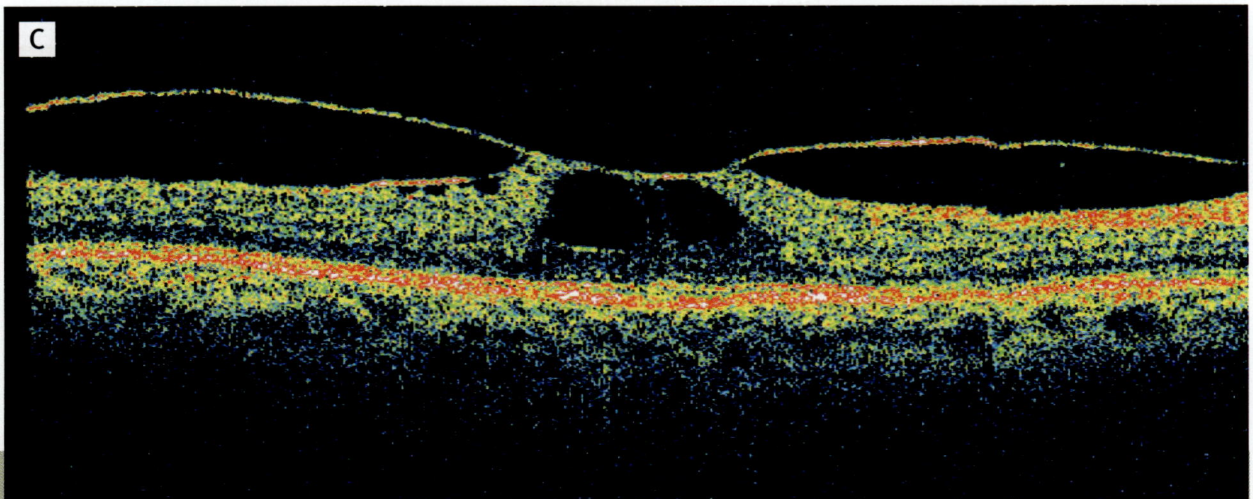

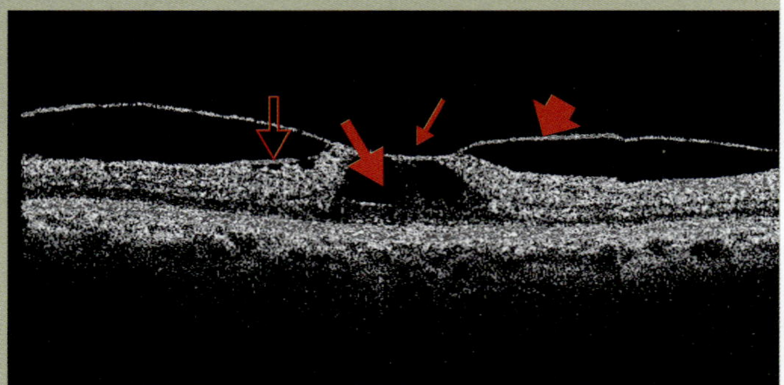

Vitreomacular traction syndrome. A. Patient with an epiretinal membrane and an obvious distortion of the retinal vessels (the arrow shows the scan direction). B. Fluorescein angiography detects mild dye leakage. C. Optical Coherence Tomography shows strong vitreomacular traction in the fovea (small arrow) with the presence of multiple cystic intraretinal formations of low reflectivity corresponding to cystoid macular edema (big arrow). The posterior cortical vitreous is detected like a thick line of high reflectivity strongly attached to the macula (thick arrow). A thin linear high reflectivity area is also detected on the retinal surface and corresponds to an epiretinal membrane that is evident on the left side of the image (empty arrow). In cases of coexistence of epiretinal membrane and thickened posterior hyaloid, Optical Coherence Tomography is the examination of choice for their identification and differentiation.

VITREOMACULAR TRACTION SYNDROME

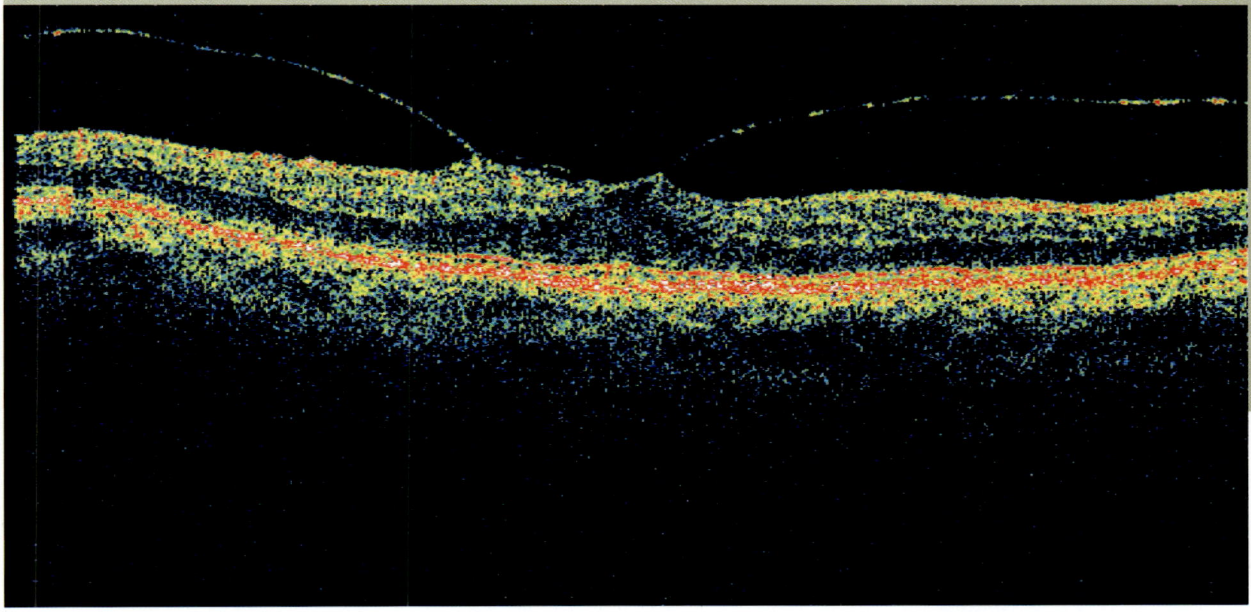

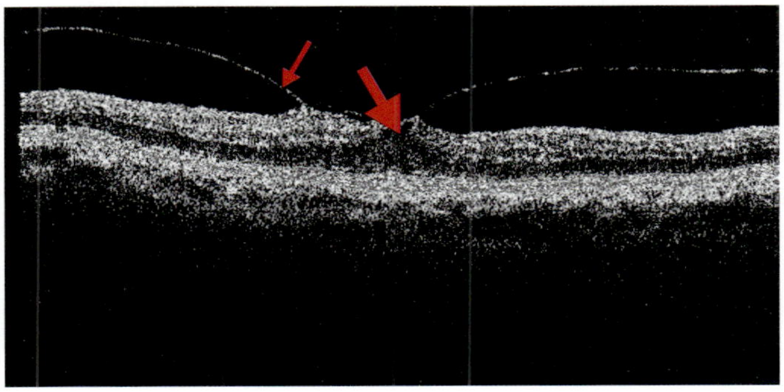

Vitreomacular traction syndrome. A linear area of high reflectivity is detected inside the vitreous cavity, connected to the fovea and corresponding to the posterior cortical vitreous that exerts strong vitreomacular traction (small arrow). There are also small cystic intraretinal formations of low reflectivity corresponding to mild cystic macular edema (big arrow).

CHAPTER 5

CENTRAL SEROUS CHORIORETINOPATHY

IOANNIS EMFIETZOGLOU

Central serous chorioretinopathy is a disease that affects most commonly healthy individuals between 20-55 years old, causing symptoms like metamorphopsia, micropsia and a positive central scotoma. Many studies report a correlation to stressful events, "Type A" personality, use of steroids and pregnancy.

The most prevalent pathophysiologic mechanism for this disease proposes an increased choroidal permeability that induces one or more localized detachments of the retinal pigment epithelium. Under that pressure the retinal pigment epithelium malfunctions diffusely or suffers breaks, through which fluid leaks to the subretinal space and causes a serous neurosensory retinal detachment.

On fundus examination there is a well delineated area of retinal detachment in the macular region. The subretinal fluid is usually clear, but in a few cases it becomes turbid because of the presence of fibrin. The areas of serous retinal pigment epithelium detachment are most commonly small and they are located within the subretinal fluid region but sometimes they can also be located outside the detached retinal area. In some cases there are yellow dot-like specks at the level of the retinal pigment epithelium that are thought to be of proteinaceous origin. Infrequently, the retinal detachment acquires such large dimensions that it may resemble a bullous detachment of the retina. Finally, at the end of the acute phase, atrophic changes may remain at the fovea[2].

Fluorescein angiography shows pooling of the dye in the retinal pigment epithelium detachment and it also depicts the leaking point. Indocyanine green angiography demonstrates the area of retinal pigment epithelium detachment and one or more hyperfluorescent areas that can be invisible on biomicroscopy or/and the fluorescein angiography or can also be present in the fellow eye. Optical Coherence Tomography offers the possibility for both qualitative and quantitative evaluation of patients with central serous chorioretinopathy.

The serous neurosensory retinal detachment is an elevation of the retinal layers above the layer of pigment epithelium and appears like a clear cavity that corresponds to the subretinal fluid. The retinal pigment epithelium, that normally is a very highly reflecting layer, can be either flat and homogeneous or locally elevated above an optically clear cavity, representing a retinal pigment epithelium detachment, or flat but non-homogeneous, demonstrating atrophic changes of the retinal pigment epithelium[1,3-5]. In some cases of long lasting or serious disturbance of the outer blood-retinal barrier, there is an increase of the thickness of the retinal layers even with the creation of cystic areas[3].

Moreover, in some cases Optical Coherence Tomography can detect an irregularity of the outer segment of the photoreceptors. This situation is correlated with a significant reduction in visual acuity and it constitutes a bad prognostic factor for the final visual acuity after the resolution of the serous macular detachment since visual acuity is improved in cases where the outer segment of the photoreceptors has been intact[6].

Recent studies confirm the increased ability of Optical Coherence Tomography to detect shallow foveal detachments in symptomatic patients, whereas clinical and angiographic signs may be missing[7]. Optical Coherence Tomography offers also the possibility of quantitative study of the retinal detachment and consequently of a careful evaluation of the course of the disease. If it is decided to follow-up the patient without treatment, the evaluation of the detachment height during this time can lead the clinician to proceed to a medical intervention (if the fluid remains stable or increases) or to continue observing the patient without medical intervention (if there is a decrease of the fluid). The quantitative study of the fluid is also important during the follow-up of the disease after a therapeutic intervention (i.e. thermal laser, photodynamic therapy).

In some cases where the age of the patient (more than 55 years old) and the results of the fluorescein angiography cannot help the ophthalmologist to draw any conclusion regarding the differential diagnosis between central serous chorioretinopathy and choroidal neovascularization, the findings of typical abnormalities at the level of the retinal pigment epithelium and choriocapillaris leads towards the age-related macular degeneration, while only the presence of serous retinal detachment makes central serous chorioretinopathy the most probable diagnosis.

CENTRAL SEROUS CHORIORETINOPATHY

1. Bek T, Kandi M. Quantitative anomaloscopy and optical coherence tomography scanning in central serous chorioretinopathy. Acta Ophthalmol Scand 2000;78(6):632-7.

2. Gass D. Stereoscopic Atlas of Macular Diseases. Diagnosis and Treatment. St. Louis Missouri: Mosby ;1997;52-70.

3. Hee MR, Puliafito CA, Wong C, Reichel E, Duker JS, Schuman JS, Swanson EA, Fujimoto JG. Optical coherence tomography of central serous chorioretinopathy. Am J Ophthalmol 1995;120(1):65-74.

4. Iida T, Hagimura N, Sato T, Kishi S. Evaluation of central serous chorioretinopathy with optical coherence tomography. Am J Ophthalmol 2000;129(1):16-20.

5. Montero JA, Ruiz- Moreno JM. Optical coherence tomography characterization of idiopathic central serous chorioretinopathy. Br J Ophthalmol 2005;89(5):562-4.

6. Piccolino FC, de la Longrais RR, Ravera G, Eandi CM, Ventre L, Abdollahi A, Manea M. The foveal photoreceptor layer and visual acuity loss in central serous chorioretinopathy. Am J Ophthalmol 2005; 139(1): 87-99.

7. Wang M, Sander B, Lund-Andersen H, Larsen M. Detection of shallow detachments in central serous chorioretinopathy. Acta Ophthalmol Scand 1999;77(4):402-5.

CENTRAL SEROUS CHORIORETINOPATHY

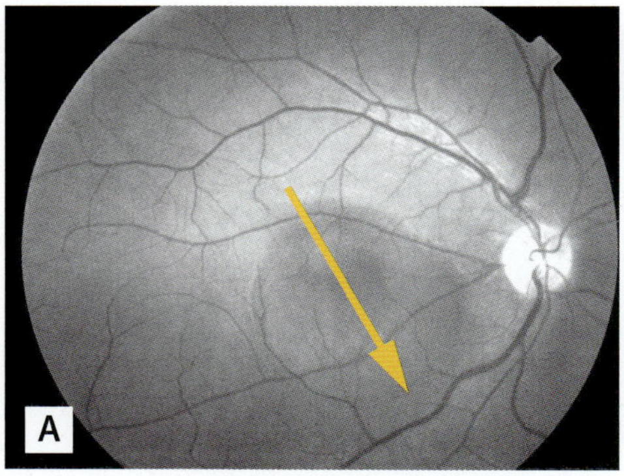

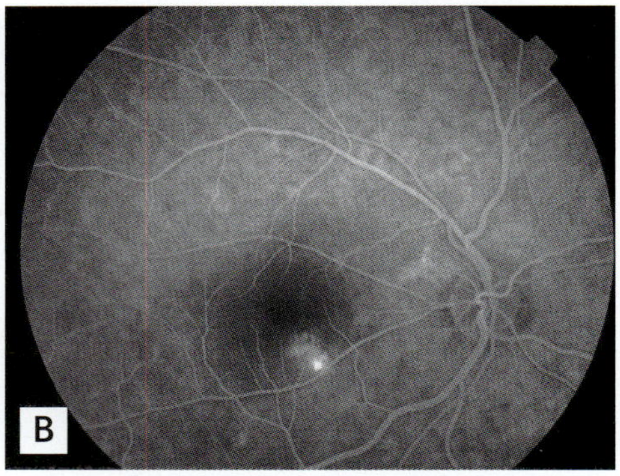

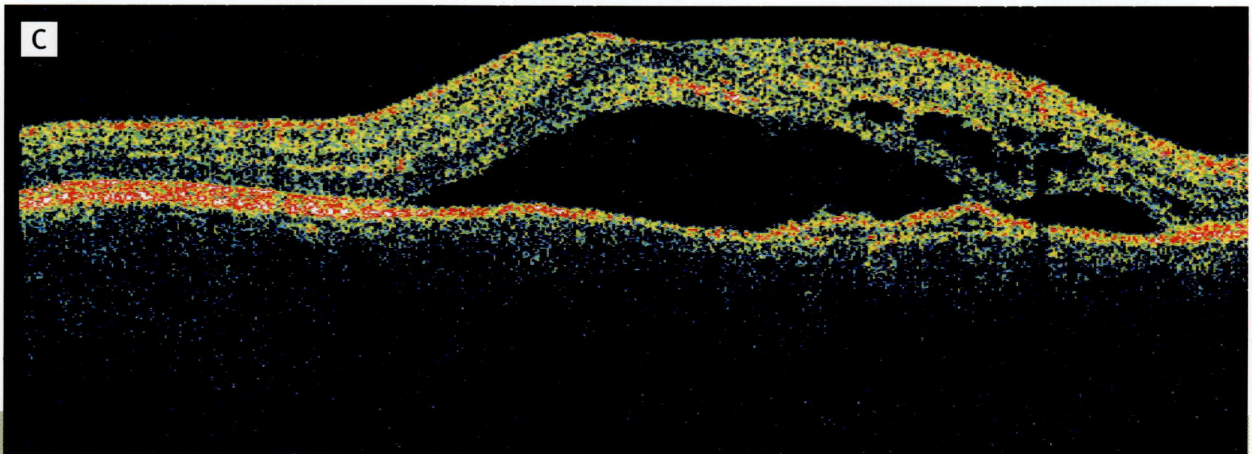

A. A 37 years old patient with the seventh episode of Central Serous Chorioretinopathy. On biomicroscopy serous detachment of the retina is detected (the arrow shows the scan direction). B. Fluorescein angiography reveals the leaking spot inferonasally to the fovea. C. Optical Coherence Tomography shows a wide area of low reflectivity between the neurosensory retina and the retinal pigment epithelium that corresponds to the subretinal fluid (small arrow). Within the retinal layers there are low signal areas that correspond to cystoid edema due to the previous episodes (big arrow). There are also two small areas of retinal pigment epithelium elevation that correspond to local detachments of the retinal pigment epithelium (thick arrows).

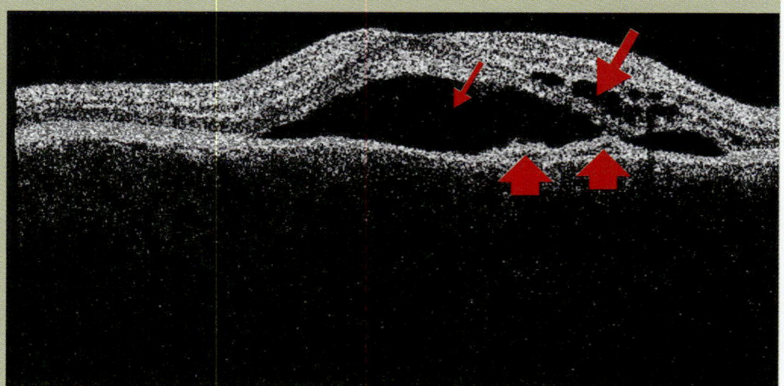

CENTRAL SEROUS CHORIORETINOPATHY

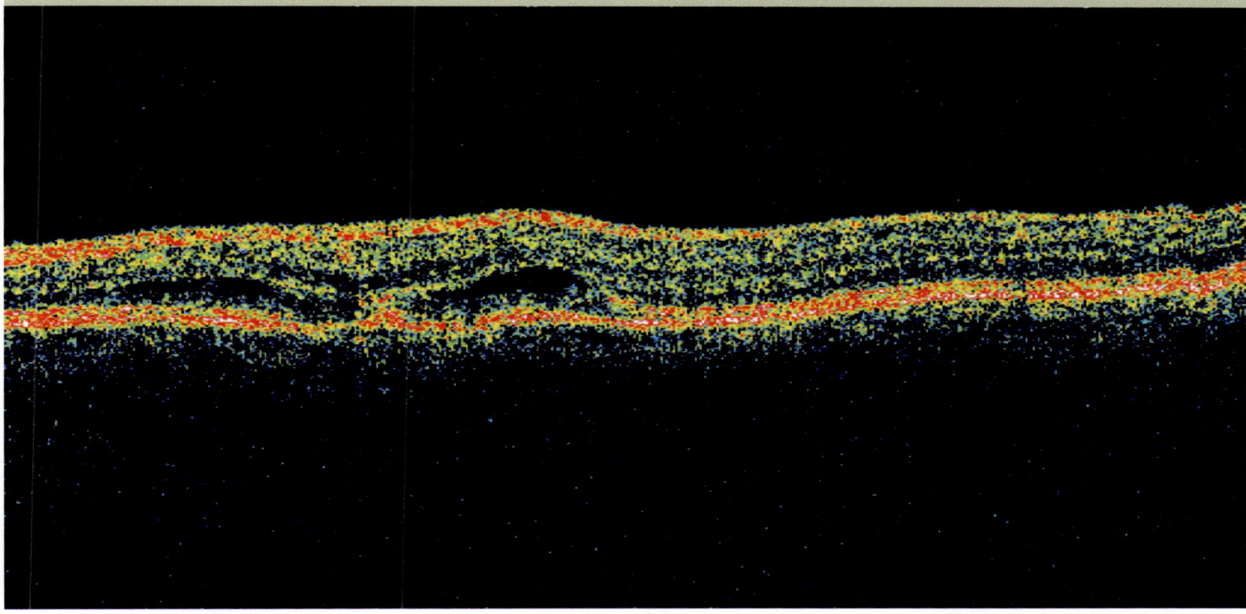

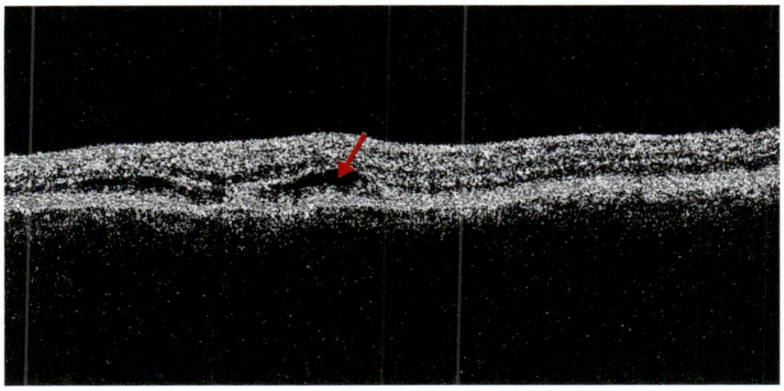

The patient of page 138 three months later. Note the resolution of the detachment and the improvement of the cystoid edema (small arrow).

CENTRAL SEROUS CHORIORETINOPATHY

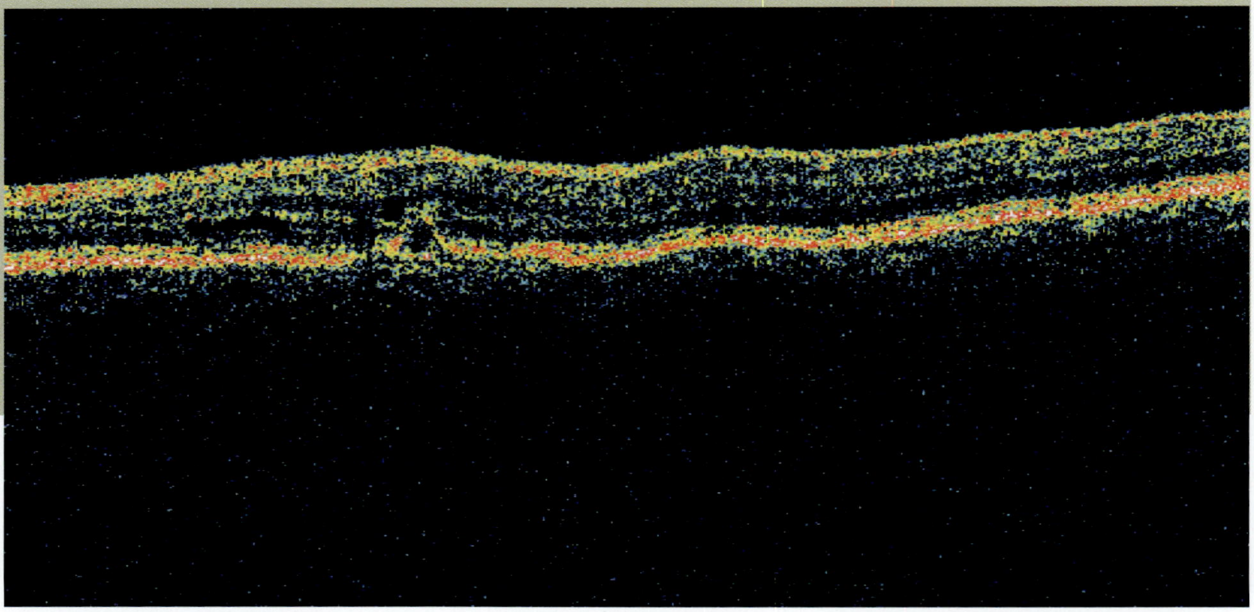

The patient of page 138 twelve months later. Note the persistence of the diffuse macular edema, even though it has been considerably reduced (chronic central serous chorioretinopathy) (arrow).

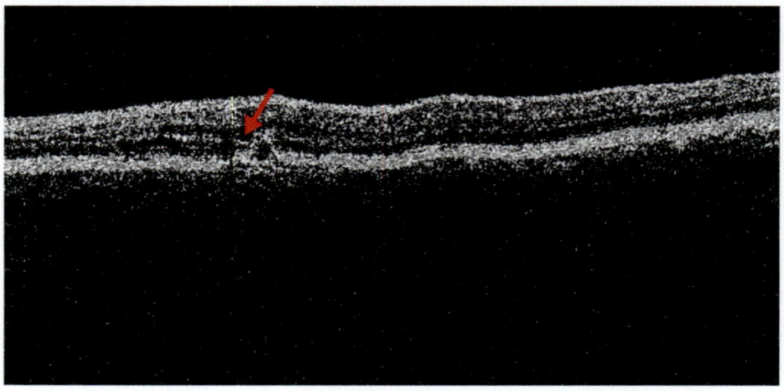

CENTRAL SEROUS CHORIORETINOPATHY

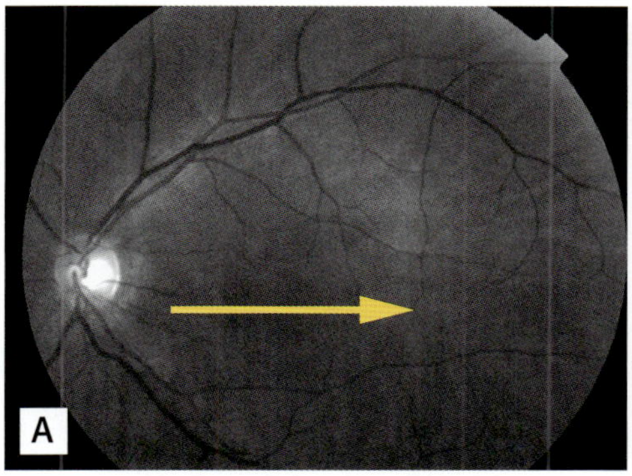

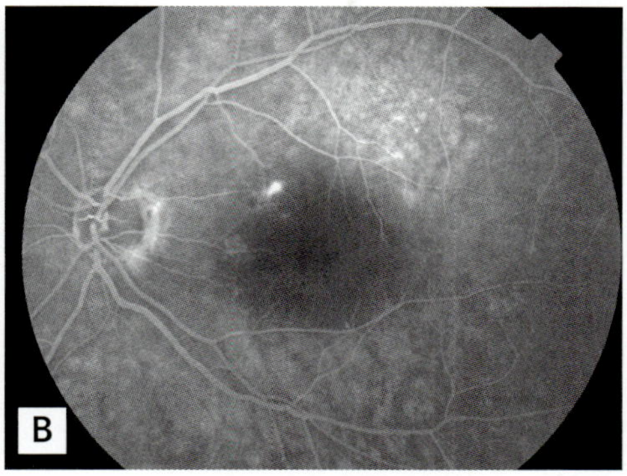

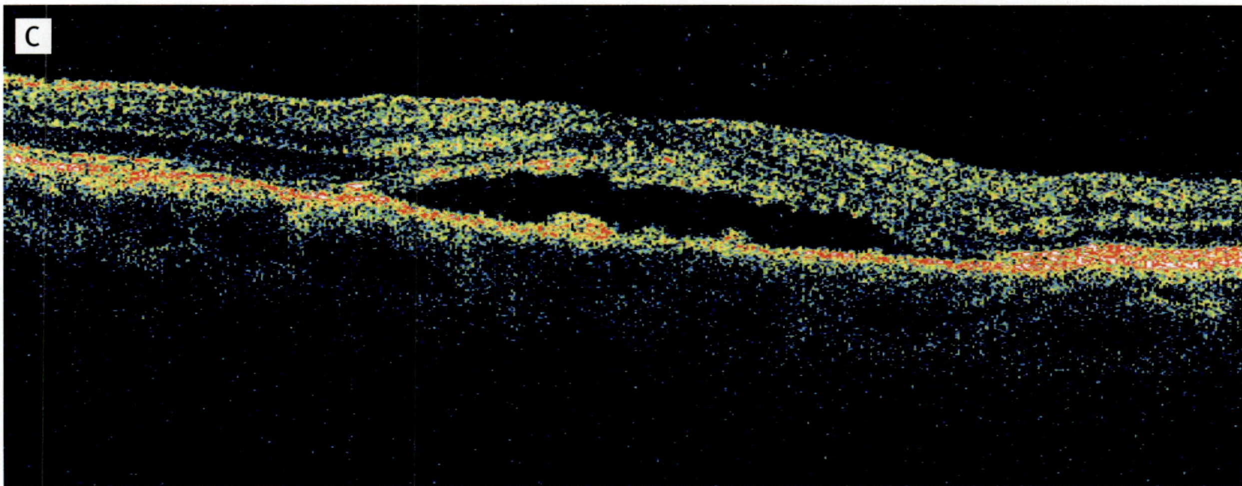

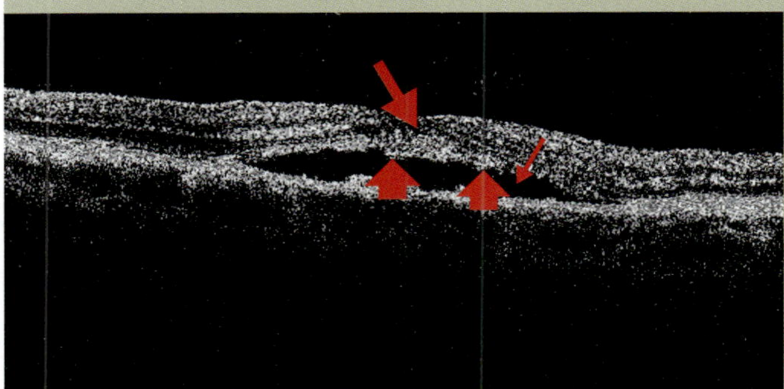

A. A 56 year old patient with Central Serous Chorioretinopathy. On fundus examination a serous detachment of the neurosensory retina is detected (the arrow shows the scan direction) B. Fluorescein angiography shows the leaking spot superiorly and nasally to the fovea. C. Optical Coherence Tomography shows an area of low reflectivity between the retina and the retinal pigment epithelium that corresponds to subretinal fluid (small arrow). There is also increased thickness of the retina due to diffuse edema (big arrow). Another characteristic finding is the irregularity of the outer surface of the retina that probably corresponds to detached parts of the photoreceptors and demonstrates chronicity (thick arrows).

CENTRAL SEROUS CHORIORETINOPATHY

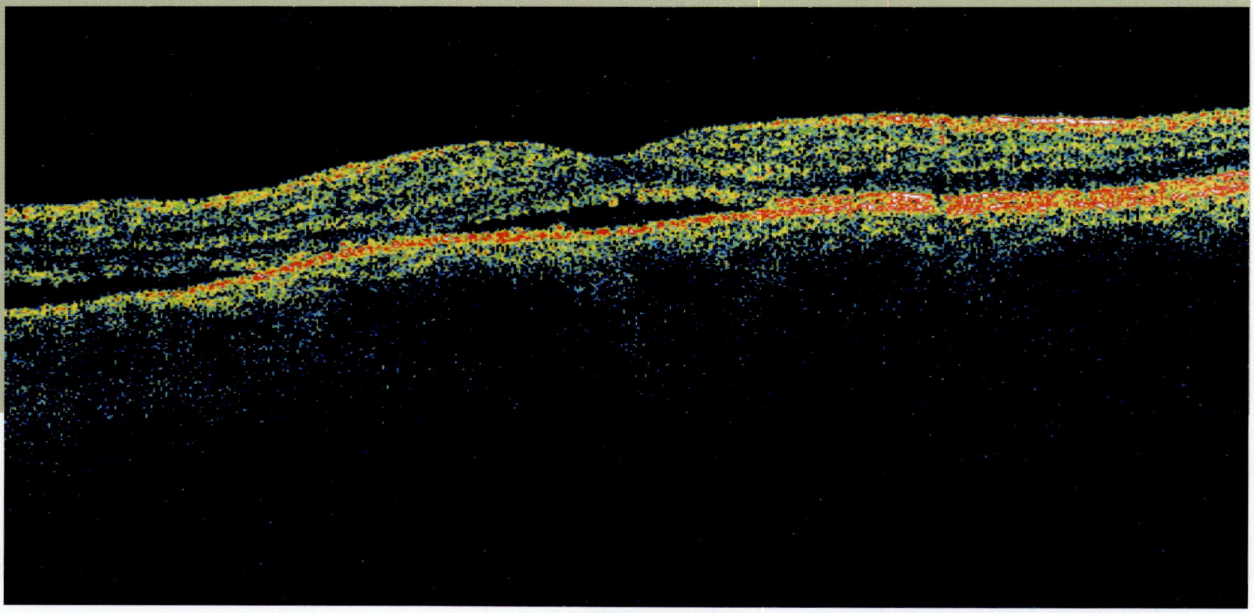

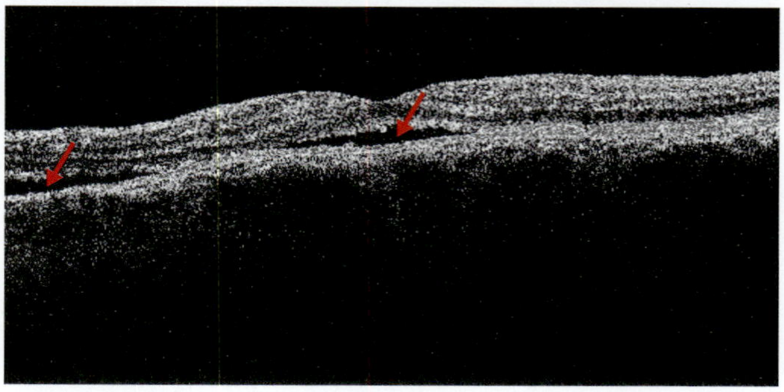

Patient with Central Serous Chorioretinopathy. There are two areas of low reflectivity between the retina and the retinal pigment epithelium, one subfoveal and the other extrafoveal, due to serous retinal detachment (arrows).

CENTRAL SEROUS CHORIORETINOPATHY

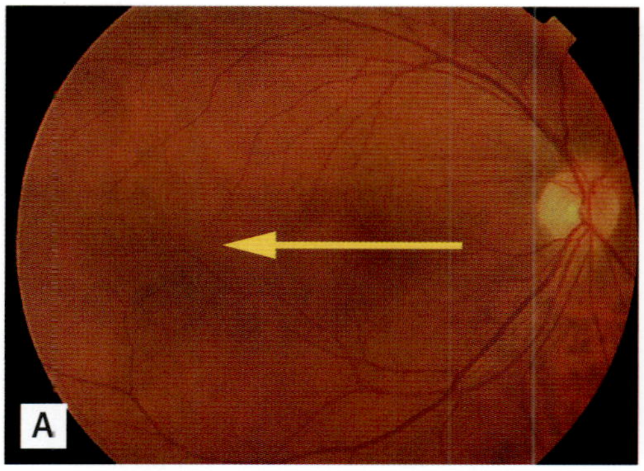

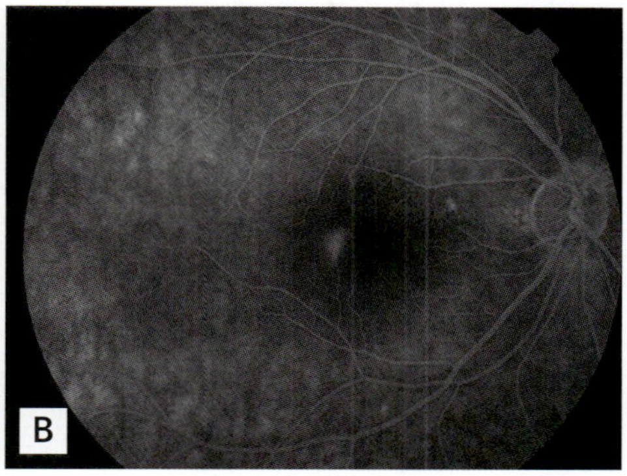

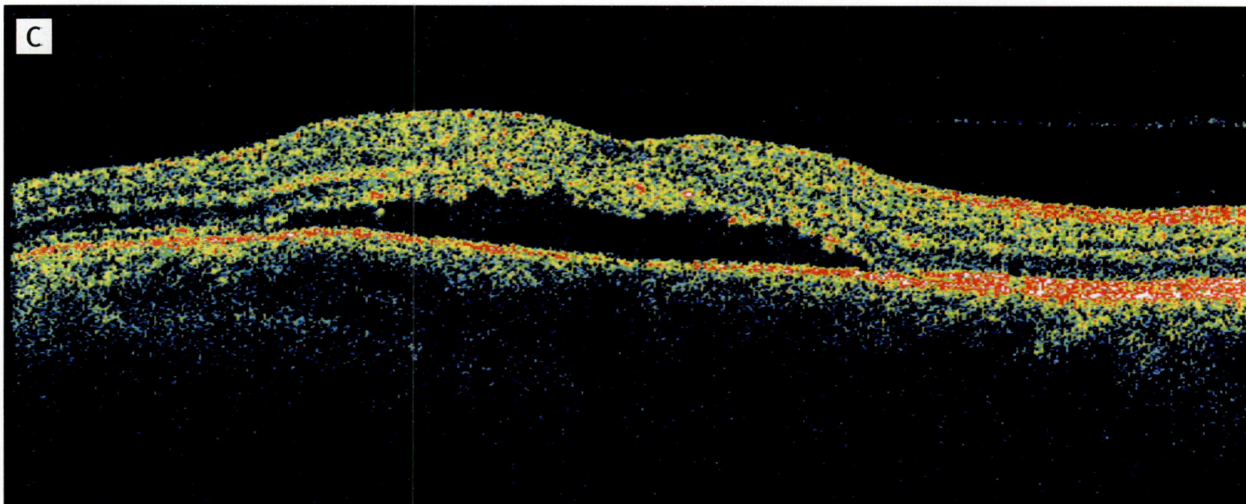

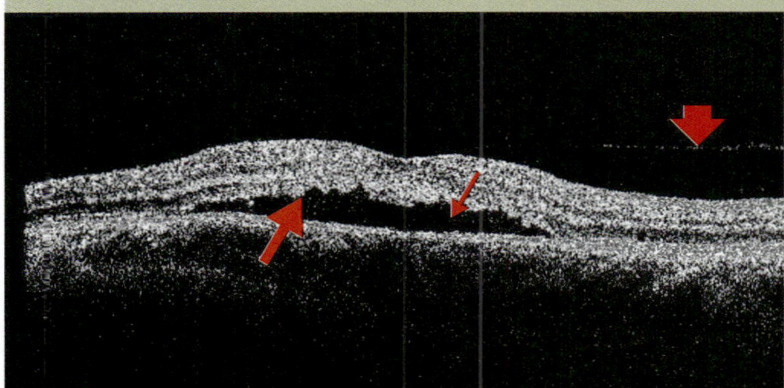

A. Patient with Central Serous Chorioretinopathy (the arrow shows the scan direction) B. Fluorescein angiography shows a smoke stack like hyperfluorescent spot. C. There is an area of low reflectivity between the retina and the retinal pigment epithelium, due to serous retinal detachment (small arrow). Observe the abnormal outer surface of the detached retina that probably corresponds to detached parts of the photoreceptors (big arrow). The vitreous is represented like a thin line of high reflectivity in the vitreous cavity that comes in contact with the retina at the foveola (thick arrow).

CENTRAL SEROUS CHORIORETINOPATHY

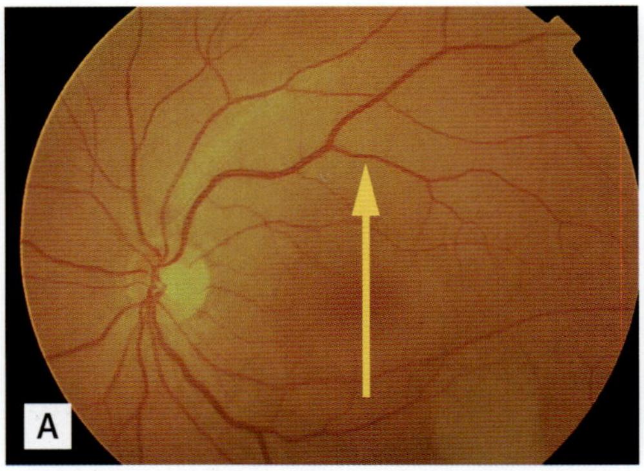

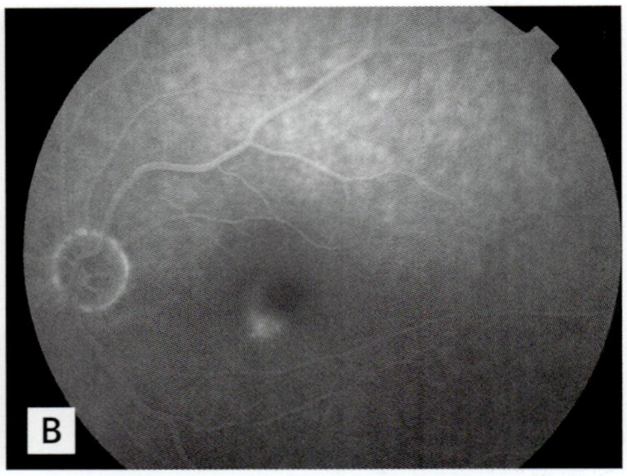

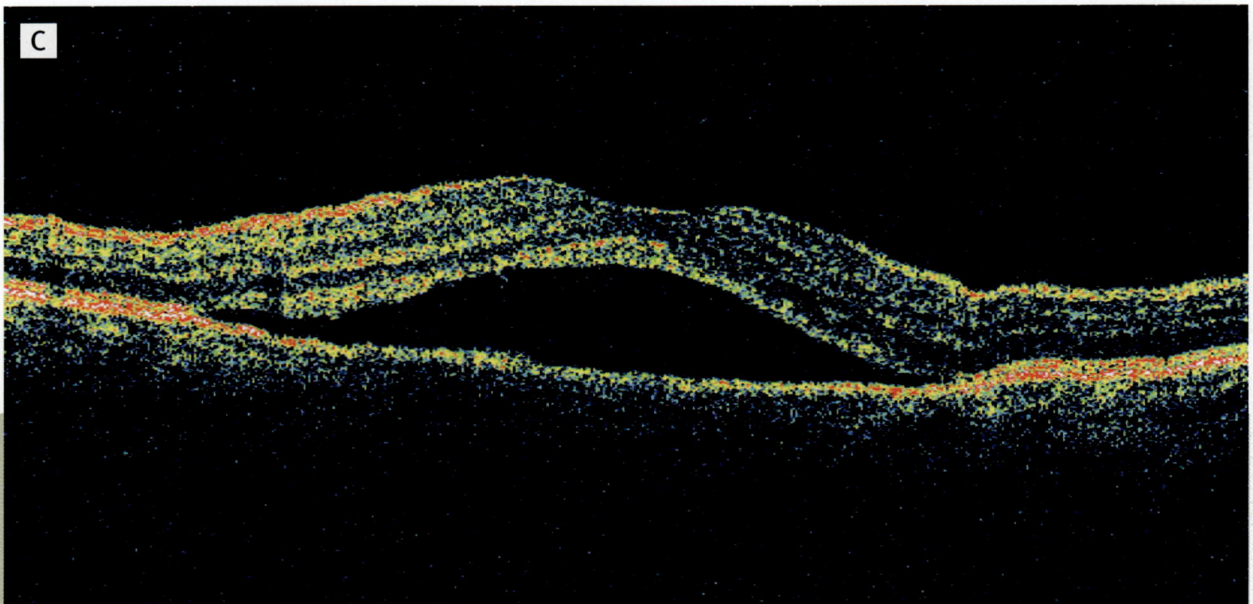

A. Patient with Central Serous Chorioretinopathy (the arrow shows the scan direction). B. Fluorescein angiography shows dye leakage like a smoke stack inferiorly and nasally to the fovea C. Optical Coherence Tomography shows an area of low reflectivity between the retina and the retinal pigment epithelium in the fovea due to a serous retinal detachment (small arrow). The outer surface of the retina is smooth (big arrow).

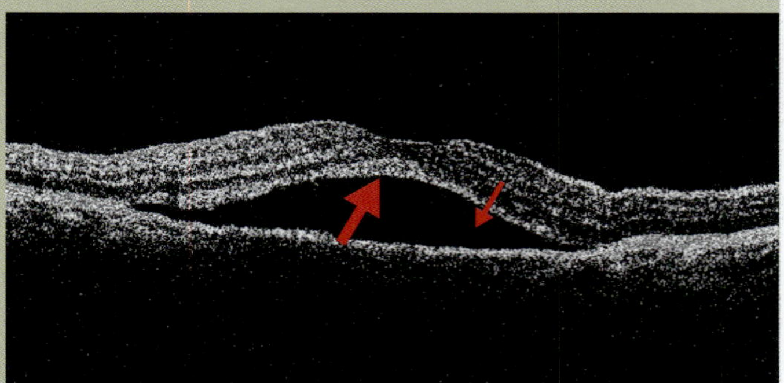

CENTRAL SEROUS CHORIORETINOPATHY

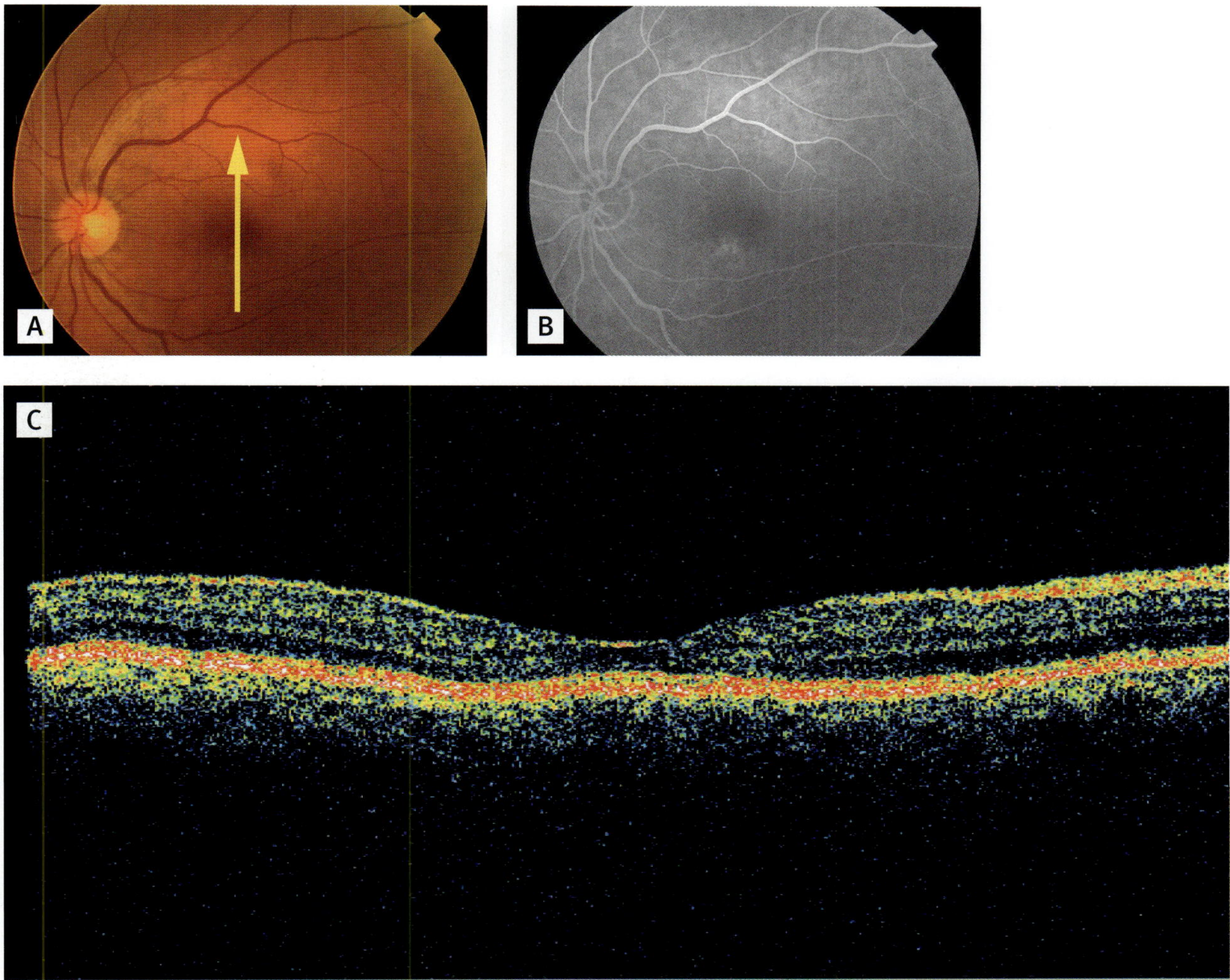

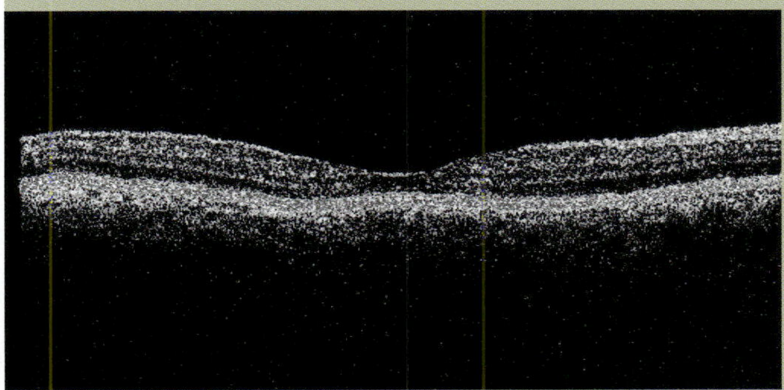

A. The patient of page 144 two years later (the arrow shows the scan direction). B. Fluorescein angiography shows an area of mild hyperfluorescence under the central fovea due to window defect that corresponds to the disrupted retinal pigment epithelium. C. The subretinal fluid has been absorbed and the central fovea has an almost normal configuration.

CENTRAL SEROUS CHORIORETINOPATHY

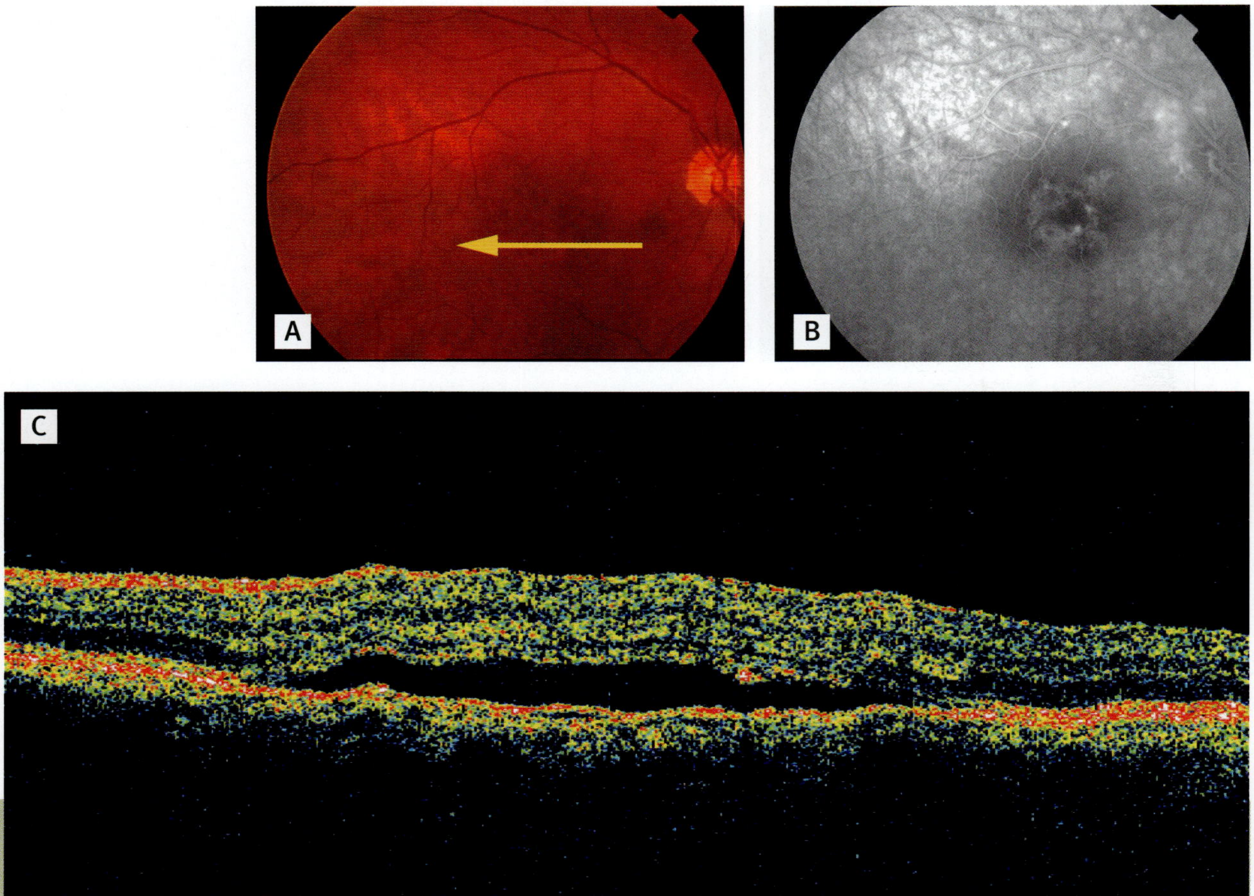

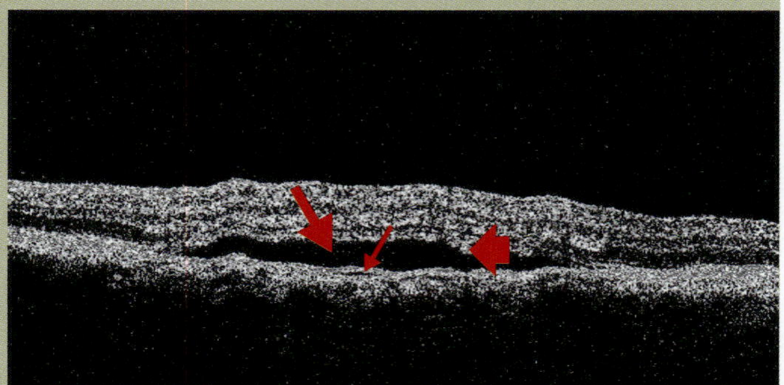

A. Patient with a history of Central Serous Chorioretinopathy (the arrow shows the scan direction). B. Fluorescein angiography shows the leaking spot. C. Optical Coherence Tomography shows a diffuse area of low reflectivity between the retina and the retinal pigment epithelium that corresponds to the serous retinal detachment (big arrow). It also shows an area of low reflectivity under the retinal pigment epithelium due to a small detachment of the retinal pigment epithelium (small arrow). Another characteristic finding is the irregular outer surface of the detached retina (layer of photoreceptors), which usually predisposes to poor functional outcome after the resolution of the detachment (thick arrow).

CENTRAL SEROUS CHORIORETINOPATHY

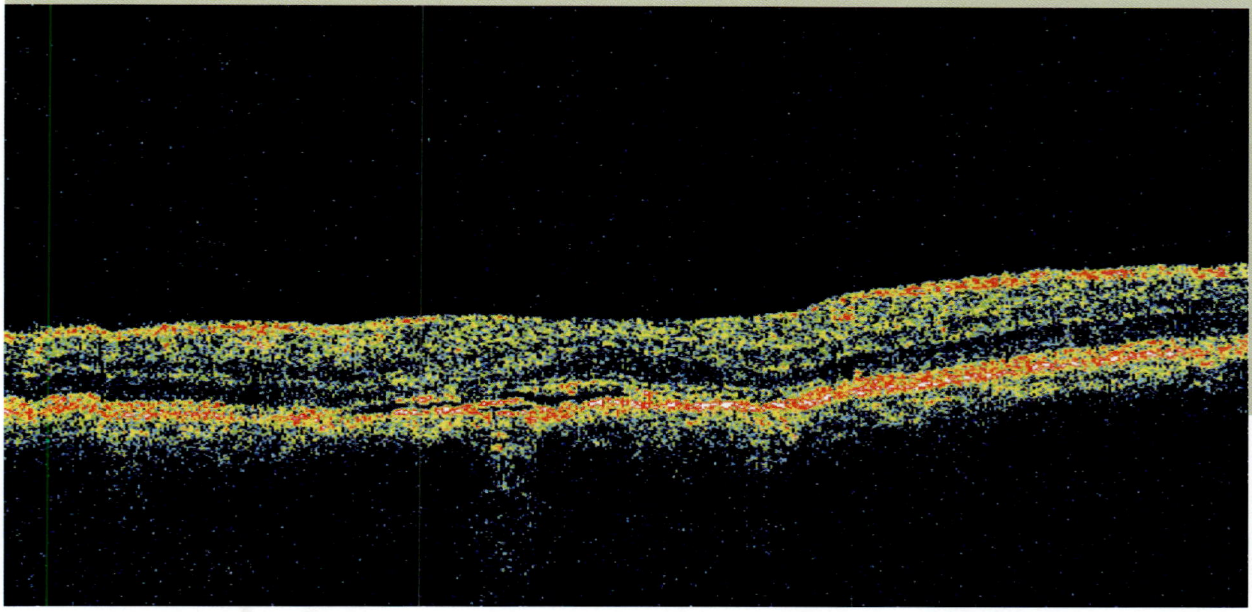

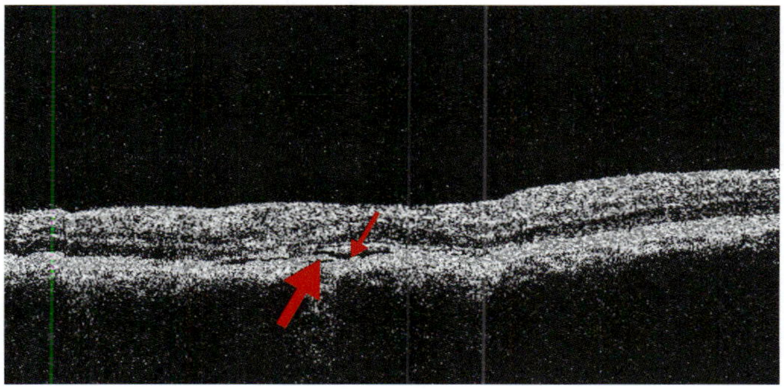

The patient of page 146 two months later. There is a significant reduction of subretinal fluid (small arrow) with persistence of the retinal pigment epithelium detachment (big arrow). The thickness of the retina is increased because of diffuse retinal edema.

CENTRAL SEROUS CHORIORETINOPATHY

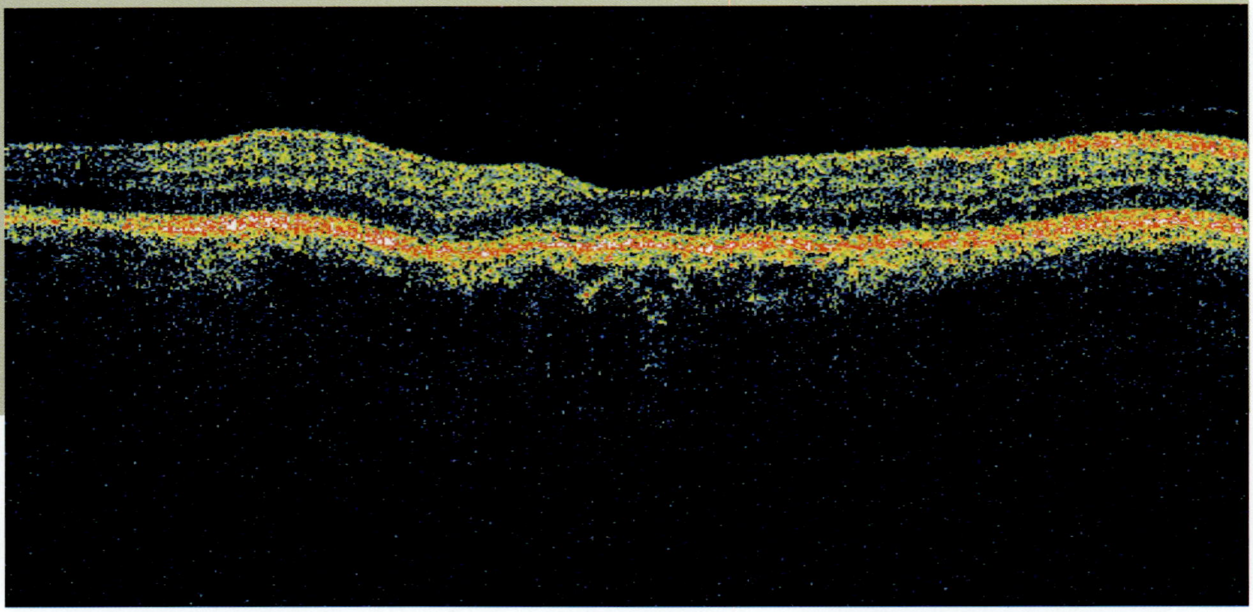

The patient of page 147 six months later. There is complete spontaneous absorption of the subretinal fluid and resolution of the retinal pigment epithelium detachment.

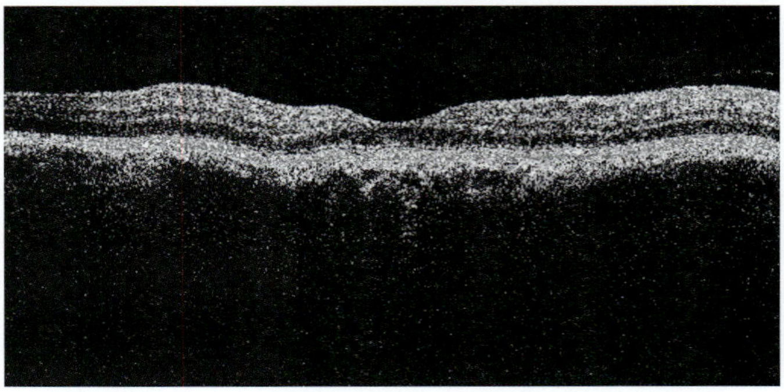

CENTRAL SEROUS CHORIORETINOPATHY

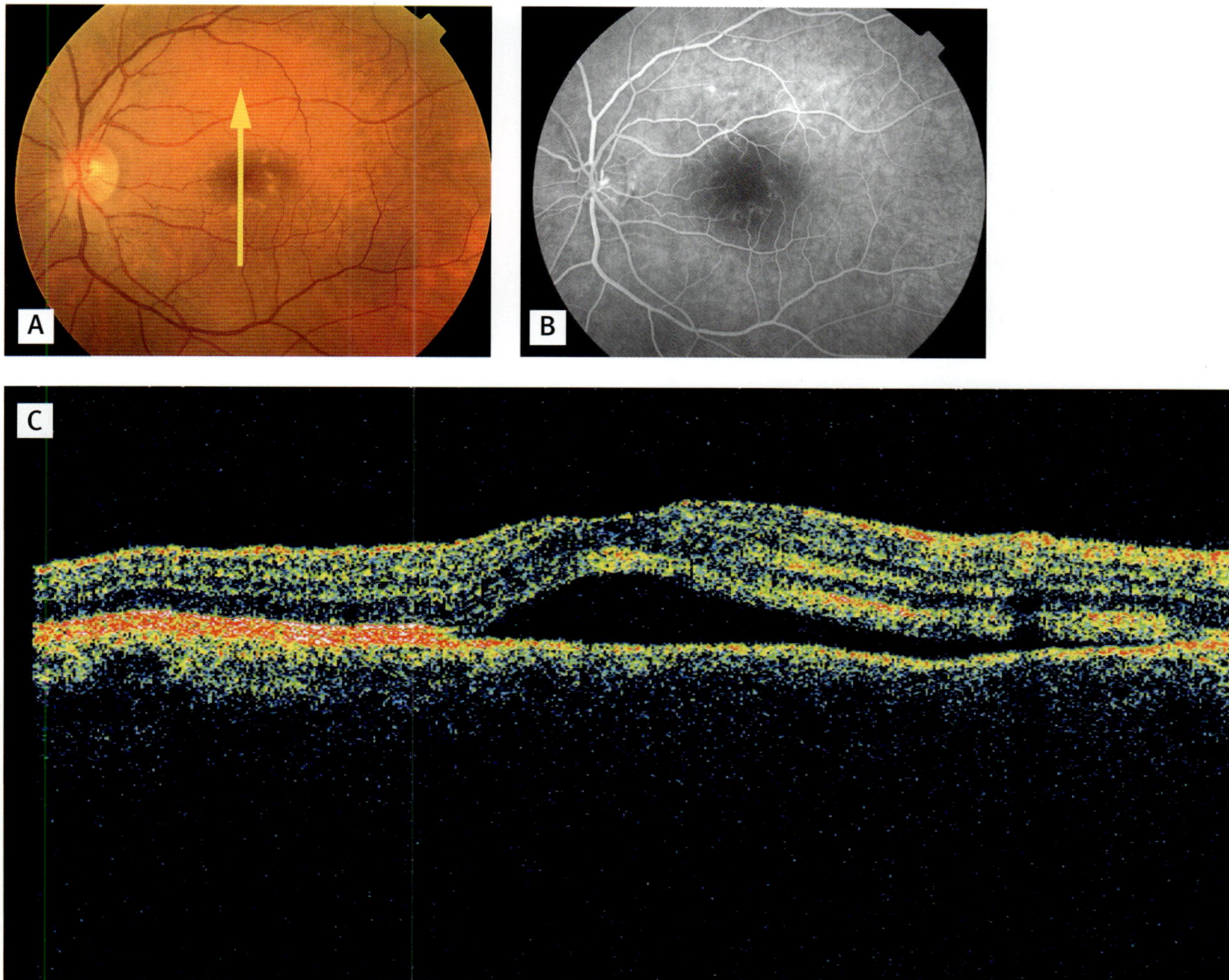

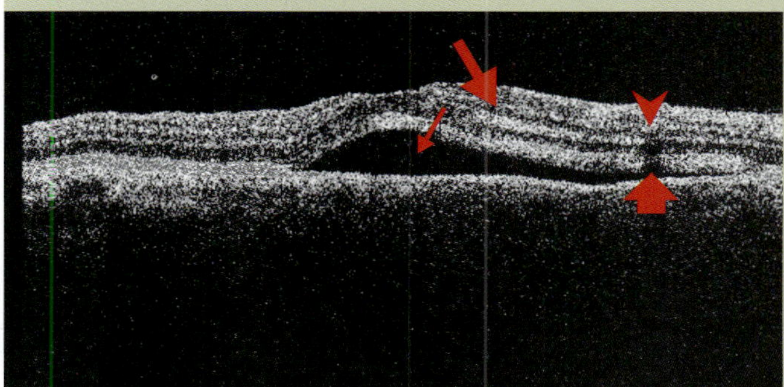

A. Patient with chronic Central Serous Chorioretinopathy (the arrow shows the scan direction). B. Fluorescein angiography doesn't show a leaking spot. C. Optical Coherence Tomography shows an area of low reflectivity between the retina and the retinal pigment epithelium due to leakage of subretinal fluid (small arrow). The thickness of the retina is increased because of the diffuse edema owed to the chronicity of the disease (big arrow). The shadow that is observed at the outer layers of the retina (thick arrow) is due to the increased reflection of a retinal vessel (arrow head).

CENTRAL SEROUS CHORIORETINOPATHY

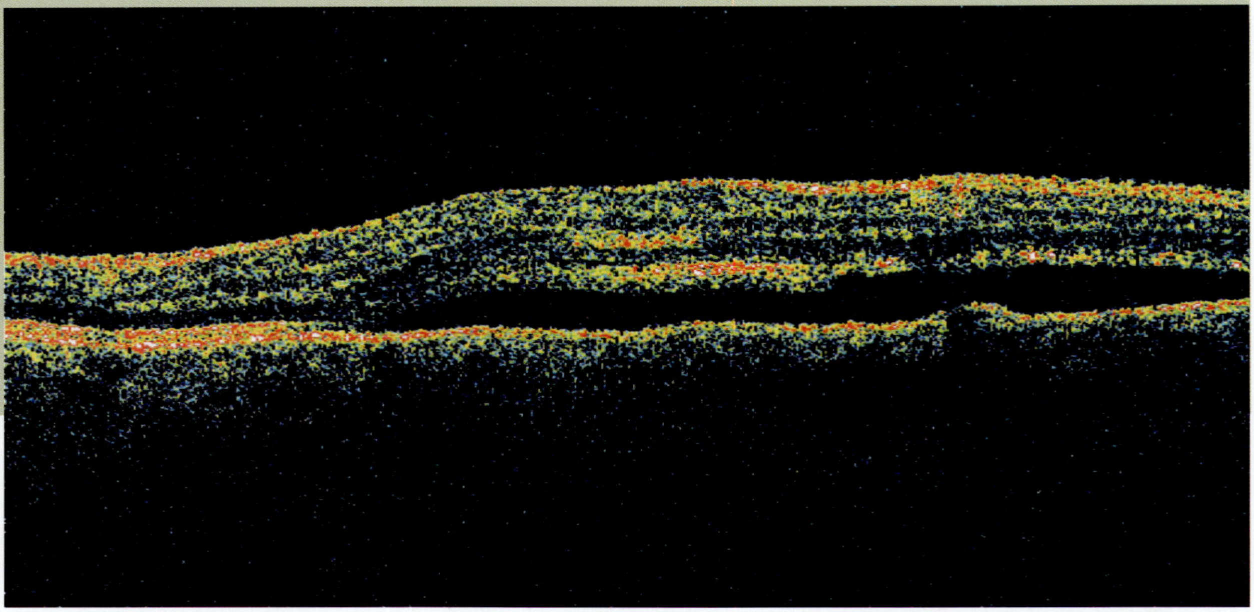

Patient with chronic Central Serous Chorioretinopathy. There is an area of low reflectivity between the retina and the retinal pigment epithelium due to leakage of subretinal fluid (small arrow). The detached outer surface of the retina is regular. The retinal thickness is increased because of the diffuse edema due to the chronicity of the disease (big arrow).

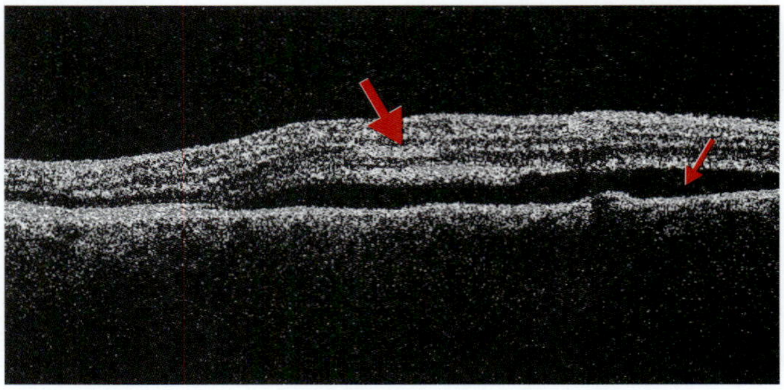

CENTRAL SEROUS CHORIORETINOPATHY

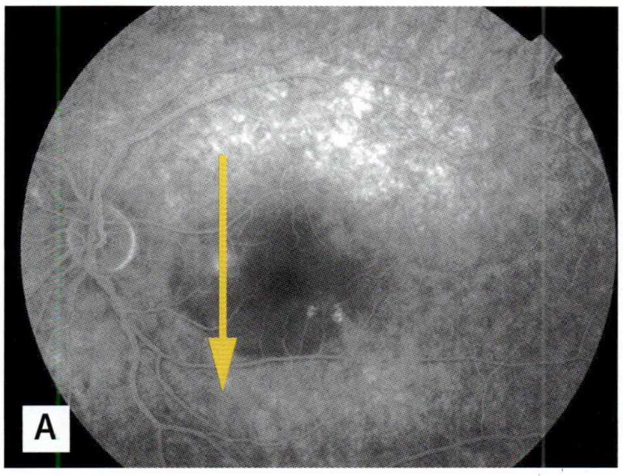

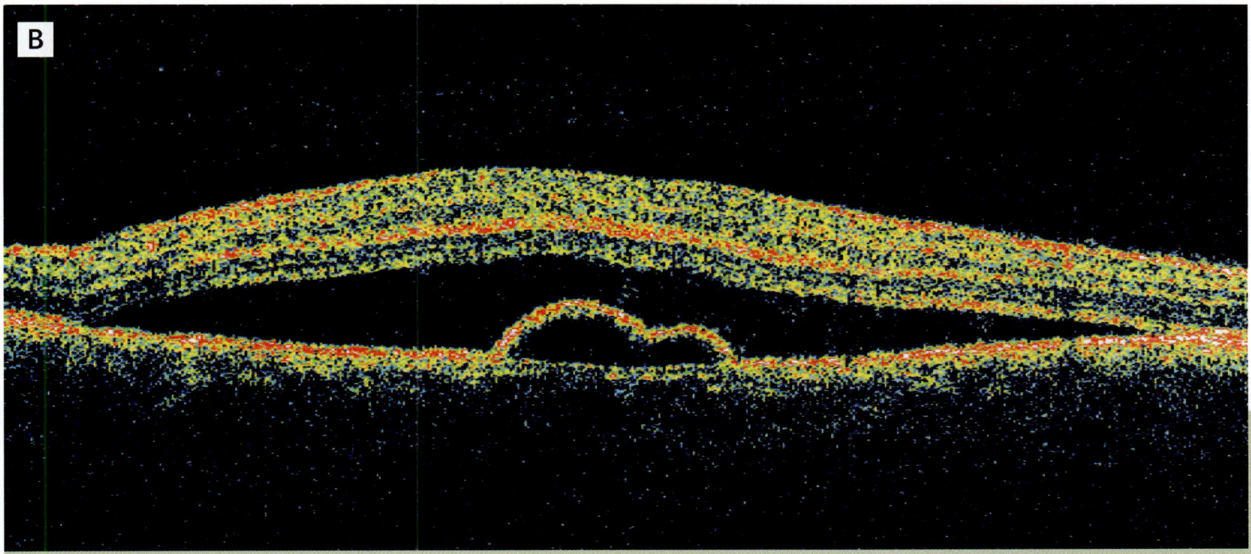

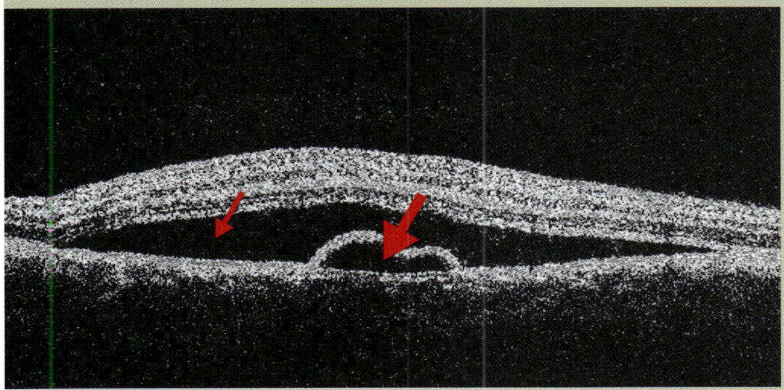

A. A 45 years old woman with Central Serous Chorioretinopathy. Fluorescein angiography shows a leaking spot nasally to the central fovea and also atrophic areas of retinal pigment epithelium inferiorly and temporally to the fovea (the arrow shows the scan direction). B. Optical Coherence Tomography shows a diffuse area of low reflectivity between the retina and the retinal pigment epithelium due to subretinal fluid (small arrow) and also a smaller area of low reflectivity under the retinal pigment epithelium that corresponds to a double-hump detachment of the retinal pigment epithelium (big arrow).

CENTRAL SEROUS CHORIORETINOPATHY

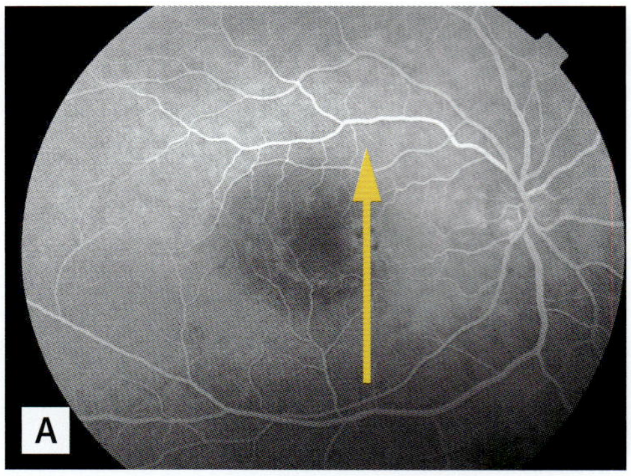

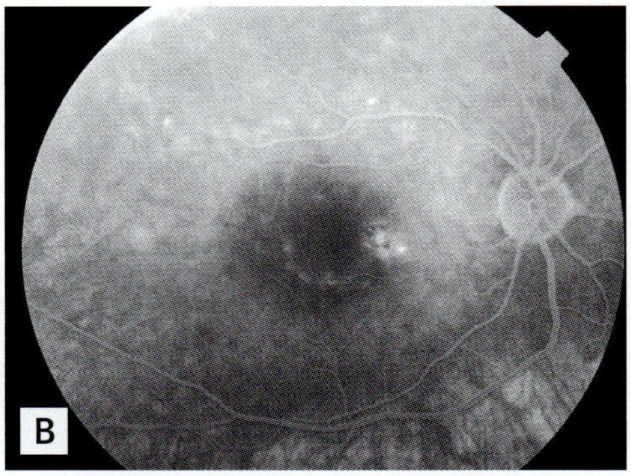

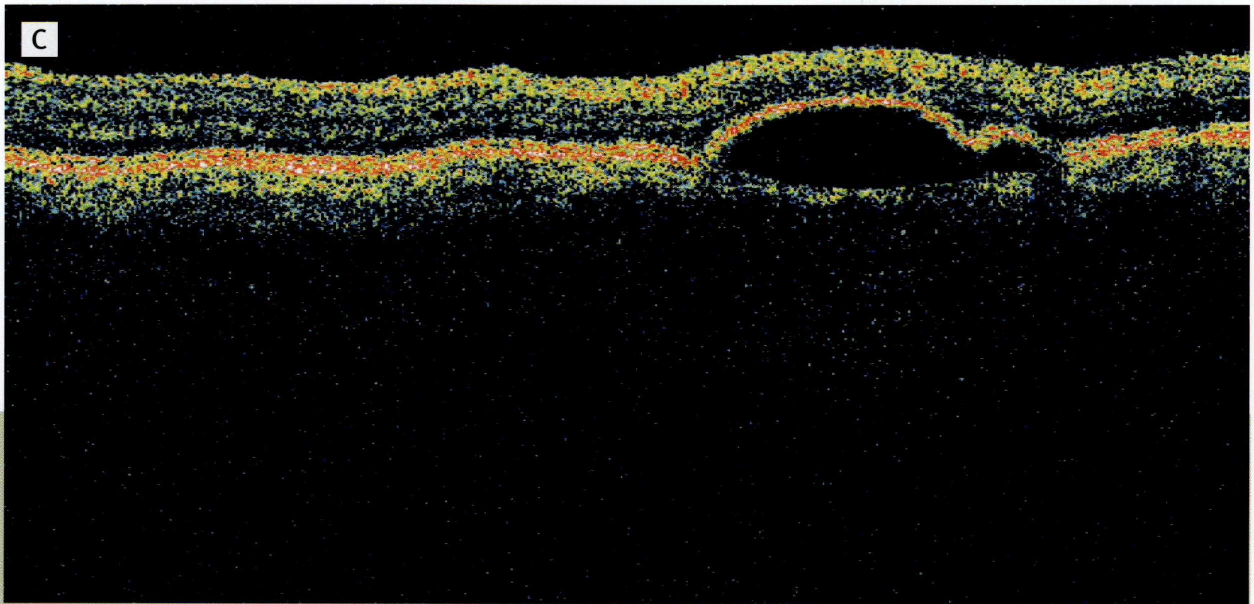

A, B. A 45 year old woman with Central Serous Chorioretinopathy (the arrow shows the scan direction). Fluorescein angiography shows the leaking spot nasally to the fovea with atrophic changes of the retinal pigment epithelium near the leaking spot and in a semicircular arrangement around the fovea where there has been subretinal fluid. C. Optical Coherence Tomography shows an area of low reflectivity under the retinal pigment epithelium due to a double-hump detachment of the retinal pigment epithelium (arrow). The subretinal fluid has been absorbed.

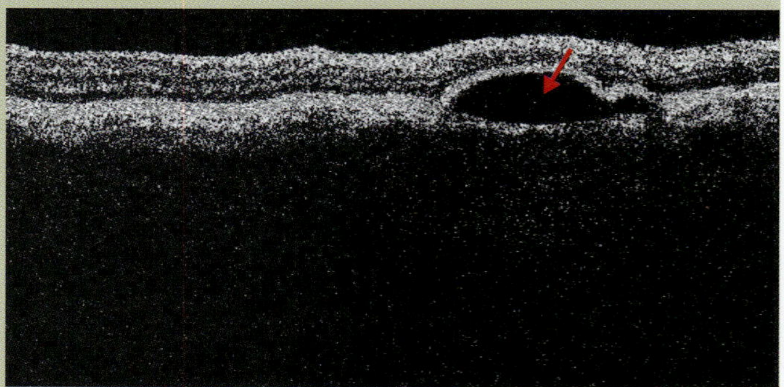

CENTRAL SEROUS CHORIORETINOPATHY

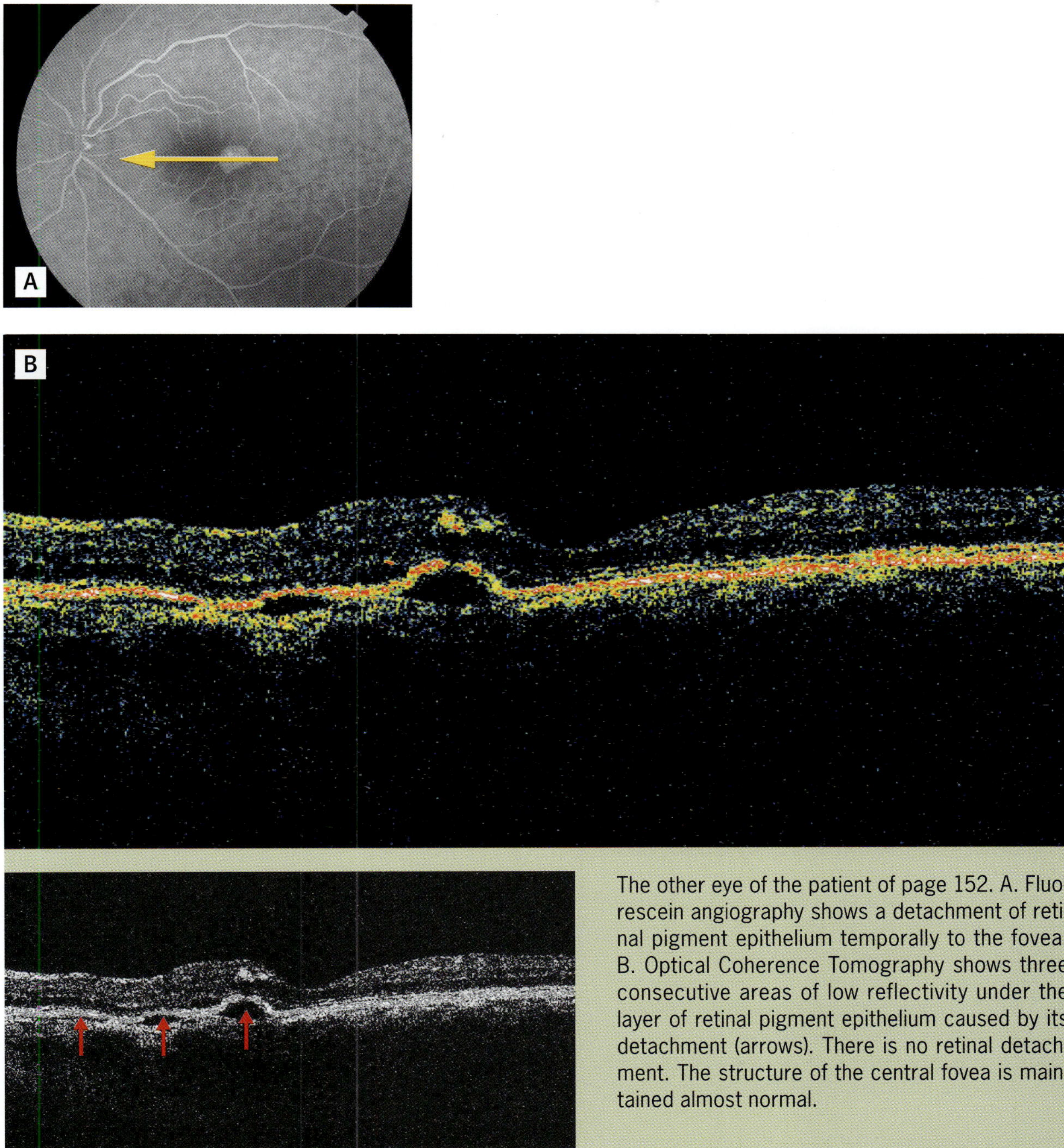

The other eye of the patient of page 152. A. Fluorescein angiography shows a detachment of retinal pigment epithelium temporally to the fovea. B. Optical Coherence Tomography shows three consecutive areas of low reflectivity under the layer of retinal pigment epithelium caused by its detachment (arrows). There is no retinal detachment. The structure of the central fovea is maintained almost normal.

CENTRAL SEROUS CHORIORETINOPATHY

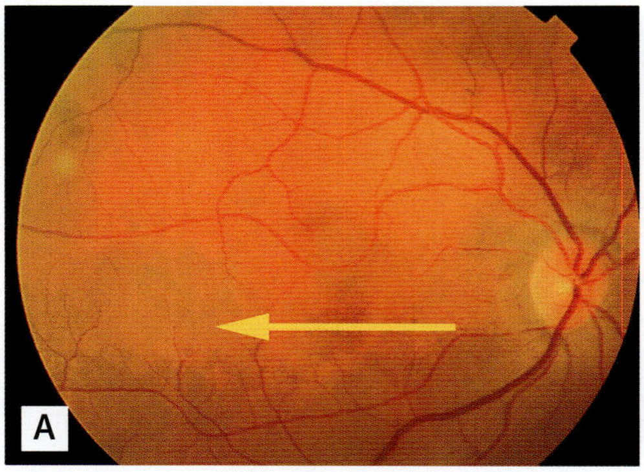

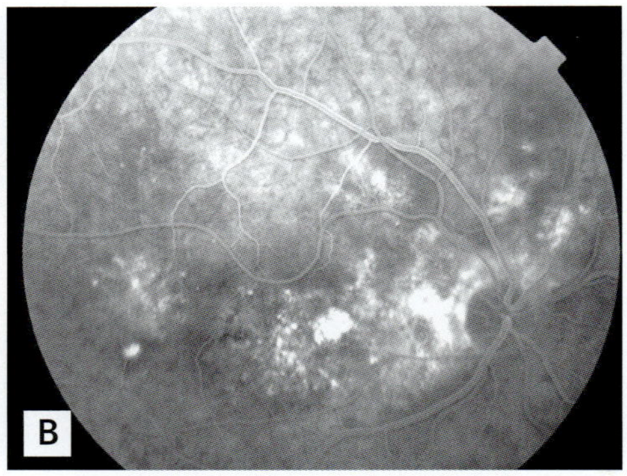

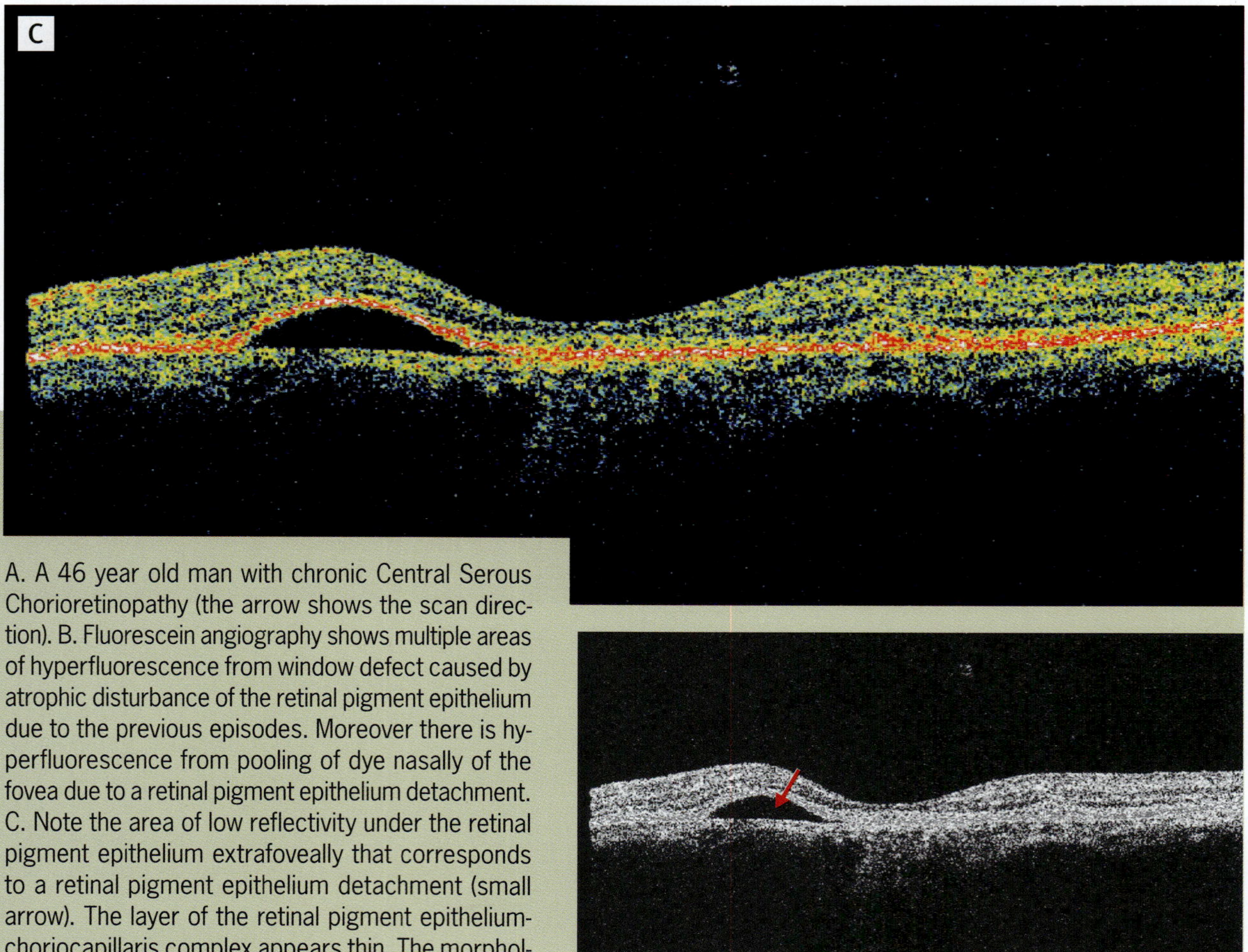

A. A 46 year old man with chronic Central Serous Chorioretinopathy (the arrow shows the scan direction). B. Fluorescein angiography shows multiple areas of hyperfluorescence from window defect caused by atrophic disturbance of the retinal pigment epithelium due to the previous episodes. Moreover there is hyperfluorescence from pooling of dye nasally of the fovea due to a retinal pigment epithelium detachment. C. Note the area of low reflectivity under the retinal pigment epithelium extrafoveally that corresponds to a retinal pigment epithelium detachment (small arrow). The layer of the retinal pigment epithelium-choriocapillaris complex appears thin. The morphology of the retina is normal.

CENTRAL SEROUS CHORIORETINOPATHY

A. The left eye of the patient of page 154. There is serous detachment of the retina inferotemporally to the macula and also perifoveal exudates (the arrow shows the scan direction). B. Fluorescein angiography shows an ink-blot area of hyperfluorescence that corresponds to the leakage of fluid and also scattered atrophic areas of the retinal pigment epithelium at the posterior pole. C. Indocyanine green angiography shows multiple areas of hyperfluorescence. D. Optical Coherence Tomography shows a diffuse area of low reflectivity at the outer retinal layers parafoveally that corresponds to cystic retinal edema (arrow).

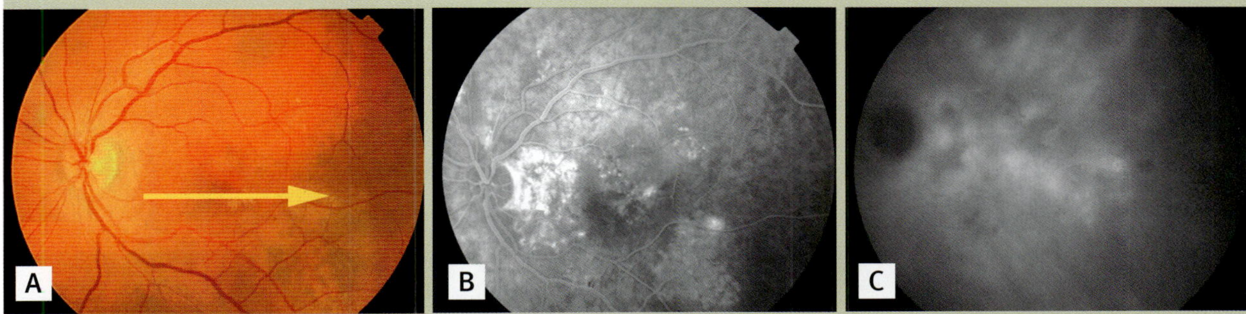

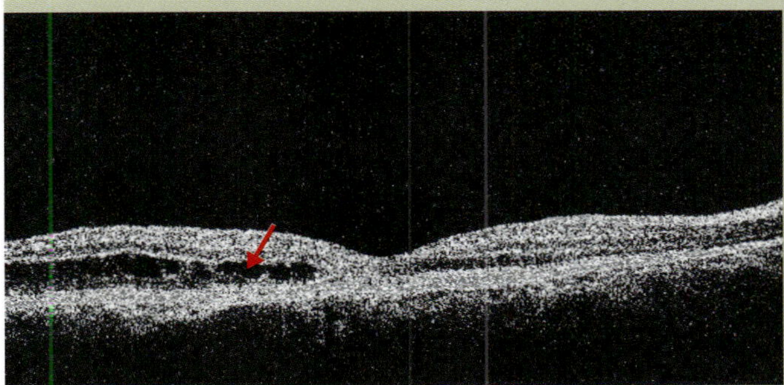

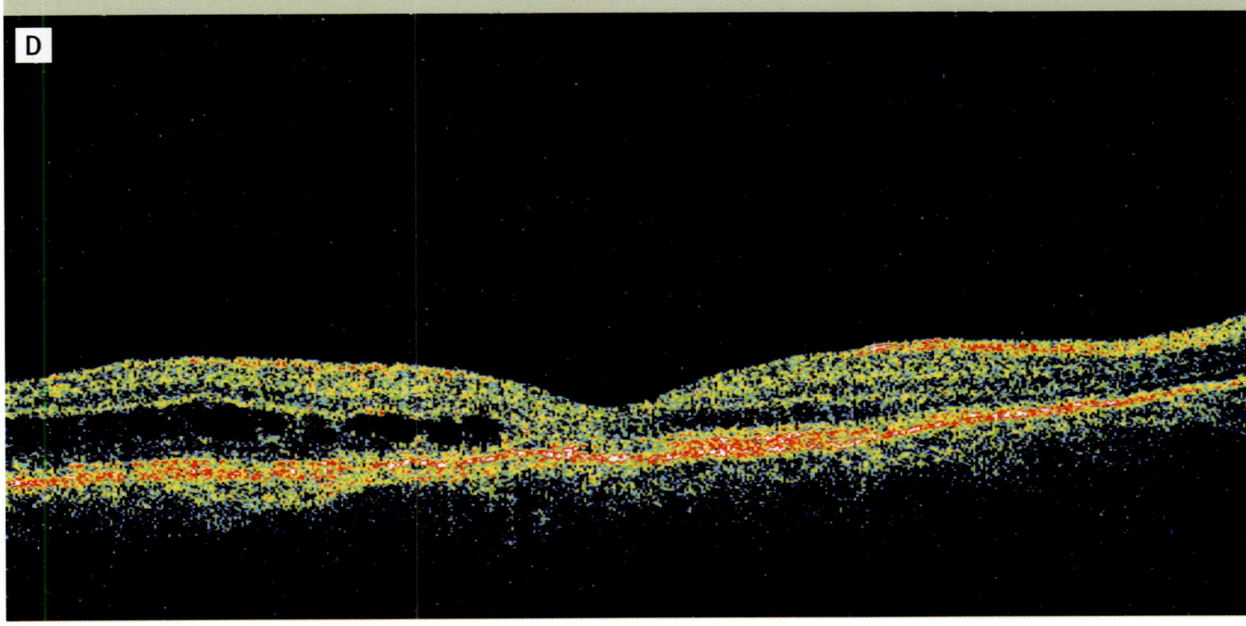

CENTRAL SEROUS CHORIORETINOPATHY

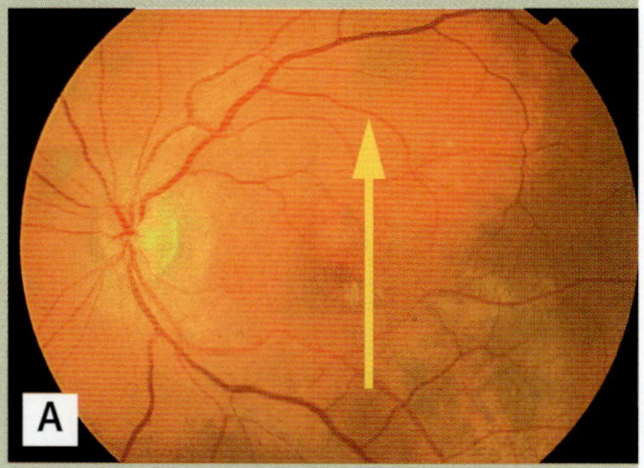

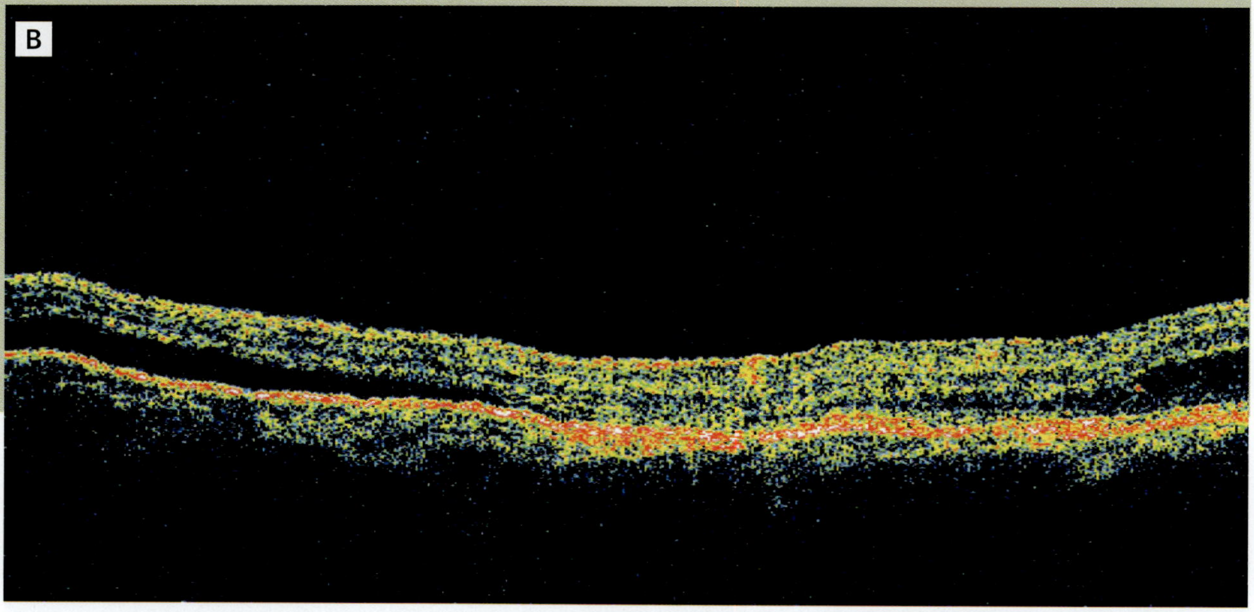

A. The same eye of the patient in page 155 in another scanning (the arrow shows the scan direction). B. Note the area of low reflectivity between the retina and retinal pigment epithelium to the left of the picture that corresponds to the retinal detachment (small arrow). To the right of the picture there is an area of low reflectivity in the outer layers of the retina that corresponds to cystic retinal edema (big arrow). In the area of cystic edema of the retina Note the existence of a thin layer of retinal tissue under the serous fluid (thick arrow) that is not found in cases of retinal detachment and constitutes a sign of differential diagnosis between retinal detachment and diffuse retinal edema.

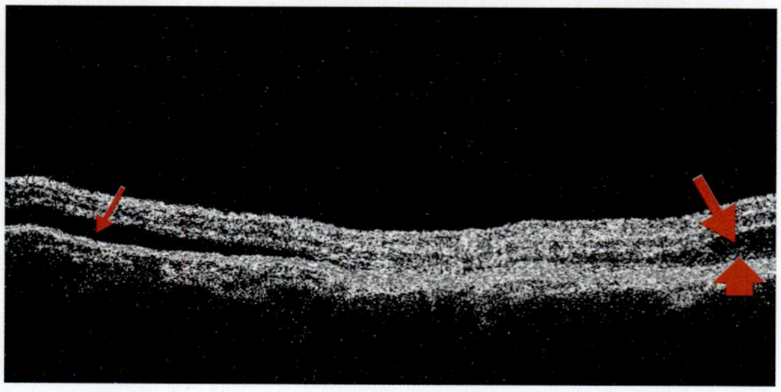

CHAPTER 6

DIABETIC RETINOPATHY

PANAGIOTIS THEODOSSIADIS

Diabetic retinopathy is one of the main causes of blindness in individuals under 60 years of age in the USA and Europe. It is a progressive disease that initially affects the retinal vessels and later causes diffuse retinal alterations, mainly in the macula, which may lead in visual acuity decrease and/or blindness.

Diabetic changes are diverse and can be classified in:
- Proliferative diabetic retinopathy
- Non-proliferative diabetic retinopathy

Proliferative diabetic retinopathy is characterized by the presence of:
- Neovascularization
- Fibrosis
- Sometimes vitreomacular traction

Neovascularization is the result of retinal ischemia which stimulates angiogenesis, new pathologic blood vessels formation and haemorrhages.

Non-proliferative diabetic retinopathy is characterized by the presence of:
- Microaneurysms
- Haemorrhages
- Soft or hard exudates
- Intraretinal microvascular abnormalities (IRMA)
- Diabetic macular edema

Diabetic macular edema is the most important cause of decrease and/or loss of central vision[10-11]. Edema can be observed in any stage of diabetic retinopathy. Optical Coherence Tomography is very important in diabetic retinopathy for the evaluation and classification of diabetic edema and for the identification of the relation between the vitreous and the retina[1-3,12]. It also contributes to the study of macular edema progression after therapeutic intervention. An important advantage of Optical Coherence Tomography is its reproducibility that is necessary for the quantitative calculation of diabetic edema and the macular thickness[4-6]. The presence of diabetic macular edema is characterized by low intraretinal reflectivity located mainly in the outer retinal layers.

Optical Coherence Tomography is important in the diagnosis and classification of macular edema, according to its morphology, in the following types: a) diffuse, b) cystic and c) cystic or diffuse with serous retinal detachment[13].

The frequent type of edema is diffuse sponge-like, followed by cystic edema and lastly by serous retinal detachment. In advanced macular edema, the cystic formations create large coalescent areas located in almost all the retinal layers and are represented as areas of low reflectivity[8,14]. The hard exudates that coexist with diabetic edema are depicted like areas of high reflectivity located in the outer retinal layers.

Optical Coherence Tomography, apart from the identification and morphology of the diabetic macular edema, measures also the thickness of the foveola and the parafoveal area. It can reveal the presence of macular edema in cases where it is not evident on biomicroscopy[17] and is also very useful in the study of diabetic macular edema accompanied by vitreous traction[7,15,16]. Vitreous traction is detected as a membrane of high reflectivity which is in closed contact to the macula. The detection of the vitreomacular traction is important to the diagnosis, surgical treatment and postoperative follow-up of the underlying diabetic macular edema[4,5,9,18-21].

Proliferative diabetic retinopathy is characterized by the presence of zones (fibrous formations) of high reflectivity located on the retinal surface and into the vitreous cavity.

DIABETIC RETINOPATHY

1. Brown JC, Solomon SD, Bressler SB, Schachat AP, DiBernardo C, Bressler NM. Detection of diabetic foveal edema: contact lens biomicroscopy compared with optical coherence tomography. Arch Ophthalmol 2004; 122: 330-335.

2. Browning DJ, McOwen MD, Bowen R Jr, O'Marah TL. Comparison of the clinical diagnosis of diabetic macular edema with diagnosis by optical coherence tomography. Ophthalmology 2004; 111: 712-714.

3. Catier A, Tadayoni R, Paques M, Erfinay A, Haouchine B, Gaudric A, Massin P. Characterization of macular edema from various etiologies by optical coherence tomography. Am J Ophthalmol 2005; 140: 200-206.

4. Goebel W, Kretzchmar-Gross T. Retinal thickness in diabetic retinopathy: a study using optical coherence tomography (OCT). Retina 2002; 22: 759-787.

5. Goebel W, Franke R. Retinal thickness in diabetic retinopathy: comparison of optical coherence tomography, the retinal thickness analyzer, and fundus photography. Retina 2006; 26: 49-57.

6. Kang SW, Park CY, Ham DI. The correlation between fluorescein angiographic and optical coherence tomographic features in clinically significant diabetic macular edema. Am J Ophthalmol 2004; 137: 313-322.

7. Karatas M, Ramirez JA, Ophir A. Diabetic vitreopapillary traction and macular oedema. Eye 2005; 19: 676-682.

8. Lattanzio R, Brancato R, Pierro L, Bandello F, Iaccher B, Fiore T, Maestranzi G. Macular thickness measured by optical coherence tomography (OCT) in diabetic patients. Eur J Ophthalmol 2002; 12: 482-487.

9. Masin P, Duguid G, Erginay A, IHaouchine B, Gaudric A, Optical coherence tomography for evaluating diabetic macular edema before and after vitrectomy. Am J Ophthalmol 2003; 135: 169-177.

10. Ozdek SC, Erdinc MA, Gurelik G, Aydin B, Bahceci U, Hasanreisoglu B. Optical coherence tomographic assessment of diabetic macular edema: comparison with fluorescein angiographic and clinical findings. Ophthalmologica 2005; 219:86-92.

11. Ozdemir H, Karacorlu M, Karacorlu S. Serous macular detachment in diabetic cystoid macular edema. Acta Ophthalmol Scand. 2005; 83: 63-66.

12. Panozzo G, Gusson E, Parolini B, Mercanti A. Role of OCT in the diagnosis and follow-up of diabetic macular edema. Semin Ophthalmol 2003; 18:74-81.

13. Panozzo G, Parolini B, Gusson E, Mercanti A, Pinachatt S, Bertoldo G, Pignatto S. Diabetic macular edema: an OCT-based classification. Semin Ophthalmol 2004; 19: 13-20.

14. Polito A, Del Borrello M, Polini G, Furlan F, Isola M, Bandello F. Diurnal variation in clinically significant diabetic macular edema measured by Stratus OCT. Retina 2006; 26: 14-20.

15. Recchia FM, Ruby AJ, Carvalho Recchis Ca. Pars plana vitrectomy with removal of the internal limiting membrane in the treatment of persistent diabetic macular edema. Am J Ophthalmol 2005; 139: 447-454.

16. Rosenblatt BJ, Shah GK, Sharma S, Bakal J. Pars plana vitrectomy limiting membranectomy for refractory diabetic macular edema without a taut posterior hyaloid. Graefes Arch Clin Exp Ophthalmol 2005; 243: 20-25.

17. Schaudig UH, Glaefke C, Scholz F, Richard G. Optical coherence tomography for retinal thickness measurement in diabetic patients without clinically significant macular edema. Ophthalmic Surg Lasers 2000; 31:182-186.

18. Sforzolini B. Optical coherence tomography findings in diabetic macular edema before and after vitrectomy. Ophthalmic Surg Lasers 2000;31: 187-191.

19. Shah SP, Patel M, Thomas D, Aldington S, Laidlaw DA. Factors predicting outcome of vitrectomy for diabetic macular oedema: results of a prospective study. Br J Ophthalmol 2006; 90: 33-36.

20. Shimura M, Saito T, Yasuda K, Tamai M. Clinical course of macular edema in two cases of interferon associated retinopathy observed by optical coherence tomography. Jpn J Ophthalmol 2005; 49: 231-234.

21. Yamamoto T, Hitani K, Tsikahara I, Yamamoto S, Kawasaki R, Yamashita H, Takeuchi S. Early postoperative retinal thickness changes and complications after vitrectomy for diabetic macular edema. Am J Ophthalmol 2003; 135: 14-19.

DIABETIC MACULAR EDEMA

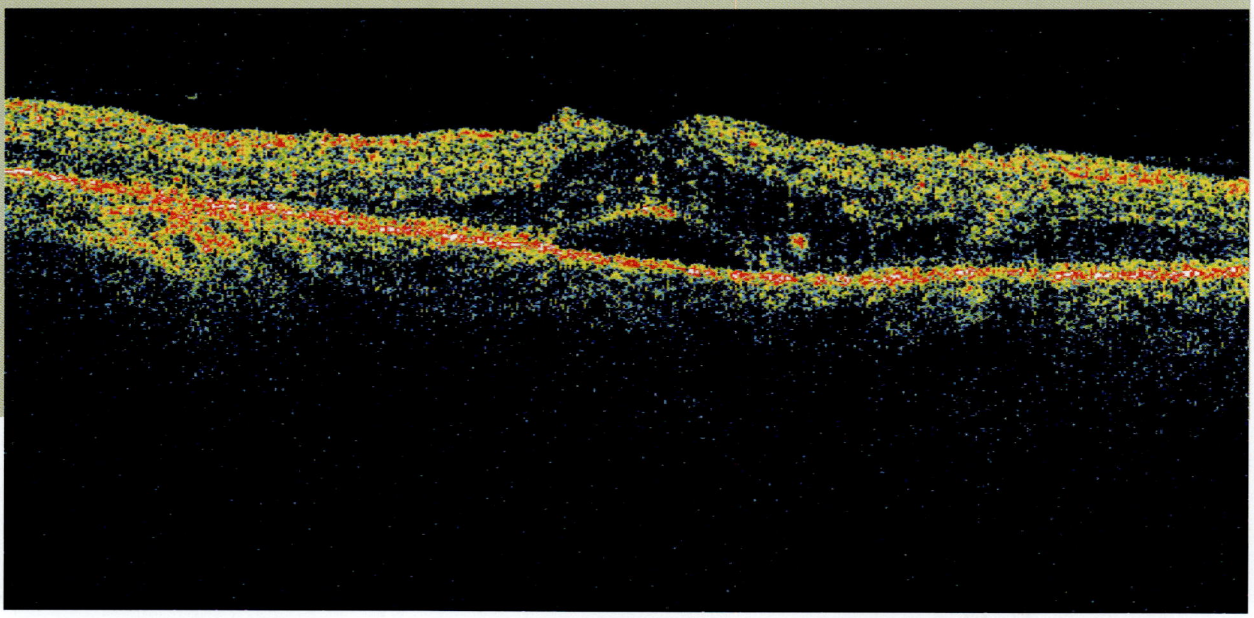

Patient with diabetic macular edema. There are multiple cystic formations in the outer retinal layers corresponding to retinal cystic edema (small arrow) and fluid accumulation between the retina and the retinal pigment epithelium corresponding to serous retinal detachment (big arrow). The vitreous appears attached on the perifoveal retina (arrow head).

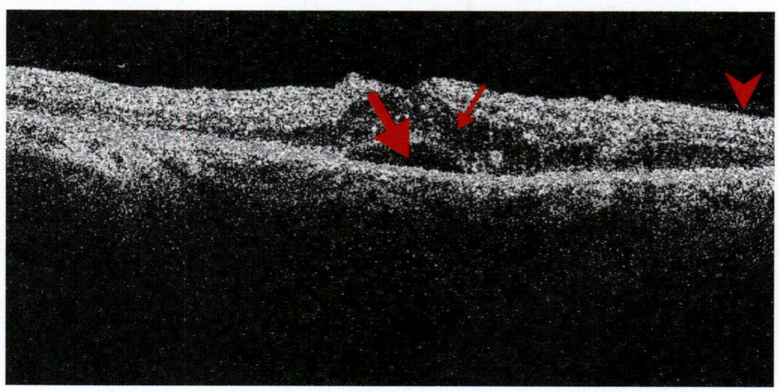

DIABETIC MACULAR EDEMA

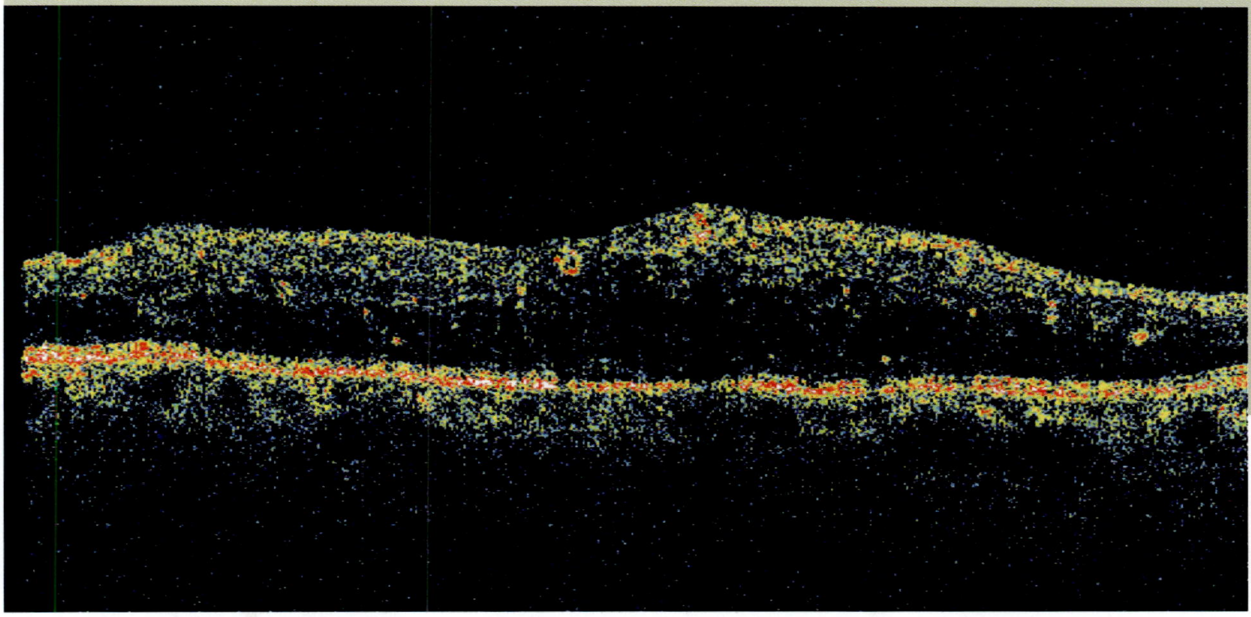

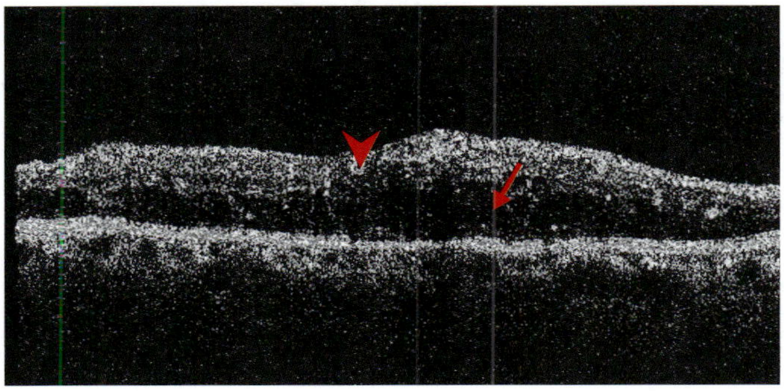

Patient with diabetic macular edema. There are multiple cystic formations in the outer retinal layers corresponding to retinal cystic edema (small arrow) that is extending under the fovea. Exudates are also clearly visible like intraretinal spots of high reflectivity (arrow head).

DIABETIC MACULAR EDEMA

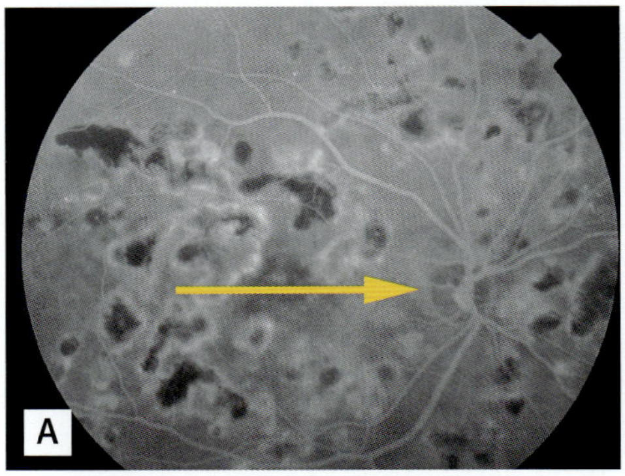

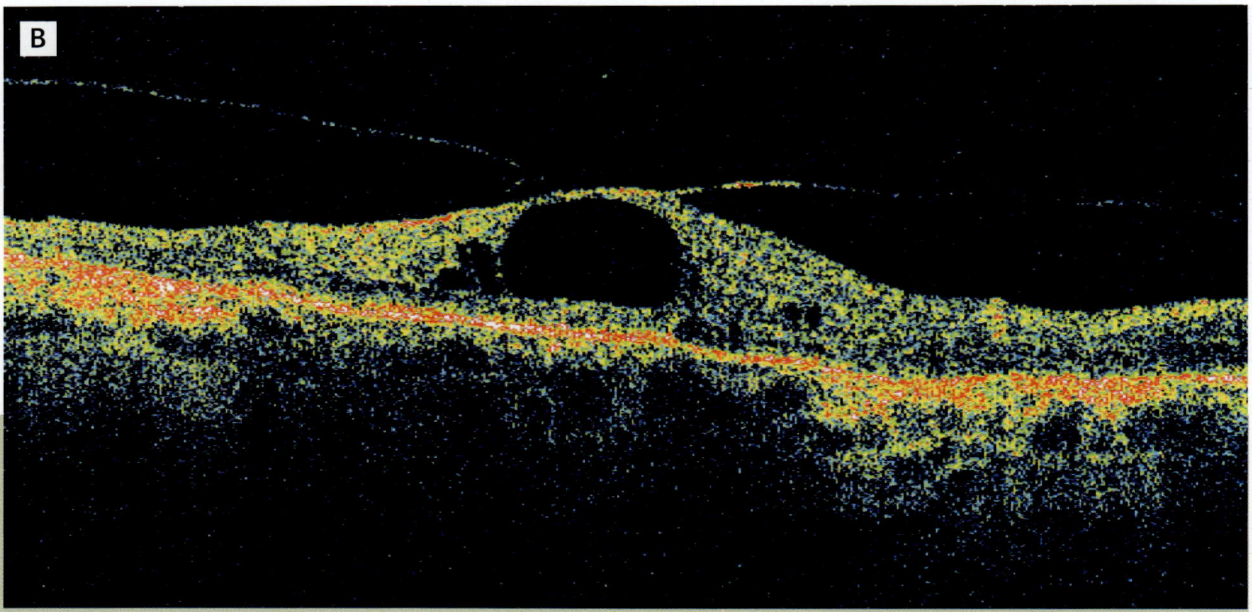

Patient with diabetic macular edema. A. Fluorescein angiography shows the scars of the previous photocoagulation treatment with persisting leakage of dye in the macular area (the arrow shows the scan direction). B. A big cystic area of low reflectivity is detected in the fovea (small arrow) corresponding to severe cystic macular edema. Vitreous is tightly attached to the fovea while it is detached in the surrounding area (big arrow).

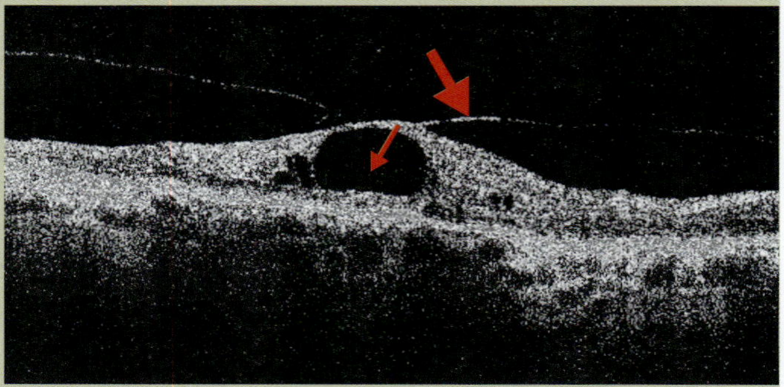

DIABETIC RETINOPATHY

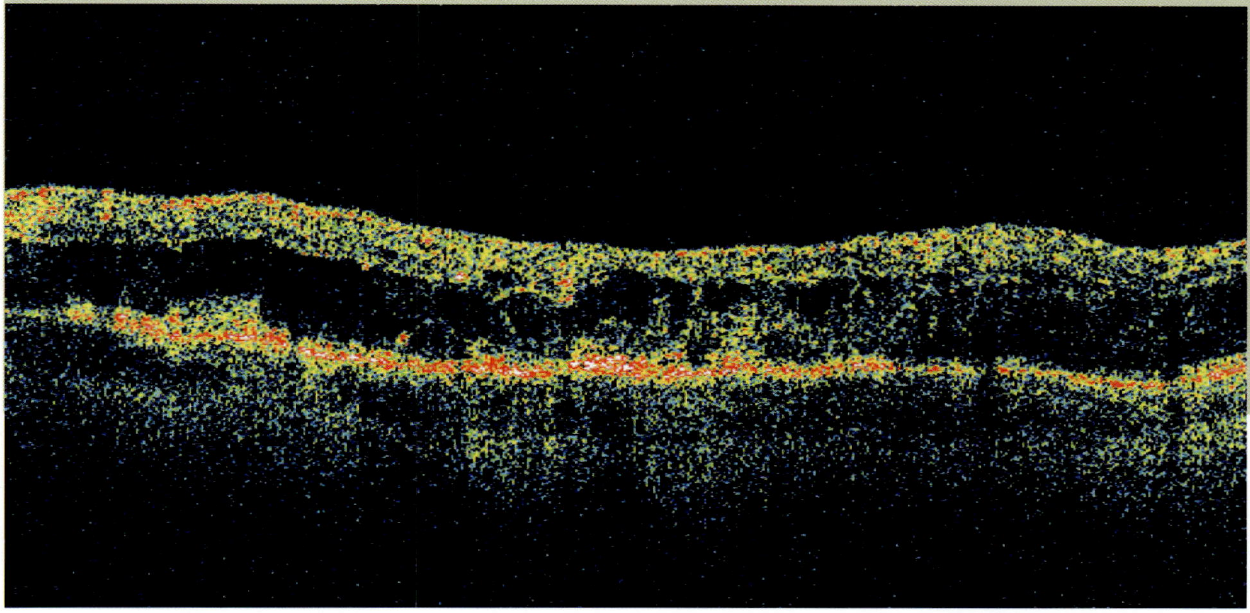

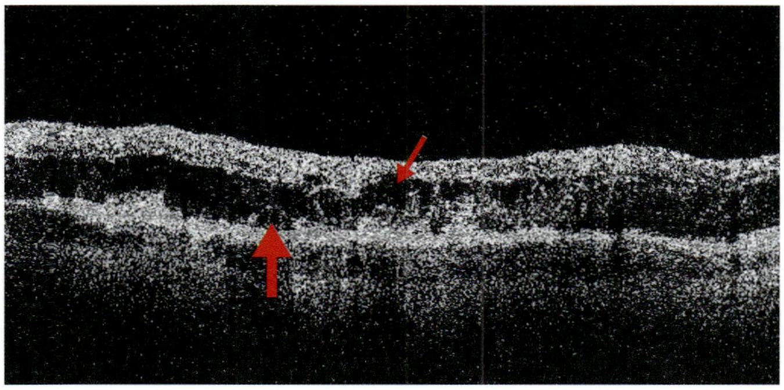

Patient with diabetic retinopathy. There are multiple coalescent cystic formations of low reflectivity corresponding to macular edema (small arrow). There is also a focal absence of the photoreceptors' layer (big arrow).

DIABETIC MACULAR EDEMA

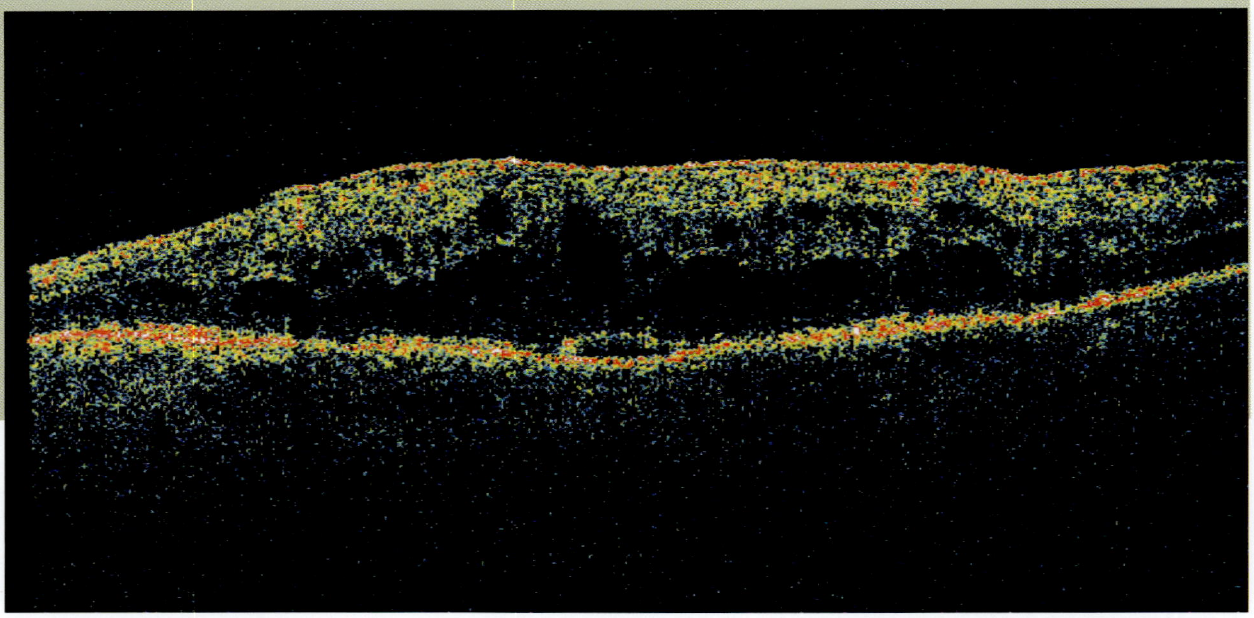

Patient with diabetic maculopathy. There are areas of low reflectivity within the retina corresponding to diffuse (thick arrow) and cystic retinal edema (small arrow). Note also the low reflectivity area between the retina and the retinal pigment epithelium due to focal retinal detachment (big arrow). Another characteristic finding is the presence of an epiretinal membrane (arrow head).

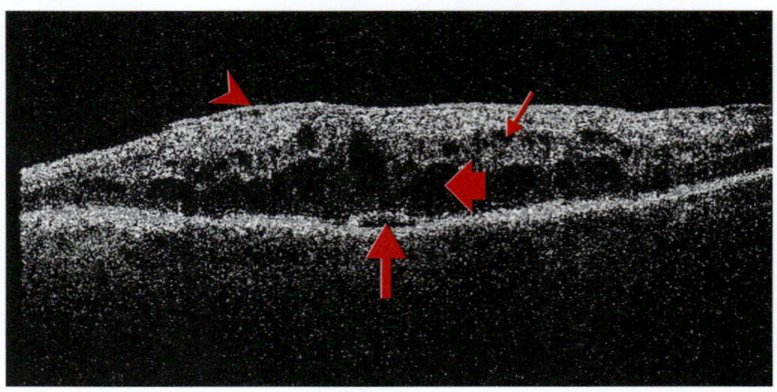

DIABETIC MACULAR EDEMA

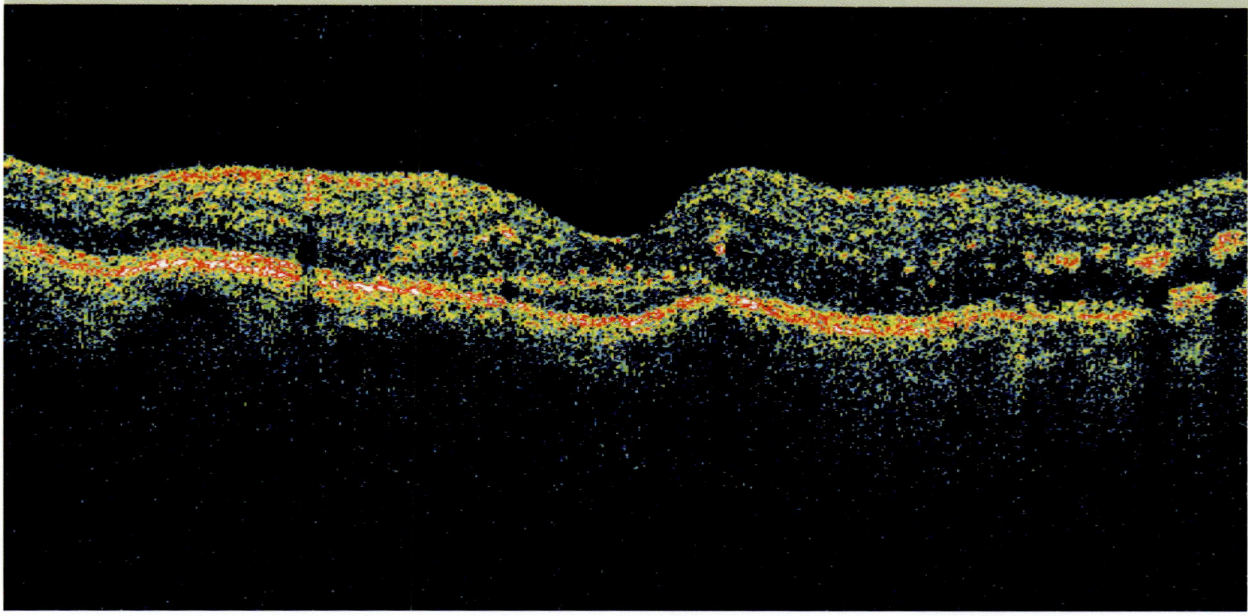

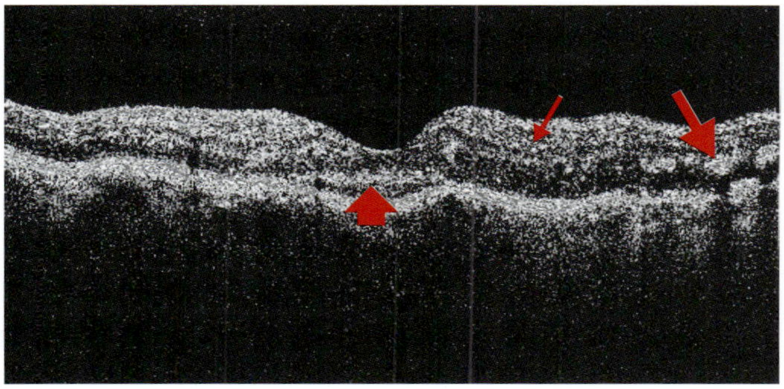

Patient with diabetic maculopathy. There is an increase of retinal thickness due to diffuse retinal edema (small arrow). The foveal depression is still detected but its thickness is increased (277μm). Elevation of the photoreceptors in the fovea is also detected (thick arrow). The round areas of high reflectivity located in the outer retinal layers correspond to hard exudates (big arrow). The light absorption explains the shadow that is Noted underneath them.

DIABETIC MACULAR EDEMA

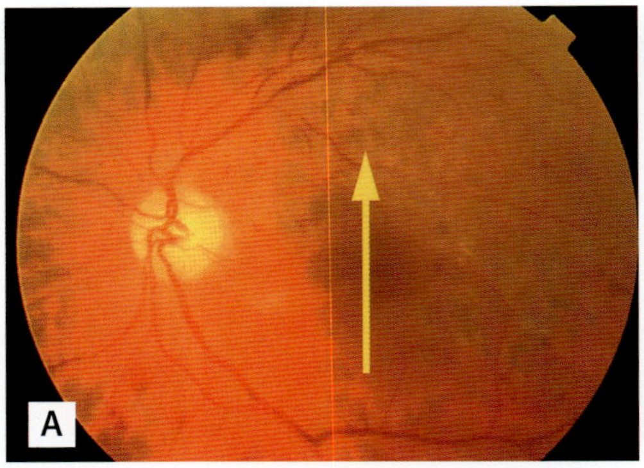

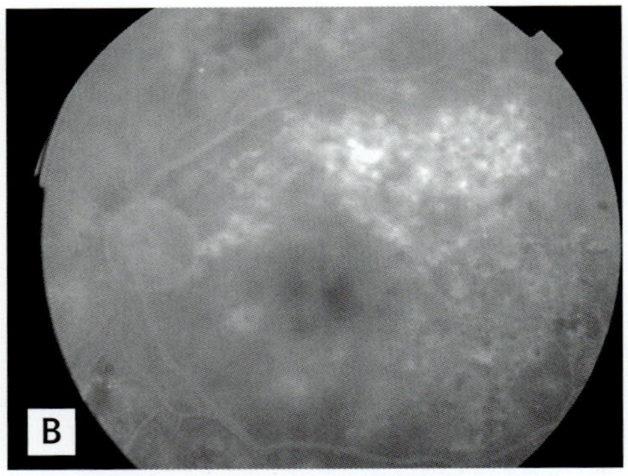

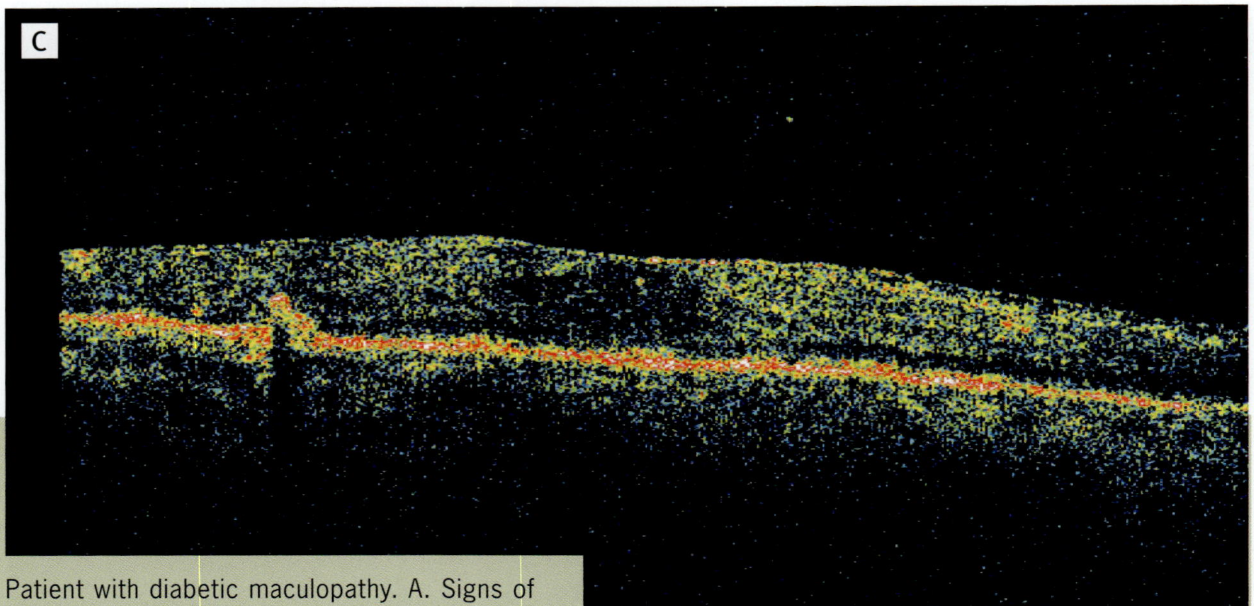

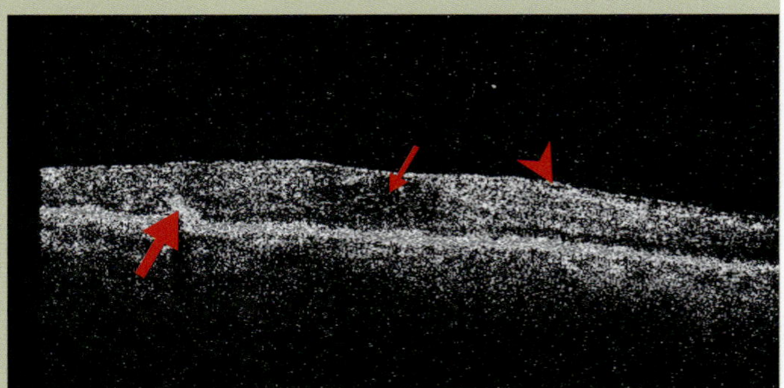

Patient with diabetic maculopathy. A. Signs of diabetic retinopathy and maculopathy previously treated by photocoagulation (the arrow shows the scan direction). B. Fluorescein angiography shows leakage of dye from microaneurysms in the macular area. C. Note increase of retinal thickness with disappearance of the foveal depression due to diffuse edema (small arrow). Coincidentally, there is a focal interruption of the retinal pigment epithelium layer (big arrow). There is also a thin line of high reflectivity on the retinal surface corresponding to an epiretinal membrane (arrow head).

DIABETIC MACULAR EDEMA

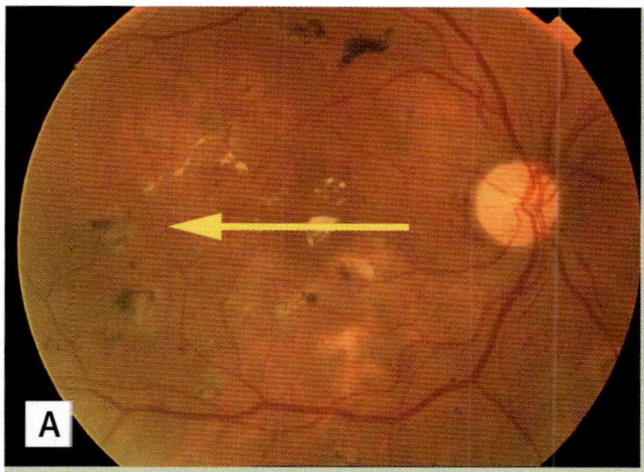

Patient with diabetic maculopathy. A. Biomicroscopy shows clinically significant edema and hard exudates in the macula with laser scars in the posterior pole (the arrow shows the scan direction). B. Optical Coherence Tomography shows increased retinal thickness in the fovea and the perifoveal area, due to diffuse edema of the central area (small arrow). Note also the area of low reflectivity between the retina and the retinal pigment

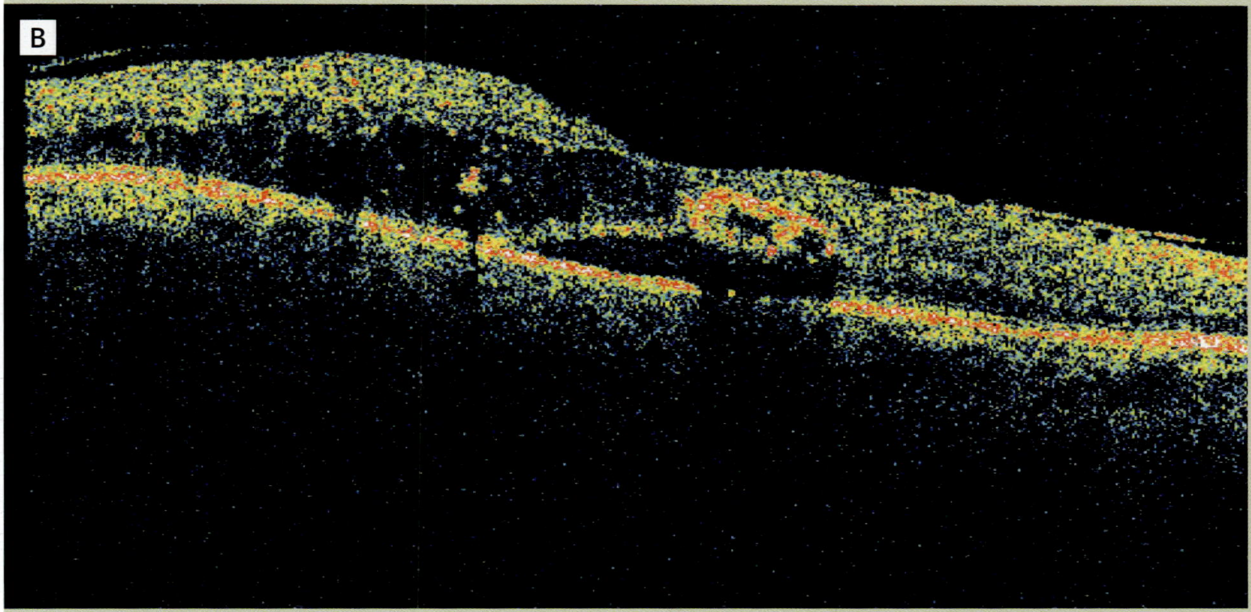

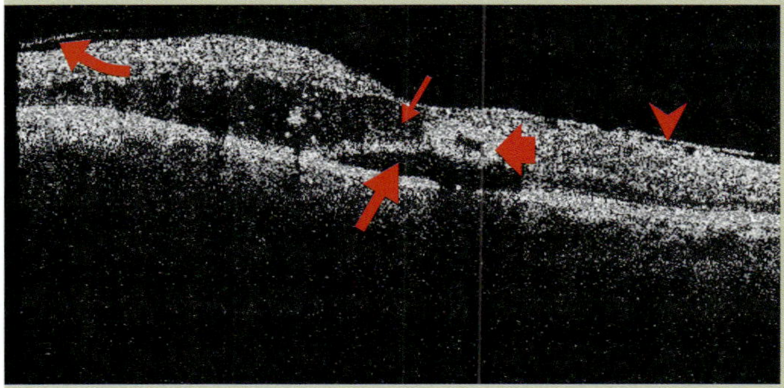

epithelium corresponding to a retinal detachment in the fovea (big arrow). The circular area of very high reflectivity that is located at the outer retinal layers corresponds to a large hard exudate (thick arrow).A thin area of high reflectivity causing retinal contraction is detected on the surface of the retina corresponding to an epiretinal membrane (arrow head). The vitreous is found attached to the retina (convex arrow).

DIABETIC MACULAR EDEMA

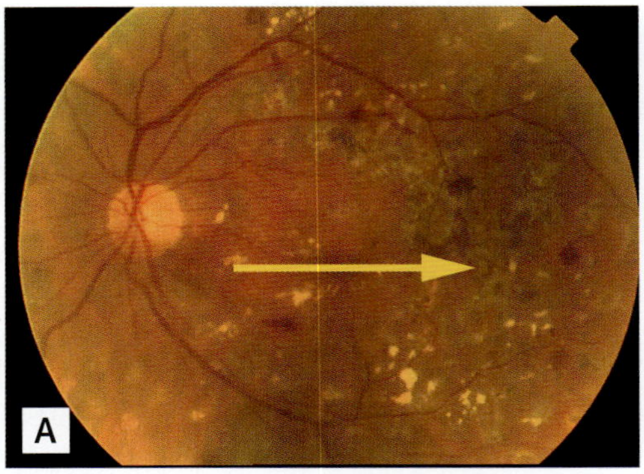

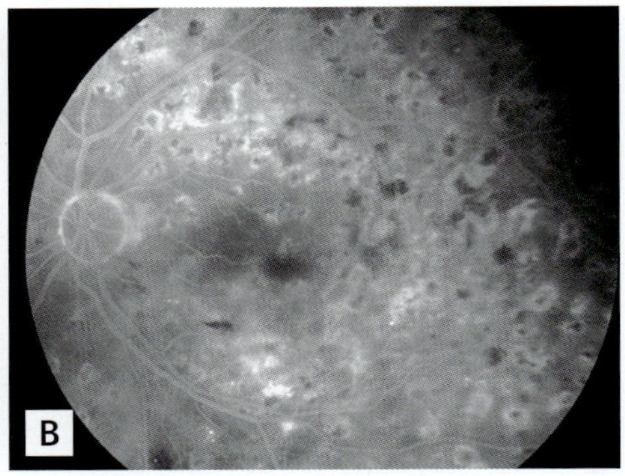

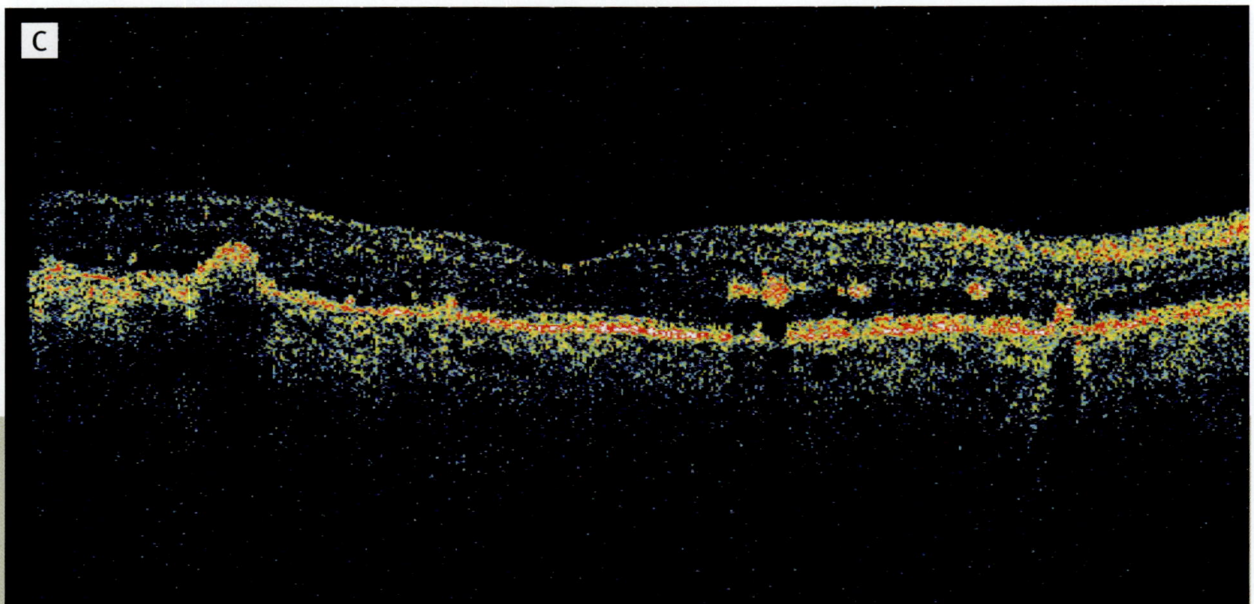

A. Diabetic maculopathy with mild macula edema, exudates and old photocoagulation scars (the arrow shows the scan direction). B. Fluorescein angiography shows absence of leakage in the fovea. C. There are multiple areas of high reflectivity, located in the outer retina layers that are due to hard exudates (small arrows). Shadowing of the underlying layers is observed beneath the larger of them. The thickness and the morphology of the fovea are preserved. The vitreous is found attached to the retina (big arrow).

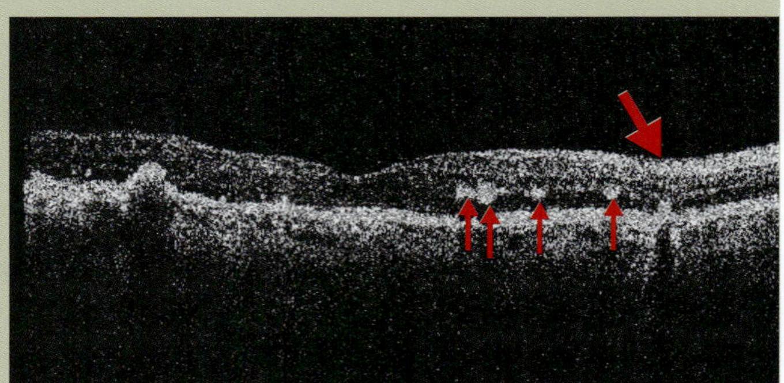

DIABETIC MACULAR EDEMA

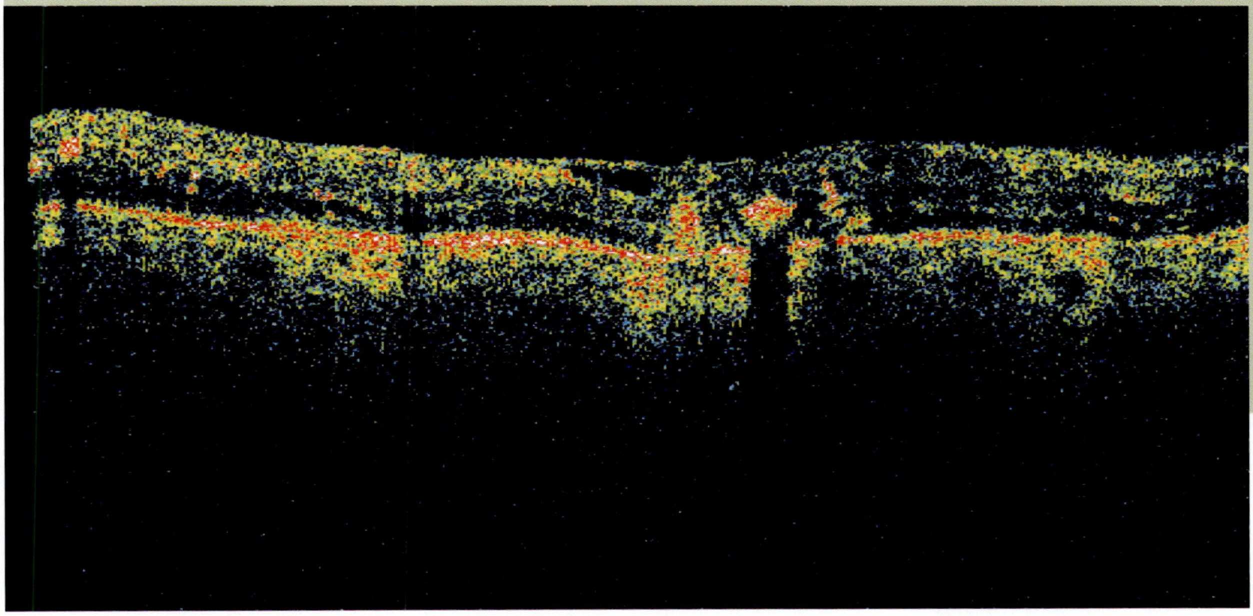

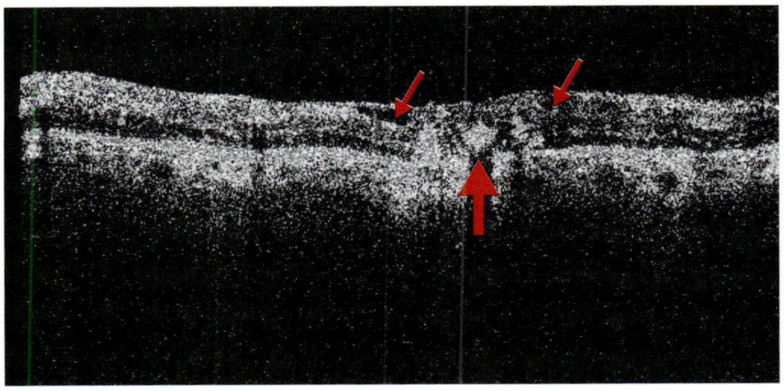

The other eye of the patient of page 170. There are multiple cystic formations of low reflectivity within the retina corresponding to cystic edema (small arrows). A high reflectivity area located inside the retina and corresponding to a big hard exudate is detected in the fovea (big arrow). The light absorption from it explains the shadow behind it.

DIABETIC MACULAR EDEMA

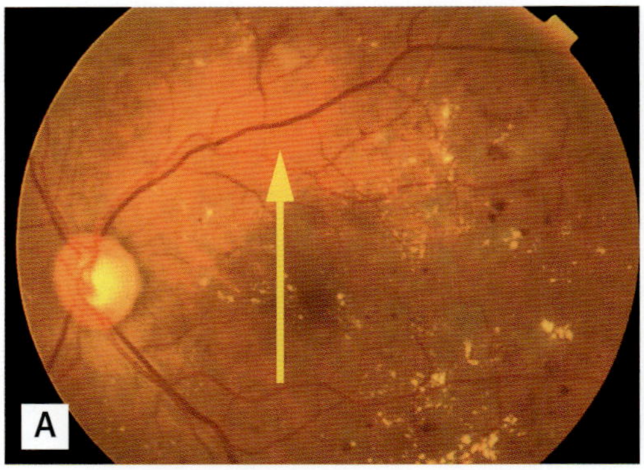

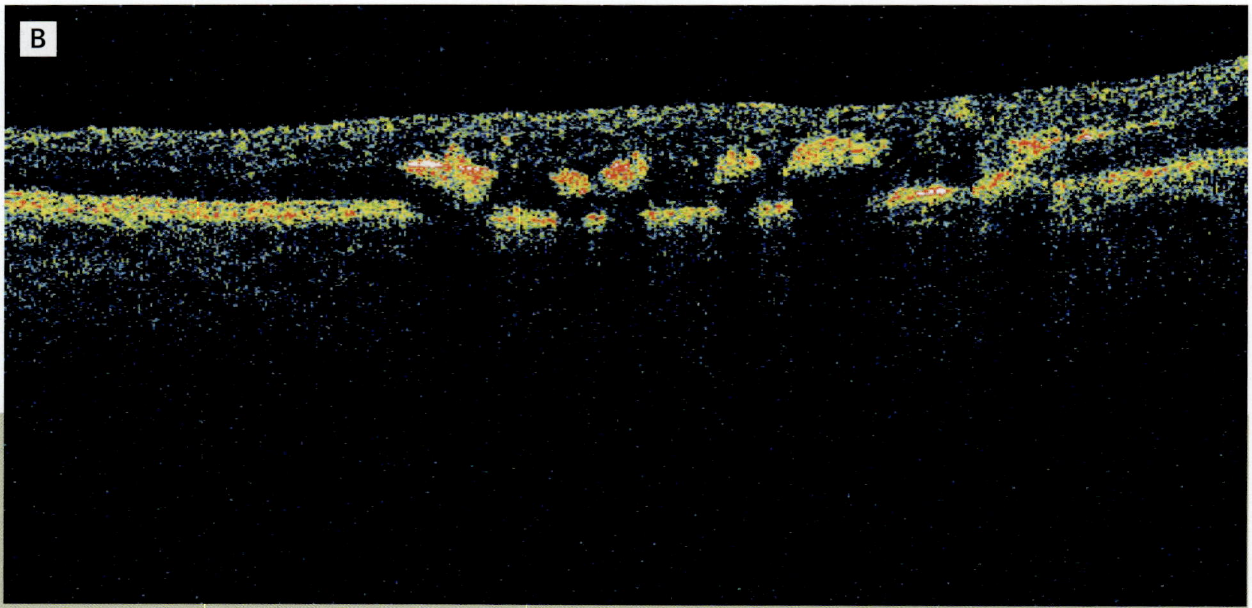

A. Diabetic maculopathy with scattered hard exudates (the arrow shows the scan direction). B. There are multiple areas of high reflectivity located in the outer retinal layers due to big hard exudates (arrows). Shadowing of the layers underneath due to light absorption is observed.

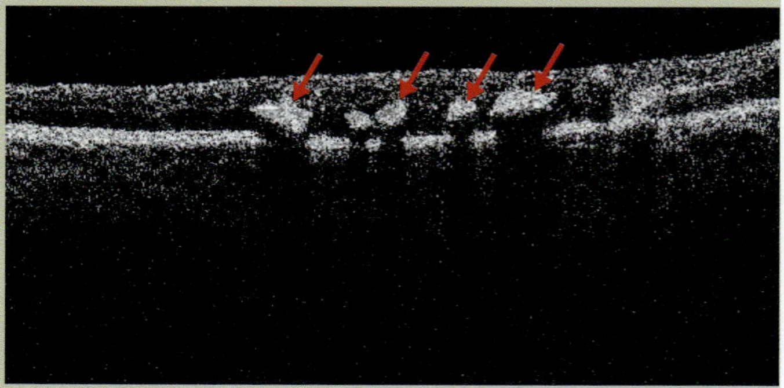

DIABETIC MACULAR EDEMA

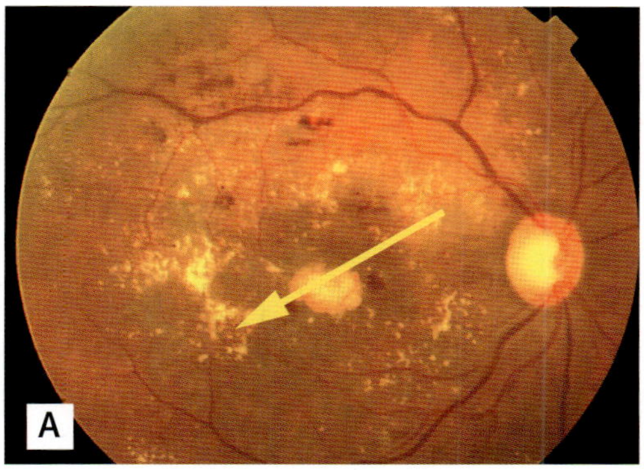

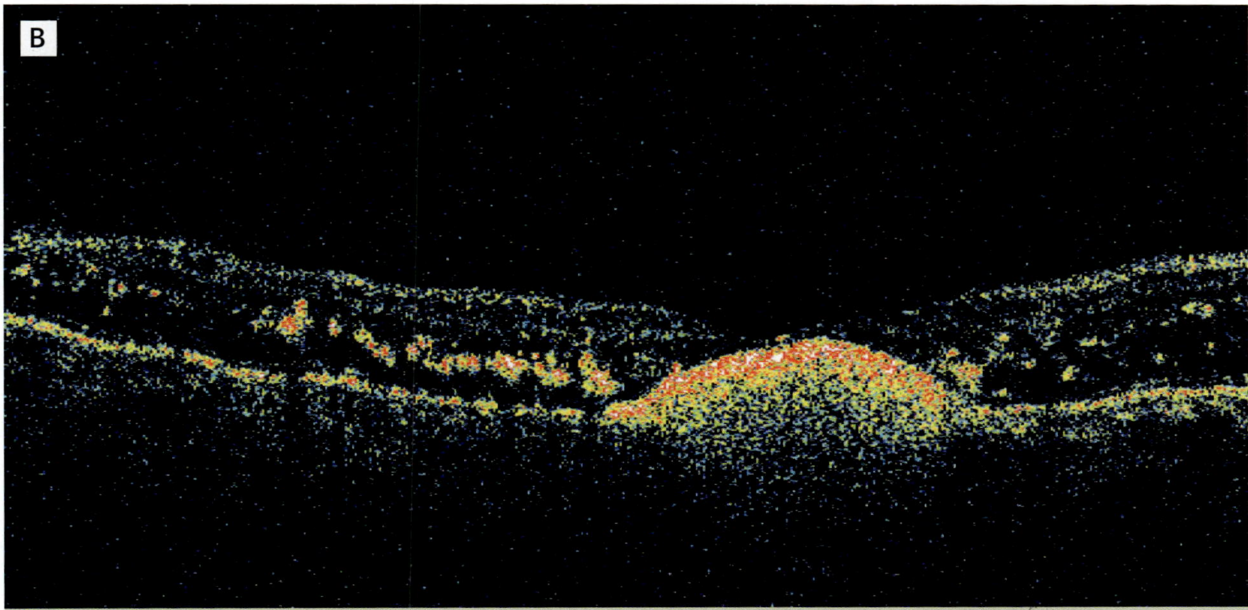

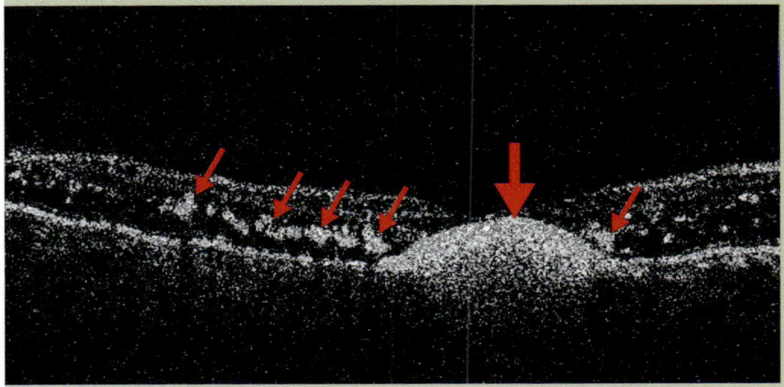

A. Diabetic maculopathy with numerous exudates and a single exudative plaque in the fovea (the arrow shows the scan direction). B. There are multiple areas of high reflectivity, located in the outer retinal layers due to hard exudates (small arrows). Note the shadowing of the layers underneath. A large area of high reflectivity corresponding to the exudative plaque is detected in the foveal area (big arrow).

DIABETIC MACULAR EDEMA

B

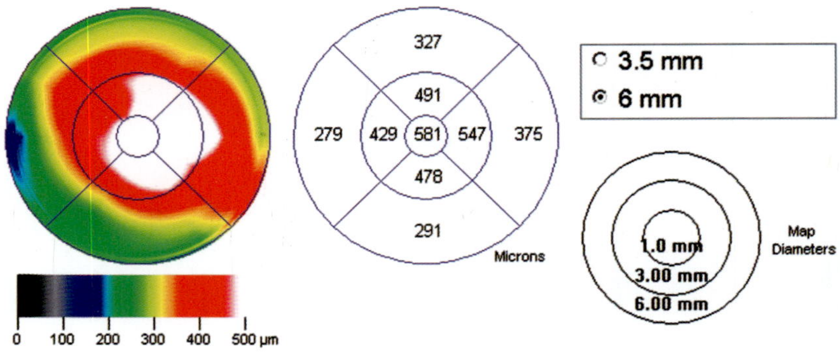

A

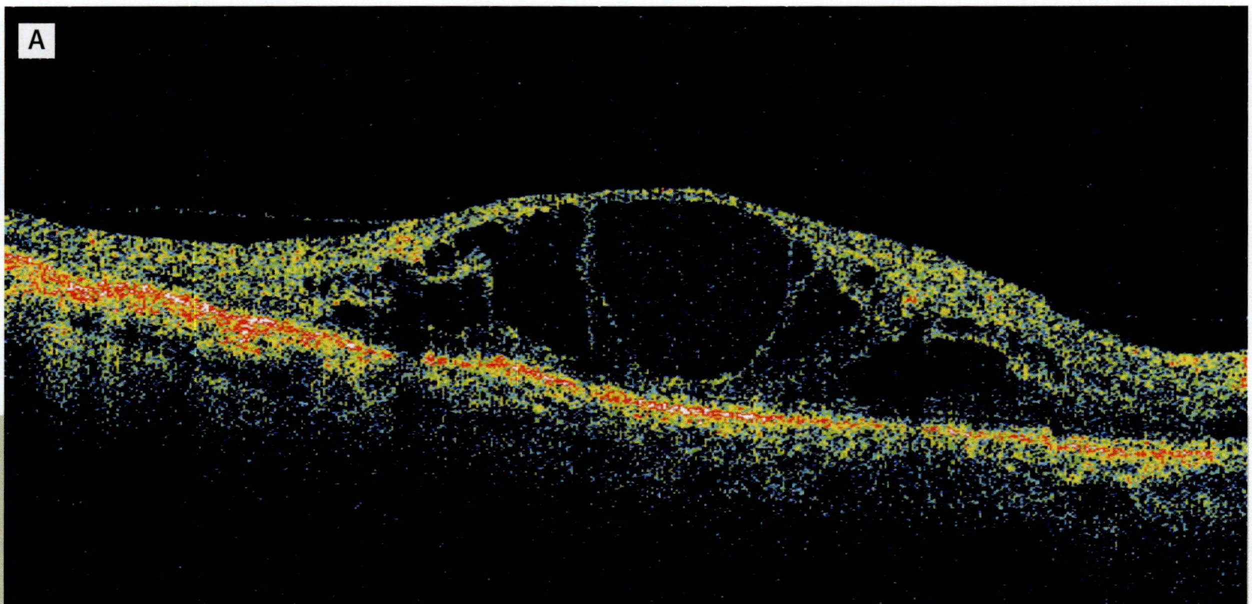

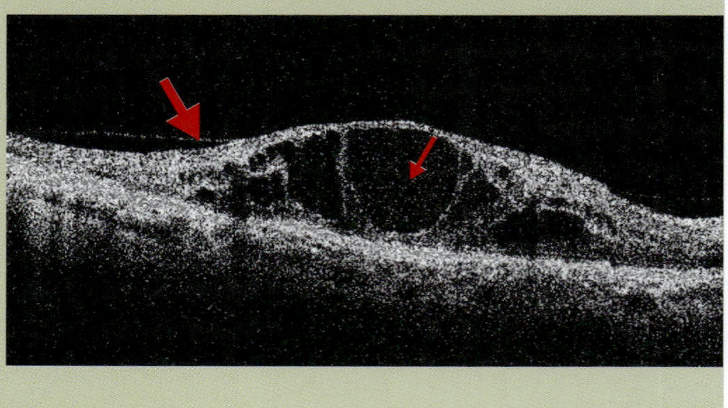

Patient with diffuse diabetic maculopathy. A. There are large cystoid formations of low reflectivity inside the retina due to cystoid edema in the fovea (small arrow). The vitreous appears attached to the retina (big arrow). B. Retinal map analysis, as created automatically from the Optical Coherence Tomography software, shows clearly the retinal thickness increase in the central area of 1mm diameter.

DIABETIC MACULAR EDEMA

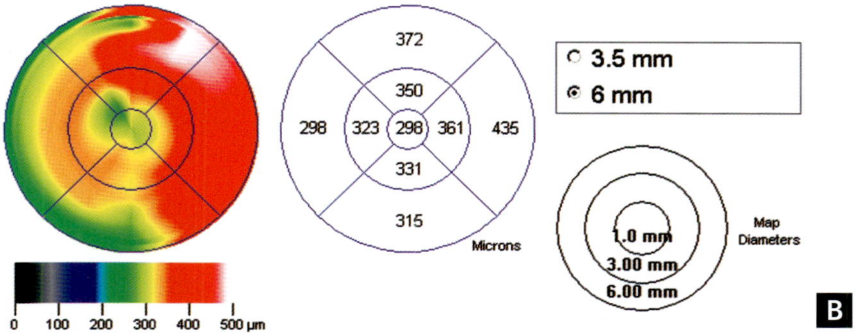

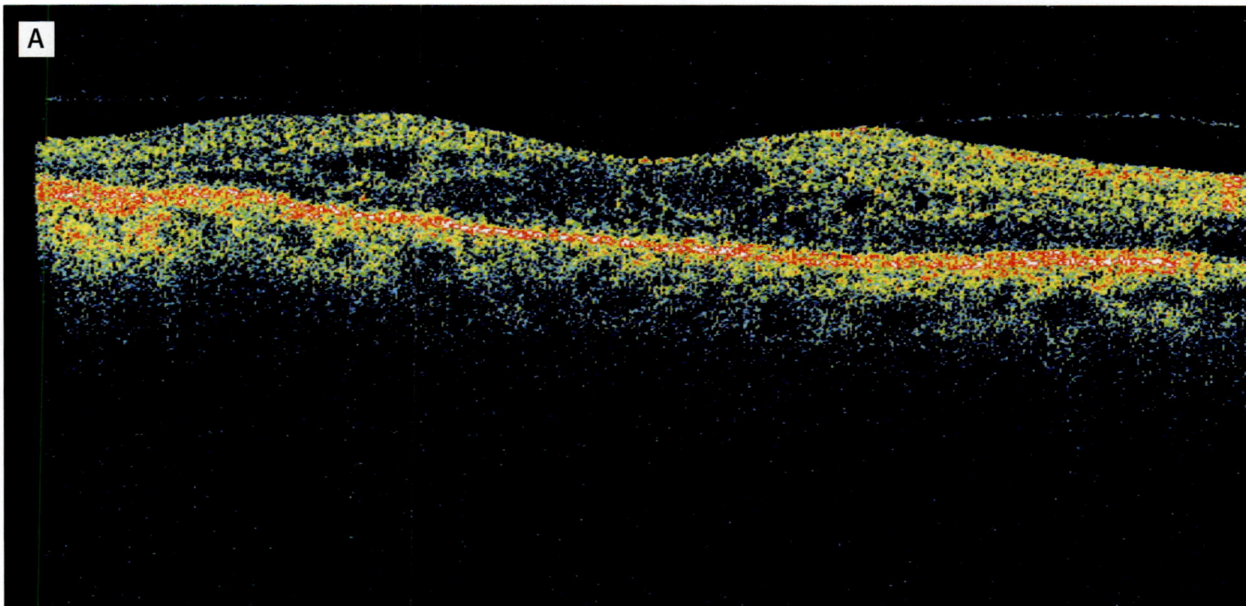

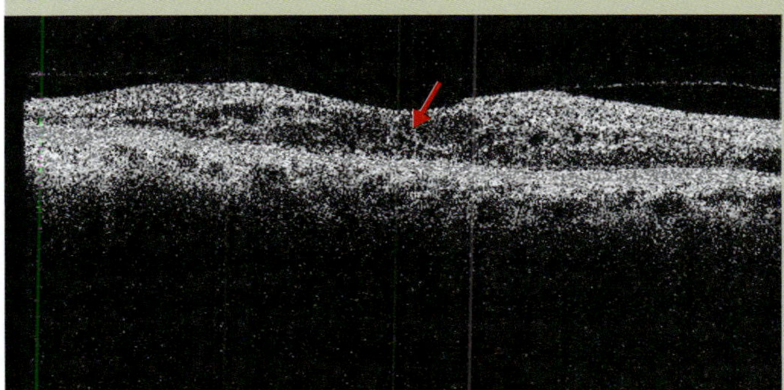

The patient of page 174 seven months after the third intravenous injection of infliximab (antagonist of Tumor Necrosis Factor). A. Note an almost complete resolution of the intraretinal cysts and a significant decrease of the retinal thickness with persistence of diffuse edema (arrow). B. This is clearly demonstrated in the retinal map as created by the Optical Coherence Tomography software.

DIABETIC MACULAR EDEMA

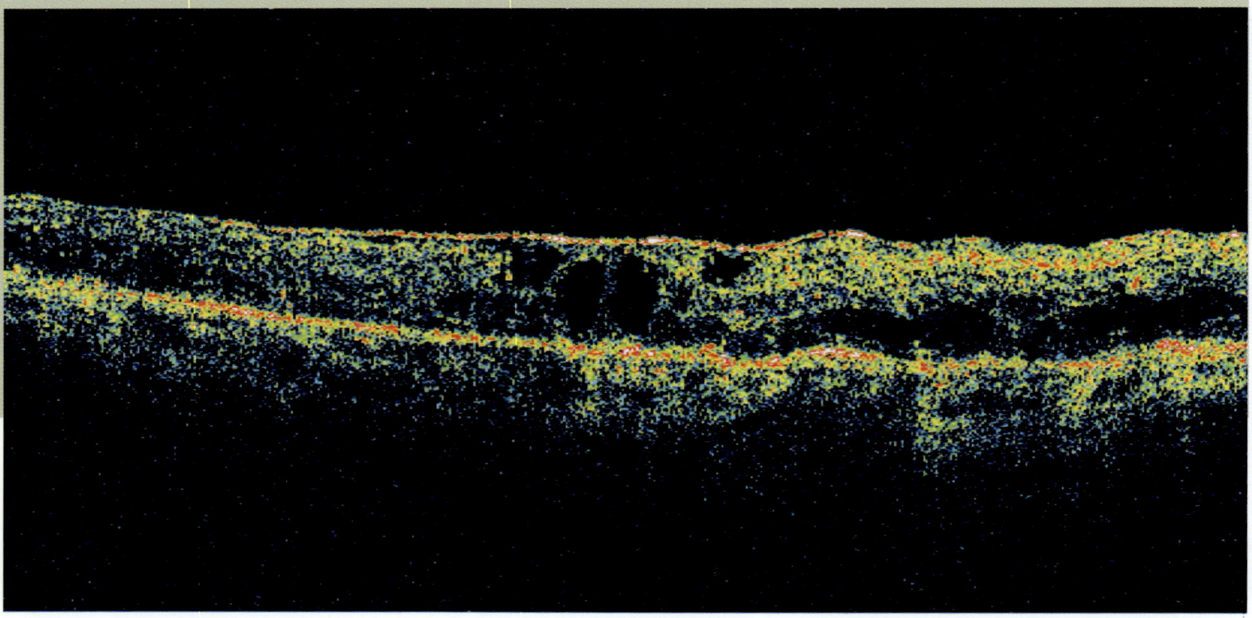

Patient with diabetic maculopathy. Note the multiple cystic intraretinal formations of low reflectivity corresponding to cystoid retinal edema (small arrow). A thin area of high reflectivity corresponding to an epiretinal membrane in the macular area is detected on the retinal surface (big arrow). Note the empty spaces detected between the membrane and the inner retinal surface (arrow head). Surgical excision of the membrane rather than laser photocoagulation will be more beneficial for this patient.

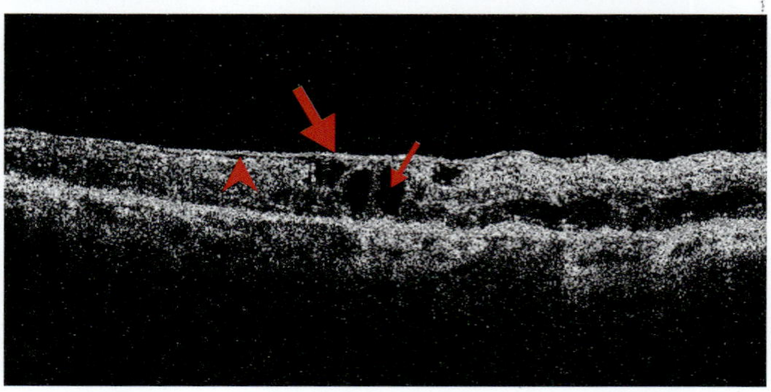

DIABETIC MACULAR EDEMA

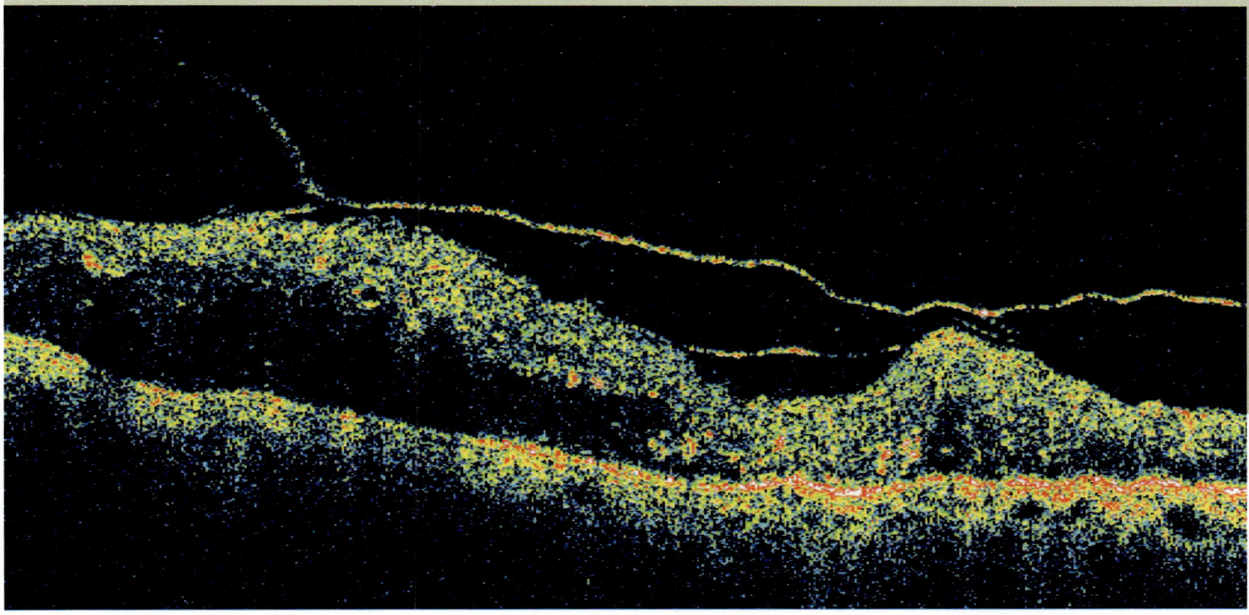

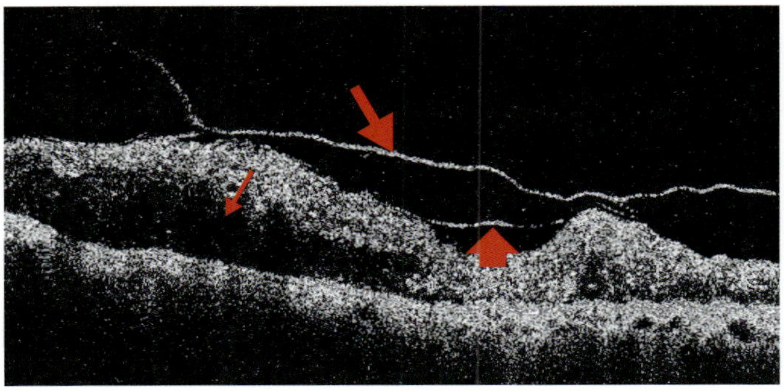

Patient with diabetic maculopathy. Optical Coherence Tomography shows a diffuse intraretinal area of low reflectivity due to diffuse intraretinal edema (small arrow). A linear formation of high reflectivity is detected inside the vitreous cavity and corresponds to a thick posterior hyaloid causing traction on the retina (big arrow). An epiretinal membrane is detected as a second line of high reflectivity between the first line and the retina (thick arrow). For this patient surgical excision is the obvious treatment.

PROLIFERATIVE DIABETIC RETINOPATHY

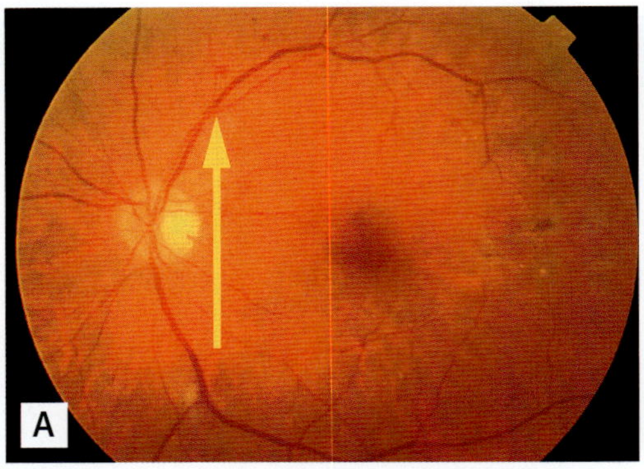

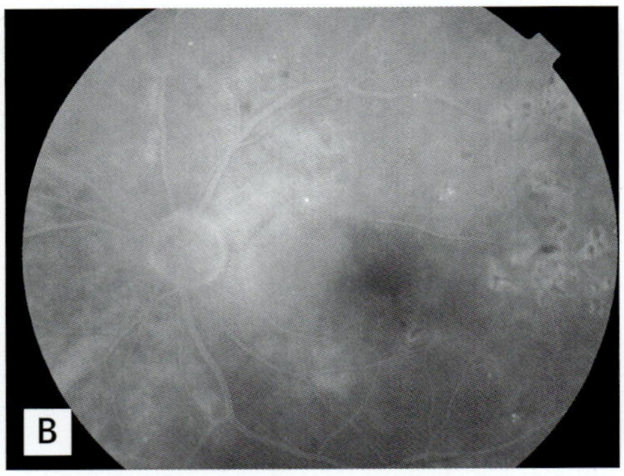

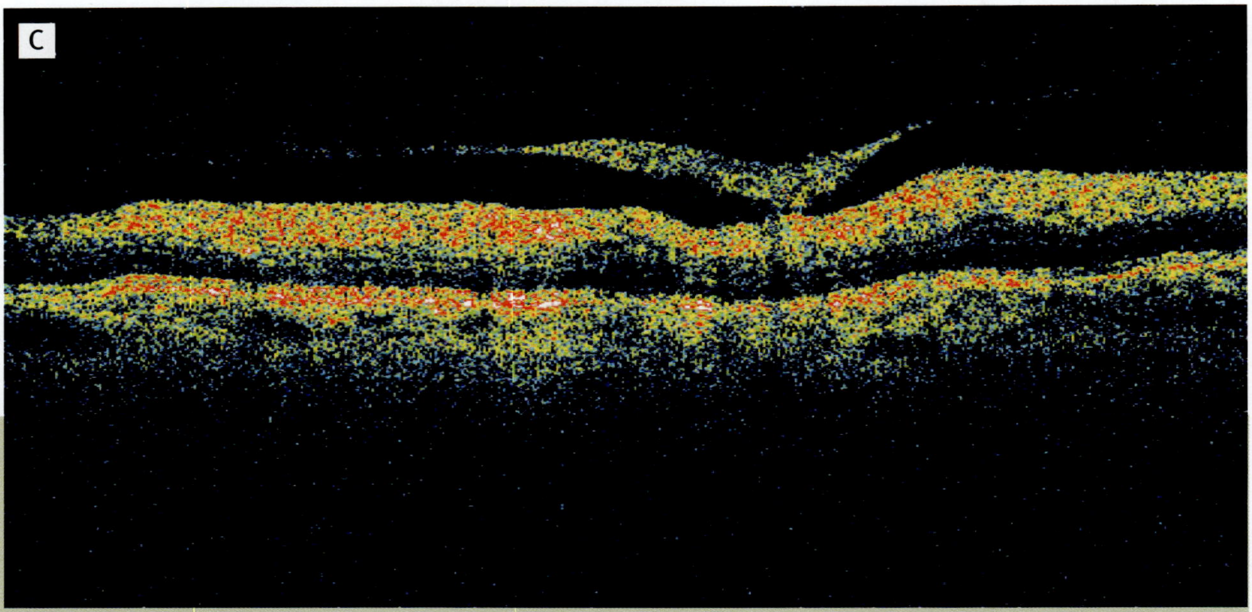

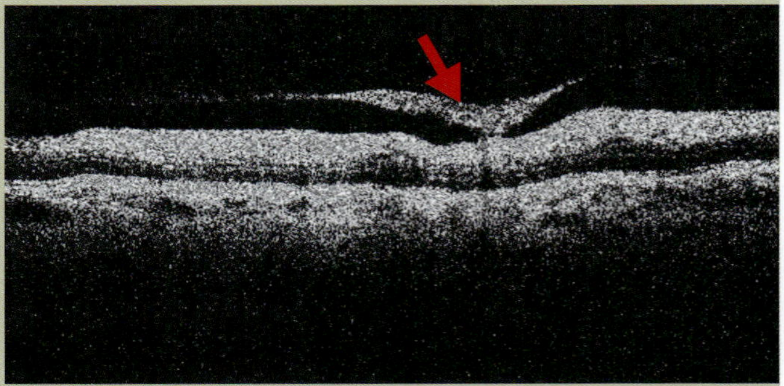

A. Patient with proliferative diabetic retinopathy. Biomicroscopically an elevated new vessel temporally to the optic disc is observed (the arrow shows the scan direction). B. Optical Coherence Tomography shows a thick linear area of high reflectivity inside the vitreous cavity attached to the retina that corresponds to the elevated retinal new vessels (arrow).

PROLIFERATIVE DIABETIC RETINOPATHY

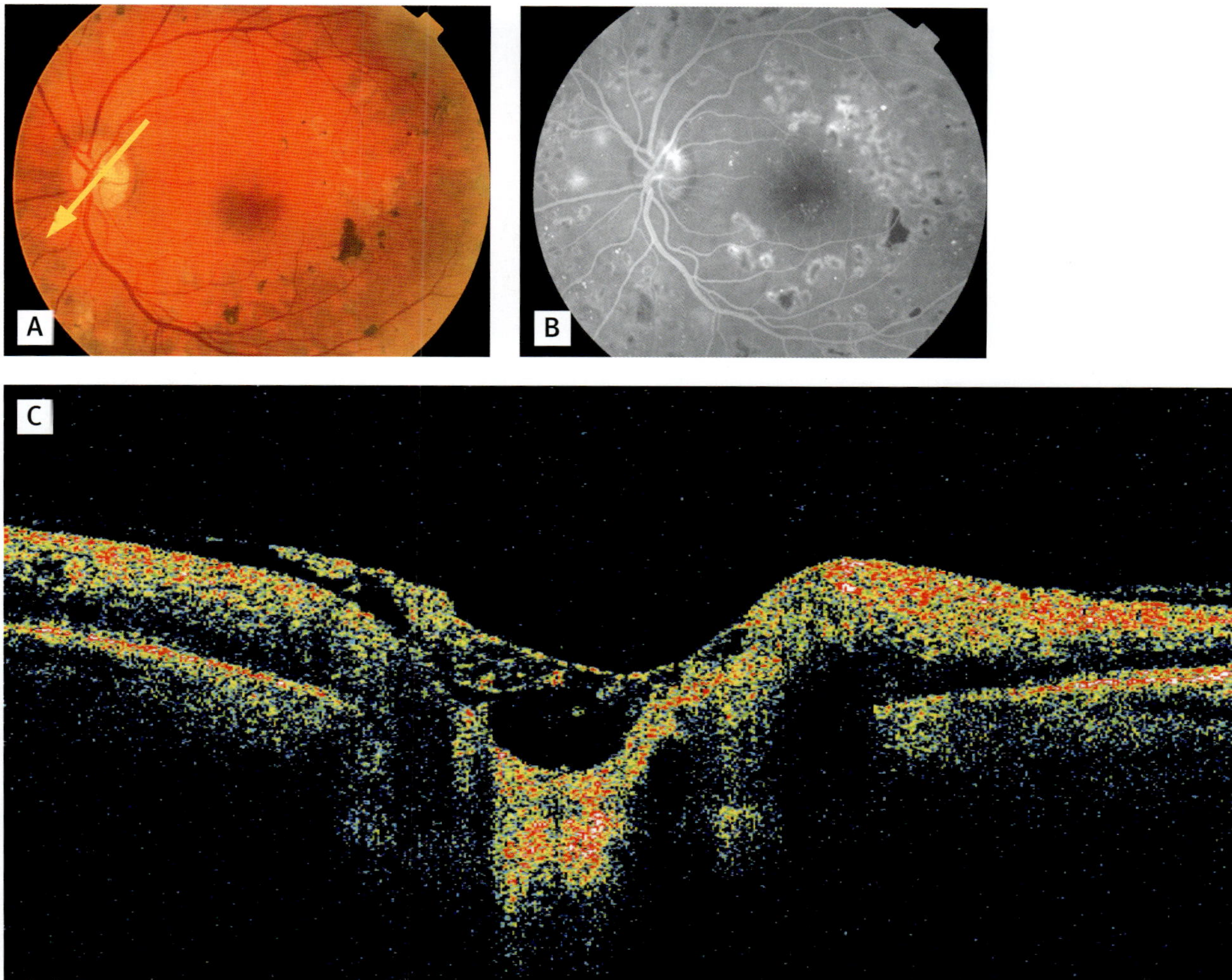

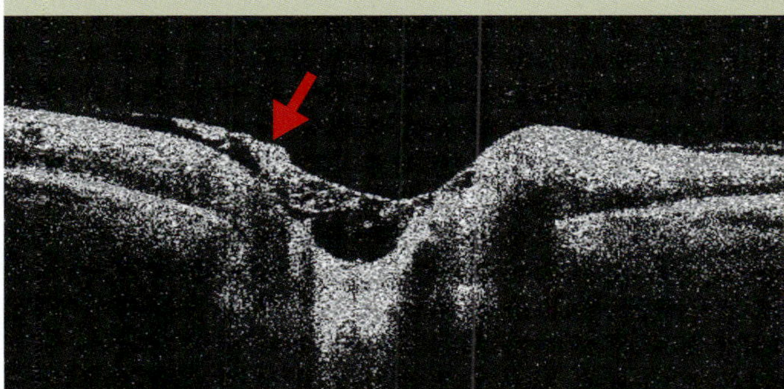

A. Patient with proliferative diabetic retinopathy. Biomicroscopically optic disc neovascularization is Noted (the arrow shows the scan direction). B. Fluorescein angiography shows leakage of dye from the neovascularization. C. Optical Coherence Tomography depicts an area of high reflectivity that is thicker towards the optic disc borders, is attached to the retinal surface and corresponds to the neovascular tissue (arrow).

CHAPTER 7

MACULAR EDEMA

VLASSIS GRIGOROPOULOS

One of the most important applications of Optical Coherence Tomography is the evaluation and follow-up of patients with macular edema. Macular edema can be due to diabetic retinopathy, retinal vein occlusion[2,4], choroidal neovascularization, intraocular surgery, inflammatory diseases, drugs or retinal dystrophies. Biomicroscopy often is not enough to evaluate macular edema and fluorescein angiography is also necessary. Optical Coherence Tomography contributes to the evaluation of macular edema and it is safer than fluorescein angiography[3]. Optical Coherence Tomography also allows for patient follow-up using quantitative criteria. In cases where Optical Coherence Tomography shows resolution of macular edema without some visual acuity recovery, further examinations may be warranted[6]. On the other hand, detection of retinal thinning in the fovea means an irreversible retinal damage with visual acuity loss and therefore, no need for further treatment.

Optical Coherence Tomography can calculate with precision and more sensitivity the retinal thickness in patients with macular edema compared to biomicroscopy. It can quantitatively assess macular edema and help in the follow-up of those patients thanks to its excellent repeatability. We are therefore able to objectively evaluate the effectiveness of the various treatment modalities (laser photocoagulation, intravitreous injection of triamcinolone or anti-angiogenic factors, intraocular systems of steroid delivery, vitrectomy etc).

Optical Coherence Tomography shows diffuse macular edema as an increase of retinal thickness with low reflectivity, mainly in the inner retinal layers, corresponding to an intraretinal concentration of fluid. Cystoid macular edema is presented as large cystic areas of low reflectivity within the inner retina. Diabetic macular edema may coexist with retinal detachment and leakage of intraretinal fluid, hard exudates and intraretinal hemorrhages (retinal areas of high reflectivity with shadowing of the underlying choroid). Optical Coherence Tomography allows us to assess the presence of vitreous traction (a thin area of high reflectivity applying traction to the retinal surface) or retinoschisis in the macular area, factors that play a crucial role in the decision for surgical treatment of diabetic macular edema.

Optical Coherence Tomography also helps to differentiate large cysts from lamellar macular holes that can be present in patients with macular edema of inflammatory origin. Finally, Optical Coherence Tomography can evaluate the presence of epiretinal membranes that cause traction on the macula and propose surgical removal as the most appropriate therapeutic option[1,5].

MACULAR EDEMA

1. Becquet F, Le Rouic JF, Zanlonghi X, Peronnet P, Hermouet-Leclair E, Pousset-Decre C, Ducournau D. Efficiency of surgical treatment for chronic macular edema due to branch vein occlusion. Fr J Ophthalmol 2003; 26: 570-576.

2. Leizaola-Fernandez C, Suarez-Tata L, Quiroz-Mercado H, Colina-Luquez J, Fromow-Guerra J, Jimenez-Sierra JM, Guerrero-Naranjo JL, Morales-Canton V. Vitrectomy with complete posterior hyaloid removal for ischemic central retinal vein occlusion: series of cases. BMC Ophthalmol 2005;20: 10.

3. Lerche RC, Schaudig U, Scholz F, Walter A, Richard G. Structural changes of the retina in retinal vein occlusion – imaging quantification with optical coherence tomography. Ophthalmic Surg Lasers 2001; 32:272-280.

4. Ozdemir H, Karacorlu M, Karacorlu S. Serous macular detachment in central retinal vein occlusion. Retina 2005 ; 25 : 561-563.

5. Patelli F, Radice P, Zumbo G, Fasolino G, Marchi S, Optical coherence tomography evaluation of macular edema after radial optic neurotomy in patients affected by central retinal vein occlusion. Semin Ophthalmol 2004;19:21-24.

6. Spaide RF, Lee JK, Klancnik JK, Gross NE. Optical coherence tomography of branch retinal vein occlusion. Retina 2003; 23: 343-347.

MACULAR EDEMA DUE TO RETINAL VEIN OCCLUSION

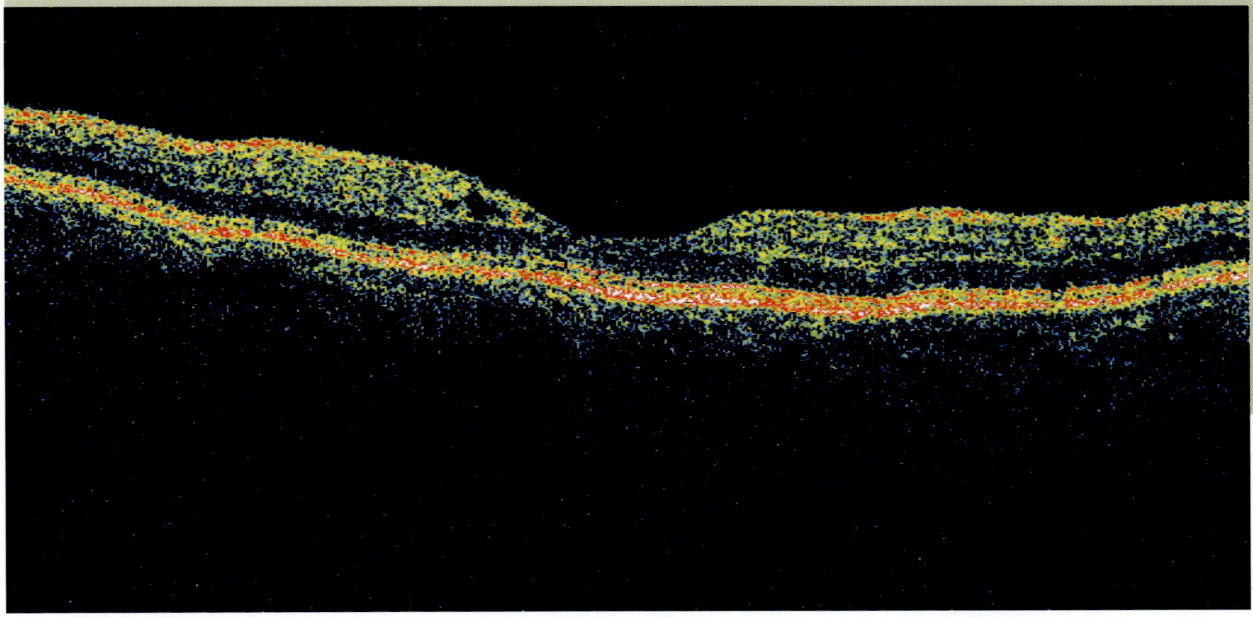

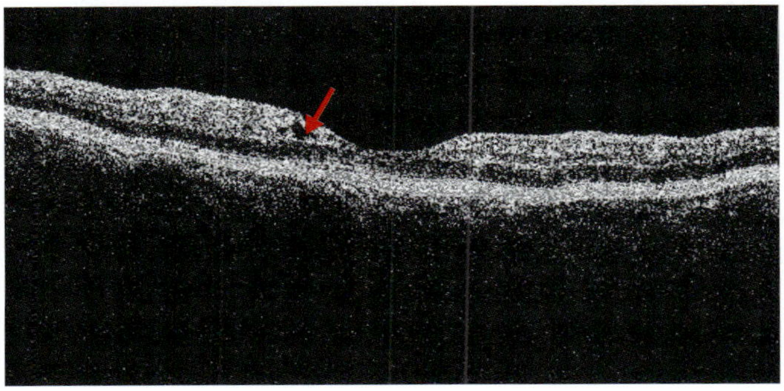

Patient with branch retinal venous thrombosis of 19 months duration. There is a small parafoveal area of low reflectivity due to mild remaining edema (small arrow). Foveal thickness and architecture are normal.

MACULAR EDEMA DUE TO RETINAL VEIN OCCLUSION

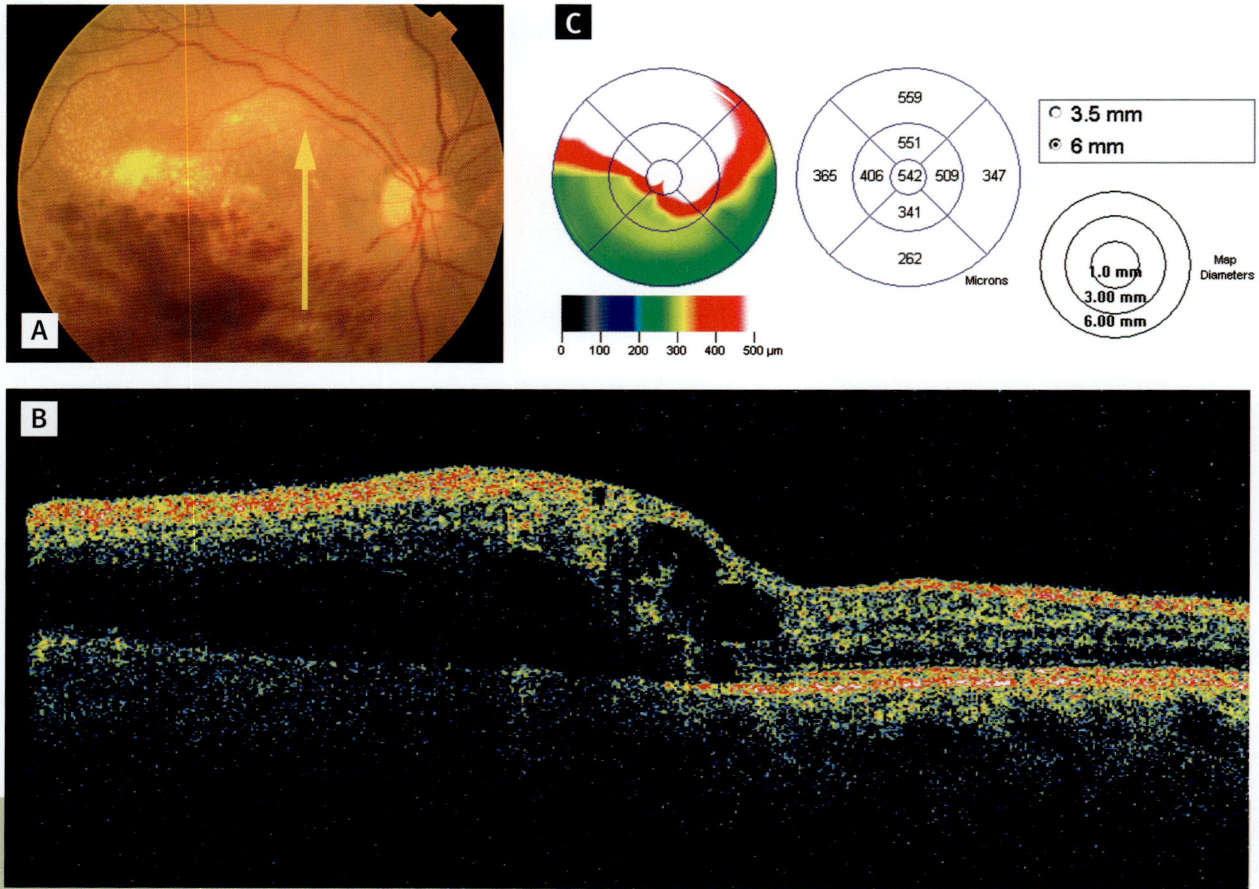

Patient with inferior temporal branch retinal venous occlusion. A. There are diffuse exudative elements around the fovea and haemorrhages in the affected area (the arrow shows the scan direction). B. High reflectivity of the inner retinal layer is detected due to blood accumulation (small arrow). Note the shadow of the underlying tissues from the increased light absorption by the blood (big arrow). Multiple intraretinal cystic formations of low reflectivity are detected in the fovea corresponding to the cystic retinal edema (thick arrow). C. The retinal map analysis shows increased retinal thickness in the central 1mm diameter area.

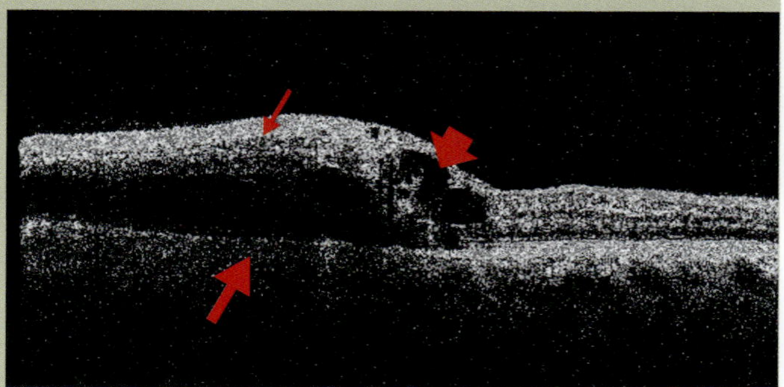

MACULAR EDEMA DUE TO RETINAL VEIN OCCLUSION

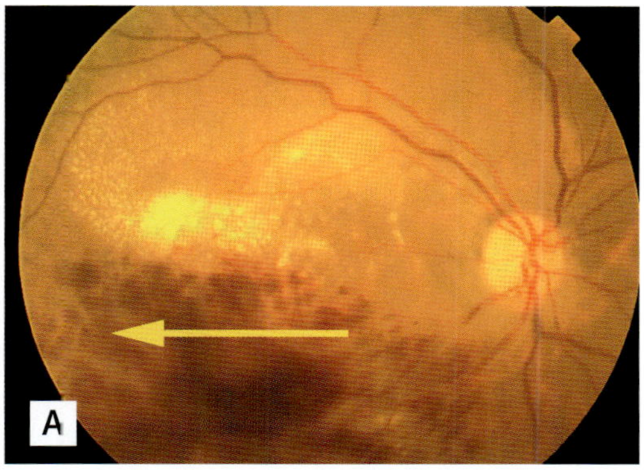

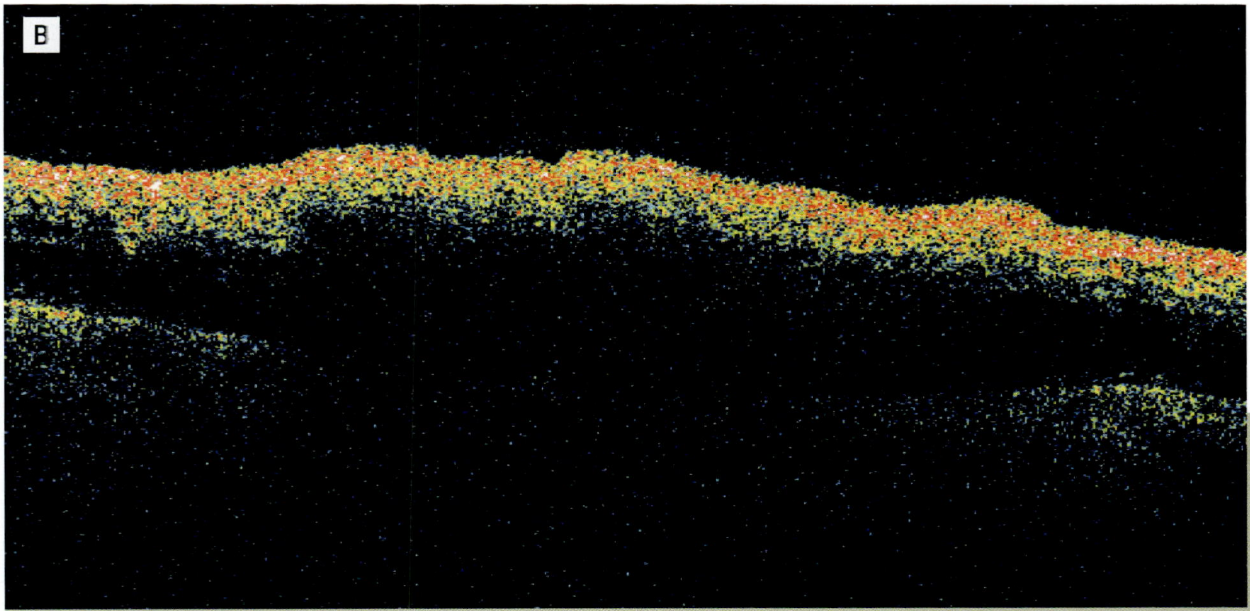

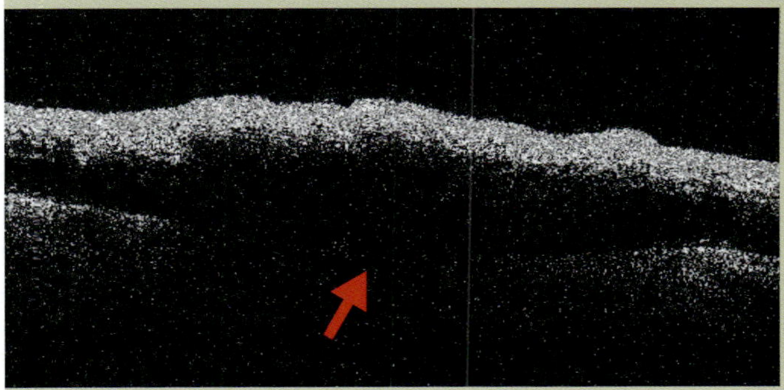

A. Patient of page 184 (the arrow shows the scan direction). B. Optical Coherence Tomography shows the diffuse haemorrhage as an area of high reflectivity in the inner retinal layers with shadowing of the underlying tissues due to the increased light absorption by the blood (arrow).

MACULAR EDEMA DUE TO RETINAL VEIN OCCLUSION

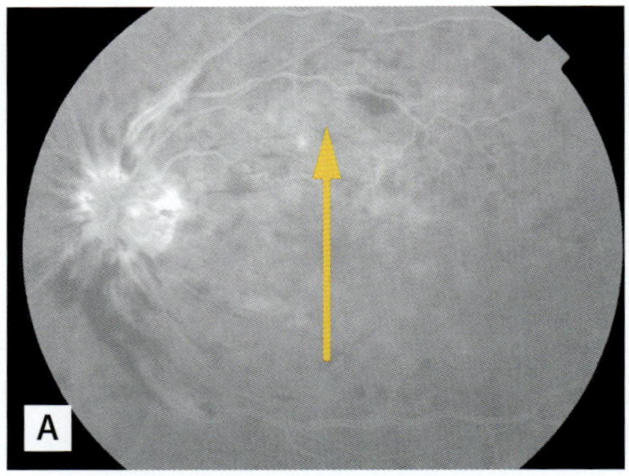

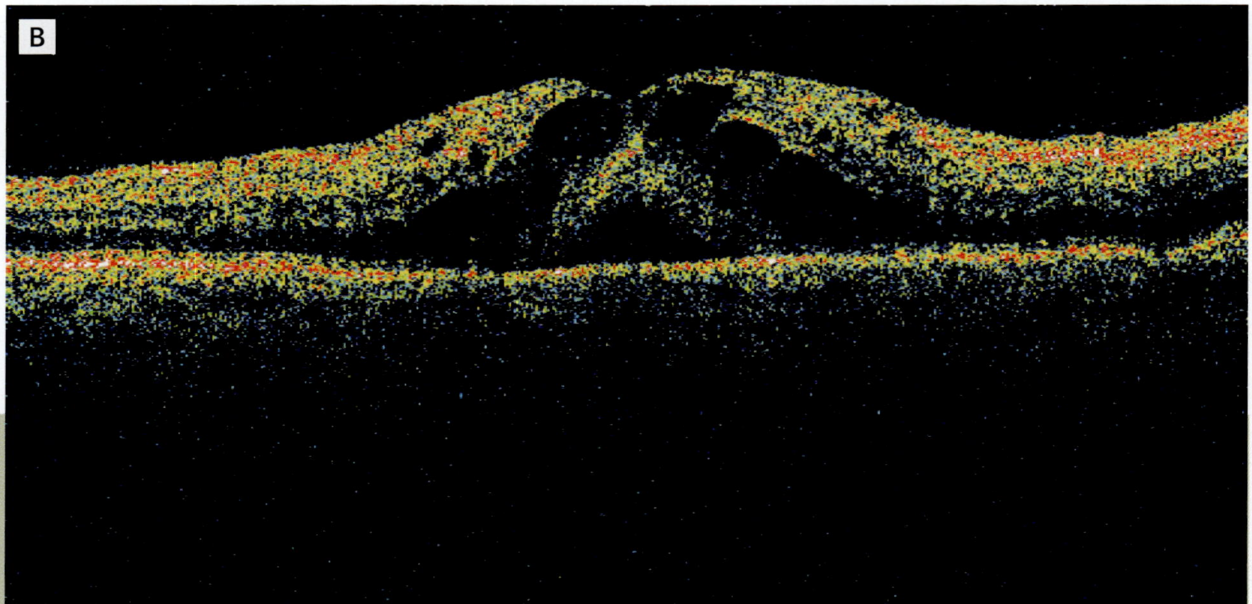

Patient six months after central retinal vein occlusion. A. Engorgement of the vein system with macular and optic disc edema (the arrow shows the scan direction). B. There are multiple intraretinal cystic formations of low reflectivity due to the cystoid edema (small arrows). In the fovea there is an area of low reflectivity between the retina and the retinal pigment epithelium corresponding to subretinal fluid accumulation (big arrow).

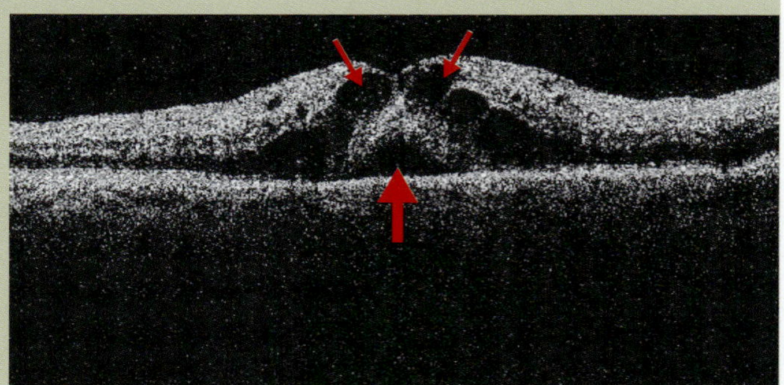

MACULAR EDEMA DUE TO RETINAL VEIN OCCLUSION

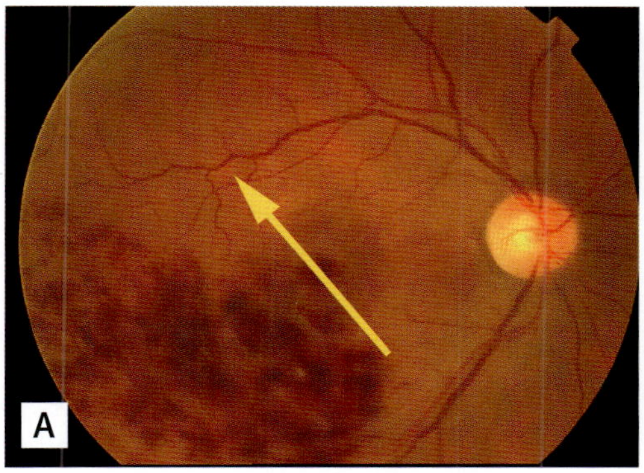

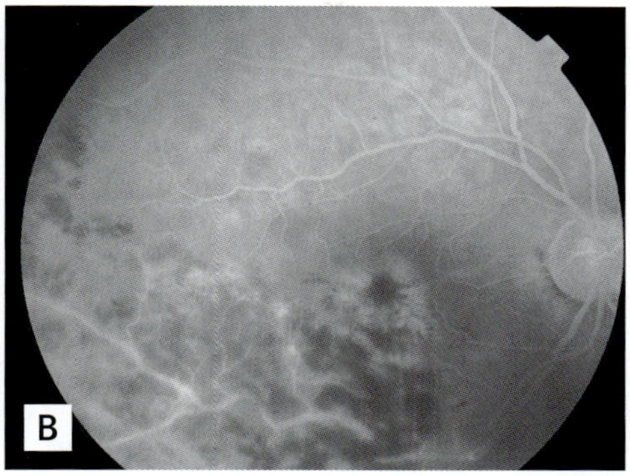

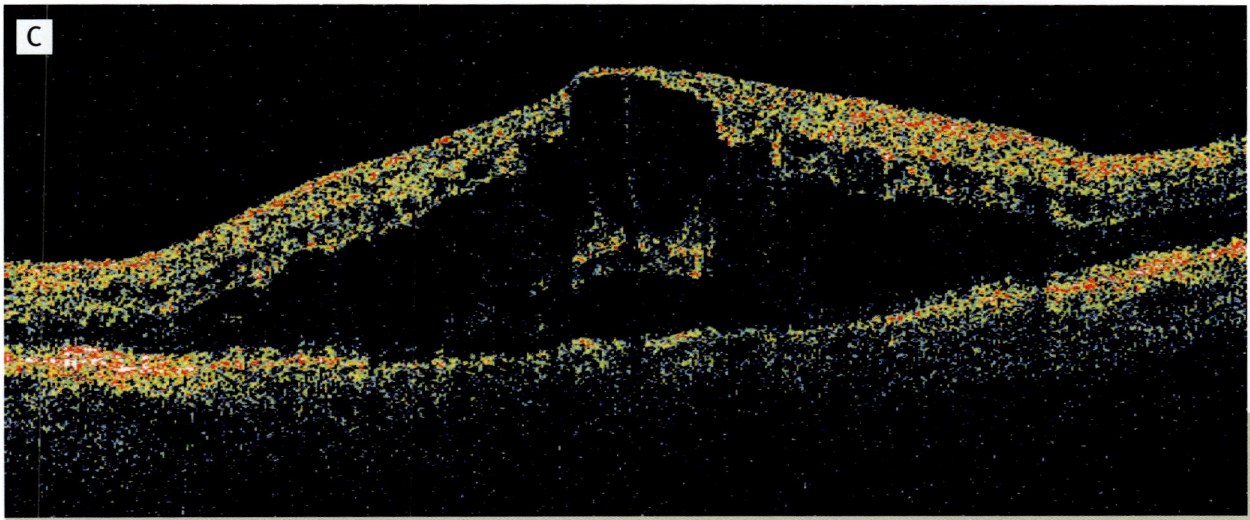

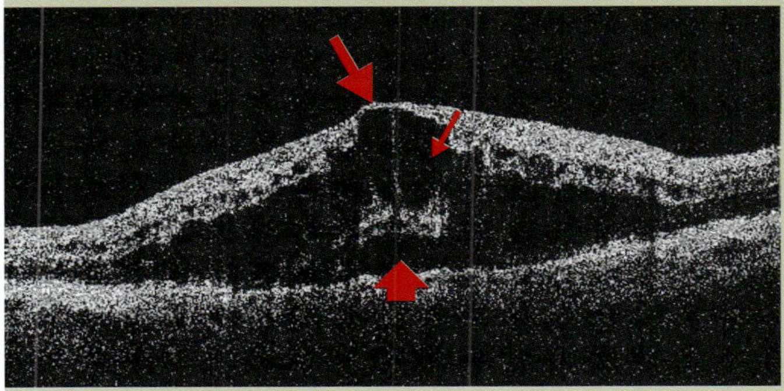

Patient with branch retinal vein occlusion. A. Note the haemorrhages and the prominent cystic macular edema (the arrow shows the scan direction). B. Fluorescein angiography shows dye leakage due to the cystic macular edema. C. A diffuse intraretinal area of low reflectivity is detected due to the diffuse cystoid edema (small arrow) and because of it the retinal tissue in the fovea is very thin (big arrow). The total foveal thickness is increased because of the significant edema. An area of low reflectivity is also detected between the retina and the retinal pigment epithelium corresponding to a focal retinal detachment (thick arrow).

POSTOPERATIVE MACULAR EDEMA

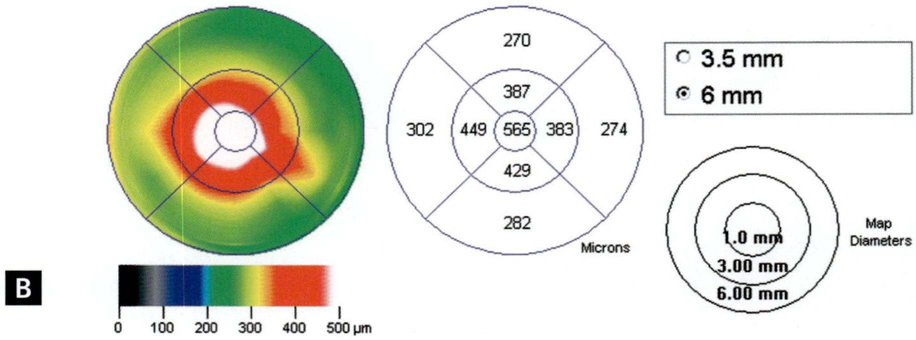

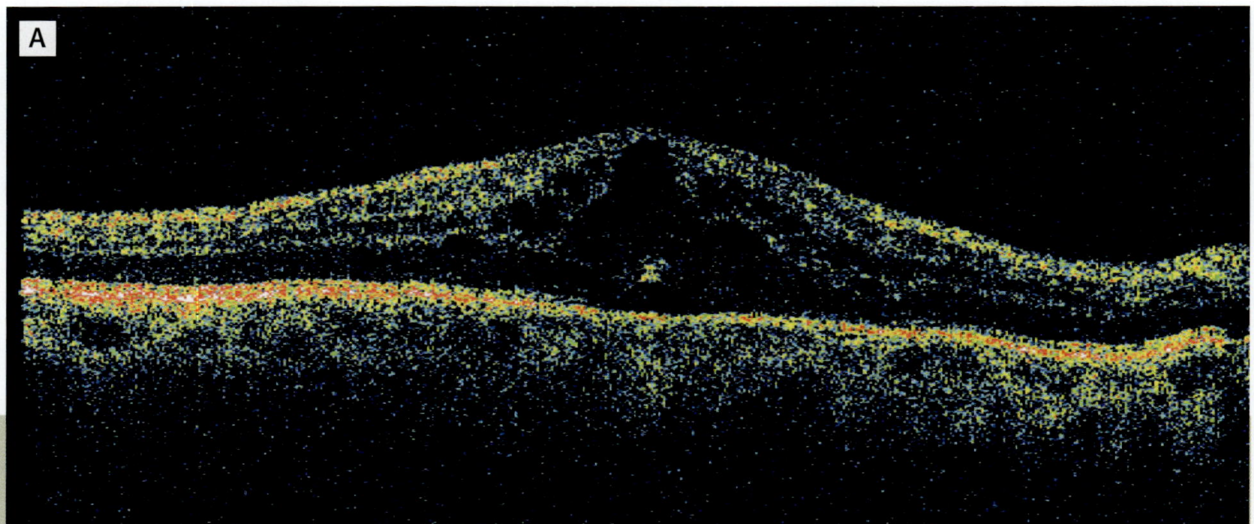

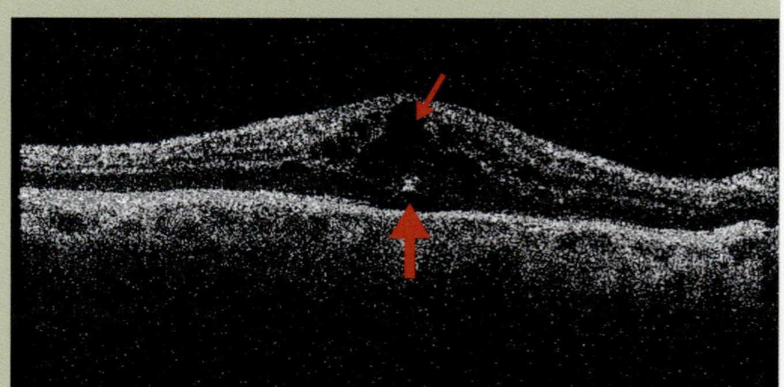

Patient 4 weeks after uneventful cataract surgery and posterior chamber intraocular lens implantation. A. There are multiple intraretinal cystic formations of low reflectivity due to the postoperative cystoid edema (Irvine-Gass) (small arrow). An area of low reflectivity between the retina and the retinal pigment epithelium is detected in the fovea and corresponds to subretinal fluid (big arrow). B. Retinal map analysis, as created automatically by the software of the Optical Coherence Tomography, shows an increased retinal thickness in the central 1mm diameter area.

POSTOPERATIVE MACULAR EDEMA

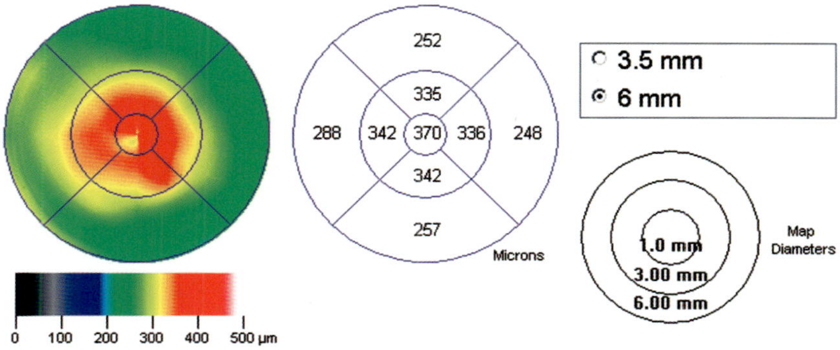

B

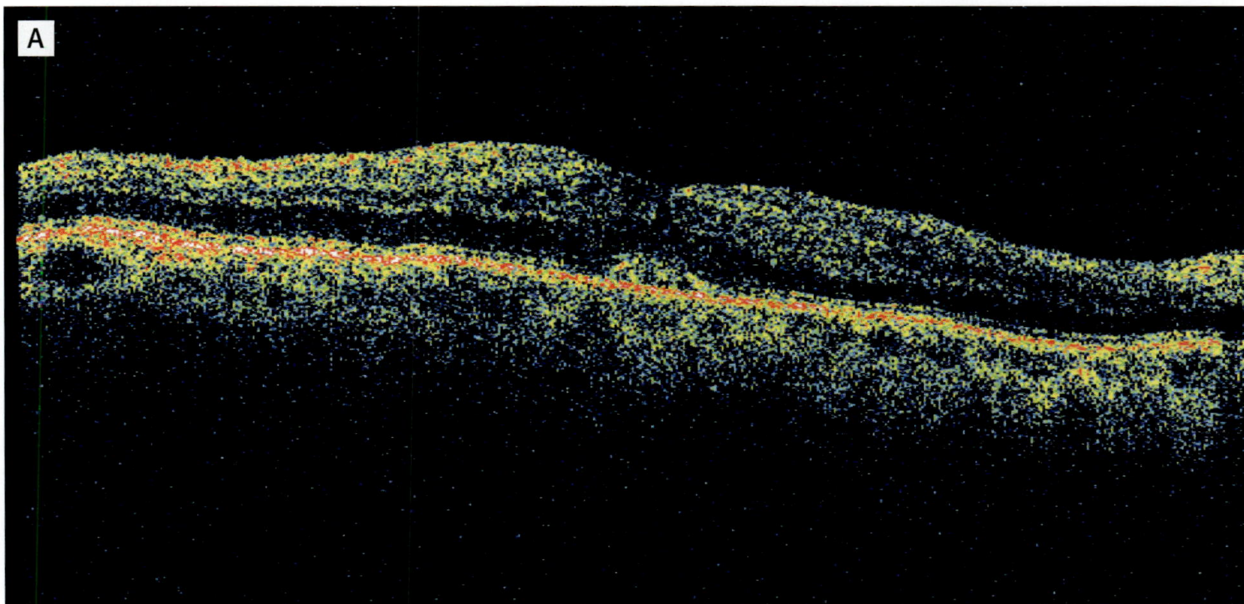

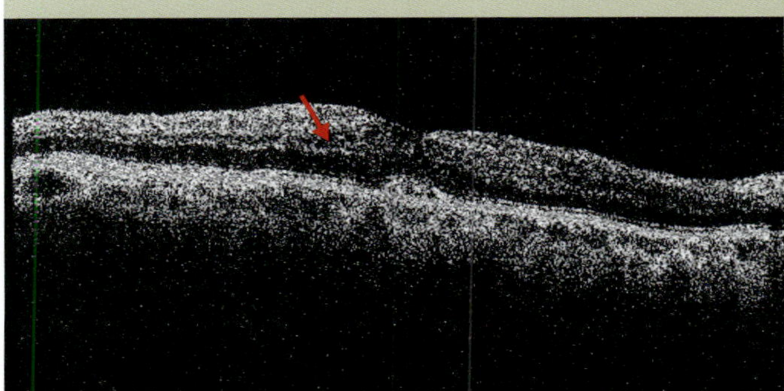

The patient of page 188 three months later.

POSTOPERATIVE MACULAR EDEMA

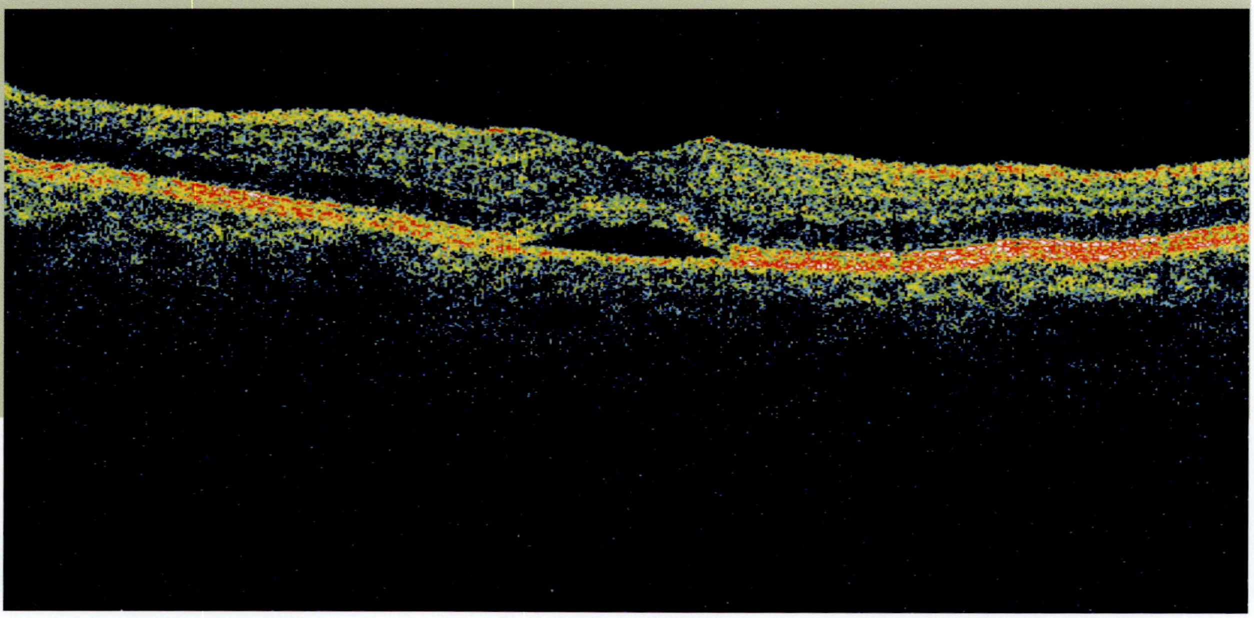

Patient with macular edema after complicated cataract surgery. There is an area of low reflectivity between the retina and the retinal pigment epithelium due to a focal retinal detachment (arrow). There is a mild increase of retinal thickness due to the diffuse edema.

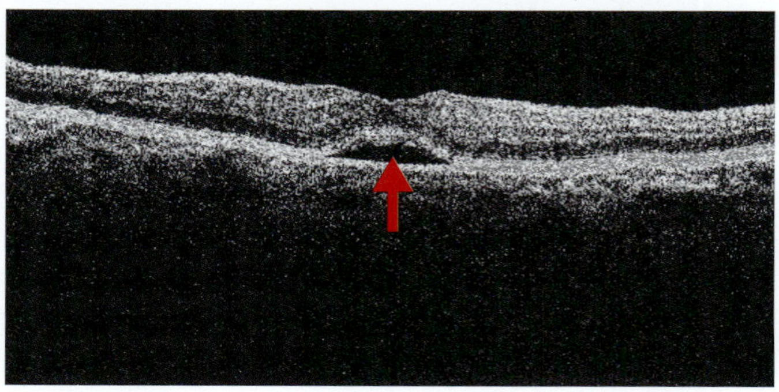

POSTOPERATIVE MACULAR EDEMA

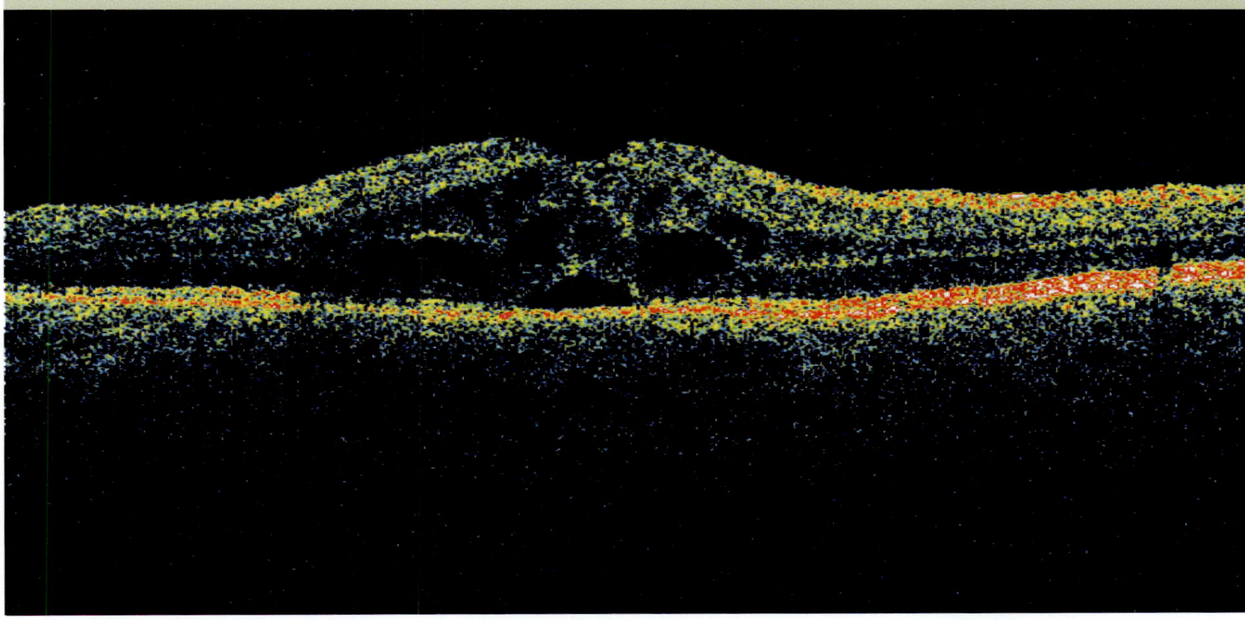

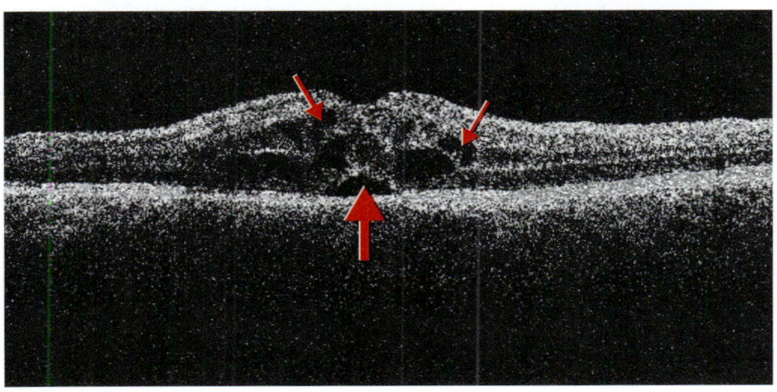

Patient with cataract surgery two years earlier and a posterior YAG capsulotomy six months before Optical Coherence Tomography examination. There are multiple cystic intraretinal formations of low reflectivity due to cystoid postoperative edema (small arrows). An area of low reflectivity is detected between the retina and the retinal pigment epithelium in the fovea corresponding to subretinal fluid (big arrow).

INFLAMMATORY MACULAR EDEMA

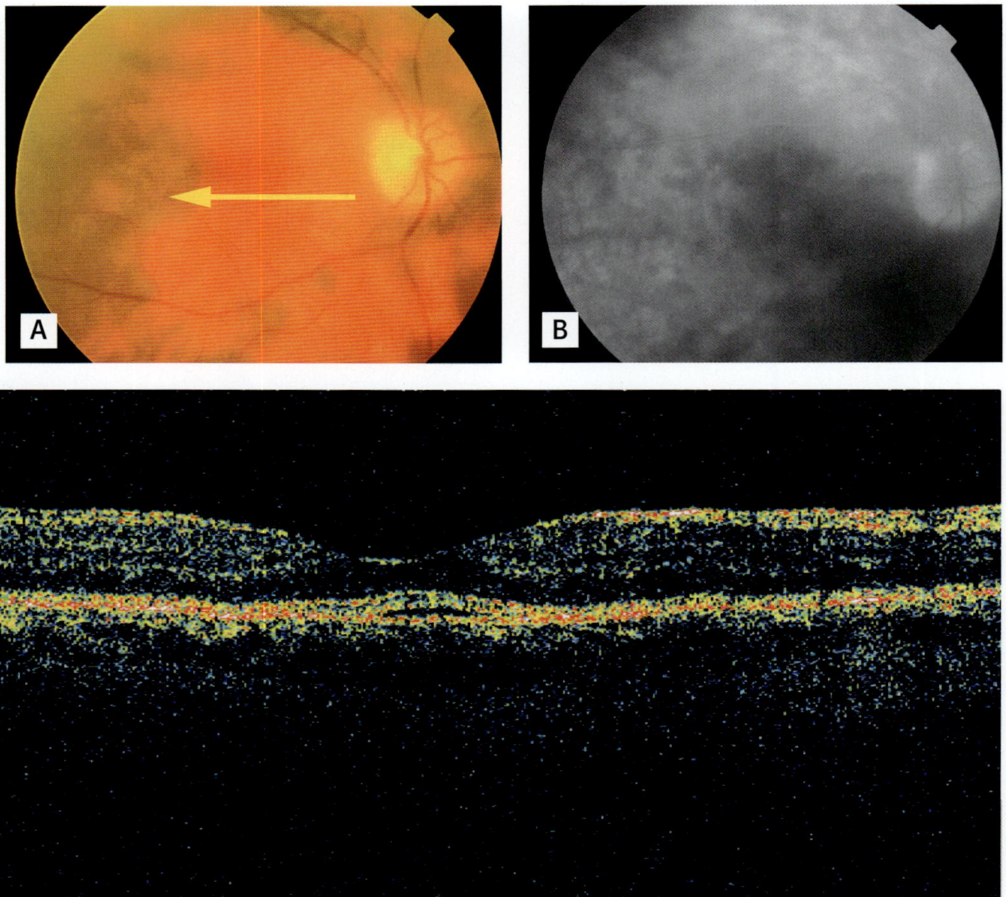

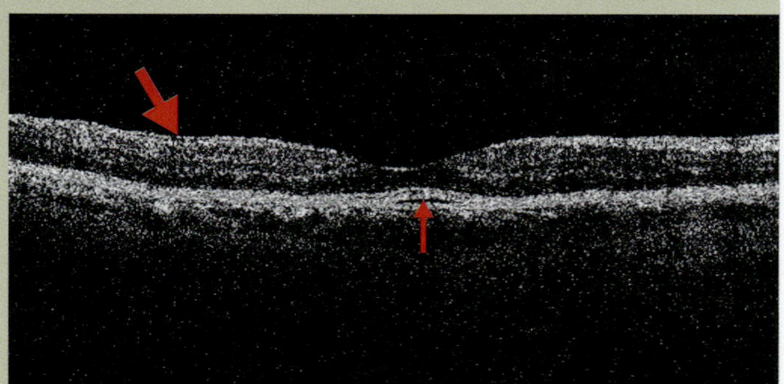

The right eye of a patient with birdshot retinochoroidopathy. A. Vitreous inflammatory reaction, optic disc edema and the characteristic creamy yellow choroidal infiltrations are observed biomicroscopically around the optic disc (the arrow shows the scan direction). B. Fluorescein angiography shows dye leakage in the optic disc (hot disk) and signs of active perivasculitis. C. Optical Coherence Tomography shows an area of low reflectivity between the retina and the retinal pigment epithelium corresponding to a retinal detachment in the foveal area (small arrow). There is also a thin line of high reflectivity on the retinal surface corresponding to an epiretinal membrane (big arrow).

INFLAMMATORY MACULAR EDEMA

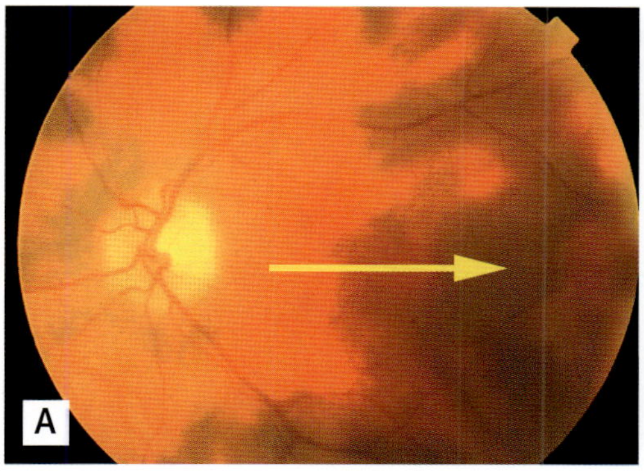

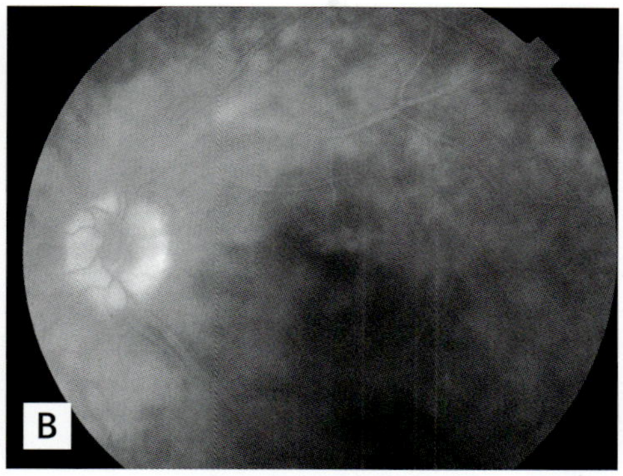

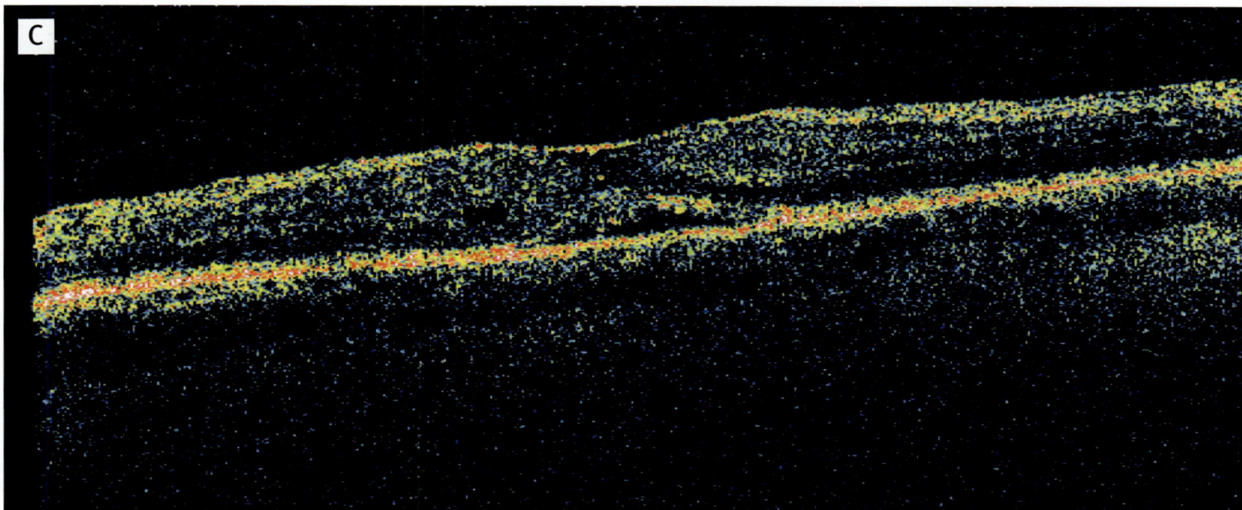

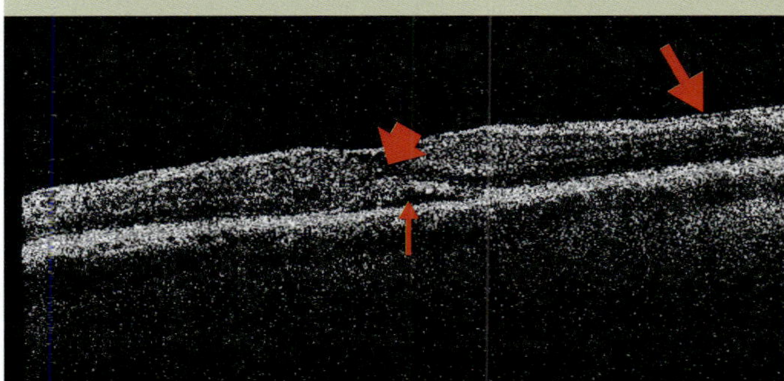

The left eye of the patient of page 192. A. Vitreous inflammatory reaction, optic disc edema and the characteristic creamy yellow choroidal infiltrations are observed biomicroscopically around the optic disc (the arrow shows the scan direction). B. Fluorescein angiography shows dye leakage in the optic disc, a few signs of active perivasculitis and macular leakage. C. Optical Coherence Tomography shows an area of low reflectivity between the retina and the retinal pigment epithelium corresponding to a retinal detachment in the foveal area (small arrow). There is also a thin line of high reflectivity on the retinal surface corresponding to an epiretinal membrane (big arrow). An increase of the retinal thickness is also detected due to diffuse edema (thick arrow).

INFLAMMATORY MACULAR EDEMA

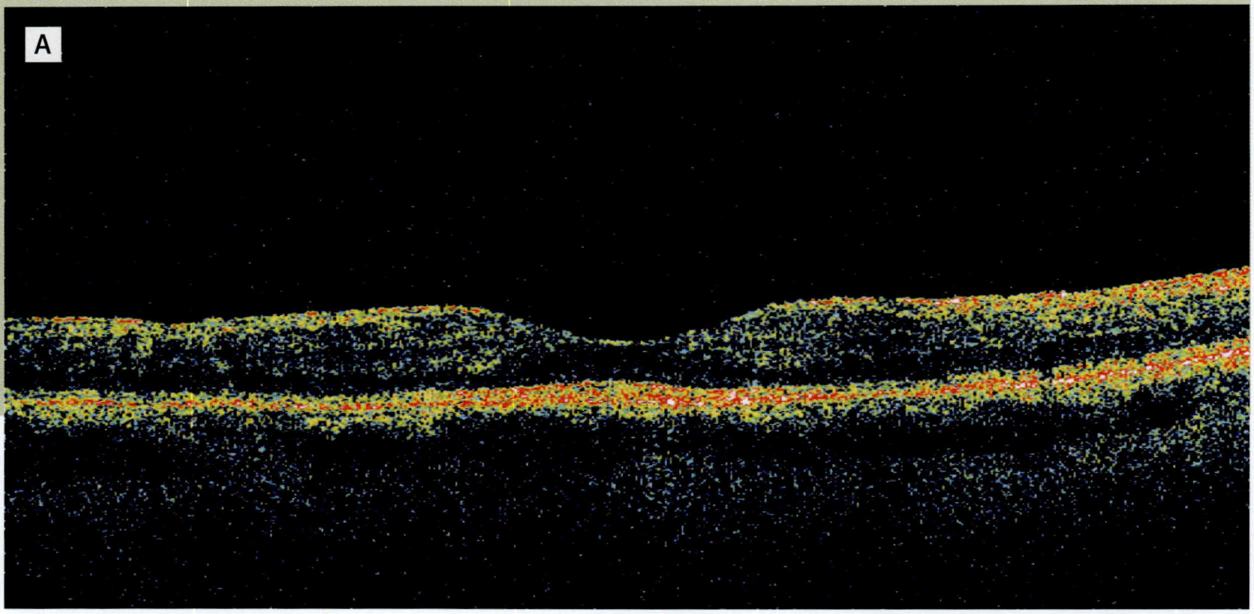

The patient of page 192 three months after initiation of corticosteroid systemic therapy. Note in the right eye (A) the resolution of the subretinal fluid and in the left eye (B) its reduction (small arrow) with a decrease in retinal edema.

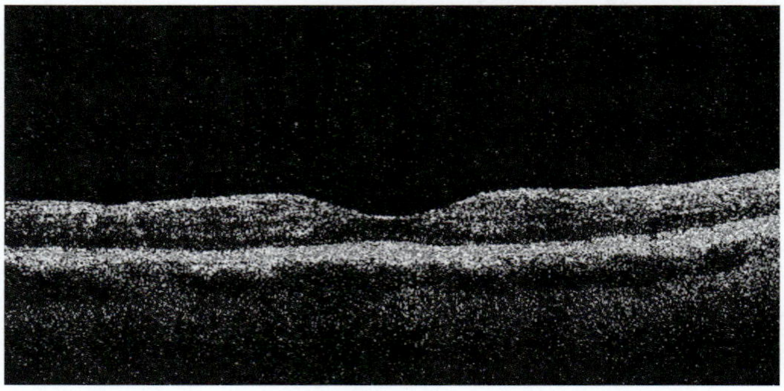

INFLAMMATORY MACULAR EDEMA

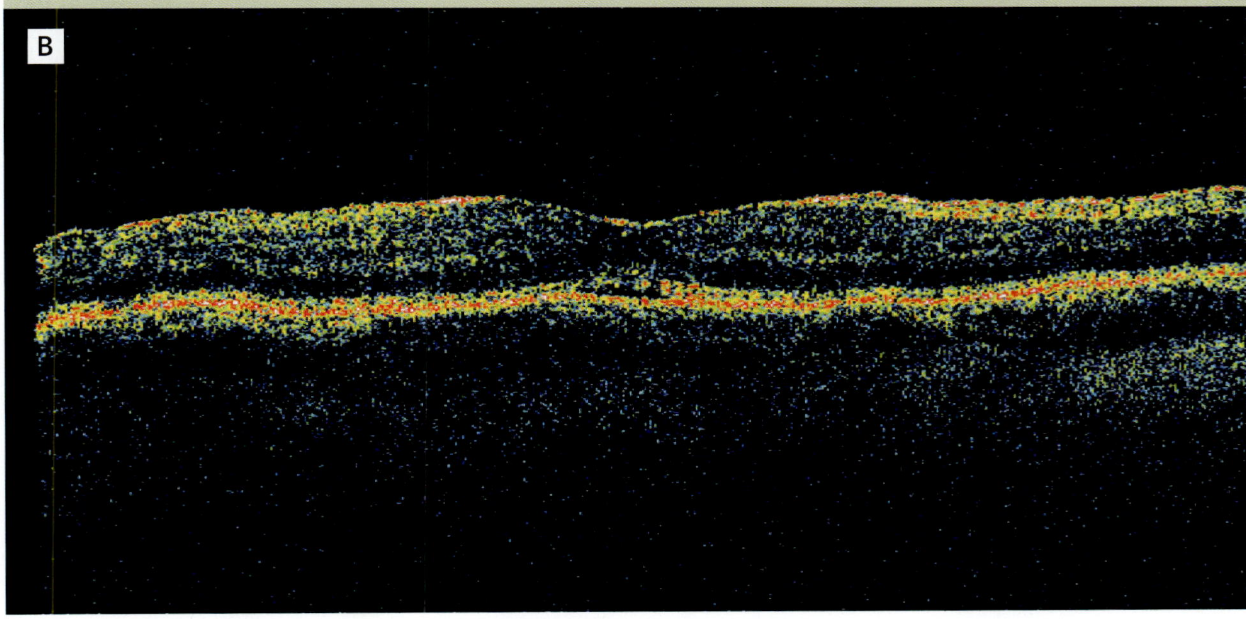

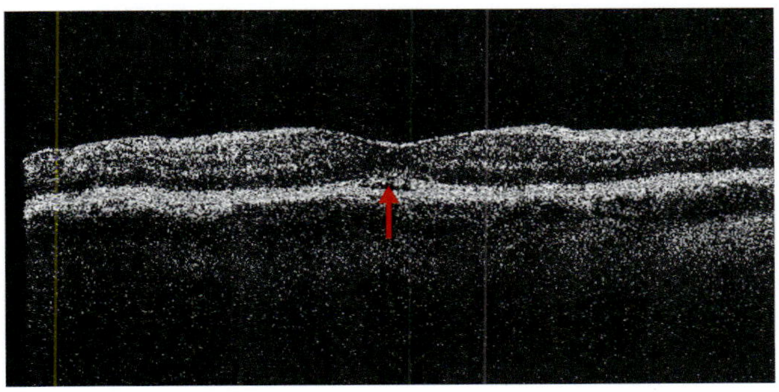

DRUG – RELATED MACULAR EDEMA

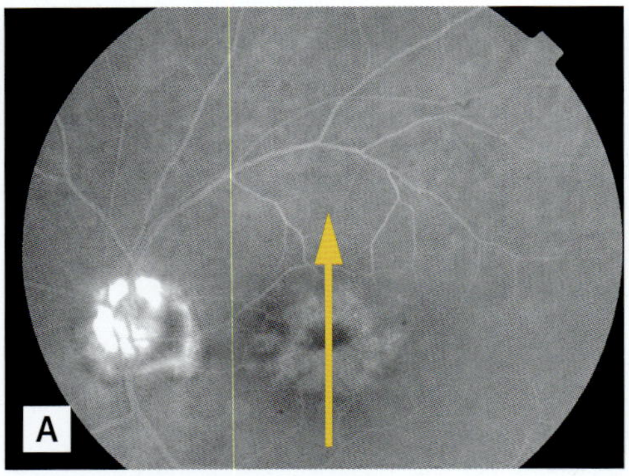

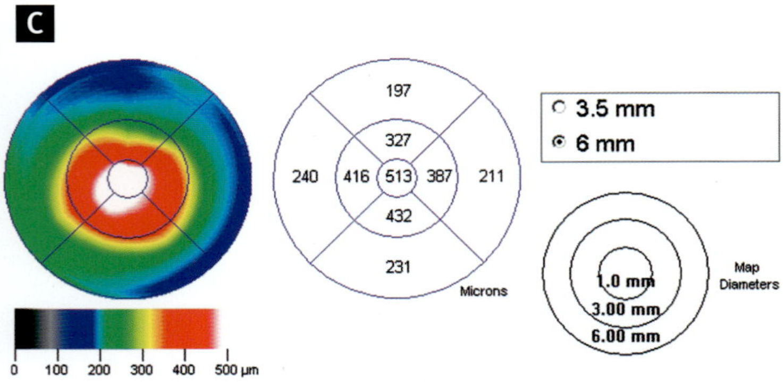

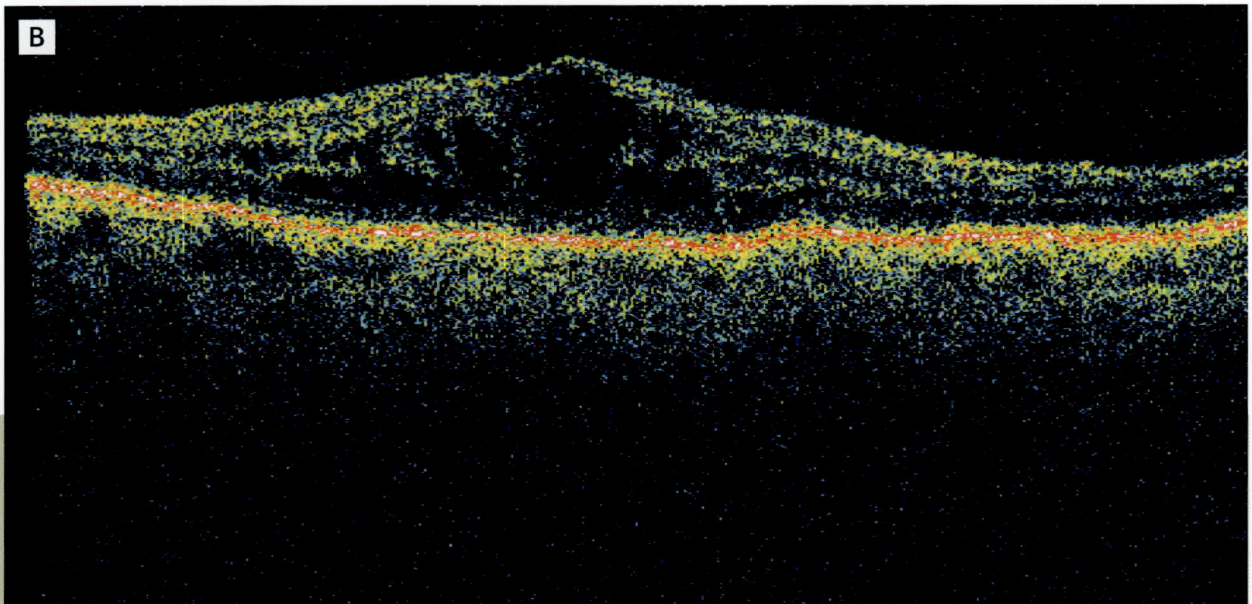

Patient with pseudophakia and posterior capsule rupture who started the topical use of prostanglandin analogue drops one day before Optical Coherence Tomography examination. The patient visited the ophthalmologist because of decreased visual acuity. A. Fluorescein angiography shows the typical cystic macular edema (arrow shows the scan direction). B. There are multiple intraretinal cystic formations of low reflectivity due to cystoid macular edema (arrow). C. Retinal map analysis shows an increase of retinal thickness in the central 1mm diameter area.

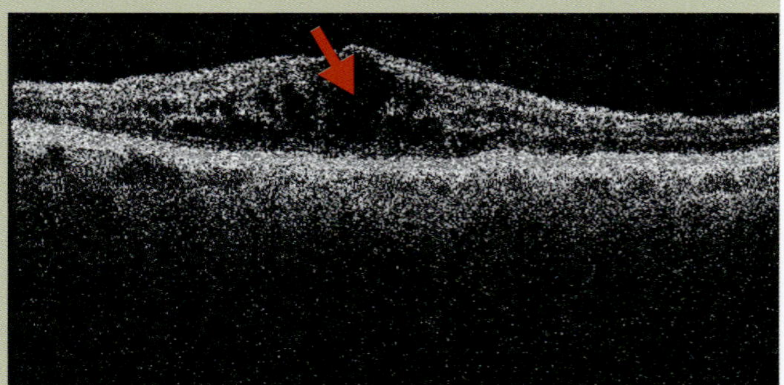

DRUG – RELATED MACULAR EDEMA

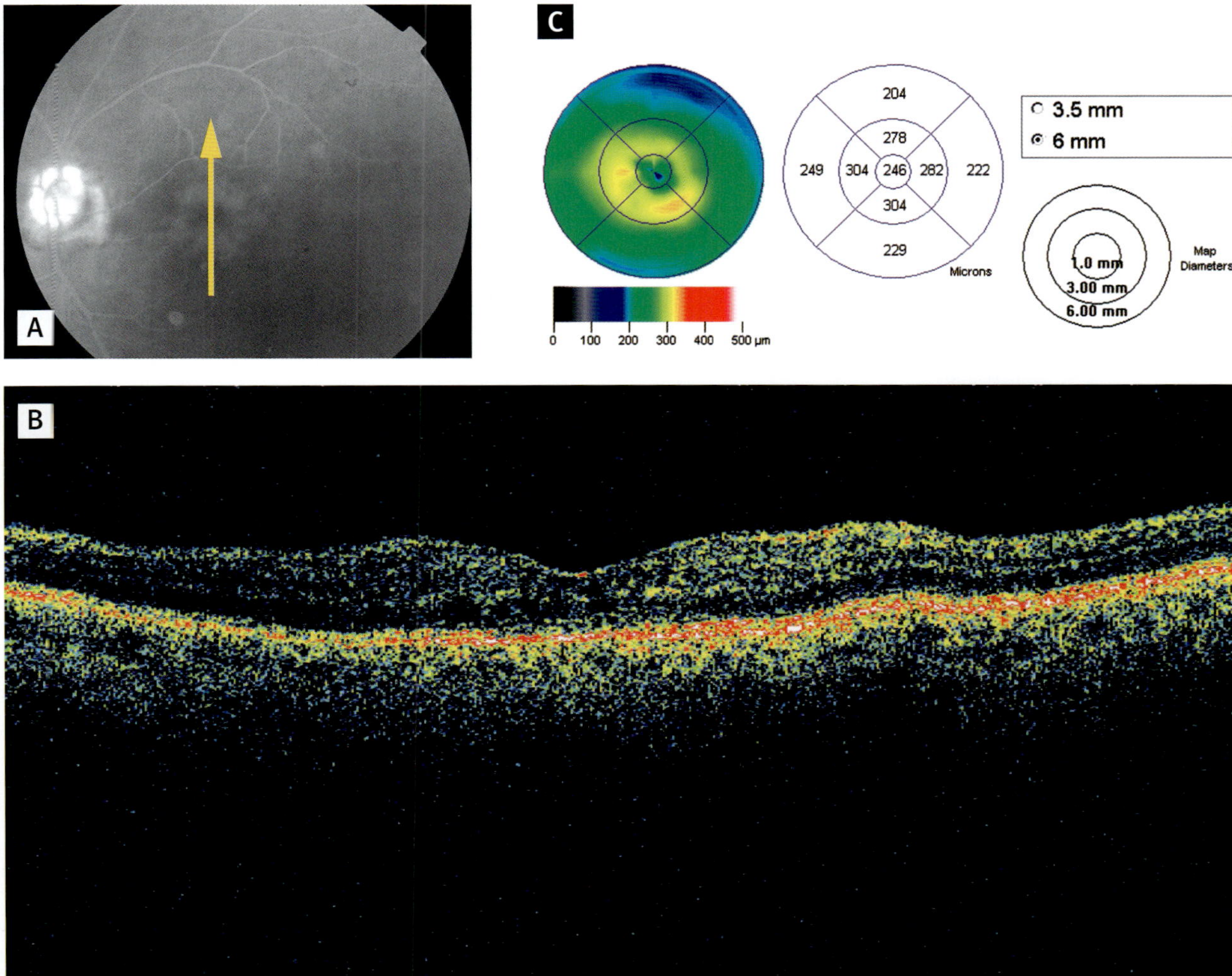

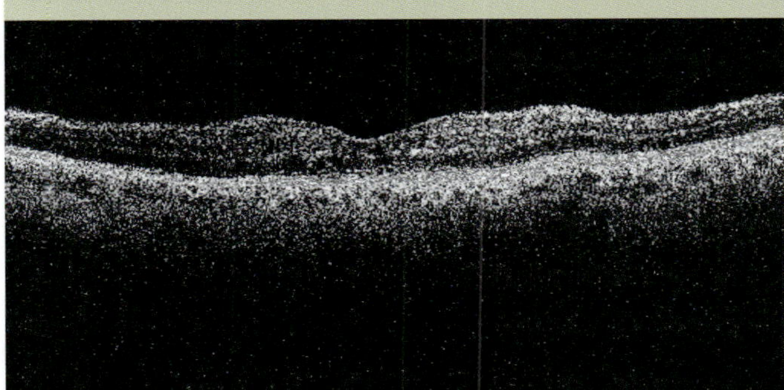

The patient of page 196 five days after discontinuation of prostanglandin analogue therapy and the initiation of topical non steroidal anti-inflammatory treatment. A. Fluorescein angiography shows a significant regression of the edema (the arrow shows the scan direction). The visual acuity is improved. B. Elimination of retinal cysts is also detected but the retinal thickness remains slightly higher because of the diffuse edema. C. This is clearly shown in the retinal map analysis.

TRAUMATIC MACULAR EDEMA

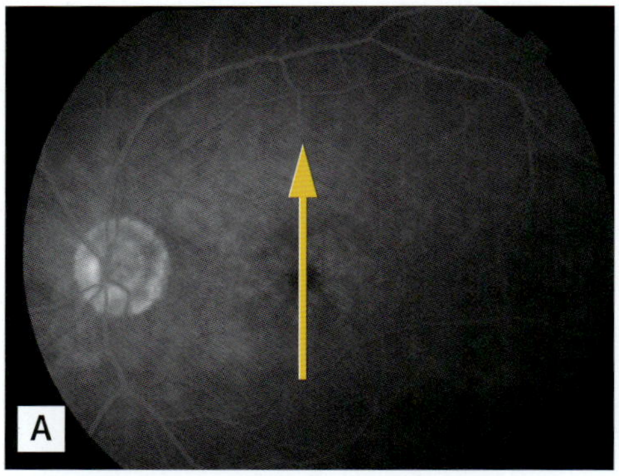

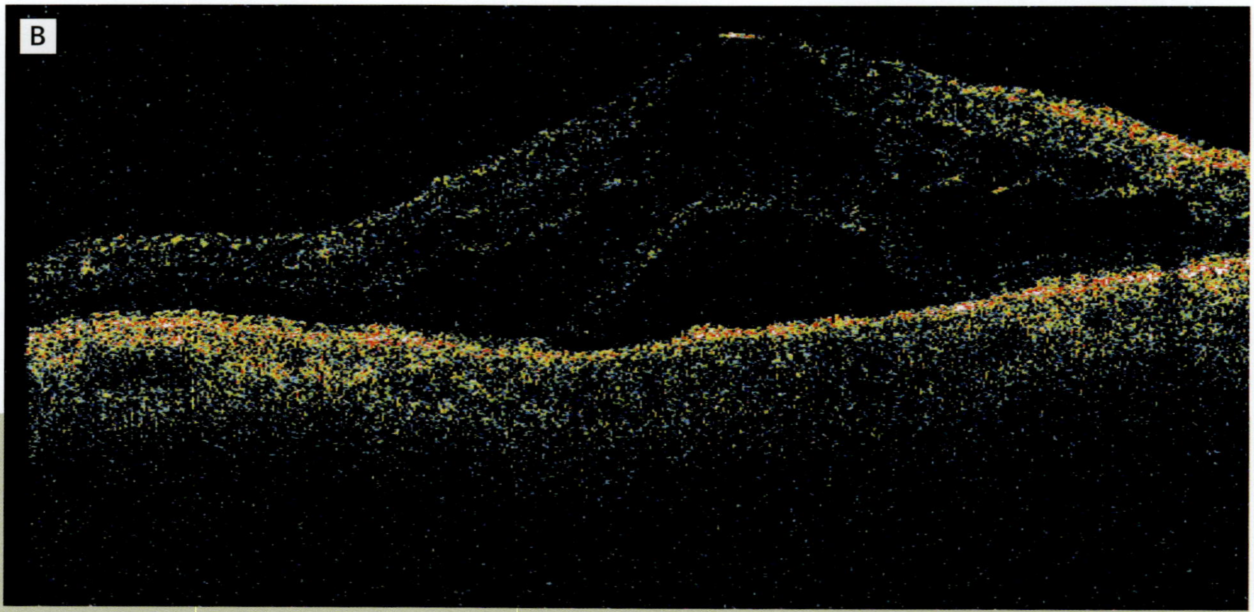

A. Patient after a blunt ocular injury. Fluorescein angiography detects cystoid macular edema (the arrow shows the scan direction). B. Optical Coherence Tomography presents multiple intraretinal cystic formations due to cystoid retinal edema (small arrow). An area of low reflectivity is detected between the retina and the retinal pigment epithelium in the fovea and corresponds to subretinal fluid (big arrow).

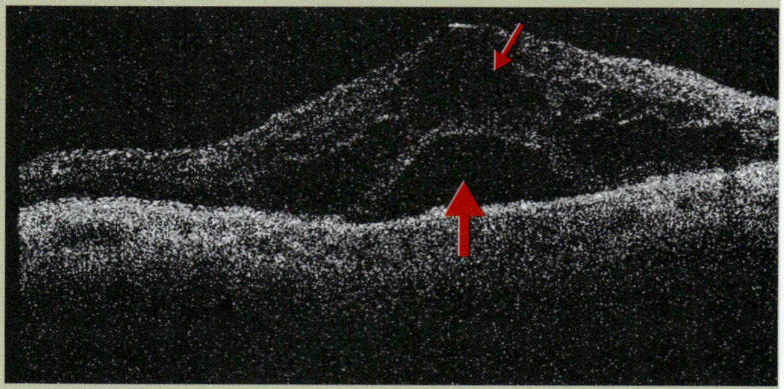

TRAUMATIC MACULAR EDEMA

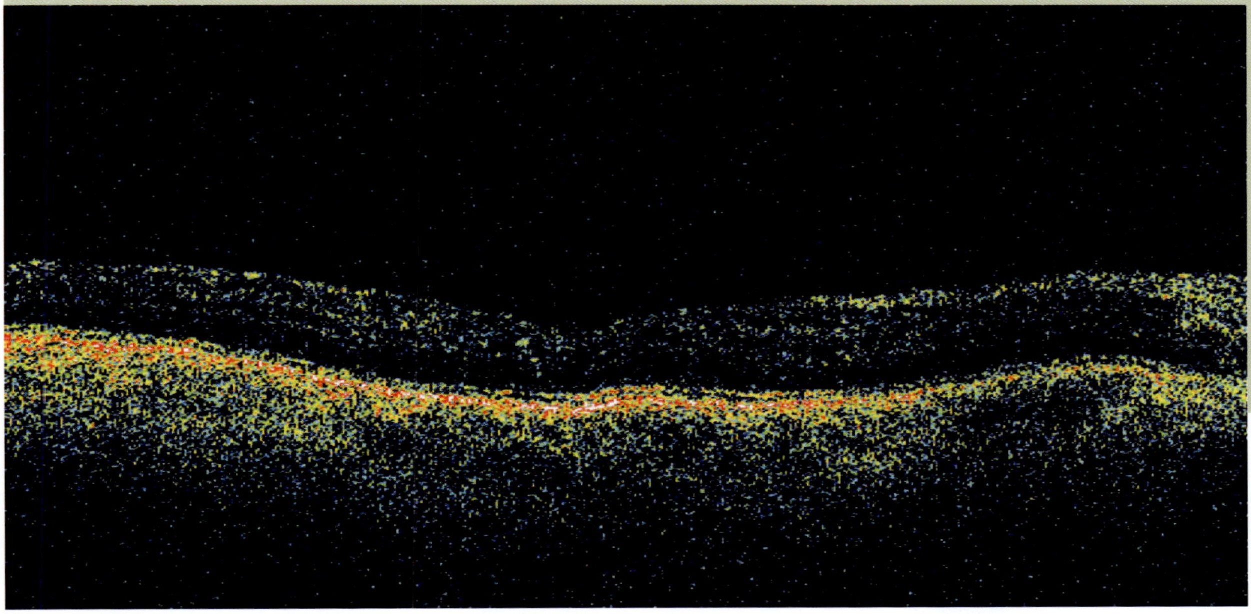

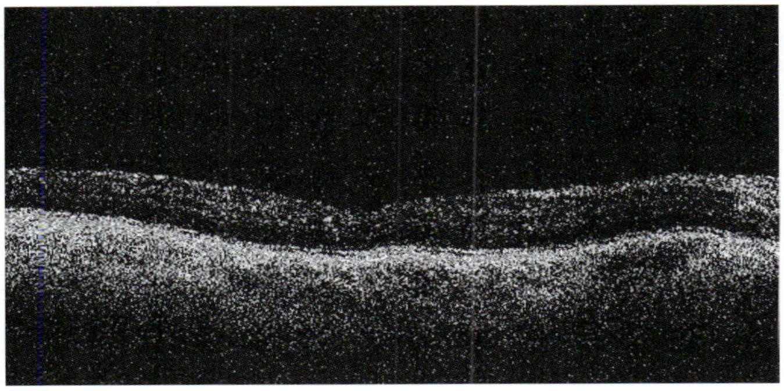

The patient of page 198 nineteen months later without any treatment. Note the significant decrease of retinal edema and the disappearance of the subretinal fluid.

CHAPTER 8

MYOPIA

PANTELIS NIKOLAIDIS, VLASSIS GRIGOROPOULOS

CHOROIDAL NEOVASCULARIZATION

Degenerative myopia is one of the main causes of blindness. Macular degeneration, which often accompanies it, is its most frequent complication. It usually appears in young people and may lead to central retinal pigment epithelium atrophy.

Important signs of macular degeneration are the rupture of Bruch's membrane (lacquer cracks), that often lead to a decrease in visual acuity, especially when complicated with hemorrhages, and type II choroidal neovascular membranes (located above the retinal pigment epithelium). In the presence of choroidal neovascular membrane Optical Coherence Tomography shows an area of high reflectivity between the neurosensory retina and the retinal pigment epithelium[1]. It is also possible to detect the subretinal fluid, located usually around the lesion, as an area of low reflectivity under the retina[3]. The choroidal shadow under the neovascular membrane varies, depending on the density and the reflectivity of the lesion. In advanced stages the reflectivity is very high due to the scar formed. Absorption of the subretinal fluid and the intraretinal edema are important signs of neovascular membrane regression.

Type I neovascular membranes are less often observed under the retinal pigment epithelium. Optical Coherence Tomography shows alterations similar to those observed in age related macular degeneration consisting in rupture and elevation of the retinal pigment epithelium with subretinal and intraretinal fluid formation. The detection of the choroidal neovascular membrane can be hindered by the presence of subretinal hemorrhages.

MACULAR HOLE

Myopia is the most common ocular refractive error. It is classified in physiologic and degenerative myopia. Physiologic myopia is considered a normal variation in ocular refractive power presented in 11-36% of the population. Degenerative myopia is characterized by a refractive abnormality of at least -6.00D and an axial length more than 26mm. It is accompanied by a progressive retinal and choroidal degeneration of the posterior pole and is present in 0.2-9.6 % of the population. Posterior staphyloma, peripapillary atrophy, early posterior vitreous detachment, retinal and choroidal thinning, Bruch's membrane rupture (lacquer cracks), retinal detachment, choroidal neovascularization and full thickness macular hole are characteristic findings in degenerative myopia.

The diagnosis of full thickness macular hole can be challenging in high myopia because of the retinal pigment epithelium and choroidal atrophy. The loss of the choriocapillaries and the decreased choroidal blood circulation may lead to a relative retinal ischemia. Moreover, posterior staphyloma also produces retinal thinning, probably due to ganglion cells layer thinning. Therefore, the resulted cystic degeneration and atrophy of the macula can lead to macular hole formation. Posterior detachment and degeneration of the vitreous that happens early in those young people may also play an important role.

Optical Coherence Tomography image of the hole is characterized by a loss of the physiologic macular anatomy and a full thickness retinal defect in the foveola. Biomicroscopy findings are classified in the same way that Gass described them in idiopathic full thickness macular hole. Stage I or impending hole is characterized by a macular detachment that appears on biomicroscopy like a yellow spot (Ia) or a yellow ring (Ib). Almost half of these holes will develop to a complete macular hole, while the rest will spontaneously resolve when the vitreous is completely detached. Stage II macular hole is characterized by a full thickness retinal defect with diameter under 400μm. In stage III there is an enlargement of the diameter of the hole above 400μm with the vitreous attached to the hole and detached around it. In stage IV there is further enlargement of the hole with a complete vitreous detachment.

Optical Coherence Tomography sometimes detects an operculum attached to one side of the hole or in front of the hole into the vitreous cavity. Gradually, a hole enlargement is observed and around it a cuff of subretinal fluid is detected located between the neurosensory retina and the retinal pigment epithelium. Also, intraretinal edema and cystic changes may be observed. Frequently, the operculum is clearly detached from the retina and remains in a small distance from the hole inside the vitreous cavity and attached to the posterior hyaloid. Finally, the vitreous completely detaches and withdraws into the vitreous cavity and therefore in many cases it is not visible on Optical Coherence Tomography. In high myopes the full thickness macular hole is in contact with liquefied vitreous, thus increasing the risk of retinal detachment in the posterior pole. Optical Coherence Tomography produces quantitative information related to the diameter of the hole, the diameter of the base of the hole as well as the retinal thickness around the hole. Various studies have shown that these measurements may have a prognostic value regarding the anatomical and functional results of macular hole repair.

Vitrectomy is the treatment of choice for a full thickness macular hole. Optical Coherence Tomography offers the possibility to observe the development and anatomical results after the surgical repair of a macular hole. Nevertheless, functional results may be poor even in cases of successful surgery because these patients frequently have already compromised vision due to the high myopia and its complications.

RETINAL SCHISIS

Patients with high myopia may develop retinoschisis in the macula. The role of vitreous traction on the macula cannot be ignored in cases of macular schisis. Retinal pigment epithelium and choroidal atrophy, together with choriocapillaries' loss and reduced choroidal blood circulation, can lead to relative retinal ischemia. It is possible that retinal ischemia combined with the vitreous traction may create macular schisis[2]. The macular area maintains some functionality, probably because of neural elements that remain attached to the inner and the outer retinoschisis layer, as opposed to degenerative retinoschisis.

Optical Coherence Tomography shows retinoschisis as a large area of low reflectivity in the outer retinal layers that resembles a retinal elevation but is differentiated by the clear appearance of a thin layer of retinal tissue over the retinal pigment epithelium. Lamellar macular hole and epiretinal membrane can also be detected. In some cases, instead of one schisis cavity, multiple elongated thin areas of low reflectivity parallel to the retinal surface are detected occupying the entire retinal thickness.

MYOPIA

1. Baba T, Ohno-Matsui K, Yoshida T, Yasuzumi K, Futagami S, Tokoro T, Mochizuki M. Optical Coherence Tomography of choroidal neovascularization in high myopia. Acta Ophthalmol Scand 2002;80(1):82-7.

2. Benhamou N, Massin P, Haouchine B, Erginay A, Gaudric A. Macular Retinoschisis in highly myopic eyes. Am J Ophthalmol 2002;133(6):794-800.

3. Montero JA, Ruiz-Moreno JM. Macular thickness in patients with choroidal neovascularization determined by RTA and OCT3: comparative results. Eye 2005;19(1):72-6.

MYOPIC CHOROIDAL NEOVASCULAR MEMBRANE

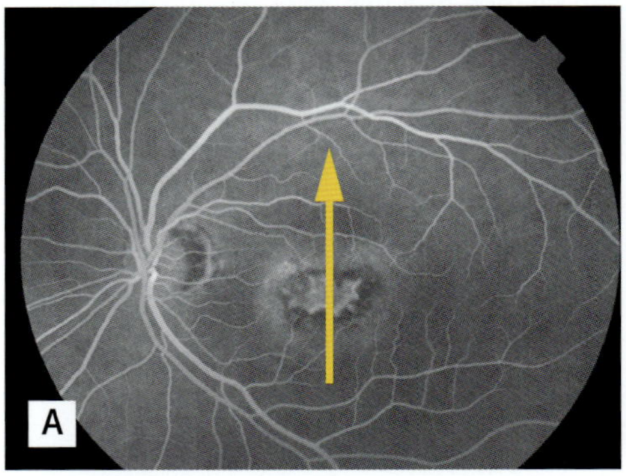

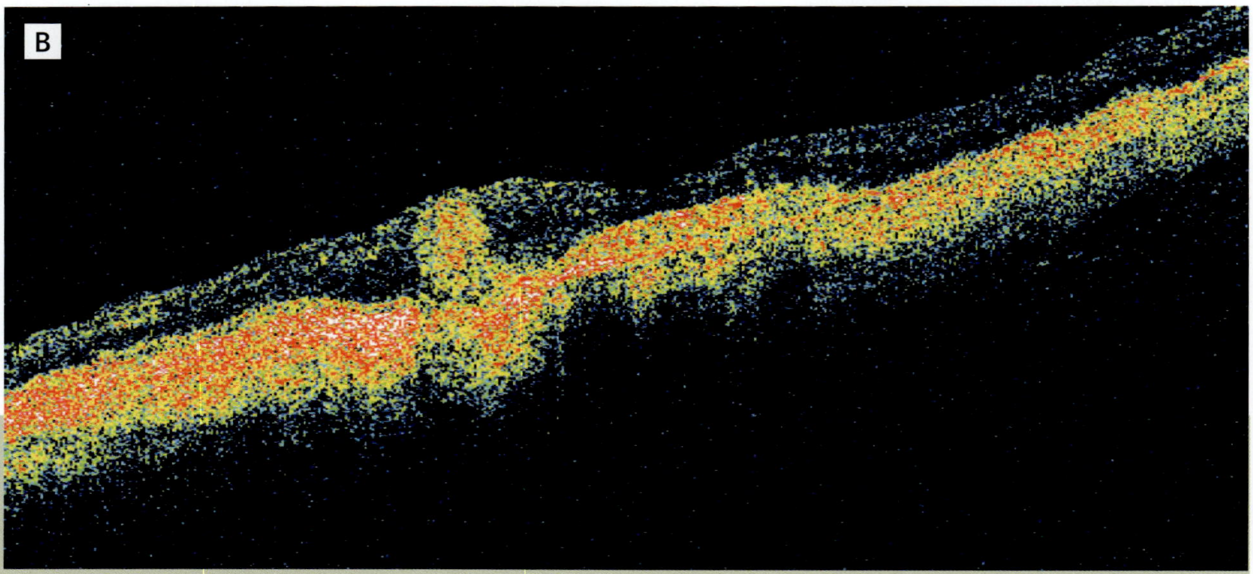

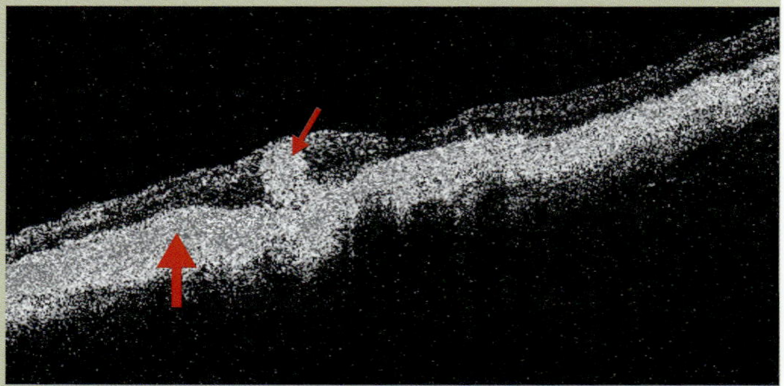

Patient with high myopia. A. Fluorescein angiography shows the presence of a choroidal neovascularization (the arrow shows the scan direction). B. Optical Coherence Tomography shows an area of high reflectivity above the retinal pigment epithelium, due to a type II choroidal neovascularization (small arrow). There is also increased reflectivity from the retinal pigment epithelium-choriocapillaries complex in both sides of the lesion that is due to retinal thinning (big arrow). A usual finding of choroidal neovascularization associated with myopia is the absence of subretinal fluid.

MYOPIC CHOROIDAL NEOVASCULAR MEMBRANE

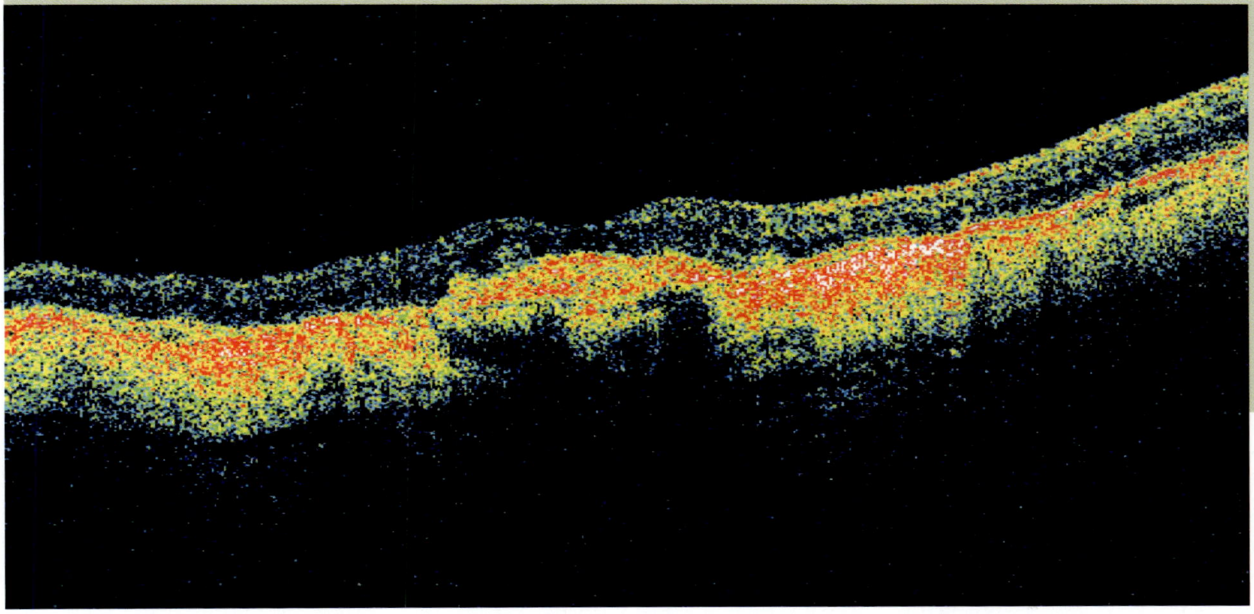

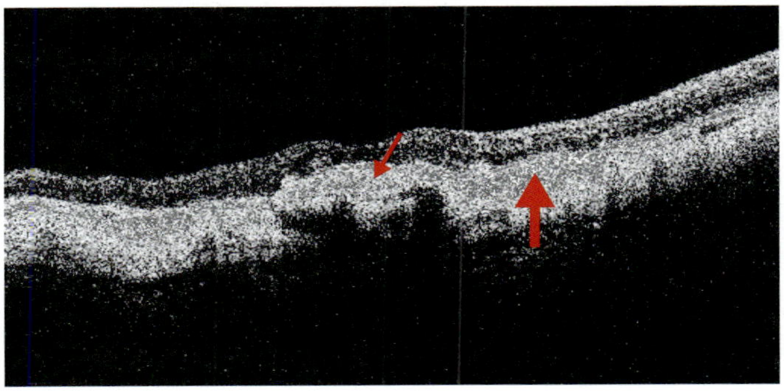

Patient with high myopia. An area of high reflectivity is detected in the macula above the retinal pigment epithelium due to a type II choroidal neovascularization (small arrow). An area of increased reflectivity from the retinal pigment epithelium-choriocapillaries complex is detected in both sides of the lesion and is due to retinal thinning (big arrow).

MYOPIC CHOROIDAL NEOVASCULAR MEMBRANE

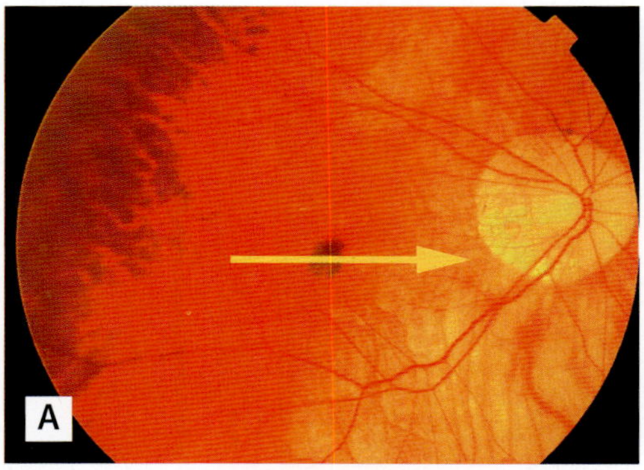

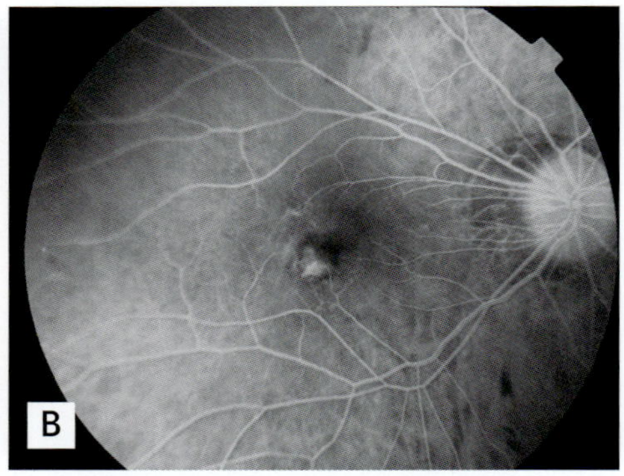

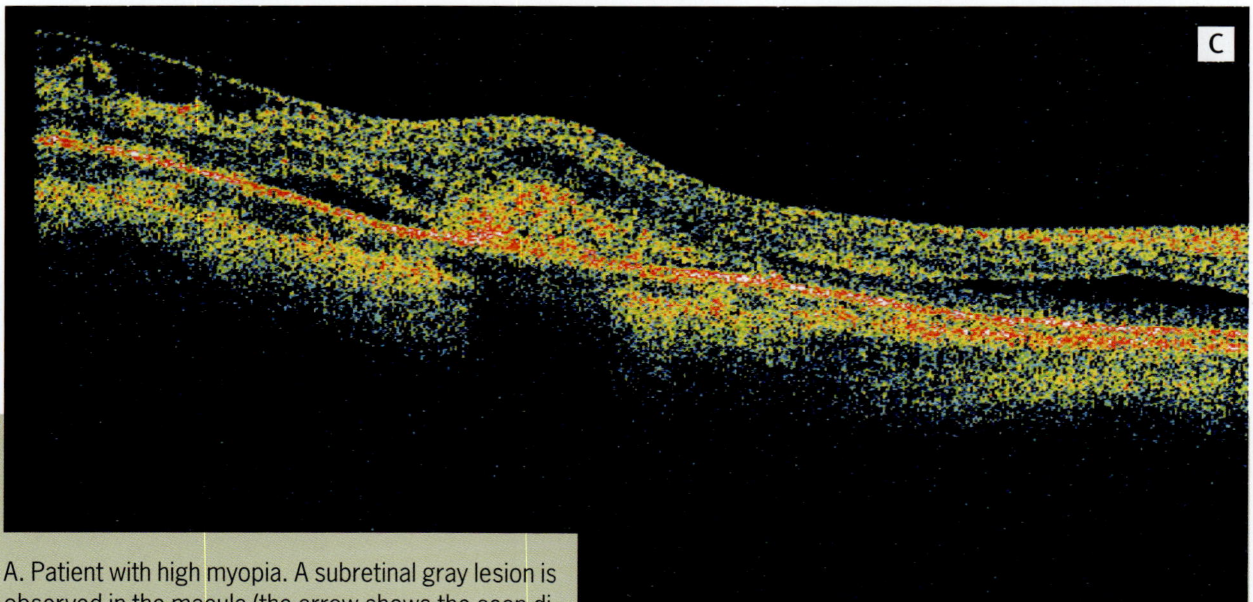

A. Patient with high myopia. A subretinal gray lesion is observed in the macula (the arrow shows the scan direction). B. Fluorescein angiography shows a choroidal neovascularization. C. Optical Coherence Tomography shows a high reflectivity area in the central fovea that is located above the pigment epithelium corresponding to a type II choroidal neovascularization (small arrow). Note the coexisting retinal edema (big arrow). A thin area of high reflectivity is detected temporally to the central fovea attached to the retina and corresponding to a partial posterior vitreous detachment (thick arrow). Subretinal fluid is detected temporally to the choroidal neovascular membrane (arrow head).

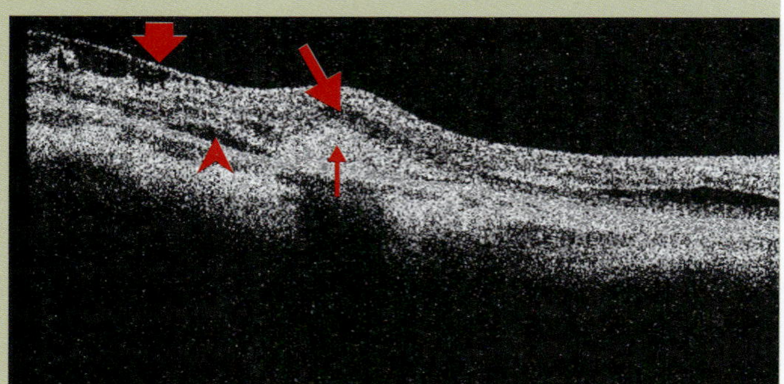

MYOPIC RETINOSCHISIS

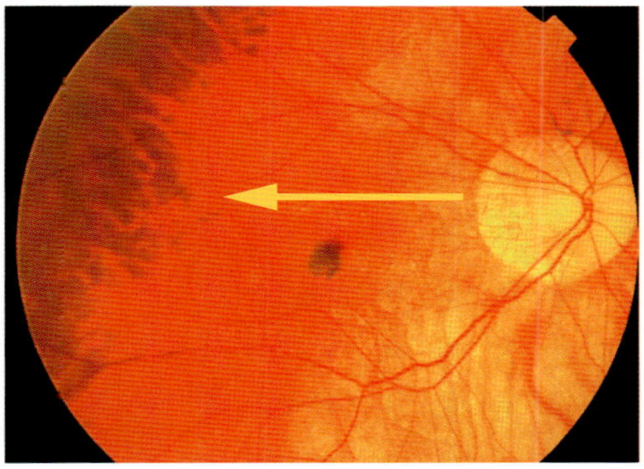

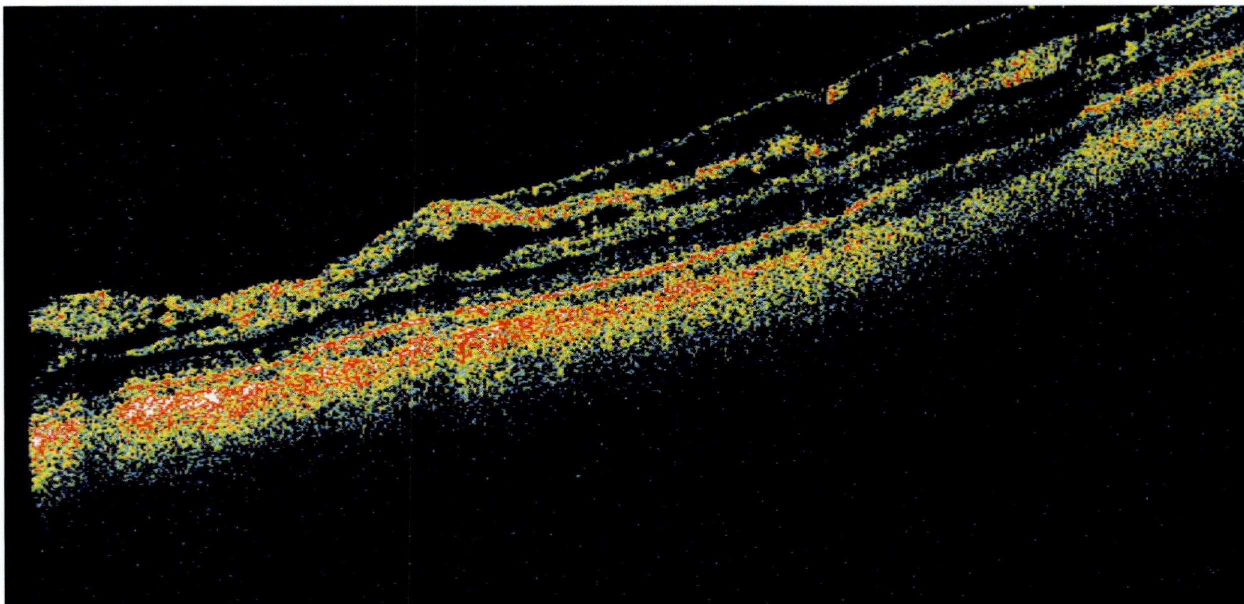

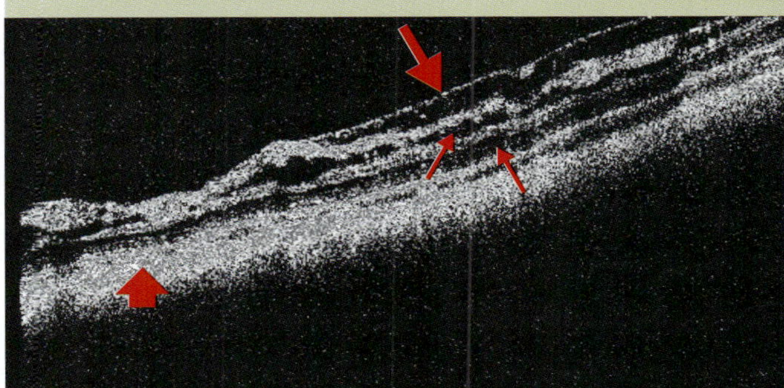

The same eye of page 206 in a papillomacular area scan. Note the presence of layers of low reflectivity within the retina (small arrows) corresponding to the retinoschisis. The posterior vitreous is detected as a line of high reflectivity with an attachment to the central area (big arrow). The area of high reflectivity represents the chorioretinal atrophy (thick arrow).

MYOPIC RETINOSCHISIS

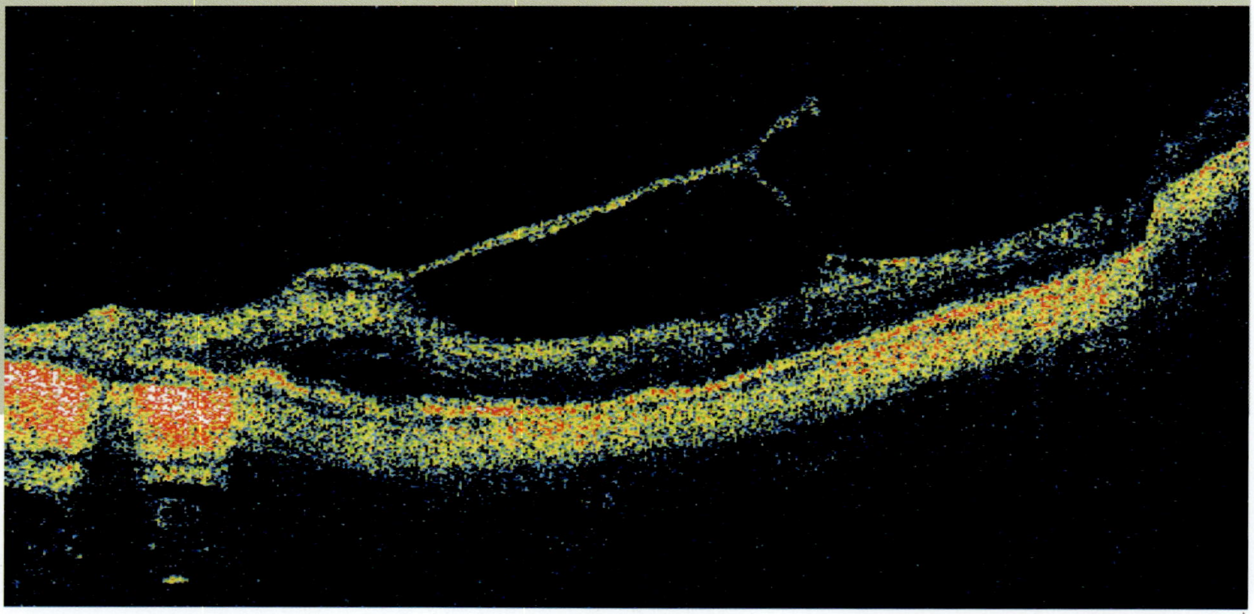

Patient with high myopia. A line of high reflectivity is detected inside the vitreous cavity (small arrow) attached to the retina and corresponding to thickened posterior vitreous. Note also the area of low reflectivity detected within the outer retinal layers and corresponding to retinoschisis (big arrow). The thin line of retinal tissue that is observed above the retinal pigment epithelium (thin layer of intermediate reflectivity) differentiates the retinoschisis from a retinal detachment (arrow head). The area of high reflectivity (thick arrow) detected around the optic nerve head corresponds to chorioretinal peripapillary atrophy.

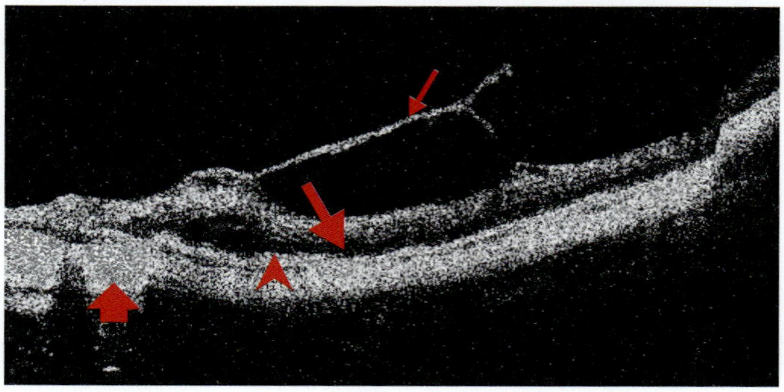

MYOPIC RETINOSCHISIS

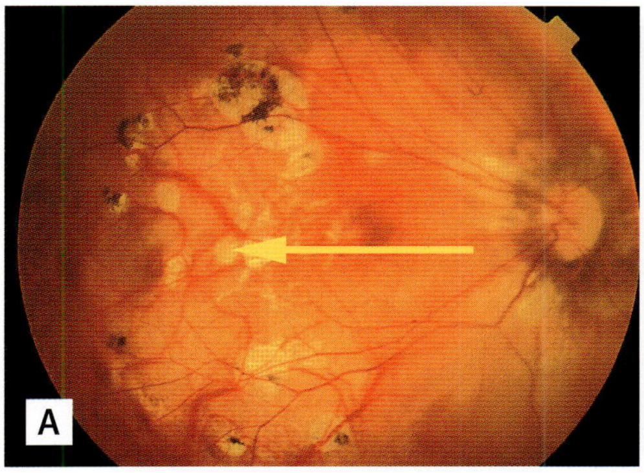

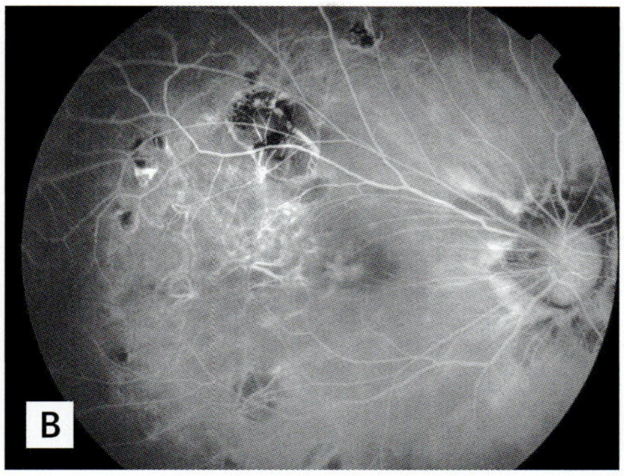

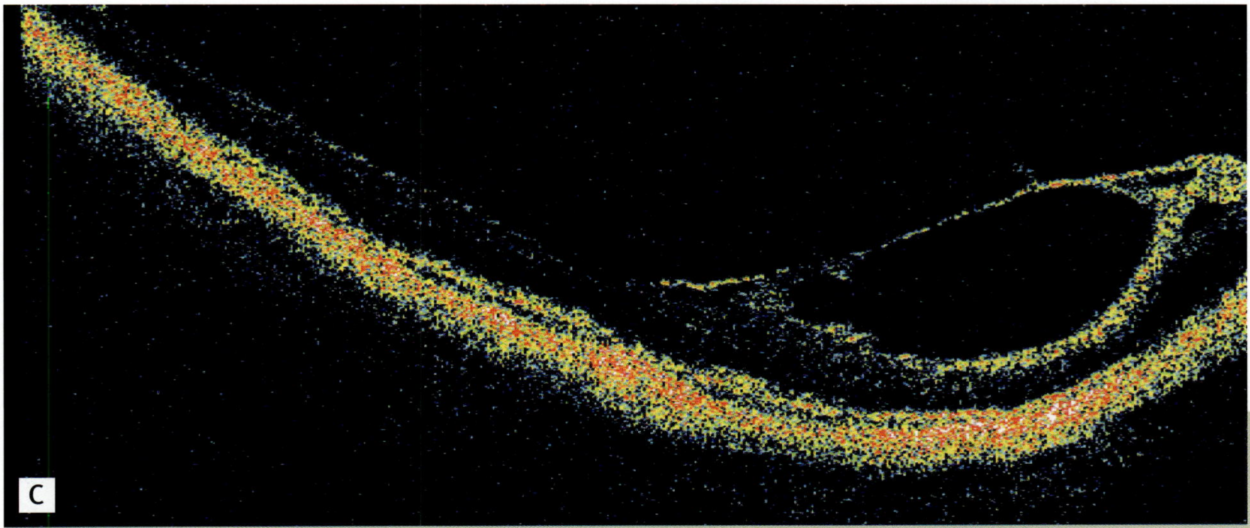

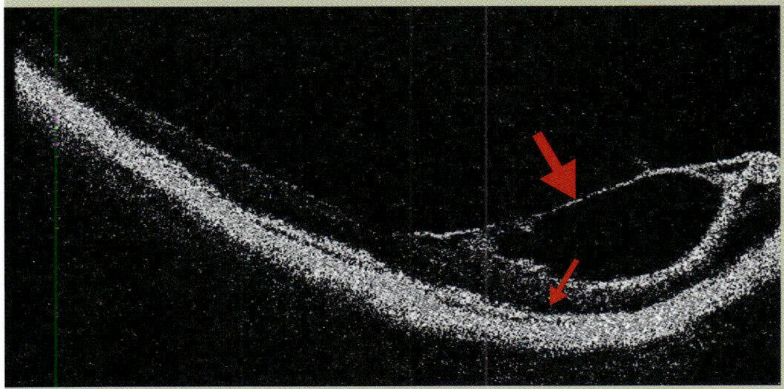

Patient with high myopia (-20D). A. Multiple chorioretinal atrophic areas and lacquer cracks are detected in the posterior pole (the arrow shows the scan direction). B. Fluorescein angiography shows a window defect type of hyperfluorescence corresponding to the lacquer cracks without active dye leakage. C. Optical Coherence Tomography detects a large area of low reflectivity in the outer retinal layers that corresponds to a macular retinoschisis (small arrow). The line of high reflectivity that is located on the retinal surface and causes significant traction on it corresponds to the cortical vitreous (big arrow). The low signal quality of the image is due to the high myopia and the large axial length of the eye.

MYOPIC RETINOSCHISIS

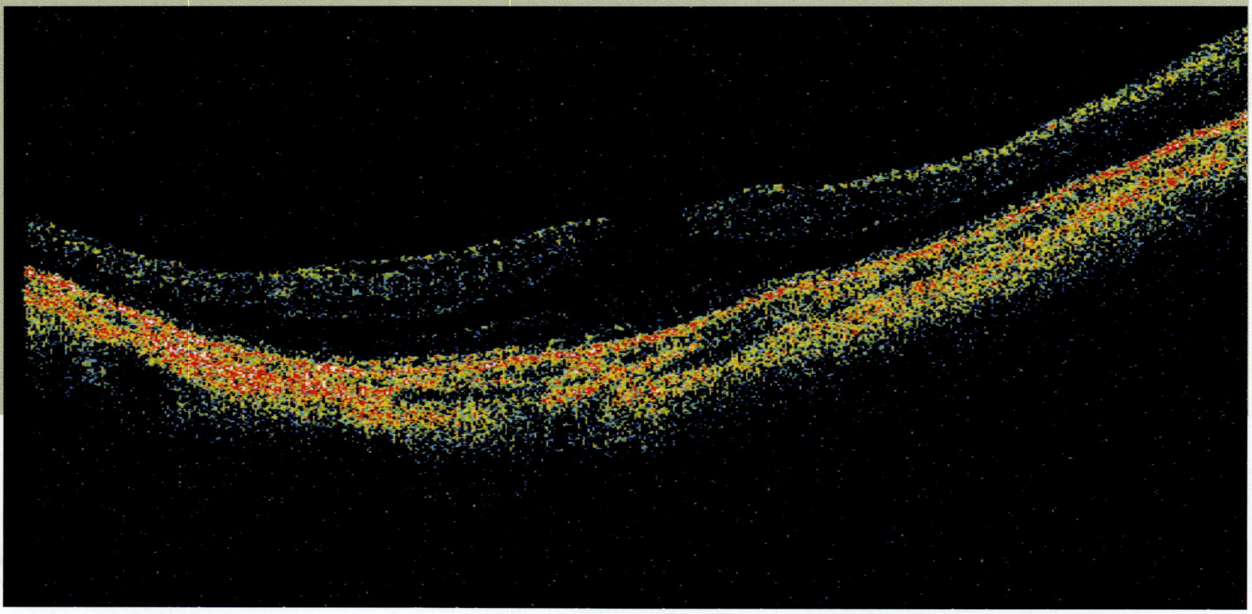

Patient with high myopia (-20D). Note the low reflectivity area in the outer retinal layers that corresponds to a macular retinoschisis (small arrow). A lamellar hole is detected in the central fovea (big arrow). There is a line of high reflectivity on the retinal surface corresponding to an epiretinal membrane (thick arrow). The low signal quality of the image is due to the high myopia and the large axial length of the eye.

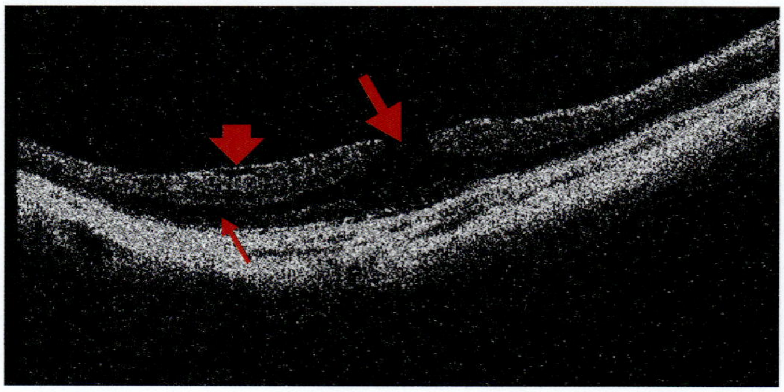

MYOPIC RETINOSCHISIS

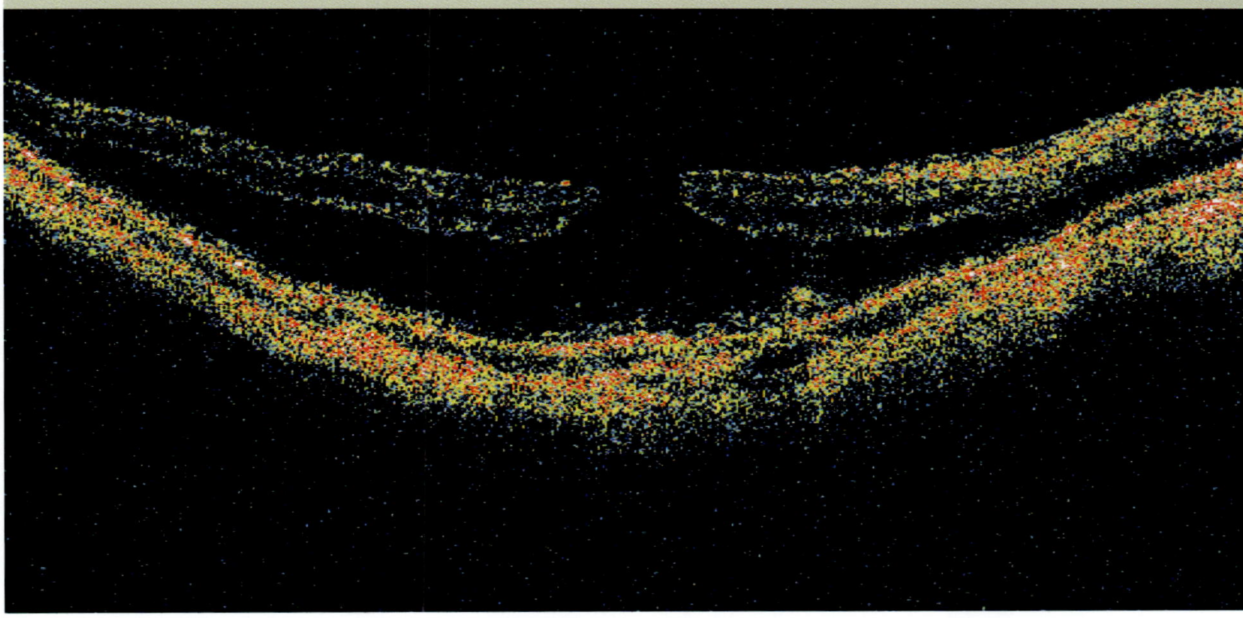

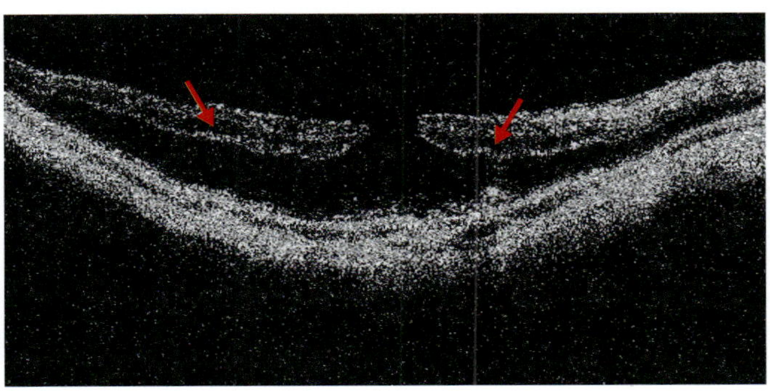

The patient of page 210 two months after vitrectomy for the removal of the epiretinal membrane. Note the increase in the size and height of the retinoschisis. Multiple small cystic areas of low intraretinal reflectivity are detected corresponding to cystic retinal edema (small arrows).

MYOPIC RETINOSCHISIS

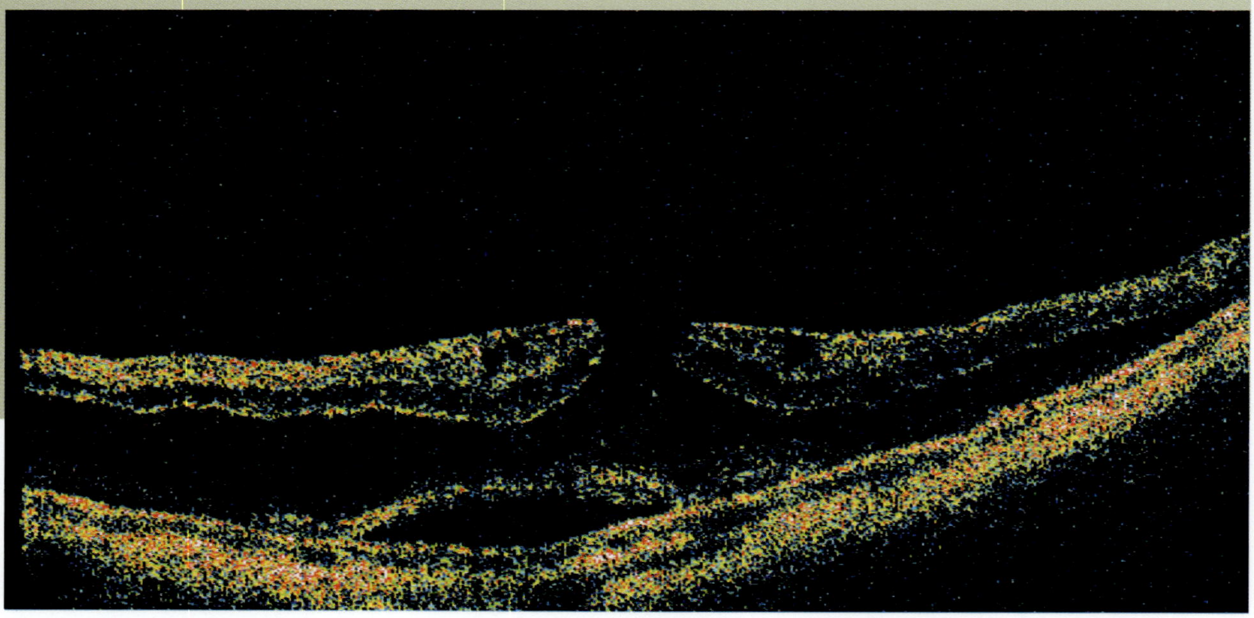

The patient of page 211 two months after the previous examination. The dimensions of the retinoschisis are further increased (big arrow) together with the cystoid retinal edema (small arrow). The opening of the lamellar hole is increased showing a tendency to become a full thickness macular hole (thick arrow). An area of low reflectivity is detected between the retina and the retinal pigment epithelium, corresponding to a retinal detachment in the fovea (arrow head). Two months later the patient developed an extensive retinal detachment from the full thickness macular hole.

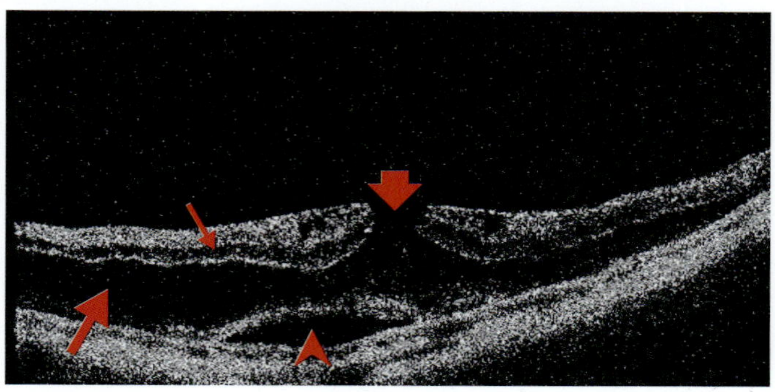

MYOPIC FULL THICKNESS MACULAR HOLE

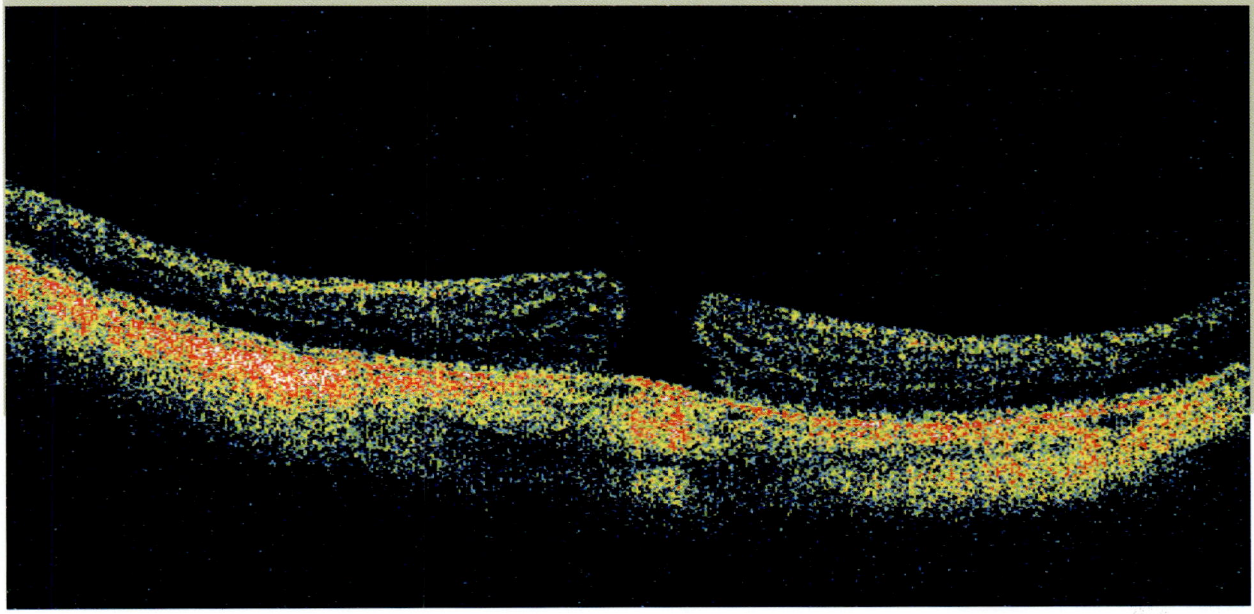

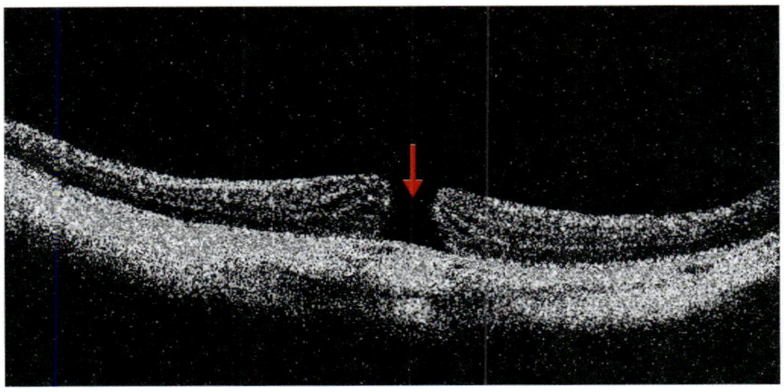

Patient with high myopia (-24D), visual acuity of 20/200 and a stage III full thickness macular hole. The hole (arrow) is not associated with significant edema or subretinal fluid around it.

MYOPIC FULL THICKNESS MACULAR HOLE

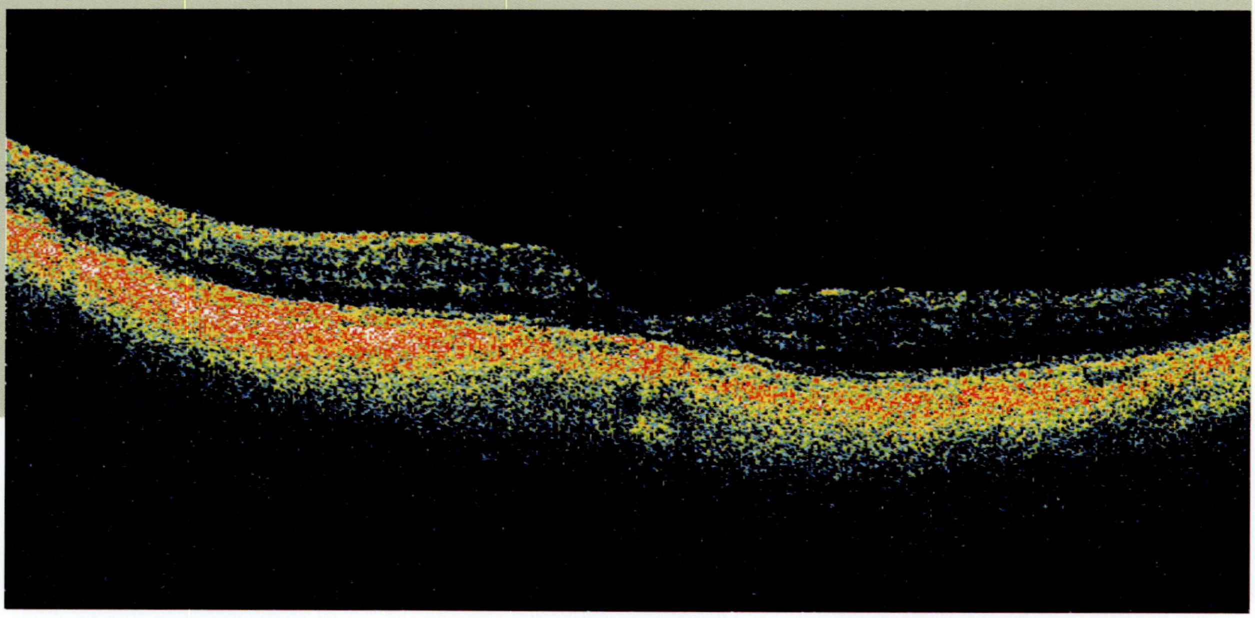

The patient of page 213 four months after surgical treatment. The visual acuity is 20/70. Note the closure of the hole and the retinal thinning in the fovea (arrow).

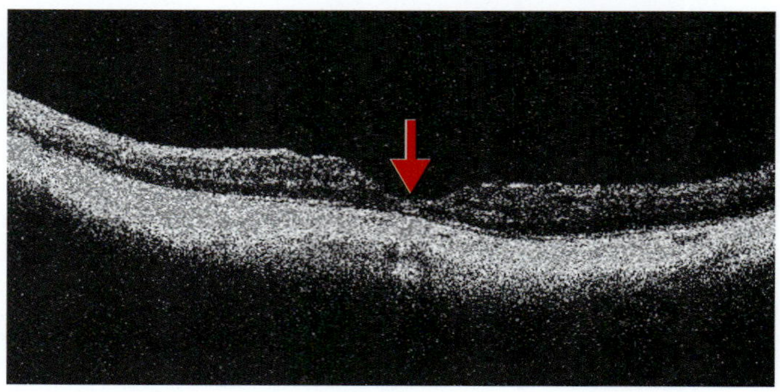

MYOPIC LAMELLAR MACULAR HOLE

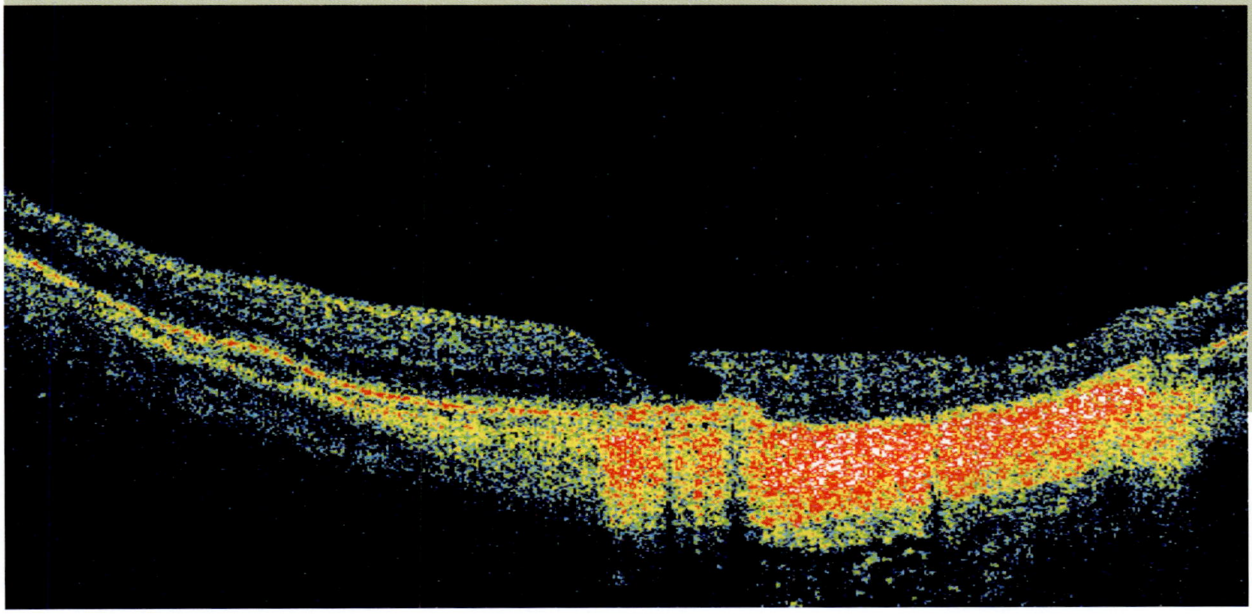

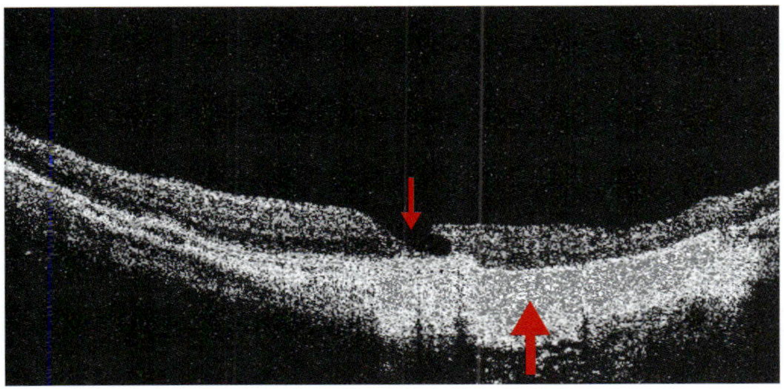

Patient with high myopia. Diffuse retinal thinning is detected in the macula. A loss of retinal tissue is detected in the fovea with maintenance of a thin retinal layer due to a lamellar macular hole (small arrow). An area of very high reflectivity is detected under the retinal pigment epithelium (big arrow) due to the high reflectivity of the sclera, which is visible because of the extensive choroidal atrophy.

CHAPTER 9

RETINAL DETACHMENT

GEORGE THEODOSSIADIS

In rhegmatogenous retinal detachment the retina is detached from the underlying retinal pigment epithelium and the space between them is occupied by fluid. The cause of the detachment is the presence of one or more retinal breaks through which fluid from the liquefied vitreous enters the subretinal space and elevates the retina.

After successful surgical treatment of a retinal detachment, the visual acuity does not always improve or if it does sometimes it may need a long time to do so. Optical Coherence Tomography can offer useful information:

• In cases with attached macula preoperatively and low postoperative visual acuity without subretinal fluid detected on biomicroscopy[8].

• In cases where complete absorption of the fluid from the macular area is delayed[1-6].

• In cases where the low postoperative visual acuity after a successful surgical treatment is due to macular atrophy, cystoid macular edema, epiretinal membrane or subretinal fibrosis[7,9,10].

Optical Coherence Tomography also offers useful information for the differential diagnosis of rhegmatogenous retinal detachment and retinoschisis, the latter being observed in the posterior pole of high myopes.

RETINAL DETACHMENT

1. Baba T, Hirose A, Moriyama M, Mochizuki M. Tomographic image and visual recovery of acute macula-off rhegmatogenous retinal detachment. Graefes Arch Clin Exp Ophthalmol 2004; 242: 576-581.

2. Gibran SK, Alwitry A, Cleary PE. Foveal detachment after successful retinal reattachment for macula on rhegmatogenous retinal detachment: an ocular coherence tomography evaluation. Eye 2006;20(11):1284-7

3. Hagimure N, Iida T, Suto K, Kishi S. Persistent foveal retinal detachment after successful rhegmatogenous retinal detachment surgery. Am J Ophthalmol 2002 ; 133 :516-520.

4. Hagimura N, Suto K, Iida T, Kishi S. Optical coherence tomography of the neurosensory retina in rhegmatogenous retinal detachment. Am J Ophthalmol 2000;129: 186-190.

5. Konno S, Akiba J, Sato E, Kuriyama S, Yoshida A. OCT in successful surgery of retinal detachment associated with optic nerve head pit. Ophthalmic Surg Lasers 2000; 31: 236-239.

6. Lecleire-Collet A, Muraine M, Menard JF, Brasseur G. Predictive visual outcome after macula-off retinal detachment surgery using optical coherence tomography. Retina 2005; 25:44-53.

7. Panozzo G, Parolini B, Mercanti A. OCT in the monitoring of visual recovery after uneventful retinal detachment surgery. Semin Ophthalmol 2003;18:82-84.

8. Theodossiadis PG, Georgalas IG, Emfietzoglou J, Kyriaki TE, Pantellia E, Gogas PS, Moschos MN, Theodossiadis GP. Optical coherence tomography findings in the macula after treatment of rhegmatogenous retinal detachment with spared macula preoperatively. Retina 2003; 23: 69075.

9. Wolfenberger TJ, Gonvers M. Optical coherence tomography in the evaluation of incomplete visual acuity recovery after macula-off retinal detachment. Graefes Arch Clin Exp Ophthalmol 2002; 240:85-89.

10. Wang Y, Li SY, Zhu M, Chen SJ, Liu Y, Men XH, Gillies M, Larsson J. Metamorphopsia after successful retinal detachment surgery: an optical coherence tomography study. Acta Ophthalmol Scand 2005;83: 168-171.

RETINAL DETACHMENT

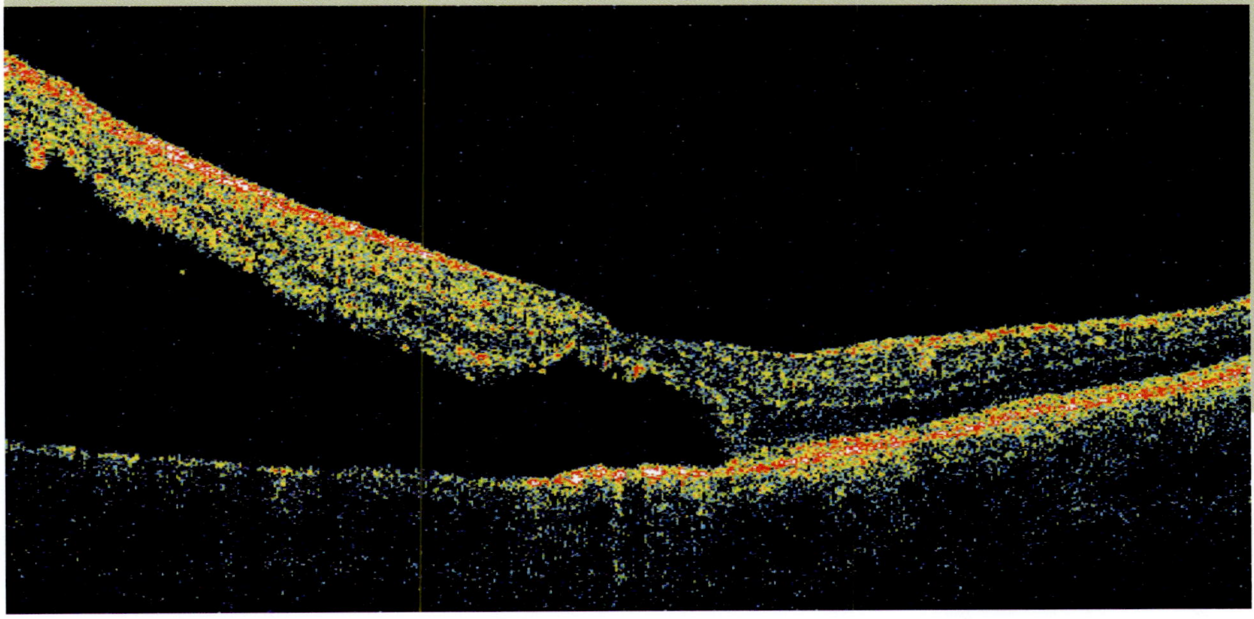

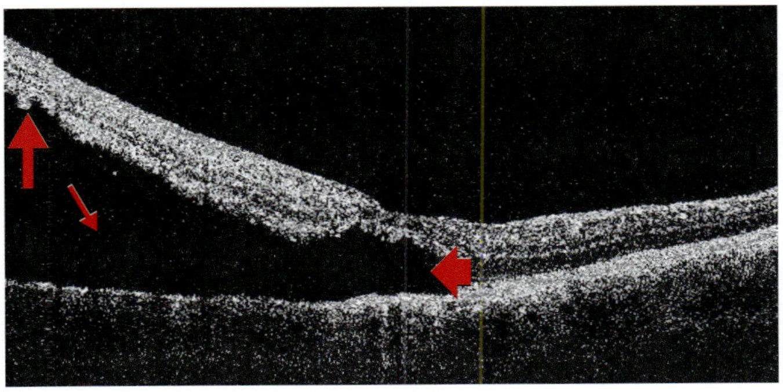

Patient with a retinal detachment and a decrease of visual acuity. A diffuse area of low reflectivity is detected between the retina and the retinal pigment epithelium (small arrow) and extends to the central area (thick arrow) due to a rhegmatogenous retinal detachment. The irregular outer surface of the detached retina (big arrow) is caused by a local photoreceptor rupture and constitutes a negative prognostic factor for the functional postoperative result.

CHAPTER 10

CHORIORETINAL INFLAMMATORY DISEASES

Pantelis Nikolaidis

VOGT KOYANAGI HARADA SYNDROME

This syndrome is characterized by posterior or anterior uveitis with exudative retinal detachment, poliosis, hearing loss, alopecia, vitiligo and meningeal signs. The syndrome evolves in 4 stages:

1. Prodromal stage: It starts a few days before the initiation of the ophthalmic signs and is characterized by headaches, ocular pain, poliosis, nausea, fever, photophobia and watering.
2. Ocular or uveitic stage: It is characterized by bilateral anterior uveitis with decrease of vision, photophobia, hearing loss and meningism. This stage can last weeks or even months. Uveitis is mainly characterized by anterior chamber reaction, posterior synechiae, optic disc edema, retinal edema[3-6], haemorrhages, exudative retinal detachment and choroidal and retinal pigment epithelium infiltrates.
3. Chronic stage: Sometimes it lasts weeks or even months. It is characterized by mild uveitis with possible intensification of neurological symptoms. In that stage retinal reattachment is possible and subretinal neovascular membrane or subretinal fibrosis may be formed.
4. Recurrent stage: Can be characterized by the presence of mutton-fat keratic precipitates, Koeppe iris nodules, posterior synechiae, cataract, glaucoma, subretinal neovascular membrane and subretinal fibrosis.

Optical Coherence Tomography can detect retinal elevation due to subretinal fluid with cystic retinal edema. The fluid can also be intraretinal, presented with mixed reflectivity due to high protein concentration.

CAT SCRATCH DISEASE – NEURORETINITIS

Cat Scratch disease is an infection caused by Bartonella (Rochalimaea) Henselae and R. Quintana. The disease can cause subacute local lymphadenitis, conjunctivitis, intermediate uveitis, vasculitis of retinal vessels, serous retinal detachment, optic disc edema and aseptic meningitis. It appears days or weeks after cat scratch or bite. The visual acuity varies and the optic disc edema can be bilateral. The disease is considered self-limited, relatively benign and without special treatment. Sometimes antibiotics like doxycycline and rifambicine are used. Optical Coherence Tomography clearly shows the optic disc edema and areas of high reflectivity located under the retina that correspond to exudates.

BIRDSHOT RETINOCHOROIDOPATHY

This disease is characterized by subretinal ovoid spots resembling birdshot scatter from a shotgun. It has many similarities with intermediate uveitis from which it is differentiated by the absence of pars plana snowbanks. It is commonly presented in the first six decades of life. Forty five per cent of patients are women while almost all patients are white. The main symptom is decreased vision and in some cases photopsia, nyctalopia, and photophobia. The syndrome is usually bilateral; the visual acuity ranges between 20/20 and 20/800 with the mean visual acuity being 20/50 or better. Ninety per cent of patients have cell infiltrates in the vitreous and characteristic choroidal infiltrations that are usually presented in radial distribution around the optic disc. Macular cystic edema and epiretinal membranes are also usual findings[1,2]. Optical Coherence Tomography can detect thickening or thinning of the retina and even the presence of an epiretinal membrane.

CHORIORETINAL INFLAMMATORY DISEASES

1. Antcliff RJ, Stanford MR, Chauhan DS, Graham EM, Spalton DJ, Shilling JS, Ffytche TJ, Marshall J. Comparison between optical coherence tomography and fundus fluorescein angiography for the detection of cystoid macular edema in patients with uveitis. Ophthalmology 2000; 107; 593-599.

2. Catier A, Tadayoni R, Paques M, Erginay A, Haouchine B, Gaudric A, Massin P. Characterization of macular edema from various etiologies by optical coherence tomography. Am J Ophthalmol 2005; 140: 200-206.

3. Chan A, Duker JS. A standardized method for reporting changes in macular thickening using optical coherence tomography. Arch Ophthalmol 2005;123: 939-943.

4. Guex-Crossier Y. The pathogenesis and clinical presentation of macular edema in inflammatory diseases. Doc Ophthalmol 1999;97: 297-309.

5. Markomichelakis NN, Halkiadakis I, Pantelia E, Peponis V, Patelis A, Theodossiadis P, Theodossiadis G. Patterns of macular edema in patients with uveitis: qualitative and quantitative assessments using optic coherence tomography. Ophthalmology 2004; 111: 946-953.

6. Reinthal EK, Volker M, Freusenthaler N, Grub M, Zierhut M, Schlote T. Optical coherence tomography in the diagnosis and follow-up of patients with uveitis macular edema. Ophthalmologe 2004; 101: 1181-1188.

CAT SCRATCH DISEASE

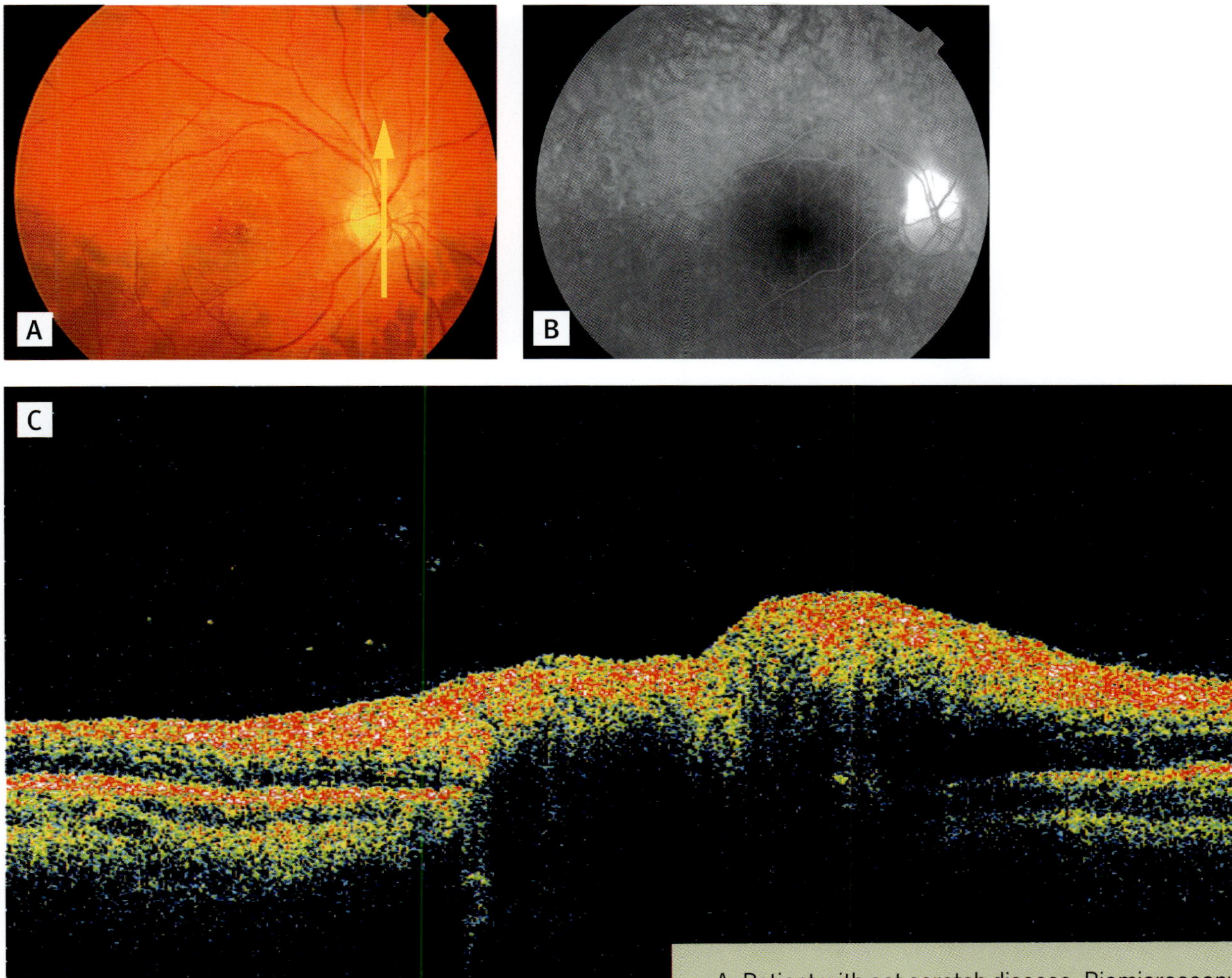

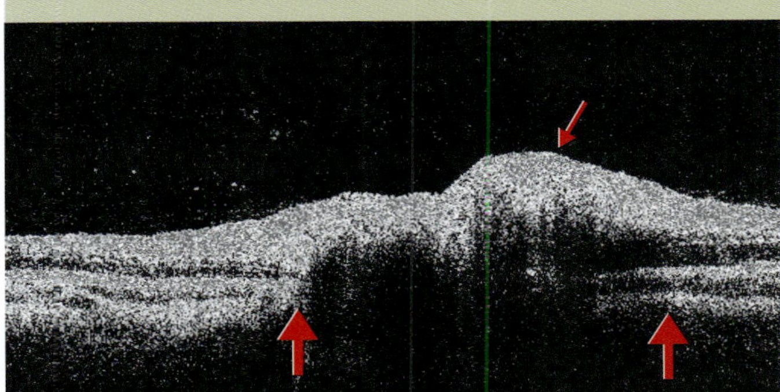

A. Patient with cat scratch disease. Biomicroscopy reveals the presence of localized edema in the superior part of the optic disc as well as a macular star at the posterior pole (the arrow shows the scan direction). B. Fluorescein angiography shows dye leakage corresponding to the edematous area in the upper margins of the optic disc. C. Optical Coherence Tomography shows an elevated area of high reflectivity corresponding to the edema of the optic disc (small arrow) with shadowing of the underlying tissues. The optic disc borders are shown (big arrows). Optical Coherence Tomography findings are not diagnostic for this disease.

CAT SCRATCH DISEASE

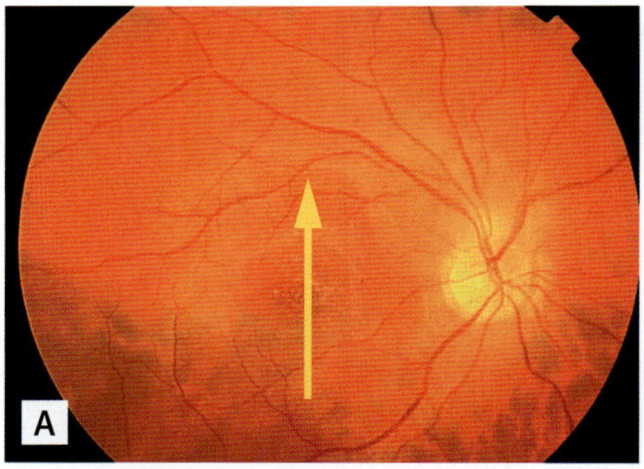

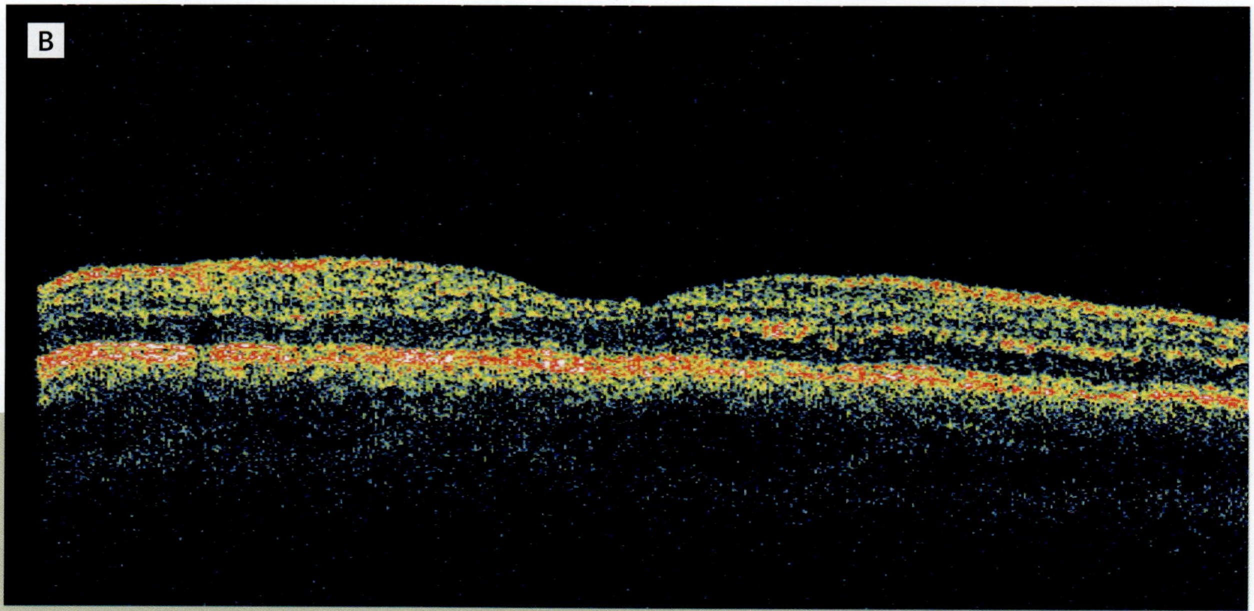

A. Another scan of the patient of page 223 (the arrow shows the scan direction). B. Multiple intraretinal small areas of high reflectivity are detected in the macular area corresponding to the hard exudates of the macular star (arrow). The foveal architecture remains normal.

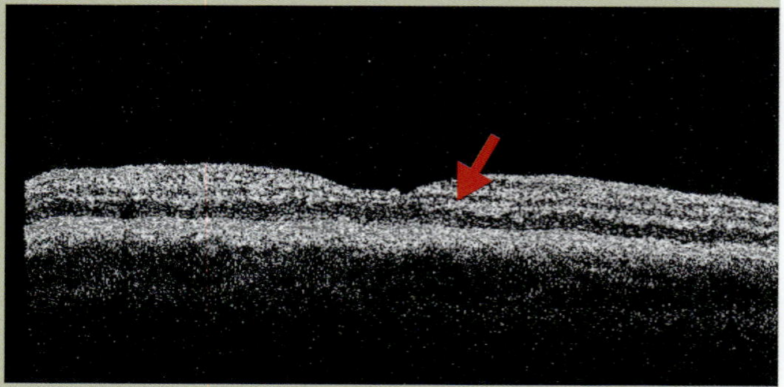

CAT SCRATCH DISEASE

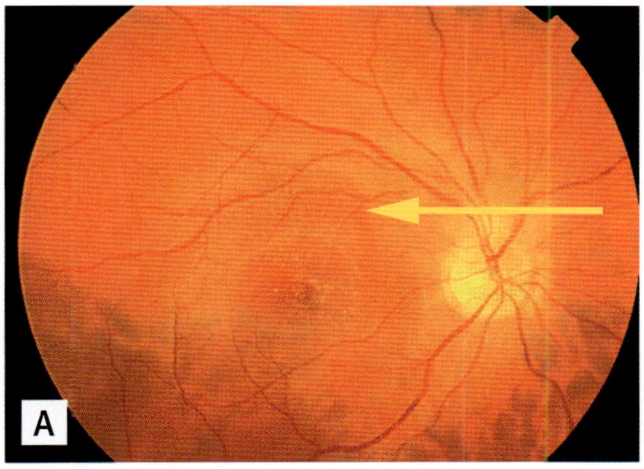

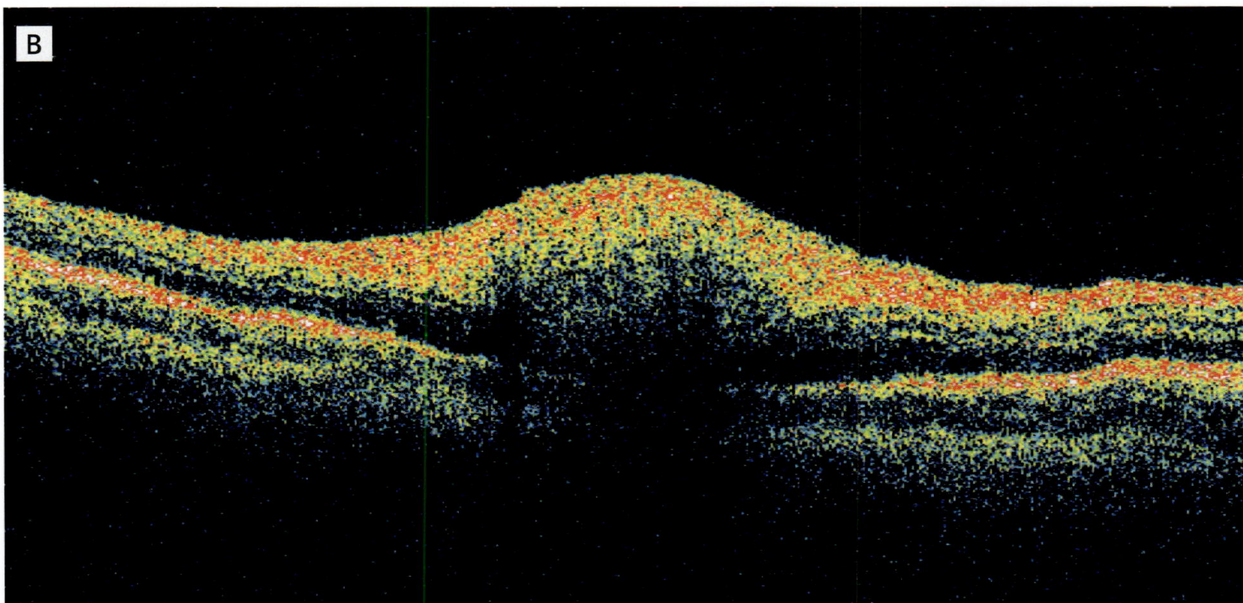

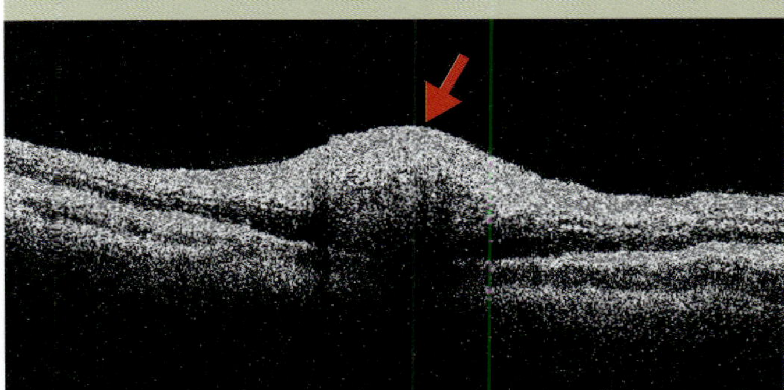

A. Another scan of the patient of page 223 that shows the retinal area above the optic disc (the arrow shows the scan direction). B. The edematous area is presented like an elevated area of high reflectivity (arrow).

BIRDSHOT CHORIORETINOPATHY

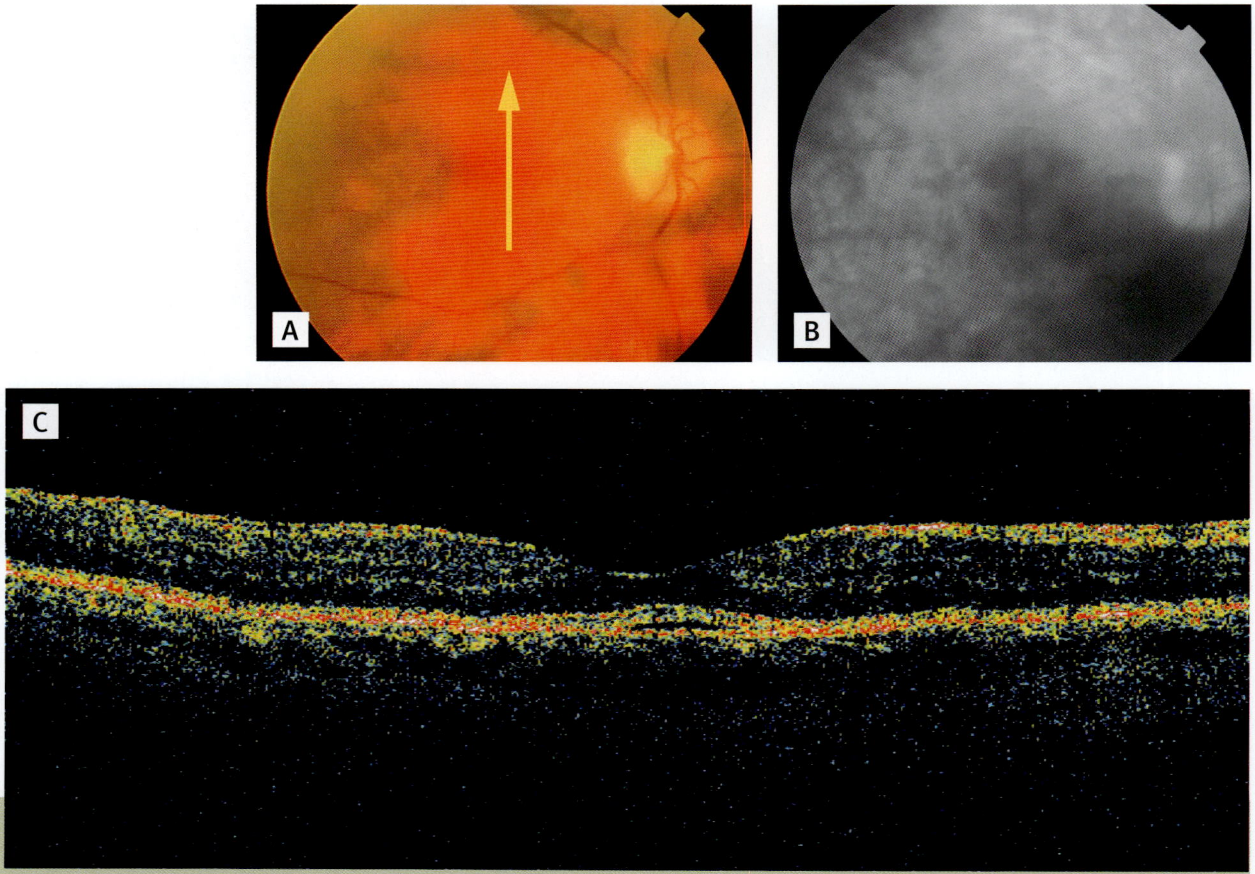

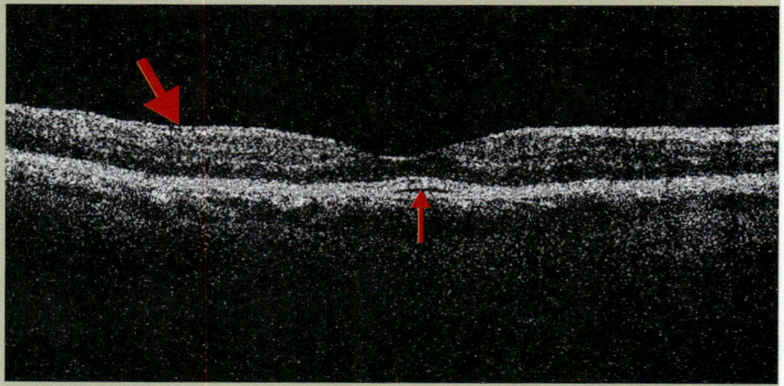

Right eye of a patient with birdshot retinochoroidopathy A. Inflammatory vitreous reaction, optic disc edema and characteristic yellow choroidal infiltrations are detected around the optic disc on biomicroscopy (the arrow shows the scan direction). B. Fluorescein angiography shows dye leakage in the optic disc (hot disc) and active perivasculitis. C. Optical Coherence Tomography shows an area of low reflectivity between the retina and the retinal pigment epithelium that corresponds to a retinal detachment in the fovea (small arrow). There is also a thin line of high reflectivity on the retinal surface corresponding to an epiretinal membrane (big arrow).

BIRDSHOT CHORIORETINOPATHY

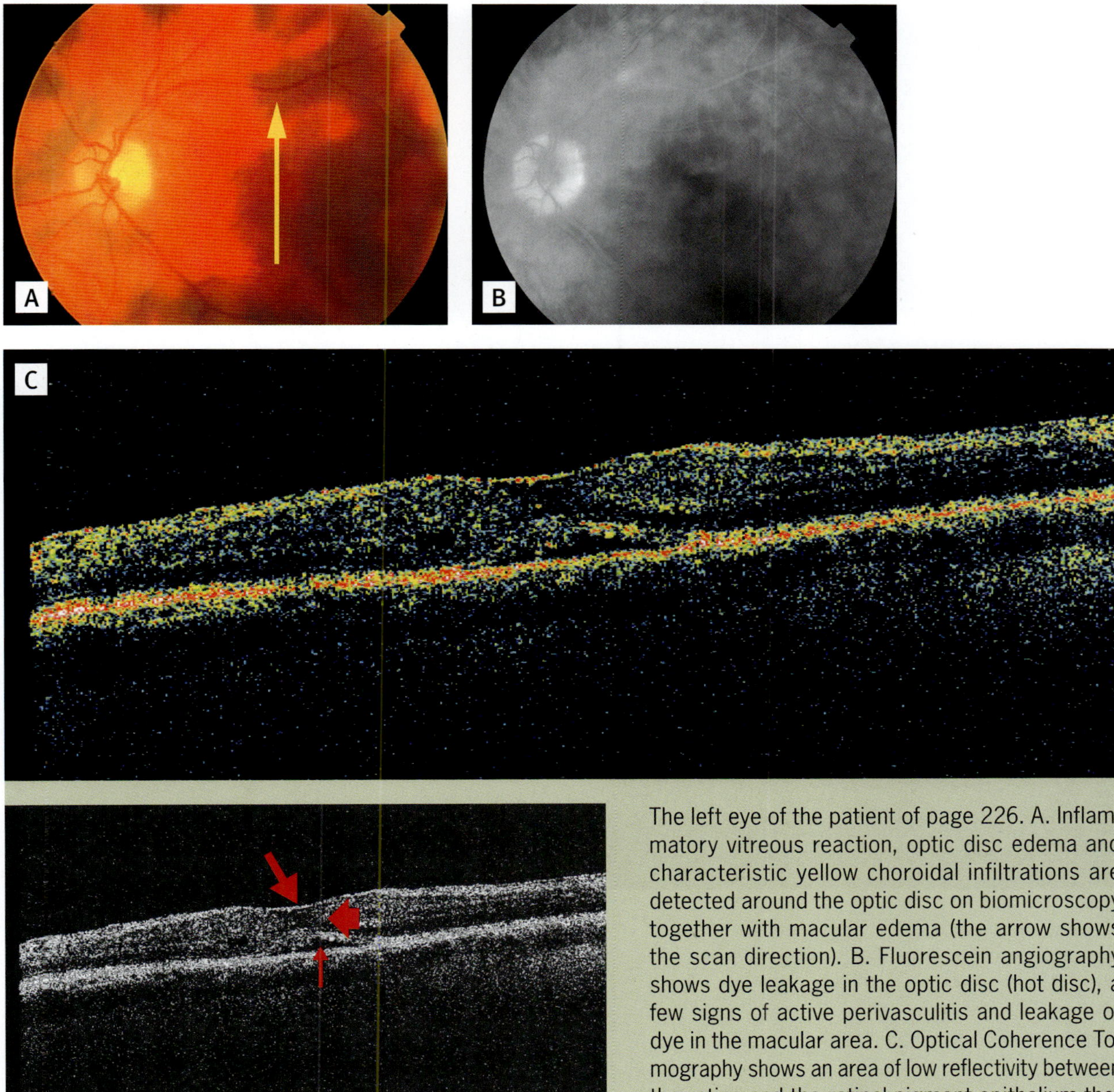

The left eye of the patient of page 226. A. Inflammatory vitreous reaction, optic disc edema and characteristic yellow choroidal infiltrations are detected around the optic disc on biomicroscopy together with macular edema (the arrow shows the scan direction). B. Fluorescein angiography shows dye leakage in the optic disc (hot disc), a few signs of active perivasculitis and leakage of dye in the macular area. C. Optical Coherence Tomography shows an area of low reflectivity between the retina and the retinal pigment epithelium that corresponds to a retinal detachment in the fovea (small arrow). There is also a thin line of high reflectivity on the retinal surface that corresponds to an epiretinal membrane (big arrow). Increased retinal thickness is detected due to diffuse retinal edema (thick arrow).

BIRDSHOT CHORIORETINOPATHY

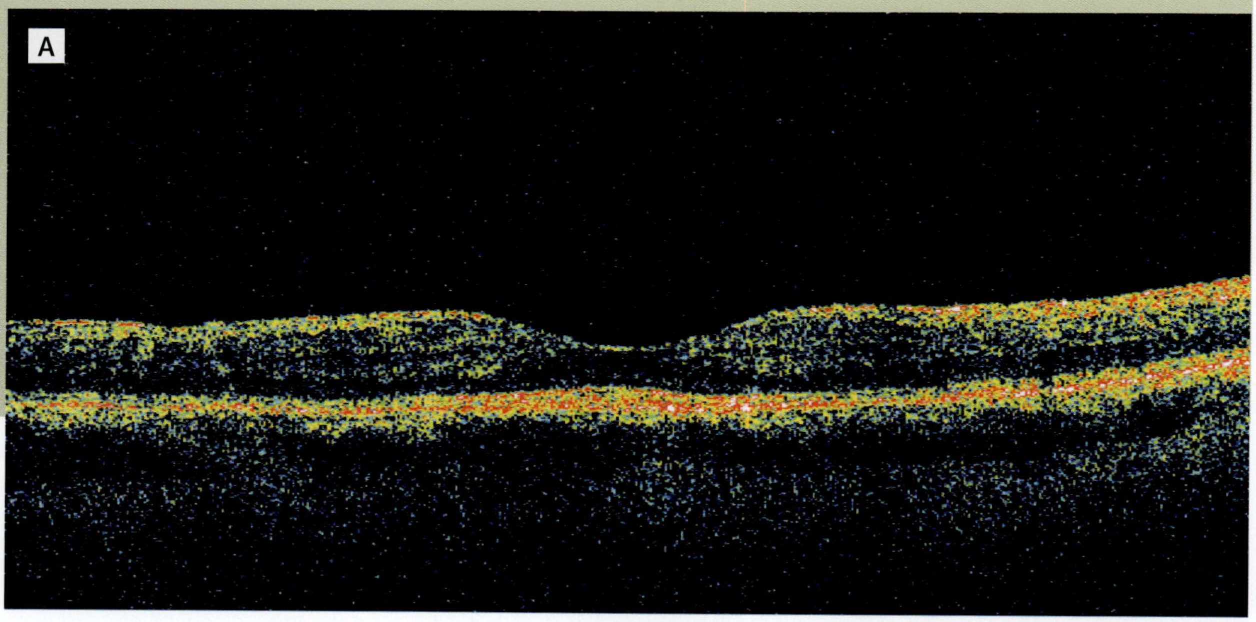

The patient of page 226 three months after initiation of systemic treatment with corticosteroids. On the right eye (A) resolution and on the left eye (B) of page 229 decrease of the subretinal fluid with decrease of retinal edema are observed.

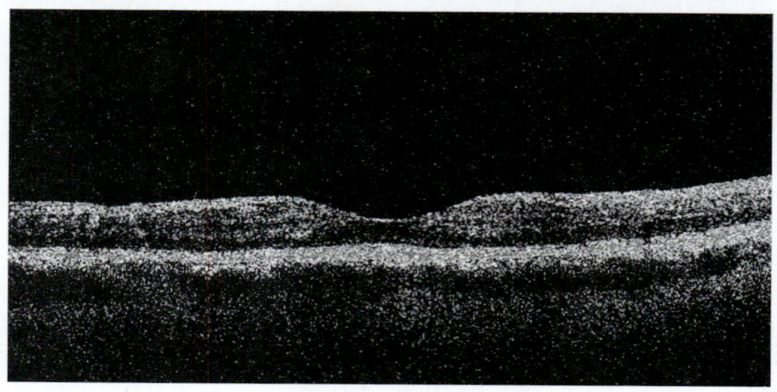

BIRDSHOT CHORIORETINOPATHY

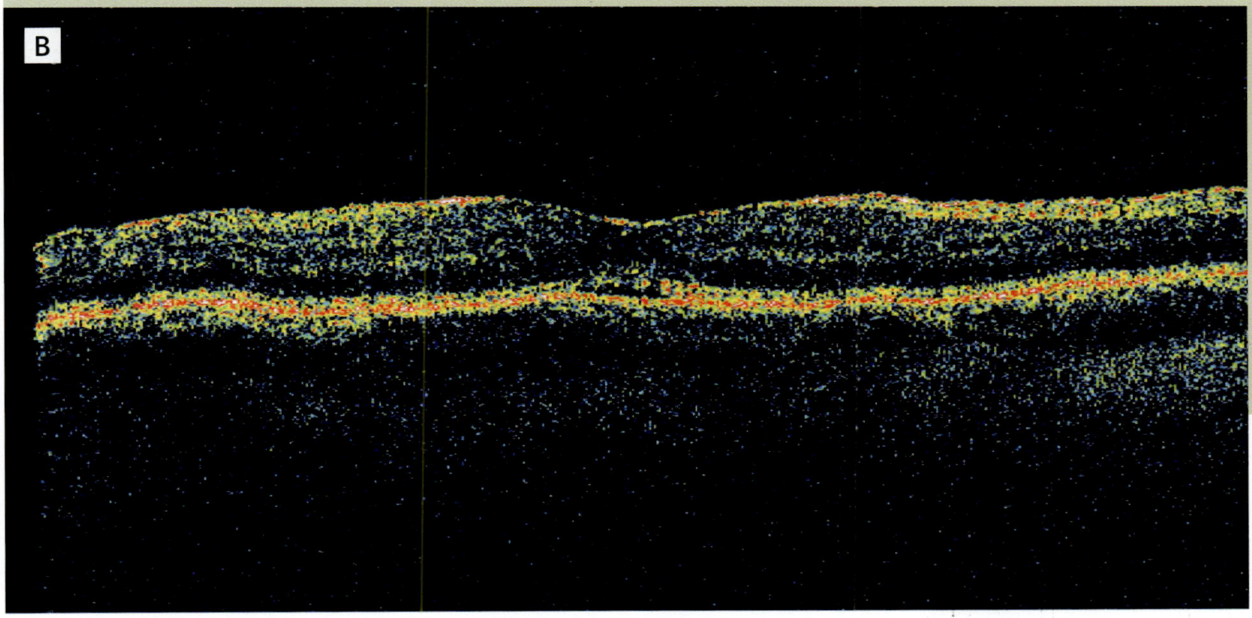

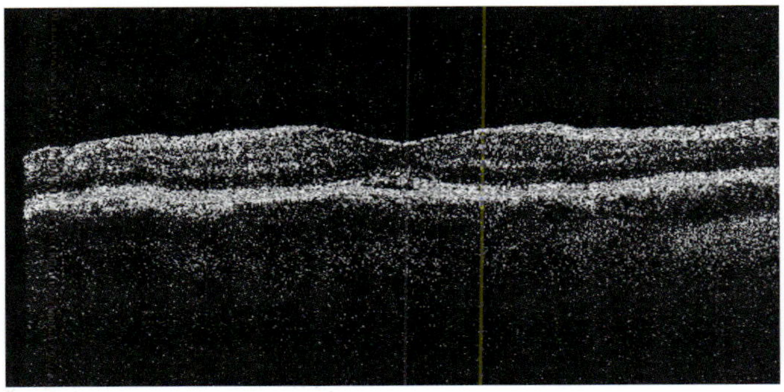

NEURORETINITIS

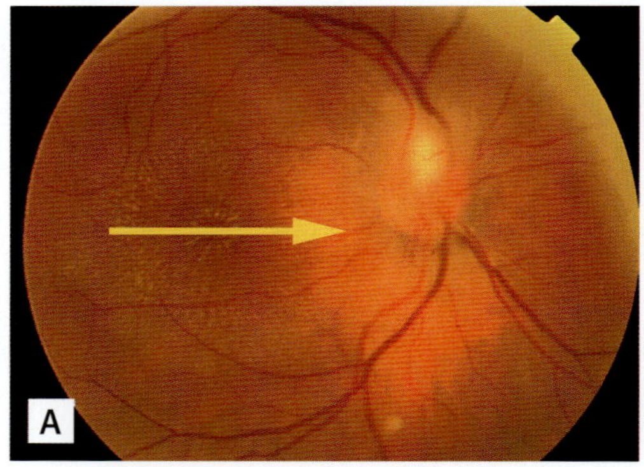

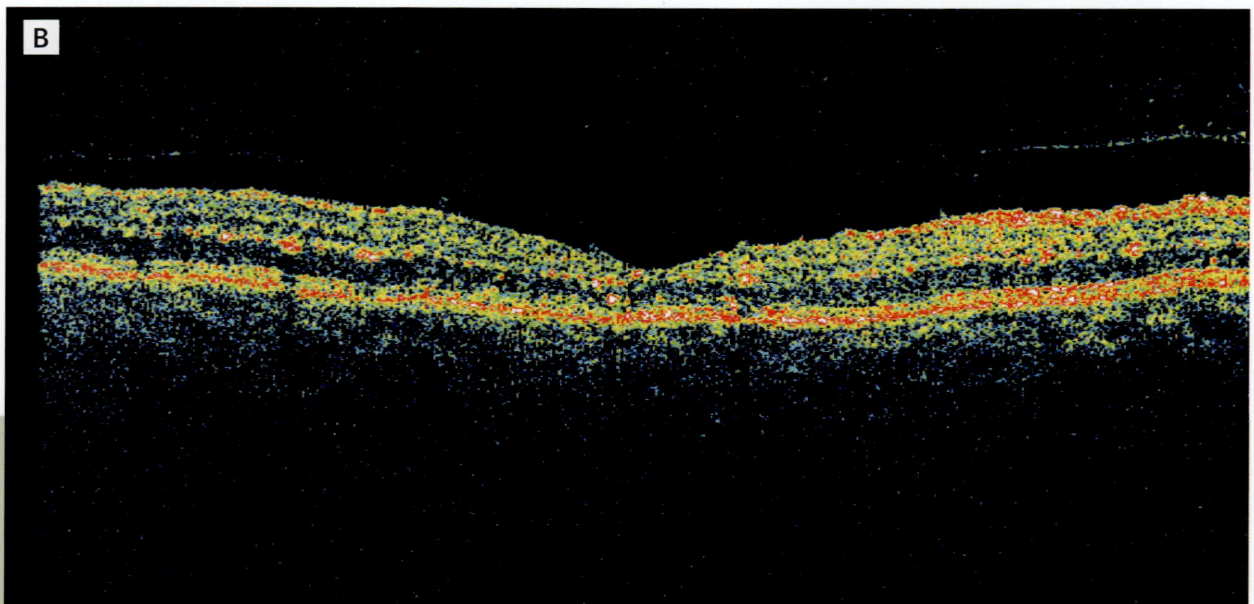

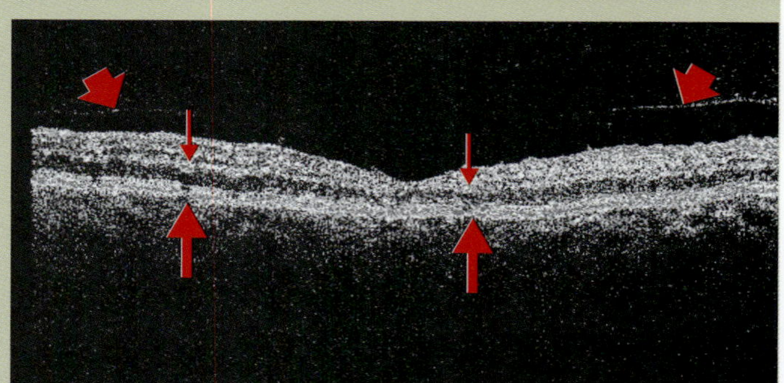

A. Patient with neuroretinitis and a macular star (the arrow shows the scan direction). B. Multiple small round areas of high reflectivity are detected in the outer retinal layers of the macula and correspond to the deposition of hard exudates forming a macular star (small arrows). Note the shadowing of the underlying layers caused by the larger exudates (big arrows). The vitreous is detected as a thin line of high reflectivity attached to the foveal area and detached around it (thick arrows).

NEURORETINITIS

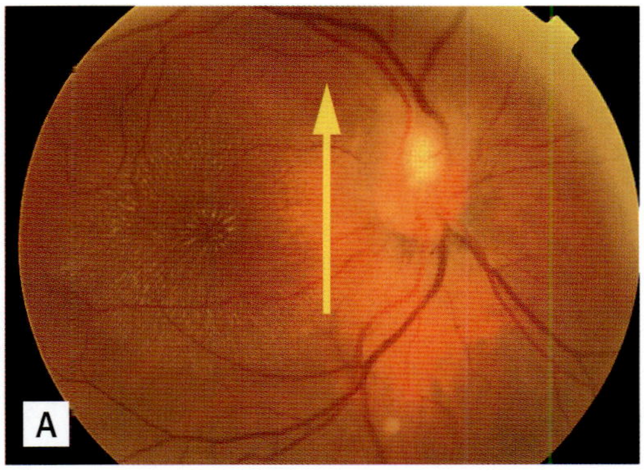

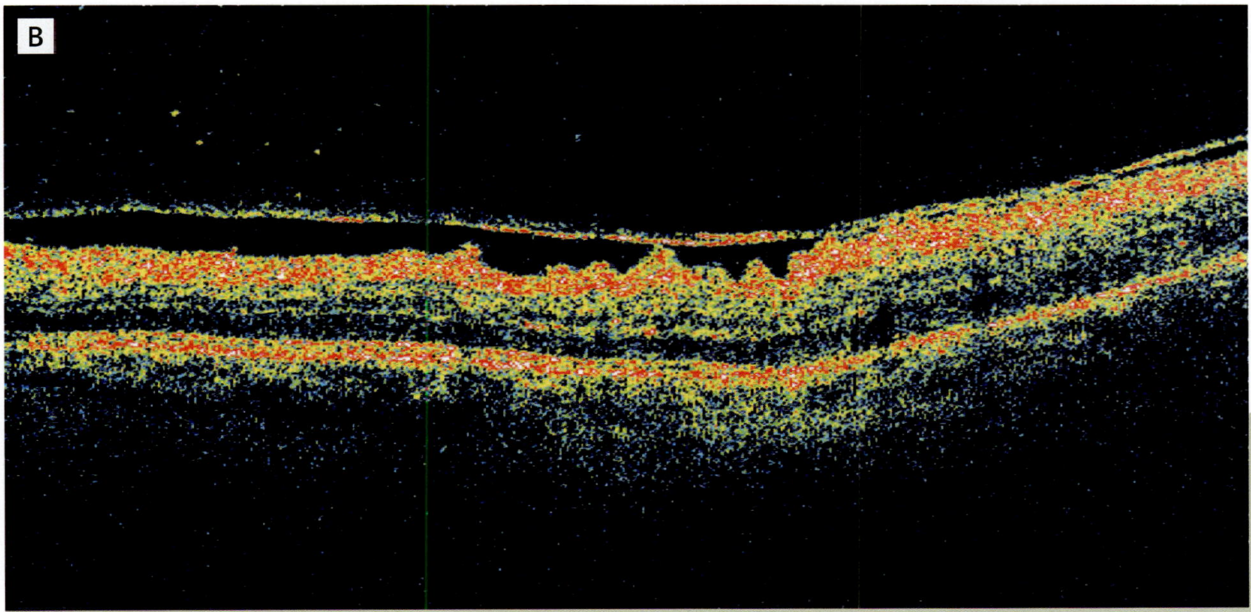

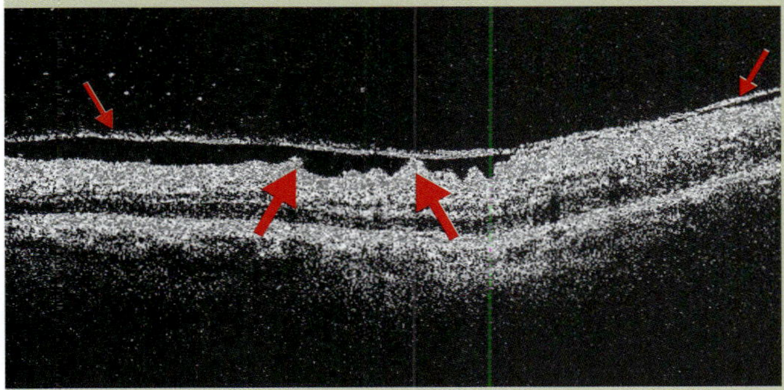

A. Vertical scan of the same eye of page 230 temporally to the optic disc (the arrow shows the scan direction). B. A line of high reflectivity with focal attachments to the retinal surface is detected (small arrows) corresponding to the posterior vitreous. Note the smooth elevations on the retinal surface that probably correspond to an epiretinal membrane (big arrows). In some cases the differentiation of the posterior vitreous face from an epiretinal membrane is difficult. In these cases it is recommended to acquire multiple scan images across the entire posterior pole.

VOGT-KOYANAGI-HARADA SYNDROME

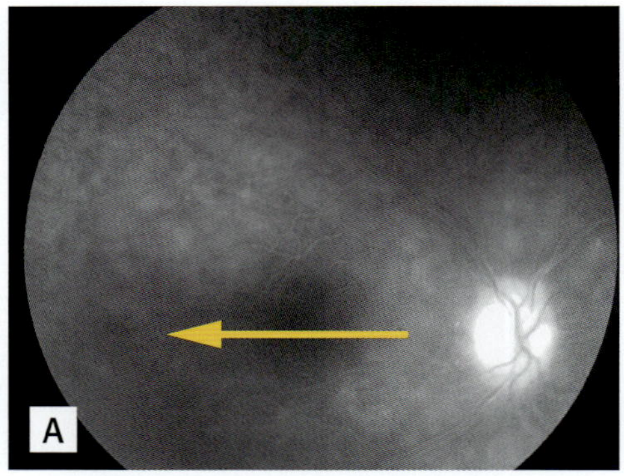

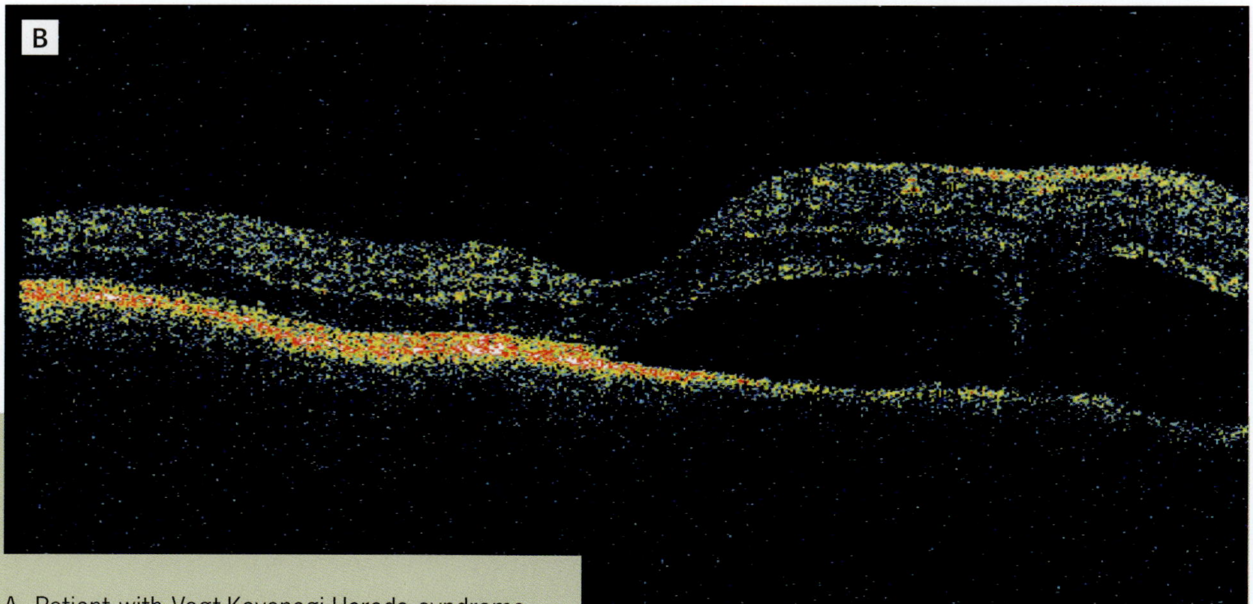

A. Patient with Vogt-Koyanagi-Harada syndrome. Retinal detachment and optic disc edema are observed biomicroscopically (the arrow scows the scan direction). Fluorescein angiography reveals multiple pin-point hyperfluorescent spots due to dye leakage as well as optic disc leakage. B. Optical Coherence Tomography shows an area of low reflectivity located between the retina and the retinal pigment epithelium in the fovea and around it that corresponds to a focal retinal detachment (small arrows) with edema of the overlying retinal layers (big arrows) in both eyes.

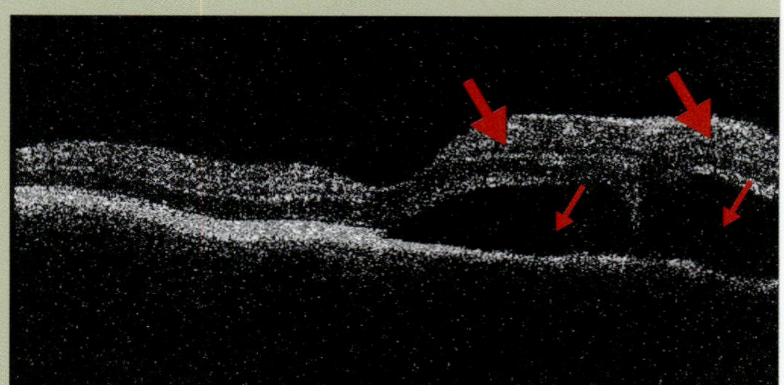

VOGT-KOYANAGI-HARADA SYNDROME

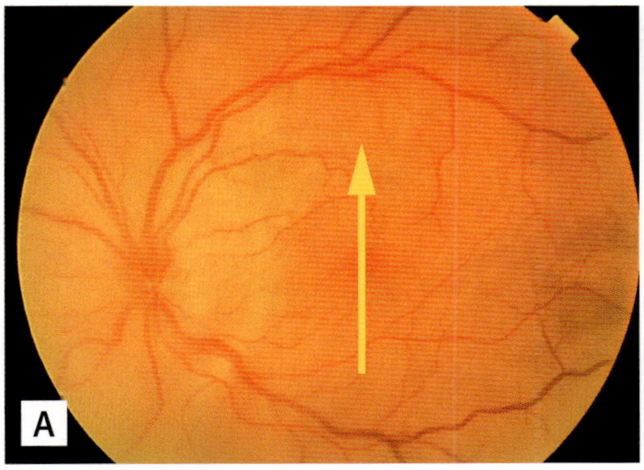

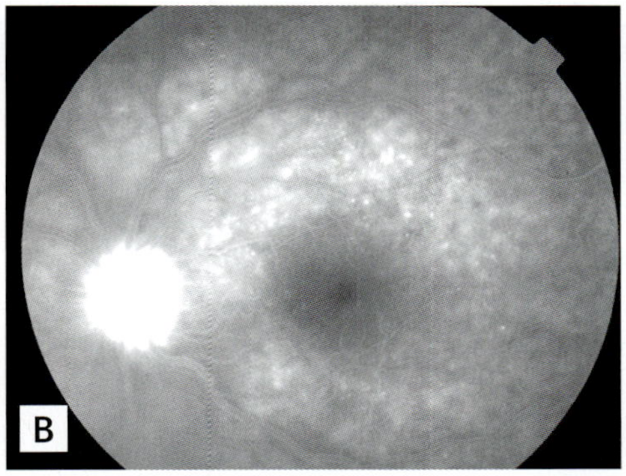

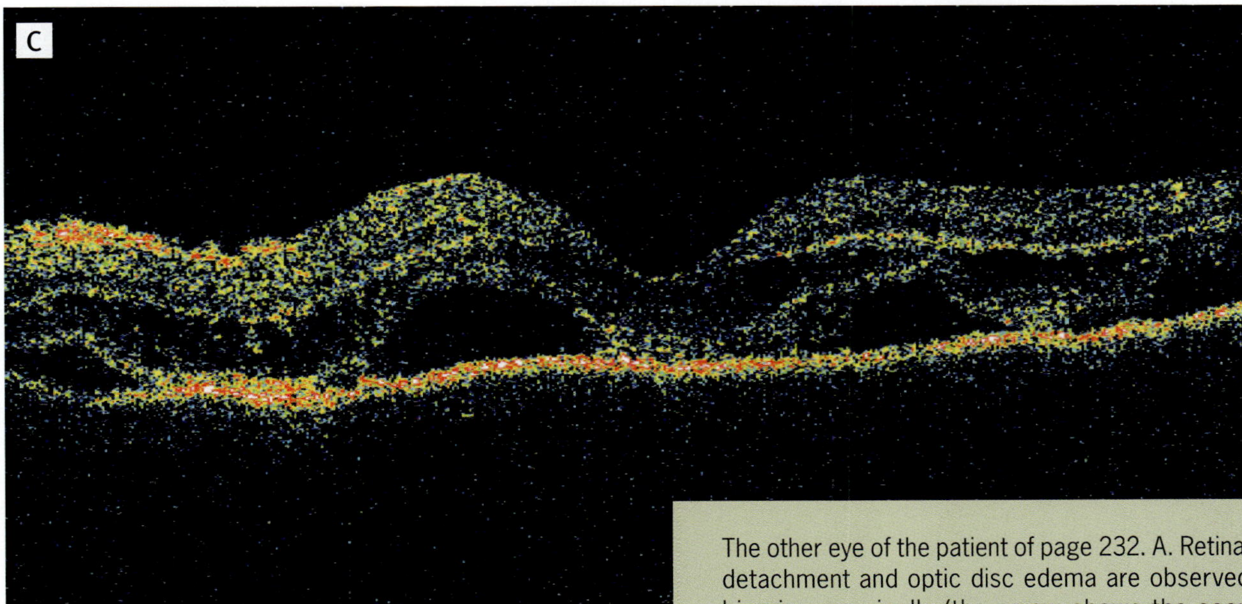

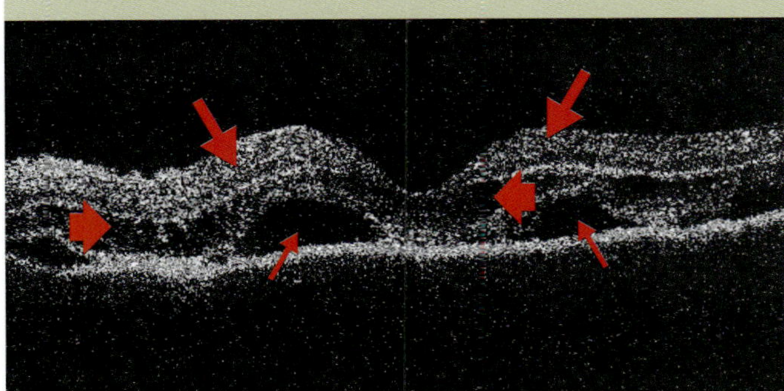

The other eye of the patient of page 232. A. Retinal detachment and optic disc edema are observed biomicroscopically (the arrow shows the scan direction).B. Fluorescein angiography shows multiple pin-point hyperfluorescent spots due to dye leakage as well as optic disc leakage. C. Optical Coherence Tomography shows an area of low reflectivity located between the retina and the retinal pigment epithelium in the fovea and around it (small arrows) with edema of the overlying retinal layers (big arrows) that corresponds to a focal retinal detachment. Note also the multiple intraretinal cystic areas of low reflectivity corresponding to cystoid retinal edema (thick arrows).

VOGT-KOYANAGI-HARADA SYNDROME

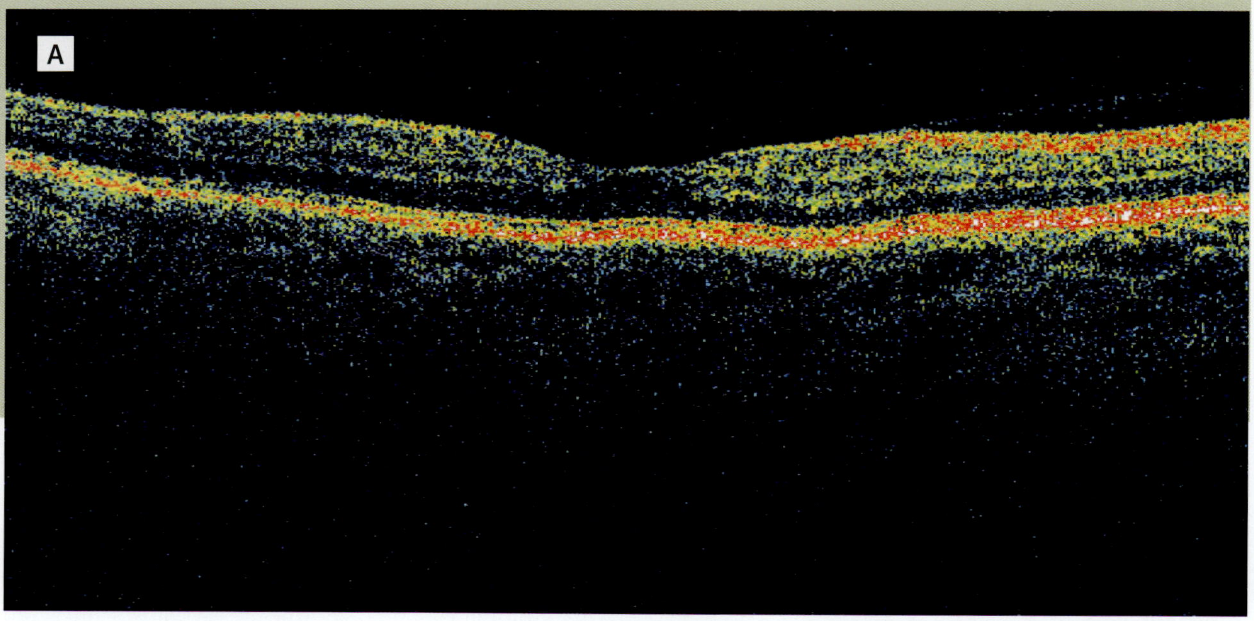

The patient of page 232 three months after systemic corticosteroid treatment. There is complete resolution of the retinal detachment and the cystoid retinal edema. The architecture of the macular area appears normal. A. Right eye. The vitreous is detected attached to the fovea (arrow).

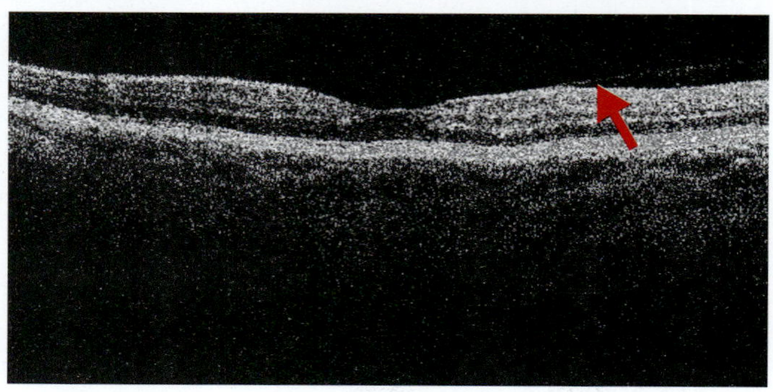

VOGT-KOYANAGI-HARADA SYNDROME

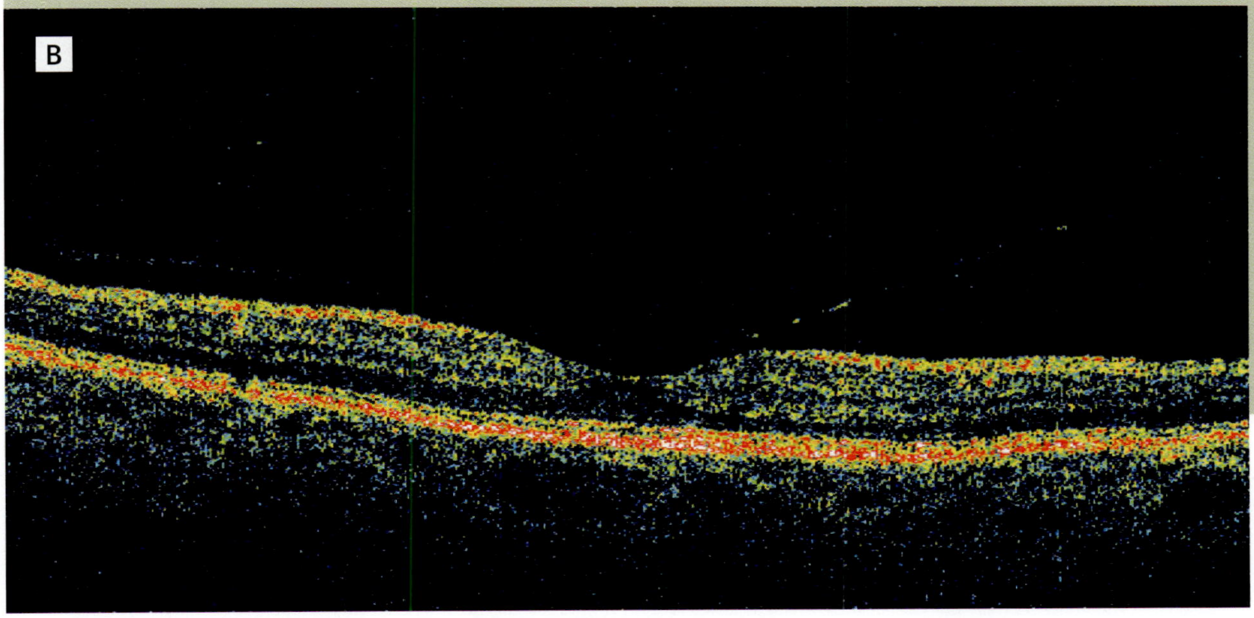

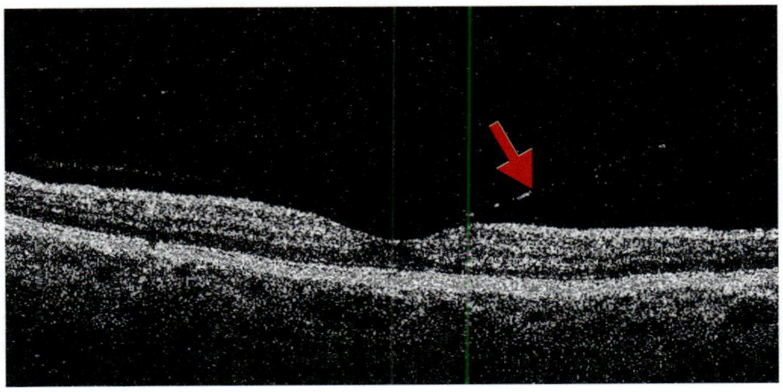

B. Left eye. The vitreous appears attached to the fovea and detached around it (arrow).

TOXOPLASMOSIS

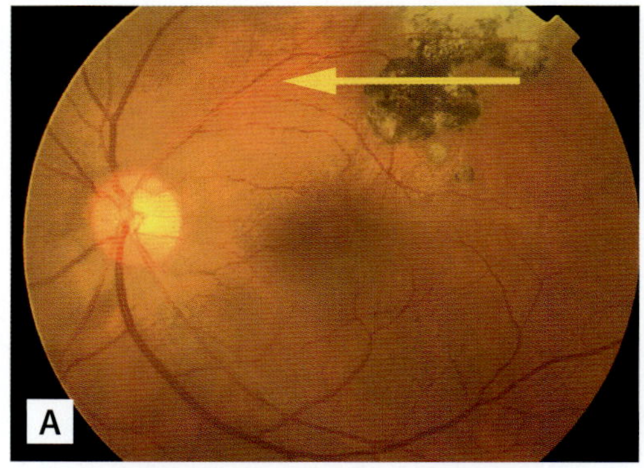

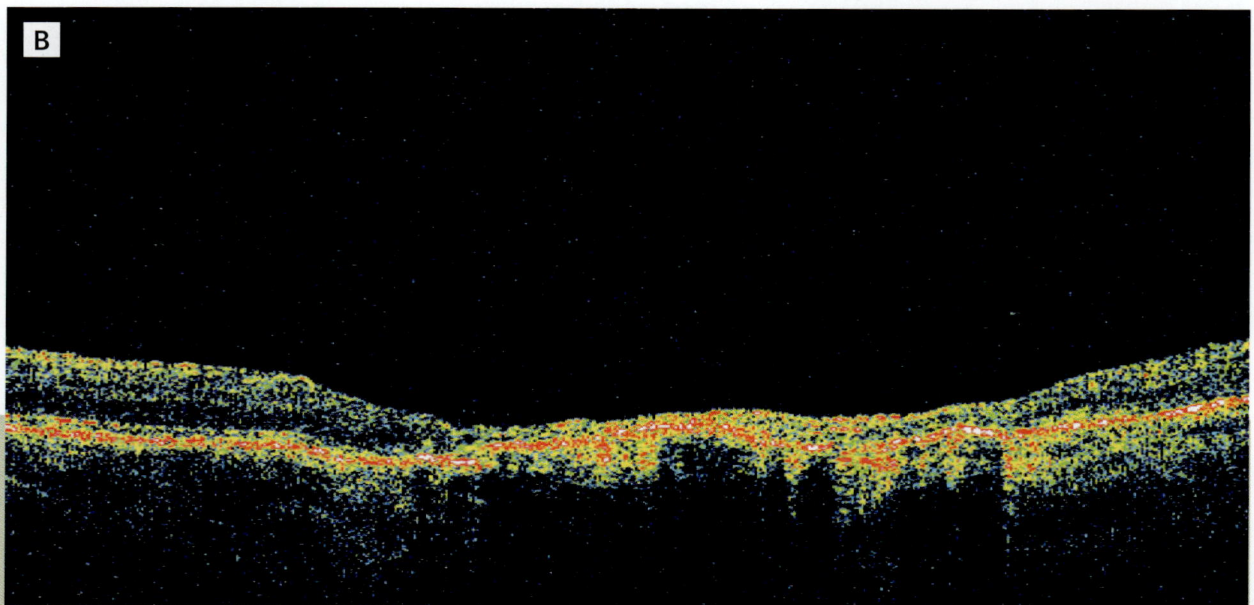

A. Patient with an old scar caused by ocular toxoplasmosis (the arrow shows the scan direction) B. Optical Coherence Tomography shows a thin area of high reflectivity corresponding to the chorioretinal scar (arrow).

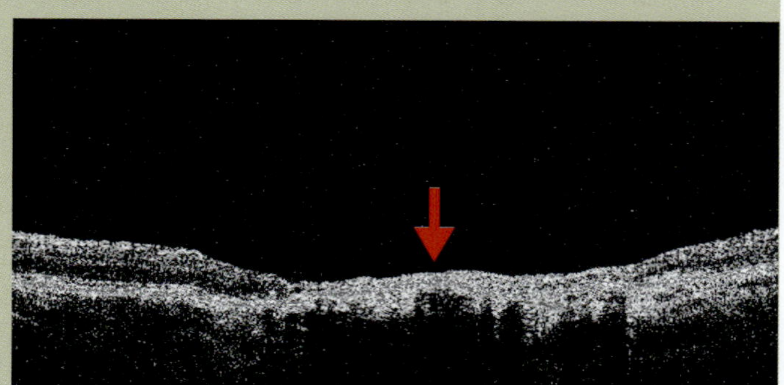

CHAPTER 11

OPTIC NERVE

George Theodossiadis, Ioannis Emfietzoglou, Pantelis Nikolaidis

OPTIC DISC PIT WITH SEROUS MACULAR ELEVATION

Optic disc pit is a congenital abnormality located in the optic nerve. The optic disc pit is accompanied by macular detachment in 50-70% of cases. Retinal elevation in the macula is characterized by the presence of retinoschisis located in the inner layers and by retinal detachment. The retinal elevation initiates temporally to the optic disc and extends towards the central area.

Optical Coherence Tomography imaging is very helpful in the diagnosis and study of the pathogenetic mechanism of the disease[3,9,10,11].

It shows the presence of retinoschisis or cystic formation in the inner retinal layers that often coexist with serous retinal detachment[6,8,12]. Both of these pathologic findings appear as areas with low reflectivity. In some cases the communication of the optic disc pit with the retinoschisis cavity of the inner retinal layers is evident[14].

Optical Coherence Tomography is also very useful in the postoperative follow-up of patients who have undergone vitrectomy[7] or scleral buckle in order to interrupt the communication between the optic disc pit and the retinal layers.
In successfully treated cases Optical Coherence Tomography shows the decrease or the disappearance of the macular detachment[1,2,4-6,13].

OPTIC DISC DRUSEN

Drusen are calcified formations, located in front or behind the lamina cribrosa within the optic disc. Those located in front of the lamina are usually bilateral and probably come from mitochondrial calcification due to alterations of the axoplasmic flow. Drusen cause enlargement of the optic disc and often resemble optic disc edema. They are idiopathic or are inherited in an autosomal dominant manner. Optical Coherence Tomography can detect changes of the nerve fiber layer in cases of optic disc edema, as opposed to the stability of the nerve fiber layer in patients with optic disc drusen. In the former the nerve fiber layer is becoming thinner with time.

OPTIC DISC PIT

1. Garcia-Arumi J, Guraya BC, Espax AB, Castillo VM, Ramsay LS, Motta RM. Optical coherence tomography in optic pit maculopathy managed with vitrectomy-laser-gas. Graefes Arch Clin Exp Ophthalmol 2004; 242: 819-826.

2. Gandorfer A, Kampik A. Role of vitreoretinal interface in the pathogenesis and therapy of macular disease associated with optic pits. Ophthalmologe 2000; 97: 276-279.

3. Hirakata A, Hida T, Ogasawara A, Iizuka N. Multilayered retinoschisis associated with optic disc pit. Jpn J Ophthalmol 2005; 49: 414-416.

4. Hirakata A, Hida T, Wakabayashi T, Fukuda M. Unusual posterior hyaloid strand in a young child with optic disc pit maculopathy: intraoperative and histopathological findings. Jpn J Ophthalmol 2005; 49: 264-266.

5. Hirakata A, Okada AA, Hida T. Long-term results of vitrectomy without laser treatment for macular detachment associated with an optic disc pit. Ophthalmology 2005; 112: 1430-1435.

6. Hassenstein A, Richard G. Optical coherence tomography in optic pit associated maculopathy. Ophthalmologe 2004; 101: 170-176.

7. Ishikawa K, Terasaki H, Mori M, Sugita K, Miyake Y. Optical coherence tomography before and after vitrectomy with internal limiting membrane removal in a child with optic disc pit maculopathy. Jpn J Ophthalmol 2005; 49: 411-413.

8. Lincoff H, Kreissig I. Optical coherence tomography of pneumatic displacement of optic disc pit maculopathy. Br J Ophthalmol 1998; 82: 367-372.

9. Lincoff H, Schiff W, Krivoy D, Ritch R. Optical coherence tomography of optic disk pit maculopathy. Am J Ophthalmol 1996; 122: 264-266.

10. Meirelles RL, Aggio FB, Costa RA, Farah ME STRATUS optical coherence tomography in unilateral colobomatous excavation of the optic disc and secondary retinoschisis. Graefes Arch Clin Exp Ophthalmol 2005; 243: 76-81.

11. Oshima Y, Emi K. Optical cross-sectional assessment of the macula by retinal thickness analyzer in optic disk pit maculopathy. Am J Ophthalmol 1999; 128: 106-109.

12. Rutledge BK, Puliafito CA, Duker JS, Hee MR, Cox MS. Optical coherence tomography of macular lesions associated with optic nerve head pits. Ophthalmology 1996; 103: 1047-1053

13. Theodossiadis GP, Theodossiadis PG. Optical coherence tomography in optic disk pit maculopathy treated by macular buckling procedure. Am J. Ophthalmol 2001; 132: 184-190.

14. Vedantham V, Ramasamy K. Spontaneous improvement of serous maculopathy associated with congenital optic disc pit: an OCT study. Eye 2005; 19: 596-599.

TILTED OPTIC DISC

Tilted optic disc is a usually bilateral condition observed in 1-2% of the general population. The disease is owed to an oblique optic nerve insertion to the globe. The optic disc usually has an ovoid appearance with an oblique vertical axis. The superotemporal part of the optic disc is located anteriorly to the inferonasal part. A meniscus of peripapillary chorioretinal atrophy, myopic astigmatism, posterior staphyloma, pigment changes of the macula and choroidal neovascularization can also exist[2]. Serous macular detachment is rarely observed without the presence of choroidal neovascularization. This condition can be detected only by Optical Coherence Tomography, since in most cases there are no fluorescein angiographic findings[1]. In tilted optic discs the optic disc level is oblique in respect to the area of the Optical Coherence Tomography scan and therefore the study of the optic disc and the nerve fiber layer thickness measurement may be difficult to perform.

TILTED OPTIC DISC

1. Theodossiadis PG, Grigoropoulos V, Emfietzoglou J, Theodossiadis GP. Optical coherence tomography study of tilted optic disk associated with macular detachment. Graefe's Arch Clin Exp Ophthalmol. 2006;244(1):122-4.

2. Young SE, Walsh FB, Knox DL. The tilted disk syndrome. Am J Ophthalmol. 1976;82(1):16-23.

MYELINATED NERVE FIBERS

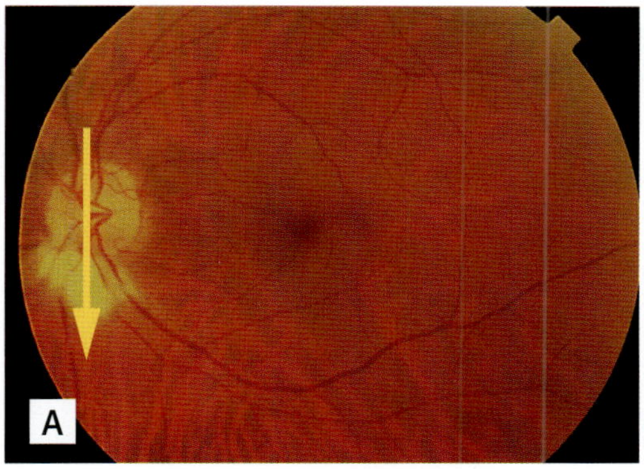

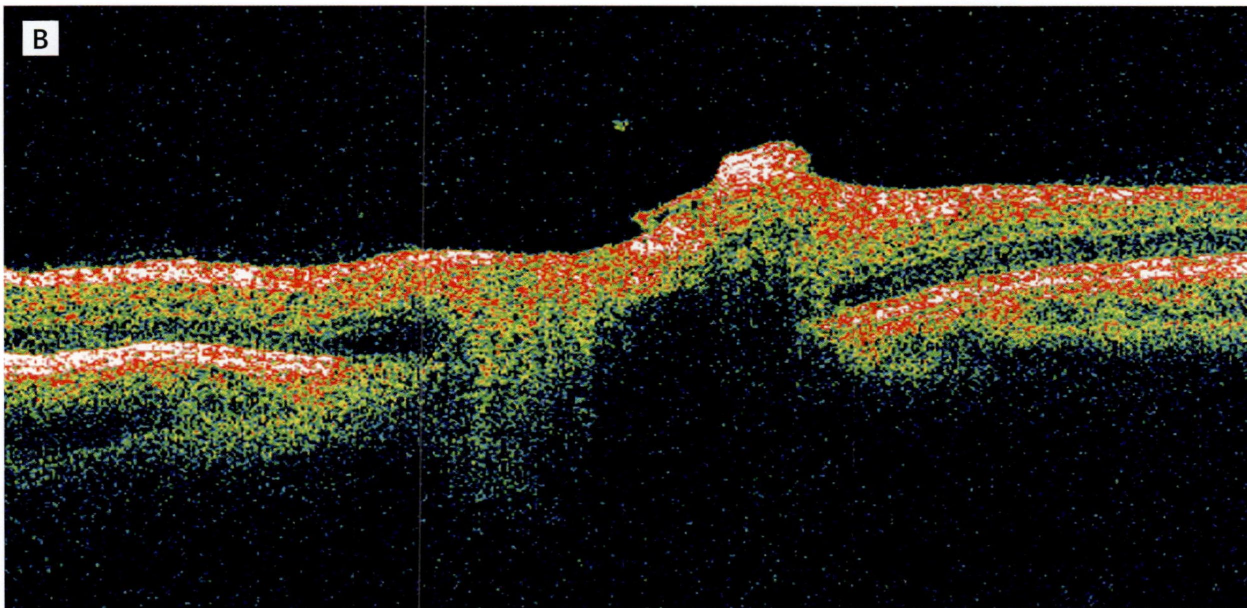

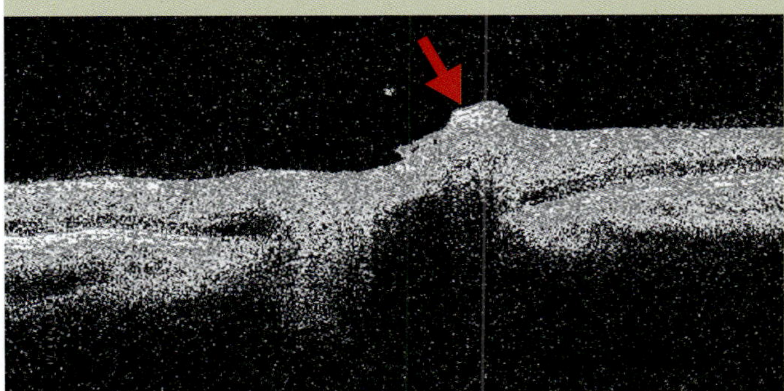

A. Patient with myelinated nerve fibers (the arrow shows the scan direction). B. Optical Coherence Tomography shows high reflectivity of the nerve fiber layer and a focal elevation due to the presence of the myelinated nerve fibers (arrow).

OPTIC DISC DRUSEN

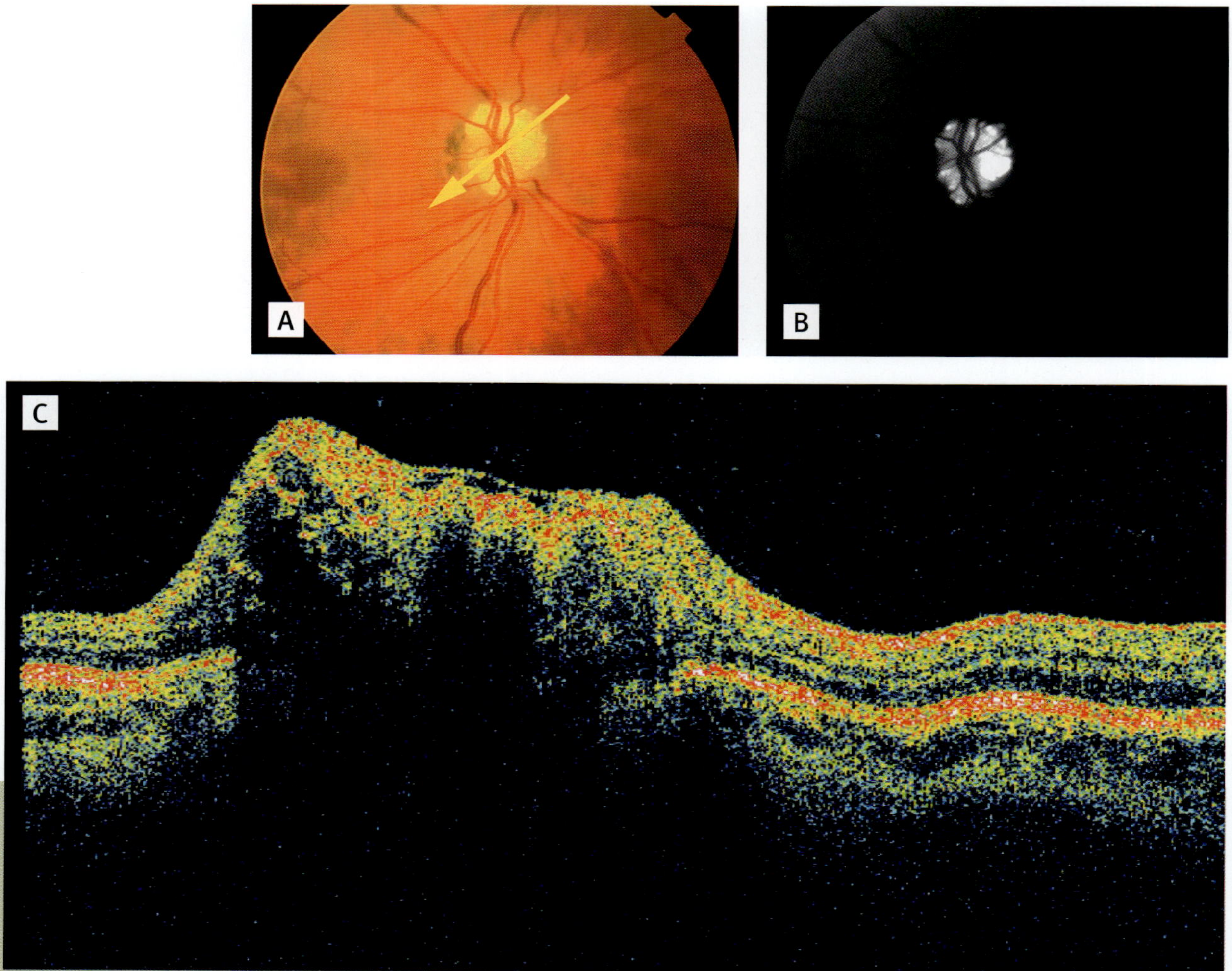

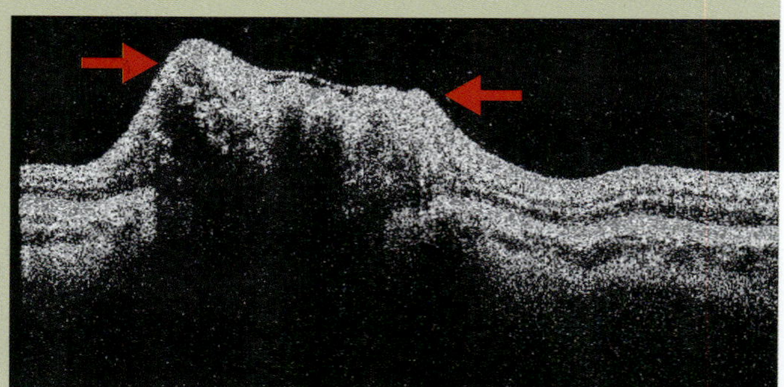

A. Right eye of a patient with bilateral optic disc drusen (the arrow shows the scan direction). B. Autofluorescence of the drusen after fluorescein angiography filters activation. C. Optical Coherence Tomography shows bilateral elevations of high reflectivity on the optic disc surface (arrows) with shadowing of the underlying tissues caused by the optic disc drusen.

OPTIC DISC DRUSEN

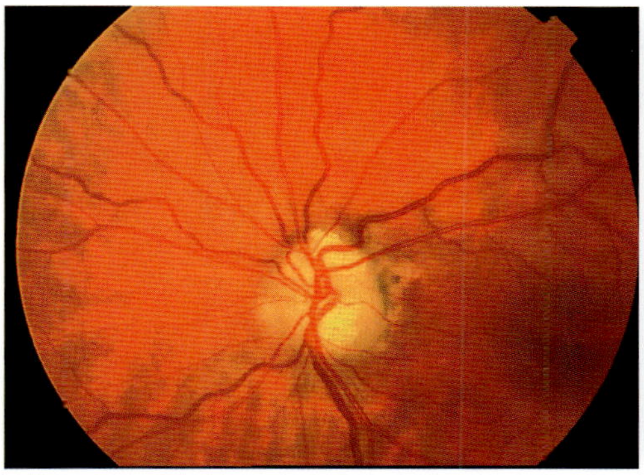

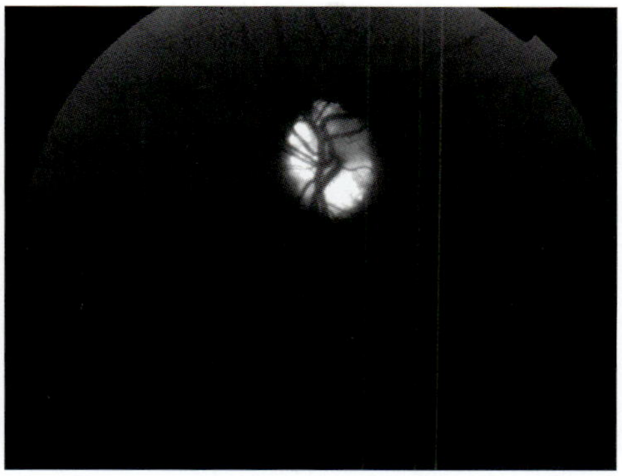

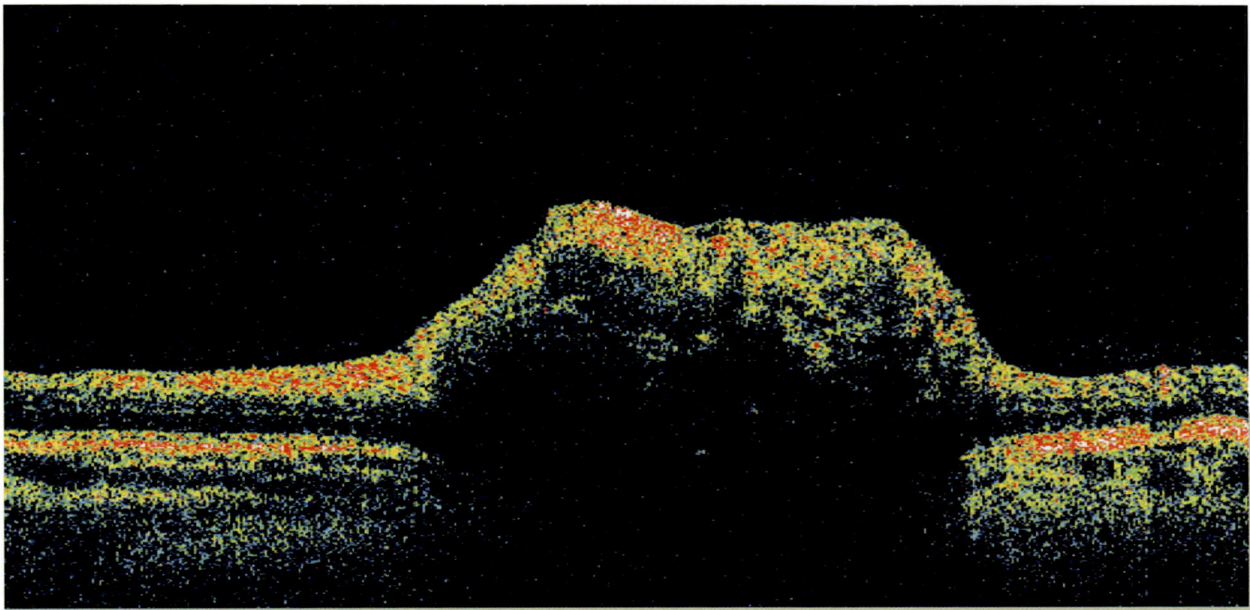

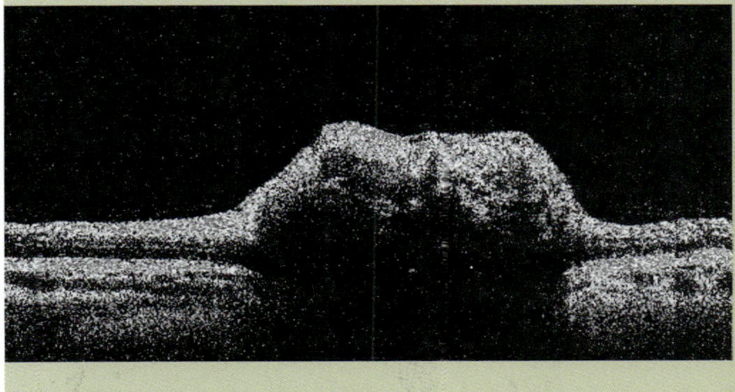

The left eye of the patient of page 244 that shares the same features.

BENIGN INTRACRANIAL HYPERTENSION

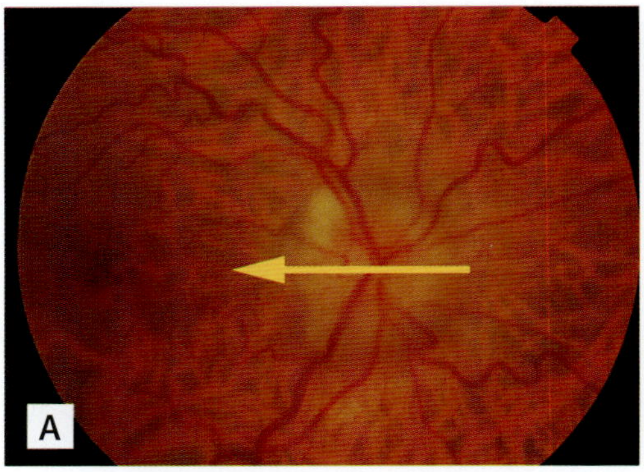

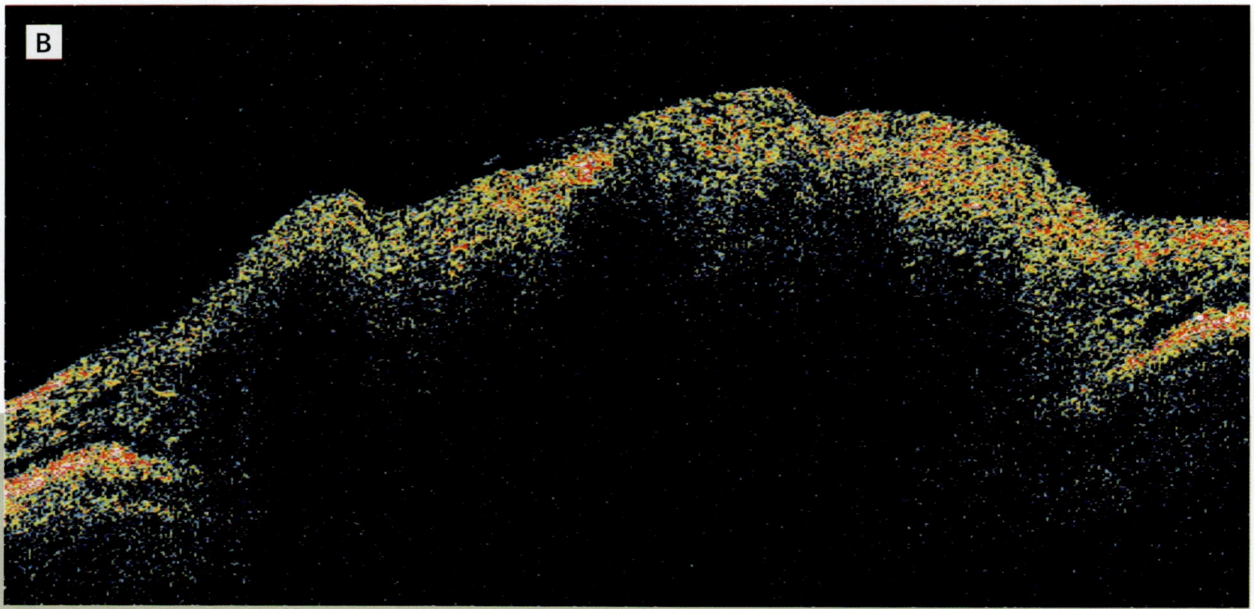

A. The right eye of a patient with bilateral optic disc edema due to increased intracranial pressure (the arrow shows the scan direction). B. Bilateral optic nerve head elevation is detected (arrow) with disappearance of its physiologic cupping.

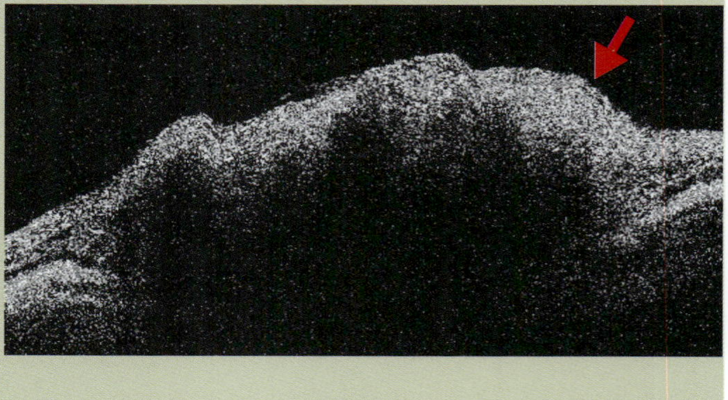

BENIGN INTRACRANIAL HYPERTENSION

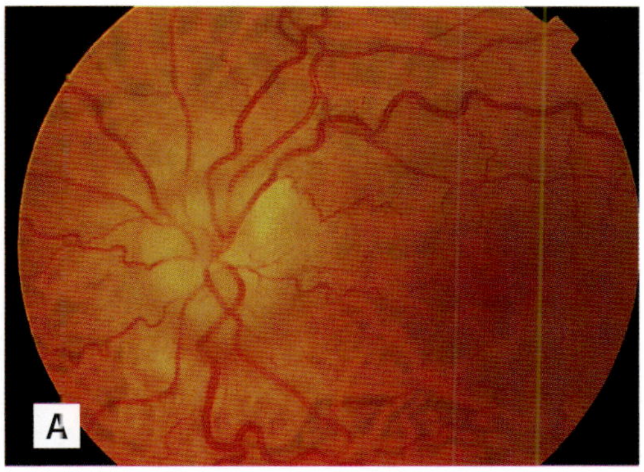

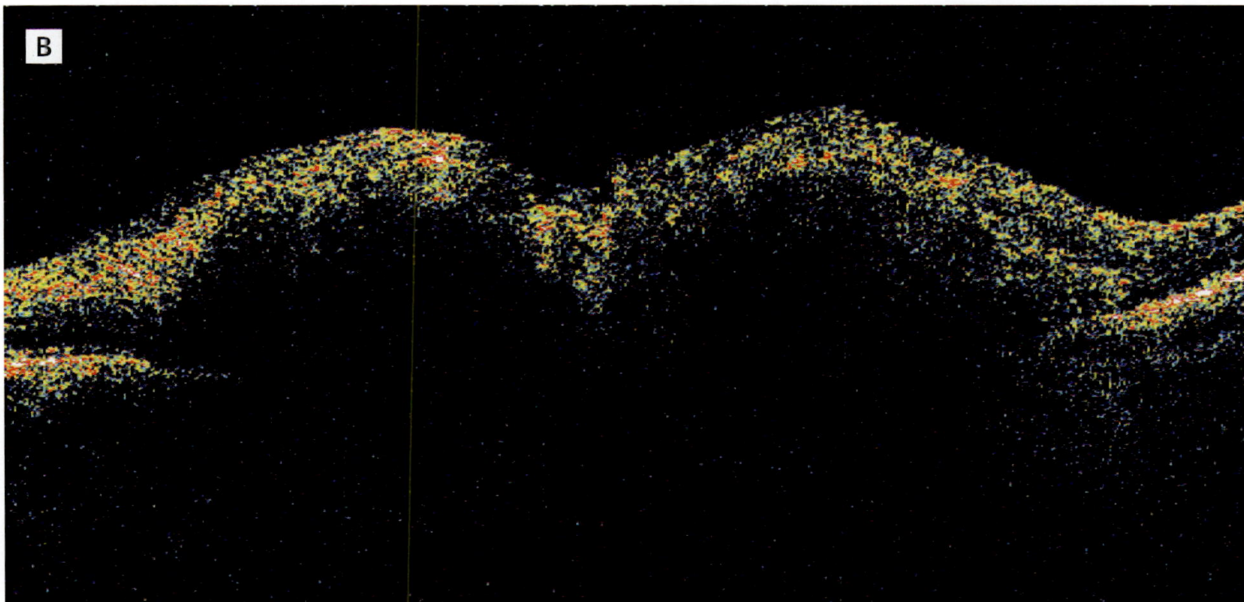

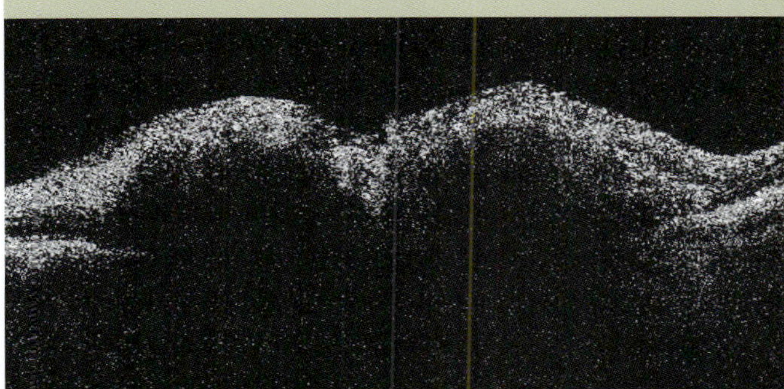

The left eye of the patient of page 246.

CONGENITAL OPTIC DISC PIT

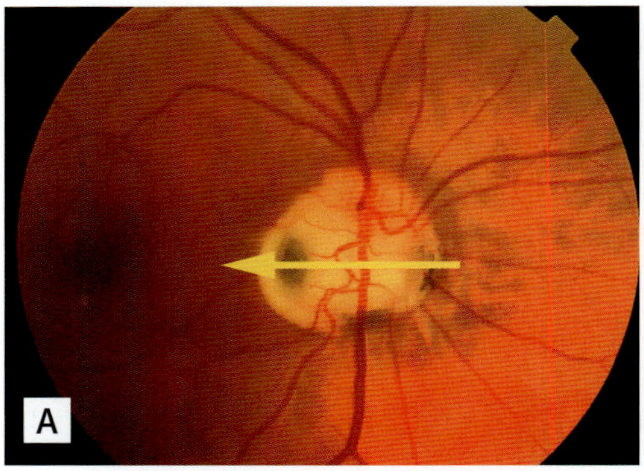

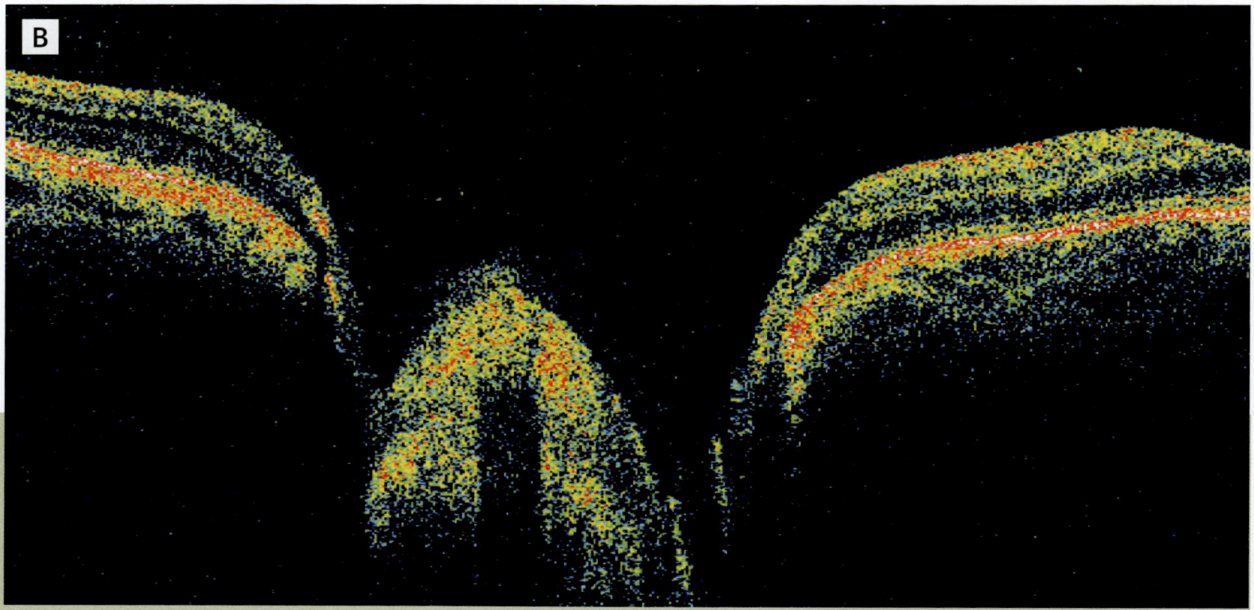

A. Patient with congenital optic disc pits without macular elevation (the arrow shows the scan direction). B. Optical Coherence Tomography shows normal architecture of the retinal layers without the presence of detachment or schisis of the retina. On both sides of the optic disc there are areas of low reflectivity that are attributed to the optic disc pits and appear to connect the optic disc surface with the deeper layers of the optic nerve (arrows).

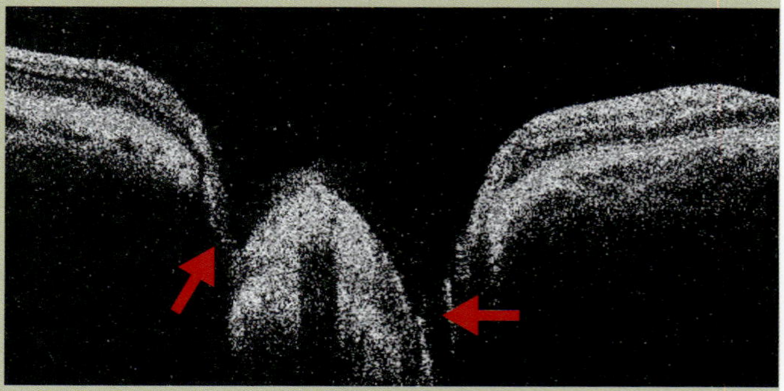

CONGENITAL OPTIC DISC PIT

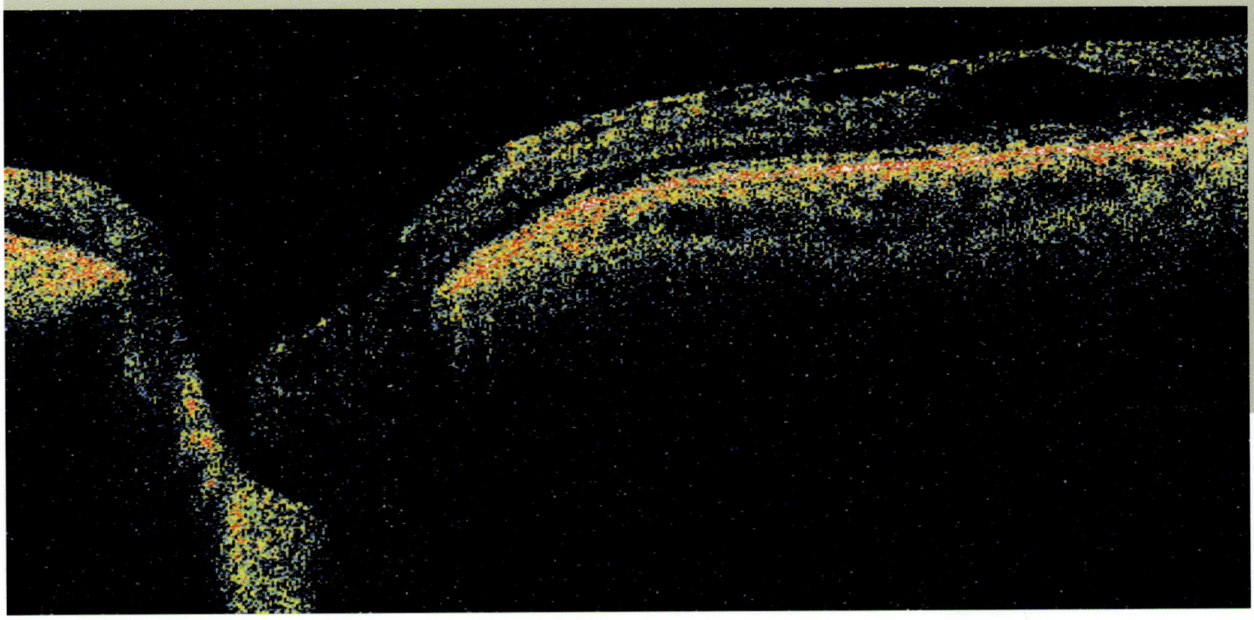

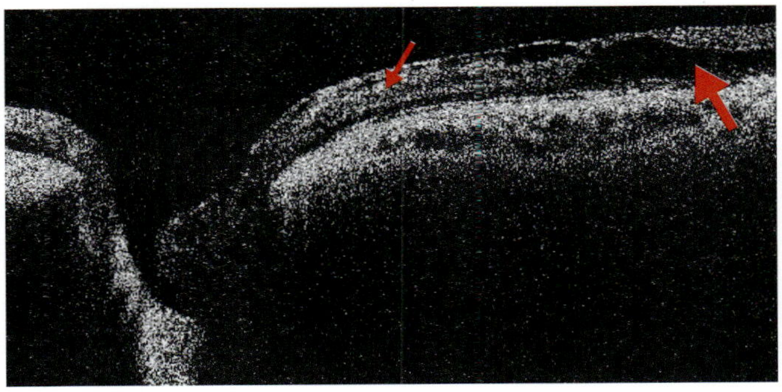

Optic disc pit. Note the low reflectivity that is located in the inner retinal layers (small arrow) and corresponds to retinal cystic oedema in the macular area. Also note the area of low reflectivity located in the outer retinal layers (big arrow) that corresponds to retinoschisis.

CONGENITAL OPTIC DISC PIT

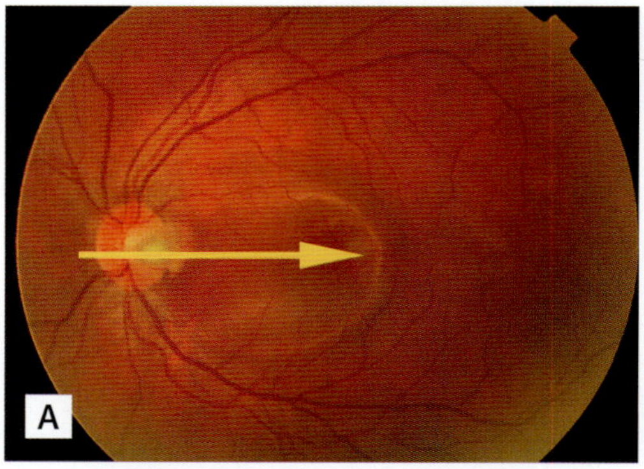

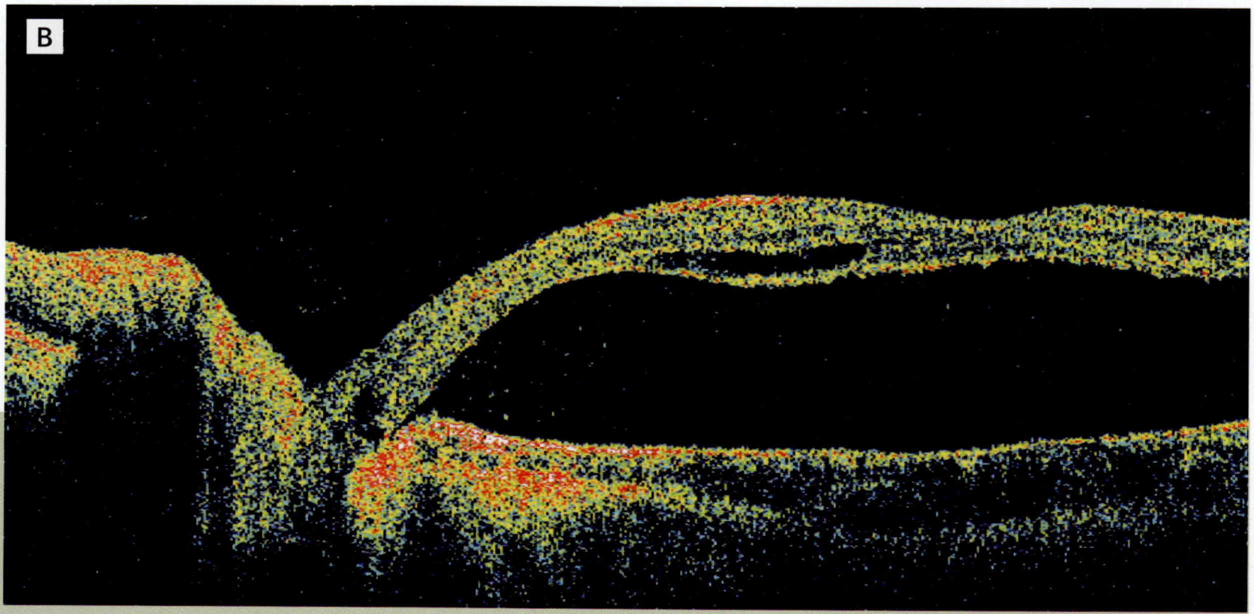

A. Optic disc pit with serous retinal detachment (the arrow shows the scan direction). B. Note the low reflectivity area located between the retina and the retinal pigment epithelium that corresponds to an extensive retinal detachment (small arrow). A cystic formation is also detected in the outer retinal layers and corresponds to cystoid retinal edema (big arrow). There is no connection observed between the optic disc pit and the serous elevation of the retina.

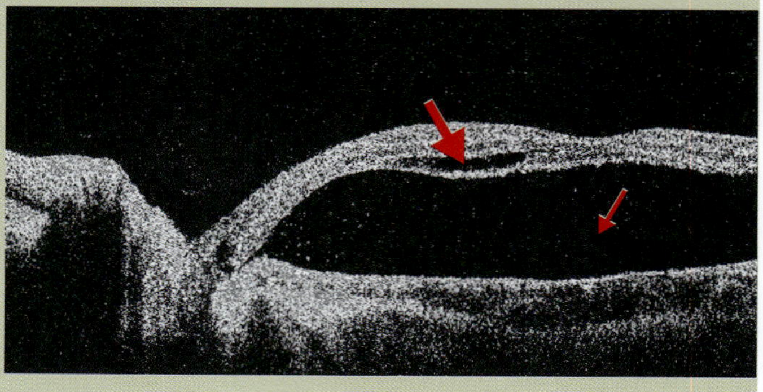

CONGENITAL OPTIC DISC PIT

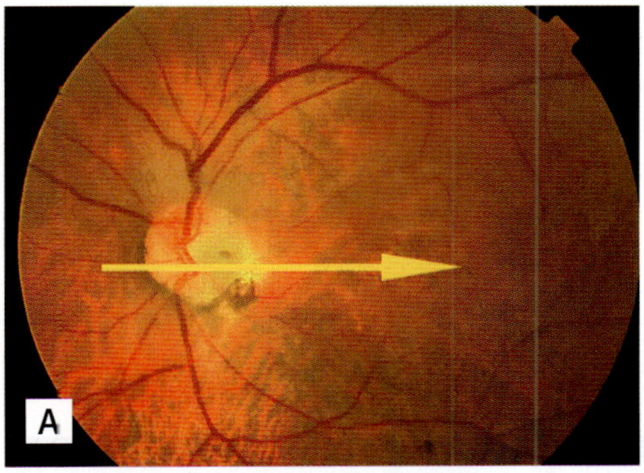

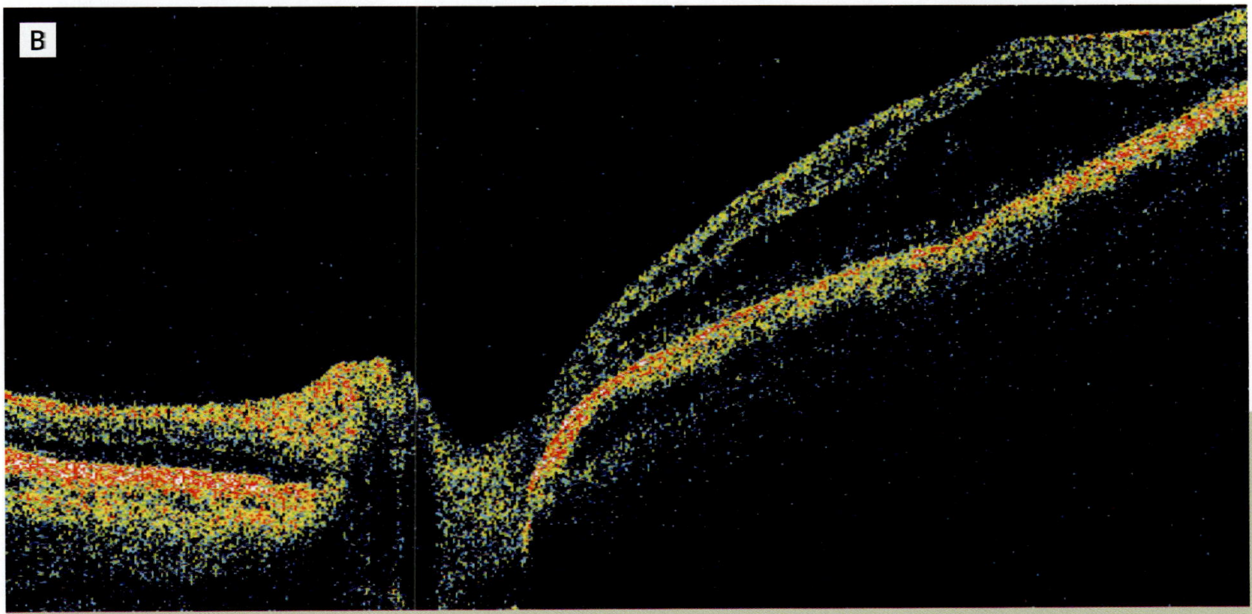

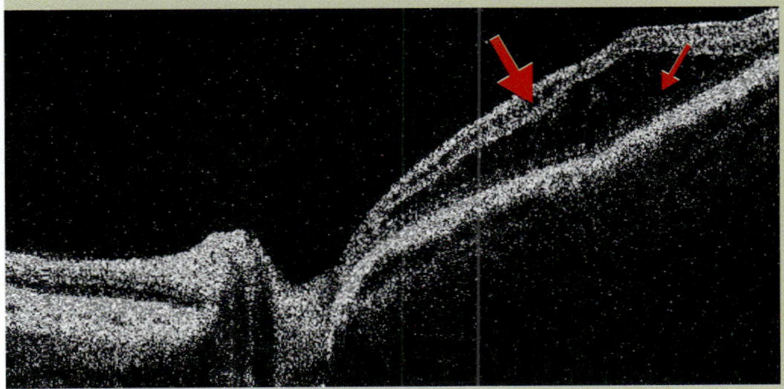

A. Centrally located optic disc pit. Chorioretinal scar and pigmentation of the inferior and temporal border of the optic disc are also evident (the arrow shows the scan direction). B. An area of low reflectivity is detected in the outer retinal layers, extending from the temporal part of the optic disc to the temporal border of the fovea and corresponds to retinoschisis (small arrow). Multiple cystic areas of low reflectivity are detected in the inner retinal layers and correspond to cystic retinal edema (big arrow). No connection between the retinoschisis and the optic disc pit is observed.

CONGENITAL OPTIC DISC PIT

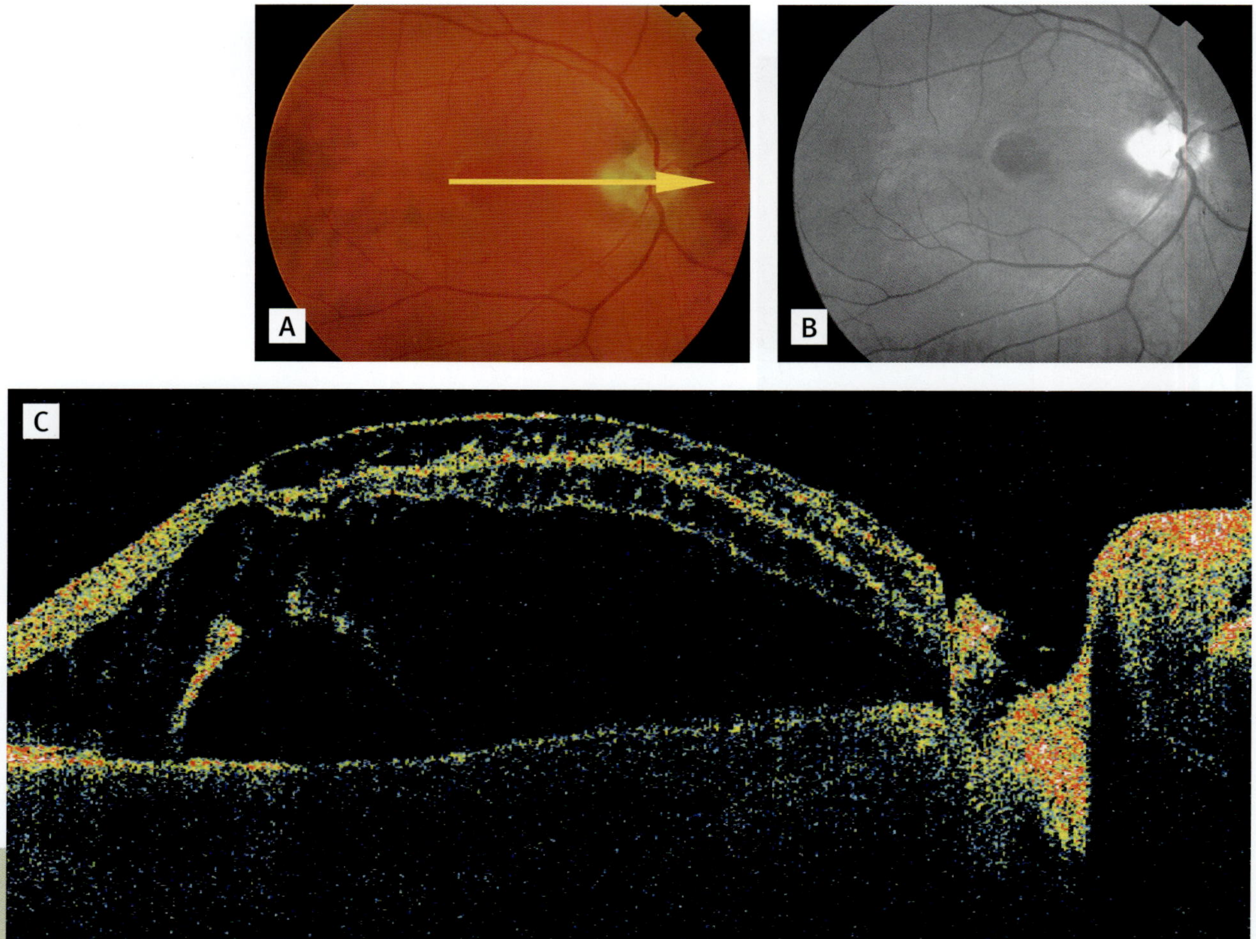

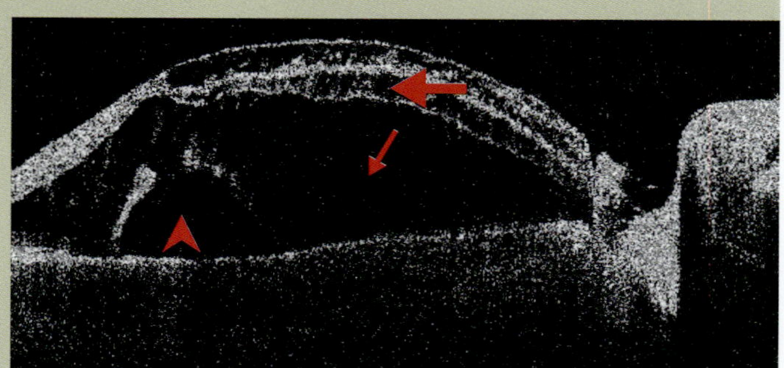

A. Patient with a temporal optic disc pit (the arrow shows the scan direction). B. Fluid accumulation in the macula is clearly visible in the red-free photograph. C. Optical Coherence Tomography shows an area of low reflectivity in the outer retinal layers that corresponds to retinoschisis (small arrow). It is accompanied by coalescent cystic formations of low reflectivity located in the inner retinal layers and corresponding to cystoid retinal edema (big arrow). An area of low reflectivity is detected in the fovea, located between the retina and the retinal pigment epithelium, corresponding to a retinal detachment (arrow head). The case is characterized by the presence of three elements of retinal elevation: retinal detachment, retinoschisis and coalescent cystic retinal formations. No connection between the optic disc pit and the retinal elevation is observed.

CONGENITAL OPTIC DISC PIT

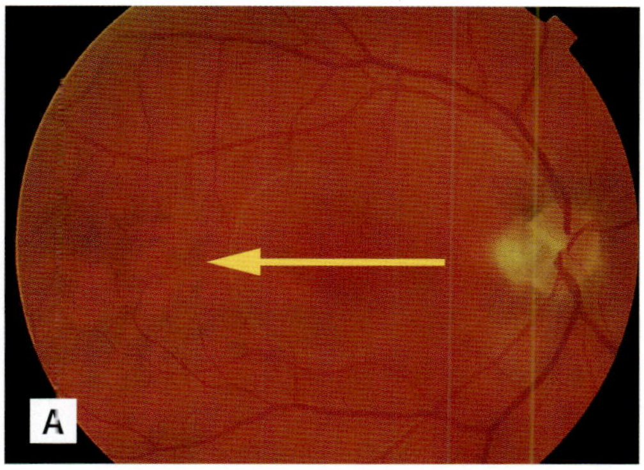

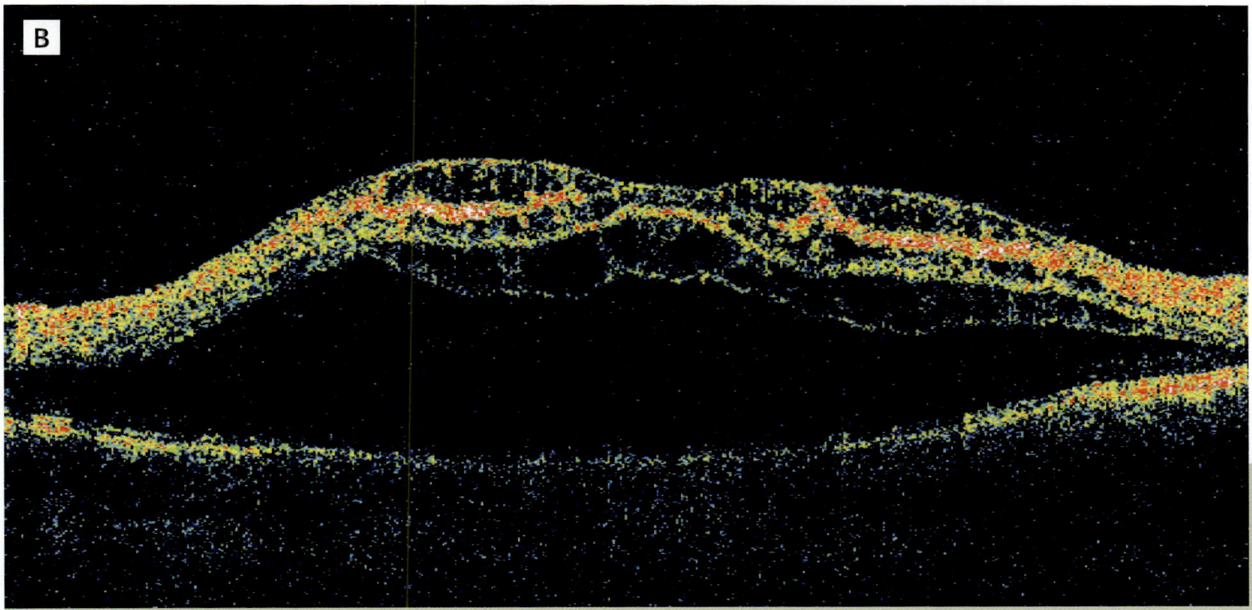

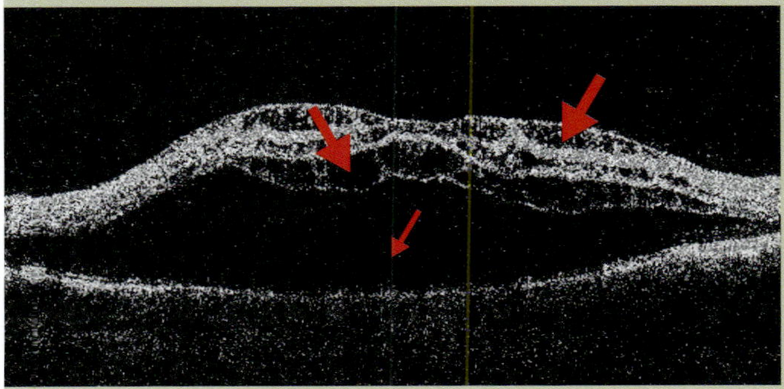

A. Patient with optic disc pit (the arrow shows the scan direction). B. An area of low reflectivity is detected in the outer retinal layers that corresponds to schisis of the fovea (small arrow). Also note the presence of big cystic areas of low reflectivity in the inner retinal layers corresponding to cystoid retinal edema (big arrows).

TILTED OPTIC DISC

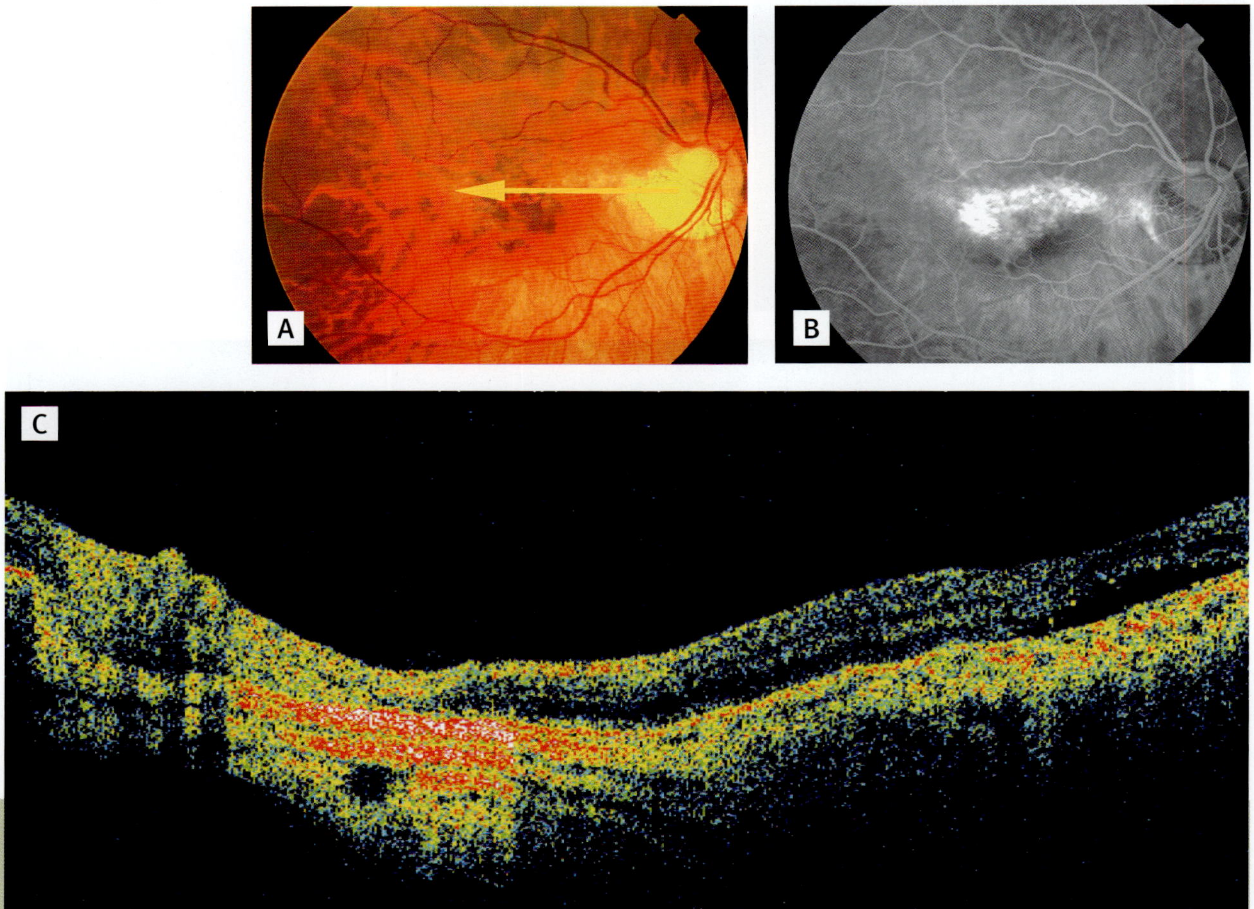

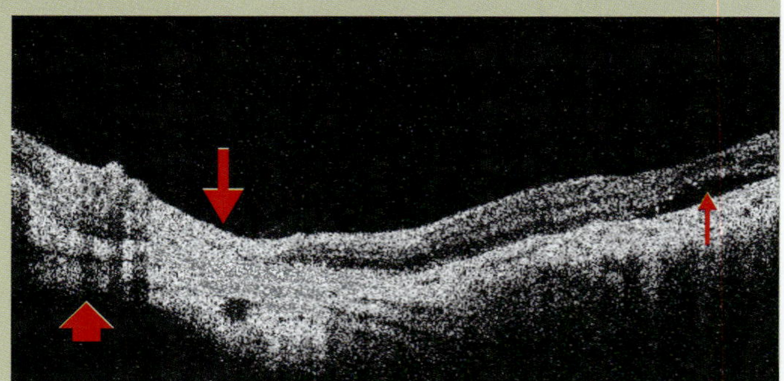

A. Patient with tilted optic disc and moderate visual acuity (the arrow shows the scan direction). B. Fluorescein angiography shows hyperfluorescence in the papillomacular area. C. Optical Coherence Tomography shows an area of low reflectivity in the fovea that corresponds to serous retinal detachment (small arrow) that is not extending to the optic disc. The presence of subretinal fluid is a rare finding of the tilted optic disc syndrome. The area of high reflectivity occupying the entire retinal thickness and the retinal pigment epithelium-choriocapillaries layer (big arrow) observed in the optic disc margins (thick arrow) is due to peripapillary chorioretinal atrophy.

TILTED OPTIC DISC

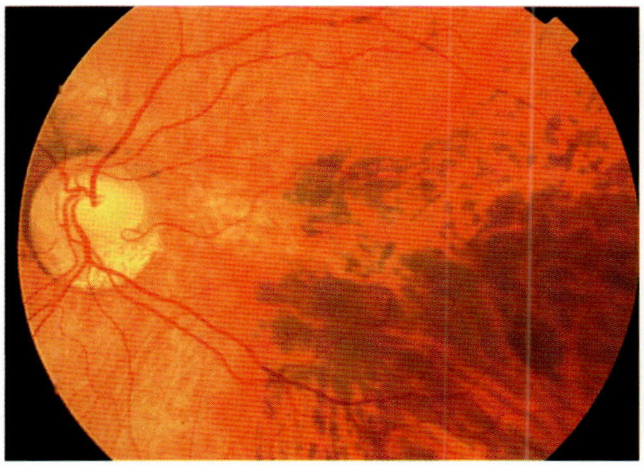
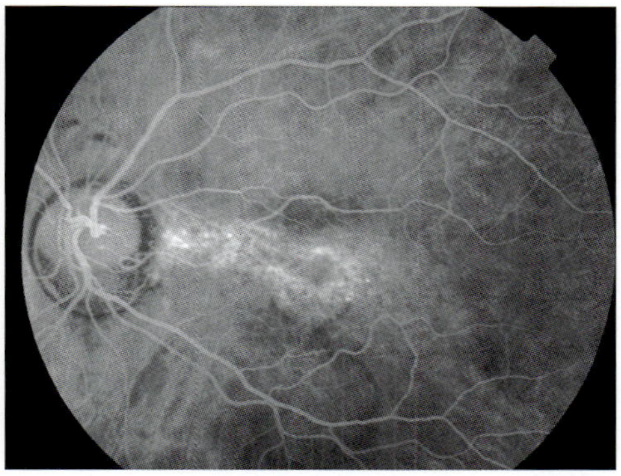
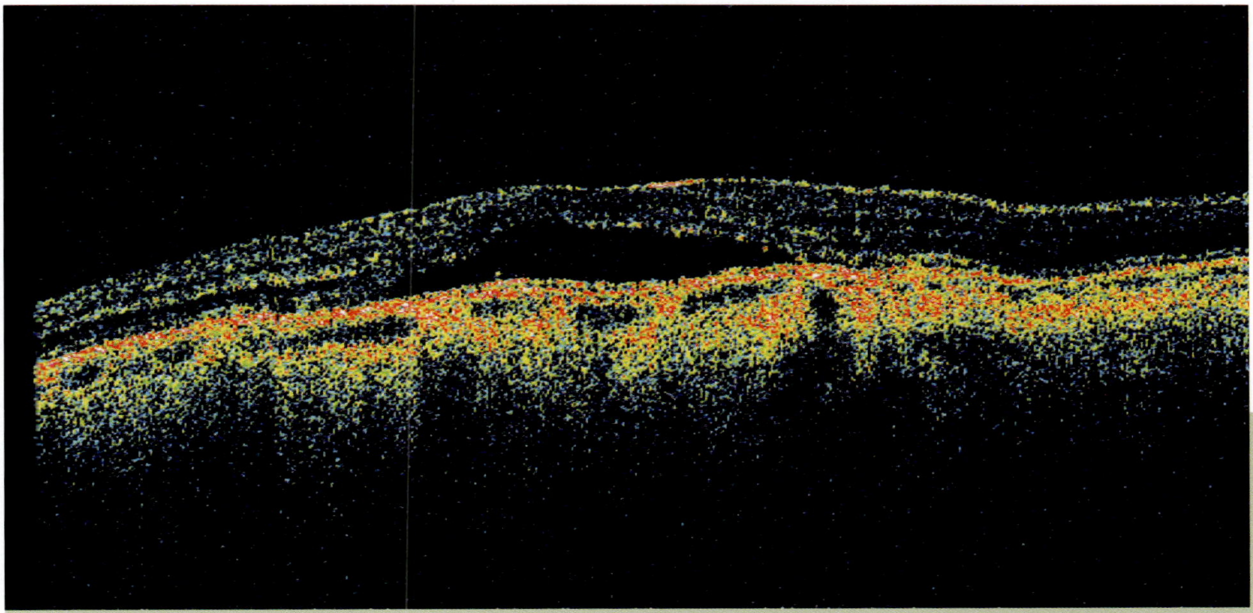
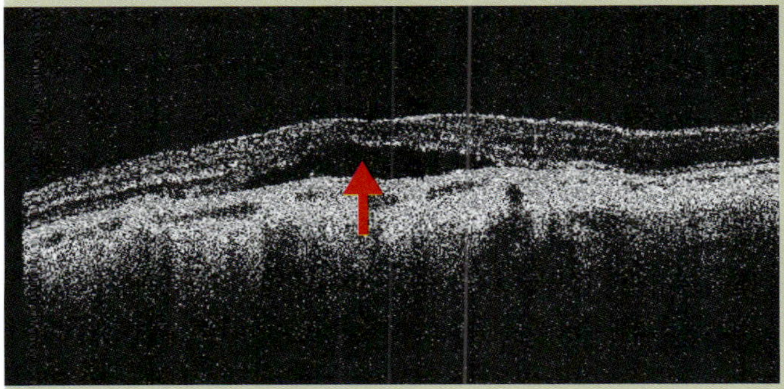

The other eye of the patient of page 254 with serous retinal elevation in the fovea (arrow).

ANTERIOR ISCHEMIC OPTIC NEUROPATHY

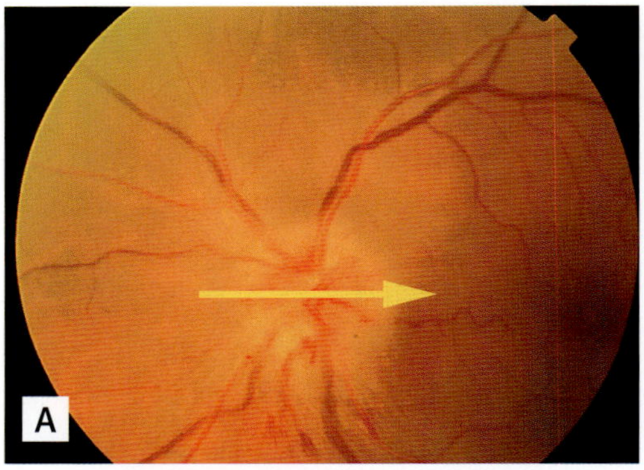

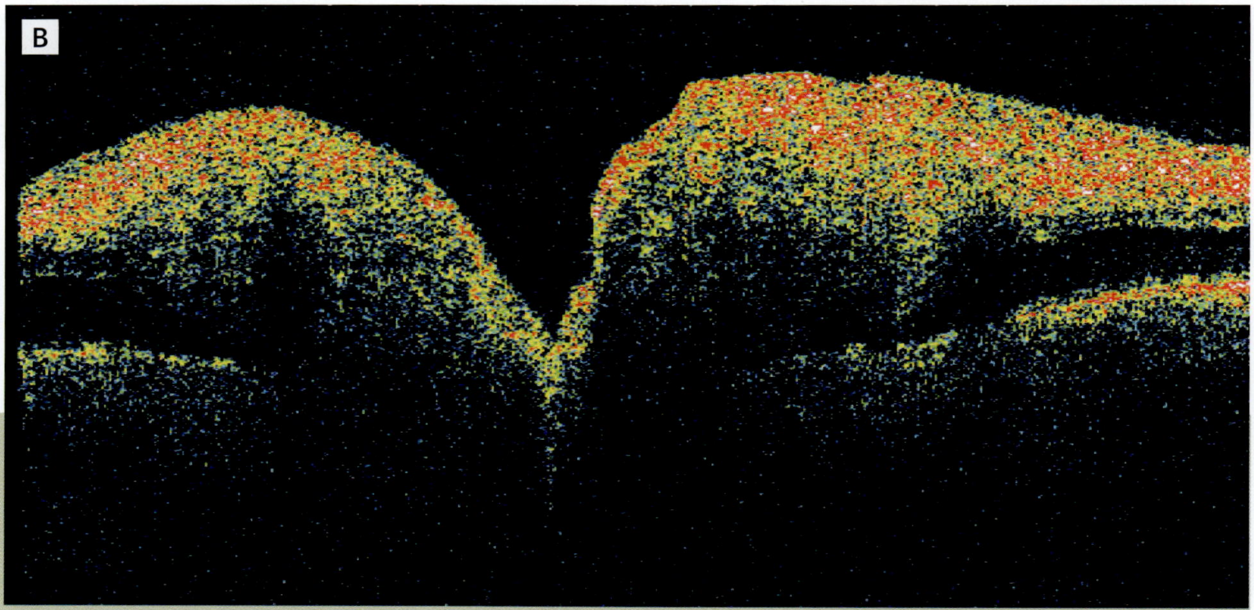

A 59 years old patient with anterior ischemic optic neuropathy. A. Optic disc edema is clearly visible (the arrow shows the scan direction). B. Optical Coherence Tomography shows the high reflectivity of the inner layer of the optic disc margins and of the surrounding retinal area as well as constriction of the optic disc cupping due to the edema (big arrows). The vitreous is attached to the peripapillary area (small arrow).

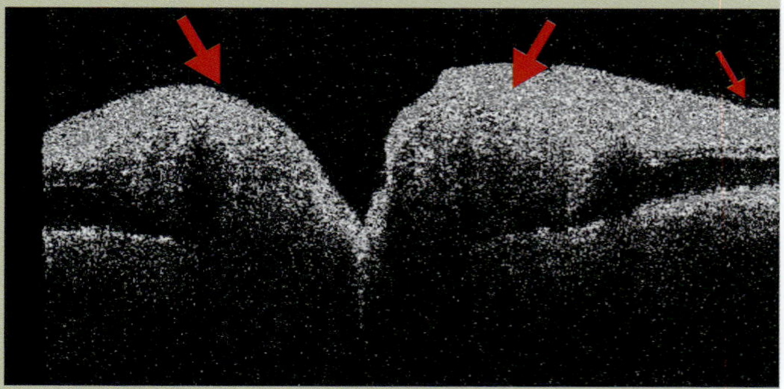

CHAPTER 12

CONGENITAL MACULAR DYSTROPHIES

GEORGE THEODOSSIADIS

Congenital dystrophies are macular diseases first presented in childhood or adolescence. The most common are:

- Stargardt's disease
- Best's disease
- Progressive cone dystrophy
- Congenital retinoschisis
- Retinitis pigmentosa

Fundus examination with biomicroscopy, fluorescein angiography and indocyanine green angiography offer useful information concerning these diseases. The examination is completed and verified with additional examinations like Optical Coherence Tomography, electrophysiology and electro-oculography.

Optical Coherence Tomography is particularly helpful in these congenital macular diseases since it contributes to:

- The detection of retinal edema and intraretinal cysts that sometimes occur during the evolution of the disease[1].
- The precise study of the retinal atrophy that is responsible for the decrease of macular thickness.
- The differentiation between the adult form and the classic form of Best's dystrophy[2-5]. In the former, a well demarcated increase of pigment epithelium thickness is observed in the macula while in Best's disease retinal detachment often appears in the macula.
- The study and the prognosis of the progression of congenital dystrophies. The measurement of the macular thickness is the most accurate index for progression of damage.

STARGARDT'S DISEASE

The disease is manifested between the 7th and the 12th year of age. It evolves quickly to a decrease and/or loss of the central vision with maintenance of the peripheral vision. It is inherited in a recessive pattern in 90% of cases.

Initially, the patient may complain of a progressive decrease of visual acuity and dyschromatopsia. Biomicroscopy reveals loss of the normal macular reflectivity. During the evolution of the disease, a granular appearance is presented while later retinal pigment epithelium atrophy of ovoid shape is often detected. Fundus flavimaculatus represents a variation of the disease, characterized by the presence of yellow-white perimacular flecks.

The diagnosis of the disease is obtained mainly by fluorescein angiography that shows a staining in the central area (Bull's eye maculopathy) and by the multifocal electroretinography that reveals low responses in the macular area even at the initial stages. In advanced stages fundus autofluorescence and indocyanine green angiography are helpful diagnostic examinations.

The adult form of the disease is rare. It is characterized by choroidal atrophy, central scotoma and occasionally by the presence of choroidal neovascularization. Histology examination reveals the presence and accumulation of lipofuscin in the retinal pigment epithelium and the loss of the retinal pigment epithelium cells as well as the photoreceptors. Optical Coherence Tomography findings confirm in vivo the histological image of the disease[1,2]. Patients with Stargardt's disease usually have thinning and disintegration of the macula with loss of the outer retinal layers. Retinal pigment epithelium atrophy permits for an increased light transmission and therefore a high choroidal reflectivity.

BEST'S DISEASE

Best's disease (vitelliform) is inherited in an autosomal dominant pattern of variable penetrance and expressivity. During the progression of the disease the following stages appear:

0. Pre-vitelliform stage. Fundus examination does not reveal macular alterations. However, electro-oculography shows retinal pigment epithelium changes.
1. Vitelliform stage. The macula has the appearance of an egg-yolk, of a size that varies from 1/2 to 2 papillary diameters. Fluorescein angiography shows hypofluorescence in the macula while the rest of the retina appears normal[2].
2. Pseudo-hypopyon stage. This stage is characterized by a) the extracellular presence and dispersion of vitelliform elements, which are initially present inside the retinal pigment epithelium cells, b) atrophy of the retinal pigment epithelium and c) a decrease in visual acuity. Extracellular accumulation of pathologic elements occupies the inferior part of the alteration, which is of ovoid shape. On fluorescein angiography the superior part of the lesion appears hyperfluorescence as opposed to the inferior hypofluorescence.
3. Scrambled-egg-appearance macular lesion.
4. Atrophic stage. This stage poses diagnostic difficulties especially in cases of negative family history and absence of previous macular examinations.
5. Cicatricial stage. It is characterized by the presence of scar tissue and low visual acuity (20/200).

Best's disease histologically is characterized by degeneration of the photoreceptors, lipofuscin aggregation in the retinal pigment epithelium and fibrous accumulation beneath it[1].

Optical Coherence Tomography images depend on the stage of the disease. It usually offers information regarding changes occurring at the retinal pigment epithelium.
An elevation of the choriocapillaries-retinal pigment epithelium complex can be initially observed with areas of low reflectivity located between the layers of the complex.

Optical Coherence Tomography also facilitates the study of the evolution of the disease.
In the atrophic stage thinning of the inner and the outer retinal borders is detected. Retinal thinning is accompanied by high reflectivity of the retinal pigment epithelium - choriocapillaries' complex. In the cicatricial stage high reflectivity is also observed due to the extended scarring of the retinal pigment epithelium.
Choroidal neovascularization may also occur.

CONE-ROD DYSTROPHY

The disease is characterized by cones' and rods' dystrophy. The affected patients suffer a decrease or loss of central vision, photosensitivity and color defects. Visual acuity varies from 20/50 to counting fingers. The disease is usually presented at the age of 20-30 years. The diagnosis is based on the electroretinogram, with both photopic and scotopic electroretinograms reduced.

It is inherited in the dominant, regressive or x-linked pattern. With progression of the disease the rods' participation becomes more evident. In advanced stages symptoms are similar to those in retinitis pigmentosa. Fundus examinations shows pigmented granules (bull's eye) or diffuse atrophy in the macula.

Optical Coherence Tomography findings are characterized by retinal thinning and loss of the photoreceptors' layer in the central area. Optical Coherence Tomography also shows a disintegration of the inner retinal layers and a decreased reflectivity of the outer nuclear layer. In some cases Optical Coherence Tomography reveals the presence of intraretinal cysts.

X-LINKED JUVENILE RETINOSCHISIS

The disease is characterized by the presence of intraretinal cysts in the macula that have the appearance of a bicycle-wheel. Juvenile retinoschisis affects only males with a few exceptions and is transmitted in an x-linked recessive pattern. The disease is usually evident in childhood or/and adolescence with decreased visual acuity, that usually ranges from 20/40 to 20/100 without leading to blindness. In some cases nystagmus, strabismus and leukocoria due to retinal detachment may rarely happen. The fundus image is characterized by the presence of multiple microcystic formations located in the inner retinal layers and are diagnosed – in addition to biomicroscopy – by fluorescein angiography, indocyanine green angiography, electroretinography and Optical Coherence Tomography.

Fluorescein angiography is usually normal but sometimes shows hyperfluorescence extending beyond the borders of the macula. Indocyanine green angiography reveals hyperfluorescence along the bicycle-wheel alterations in the late phases. Electroretinography reveals b-wave alterations while the a-wave appears normal.

Optical Coherence Tomography images are similar to the histological findings of the disease. In particular, an area of low reflectivity in the inner retinal layers due to intraretinal splitting is observed. Intraretinal splitting consists mainly of cystic formations with gradually decreasing size from the center of the macula to the periphery. In case of surgical intervention Optical Coherence Tomography is very useful for the preoperative evaluation of the lesion and the postoperative follow-up of the patient.

RETINITIS PIGMENTOSA

It is probably the more common congenital retinal disease. Patients usually complain of difficulty in dim light and loss of the peripheral visual field. The clinical findings are pale optic disc, bone-spicule pigment peripheral deposits, decrease of the lumen of the retinal vessels and atrophy of the peripheral retina that later extends centrally.

In many cases, the disease is characterized by the presence of cystic formations inside the retinal layers of the macula due to the breakdown of the blood-retinal barrier and secondarily probably to the vitreous traction on the posterior pole. In advanced stages, the disease is characterized by thinning of the retina and the choriocapillaries layer. An epiretinal membrane is often detected in the posterior pole.

Optical Coherence Tomography helps in the detection of the cystic formations in the macula and offers important information regarding the progression of the cysts after treatment with acetazolamide that seems to contribute to reduction or disappearance of the cysts[1-3]. In Optical Coherence Tomography the cystic formations are characterised by low reflectivity[3,4]. In advanced stages high reflectivity is observed in the choroidal layer due to thinning and atrophy of the retinal pigment epithelium and increased transmission of the light[5,6]. The appearance, due to low reflectivity, of the choroidal vessels like dark circles is also characteristic.

STARGARDT'S DISEASE

1. Ergun E, Hermann B, Wirtitsch M, Unterhuber A, Ko TH, Sattmann H, Scholda C, Fujimoto JG, Stur M, Drexler W. Assessment of central visual function in Stargardt's disease/fundus flavimaculatus with ultrahigh- resolution optical coherence tomography. Invest Opthalmol Vis Sci 2005 Jan;46(1):310-6.

2. Hargitai J, Zernant J, Somfai GM, Vamos R, Farkas A, Salacz G, Allikmets R. Correlation of clinical and genetic findings in Hungarian patients with Stargardt disease. Invest Opthalmol Vis Sci 2005 Dec;46(12):4402-8.

BEST'S DISEASE

1. Chan CK, Gass JD, Lin SG. Acute exudative polymorphous Vitelliform maculopathy syndrome. Retina. 2003 Aug;23(4): 453-62.

2. Benhamou N, Souied EH, Zolf R, Coscas F, Coscas G, Soubrane G. Adult – onset foveomacular Vitelliform dystrophy: a study by optical coherence tomography. Am J Ophtalmol 2003 Mar; 135(3): 362-7.

3. Do P, Ferrucci S. Adult – onset foveomacular Vitelliform dystrophy. Optometry 2006 April; 77(4):156-66.

4. Hayami M, Decock C, Brabant P, Van Kerckhoven W, Lafaut BA, DE Laey JJ. Optical coherence tomography of adult – onset vitelliform dystrophy. Bull Soc Belge Ophthalmol 2003;(289):53-61.

5. Pierro L, Tremolada G, Introini U, Calori G, Brancato R. Optical coherence tomography findings in adult – onset foveomacular Vitelliform dystrophy. Am J Ophthalmol 2002 Nov;134(5):675-80.

RETINITIS PIGMENTOSA

1. Hamada S, Yoshida K, Chihara E. Optical coherence tomography images of retinitis pigmentosa. Ophthalmic Surg Lasers 2000 May - Jun;31(3):253-6.

2. Garcia – Arumi J, Martinez V, Sararols L, Corcostegui B. Vitreoretinal surgery for cystoid macular edema associated with retinitis pigmentosa. Ophthalmology 2003 Jun;110(6):1164-9.

3. Grover S, Apushkin MA, Fishman GA. Topical Dorzolamide for the Treatment of Cystoid Macular Edema in Patients With Retinitis Pigmentosa Am J Ophthalmol. 2006;141:850-858

4. Ko TH, Fujimoto JG, Schuman JS, Paunescu LA, Kowalevicz AM, Hartl I, Drexler W, Wollstein G, Ishikawa H, Duker JS. Comparison of ultrahigh and standard resolution optical coherence tomography for imaging macular pathology. Ophthalmology 2005 Nov;112(11):1922.

5. Rumen F, Souied E, Oubraham H, Coscas G, Soubrane G. Optical coherence tomography in the follow up of macular edema treatment in retinitis pigmentosa. J Fr Ophthalmol 2001 Oct;24(8):854-9.

6. Sandlberg MA, Brockhurst RJ, Gaudio AR, Berson EL. The association between visual acuity and central retinal thickness in retinitis pigmentosa. Invest Ophthalmol Vis Sci 2005 Sep; 46(9):3349-54.

ADULT VITELLIFORM MACULAR DYSTROPHY

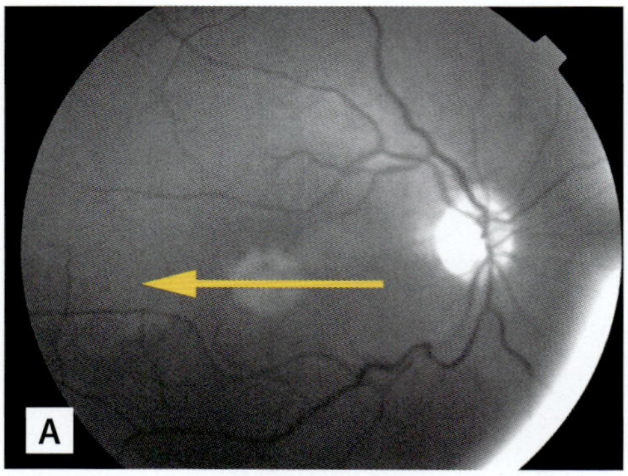

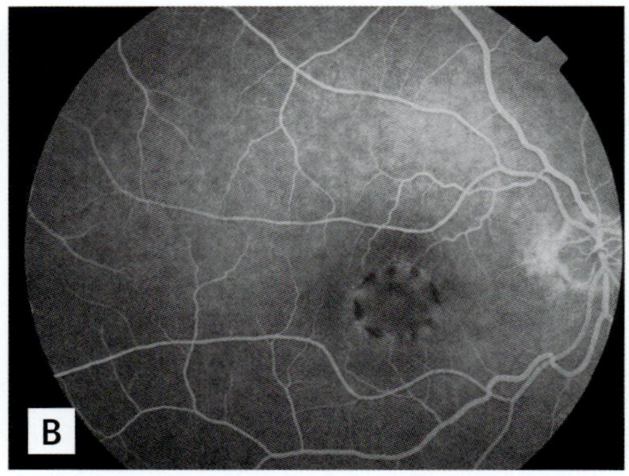

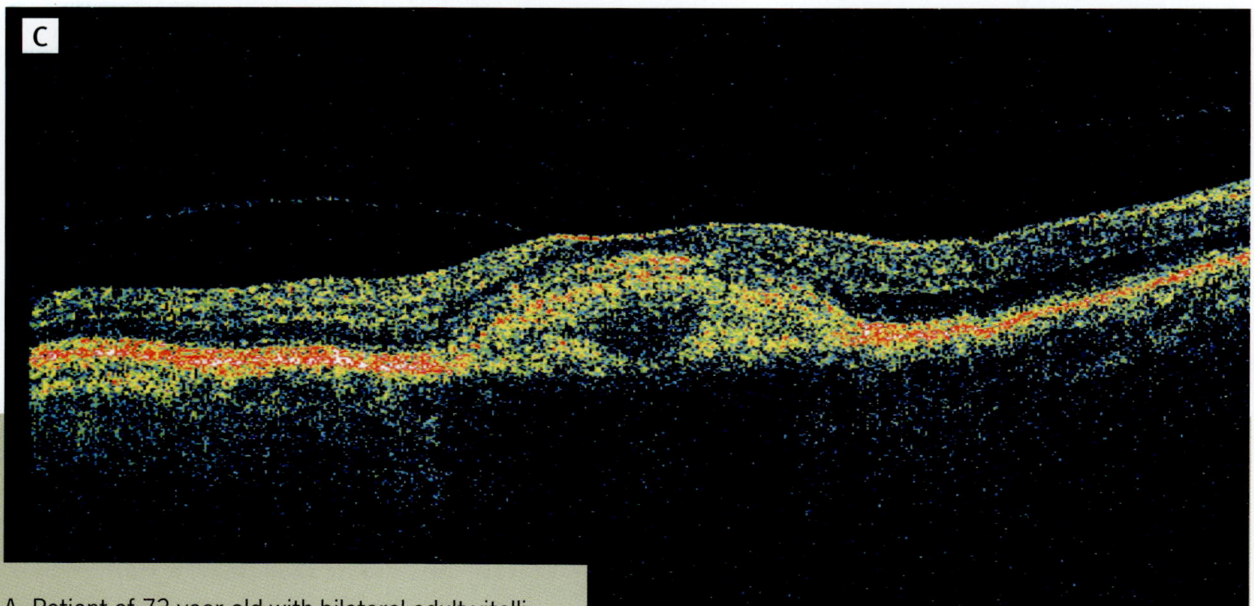

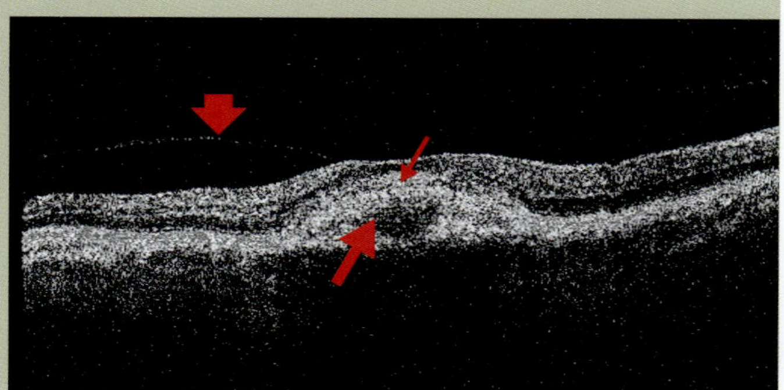

A. Patient of 73 year old with bilateral adult vitelliform macular dystrophy (the arrow shows the scan direction). B. Fluorescein angiography shows mild hyperfluorescence corresponding to the vitelliform lesion and focal areas of hypofluorescence due to pigmented alterations. C. There is a smooth elevation of high reflectivity in the retinal pigment epithelium layer and under it that causes an elevation of the fovea (small arrow) due to the deposition of the vitelliform material (big arrow). The vitreous (thick arrow) is detected attached to the fovea and detached around it.

ADULT VITELLIFORM MACULAR DYSTROPHY

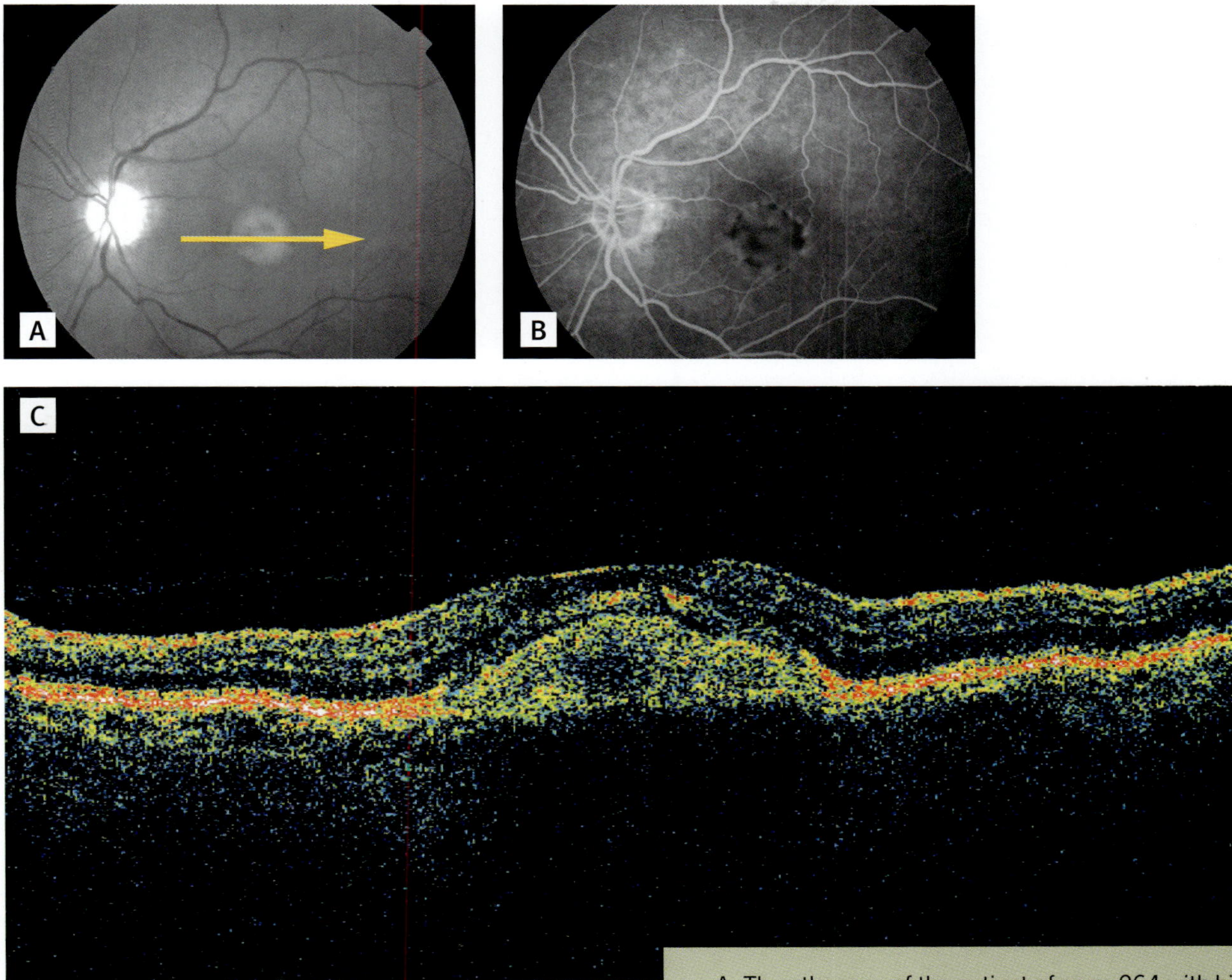

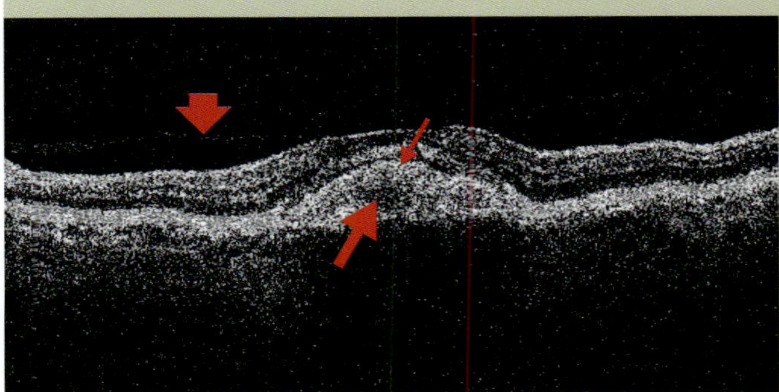

A. The other eye of the patient of page 264 with bilateral adult vitelliform macular dystrophy (the arrow shows the scan direction). B. Fluorescein angiography shows mild hyperfluorescence corresponding to the vitelliform macular dystrophy with focal areas of hypofluorescence due to the pigmented lesions. C. There is a smooth elevation of high reflectivity in the retinal pigment epithelium and under it that causes an elevation of the fovea (small arrow) due to the deposition of the vitelliform material (big arrow). The vitreous (thick arrow) is detected attached to the fovea and detached around it.

ADULT VITELLIFORM MACULAR DYSTROPHY

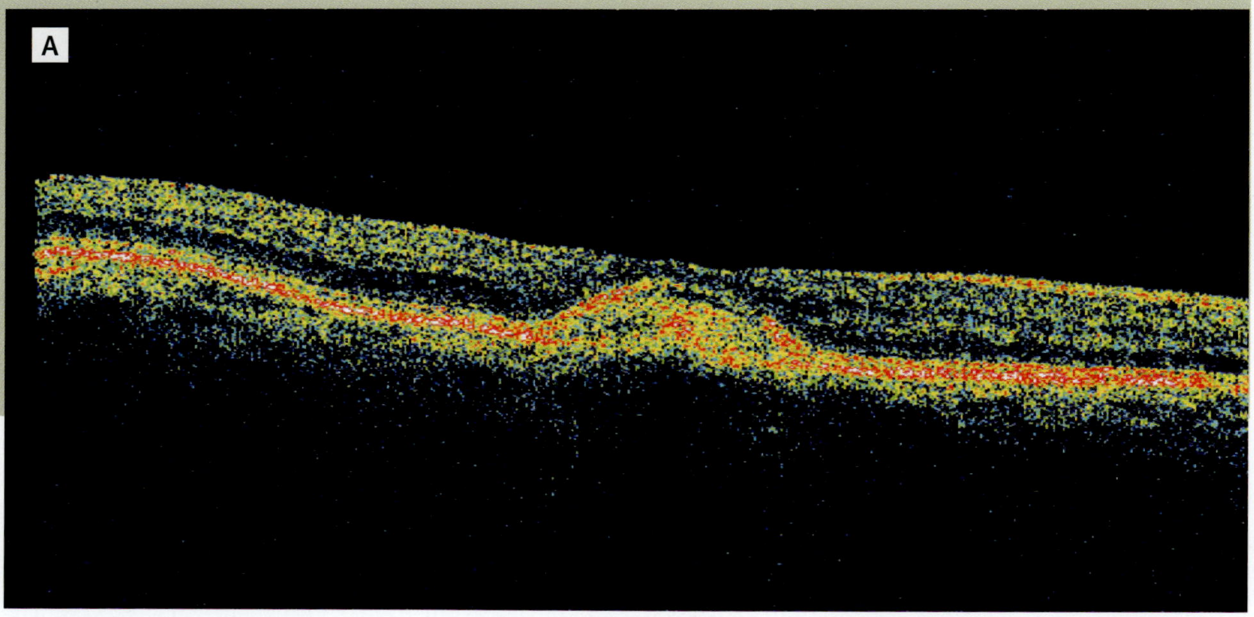

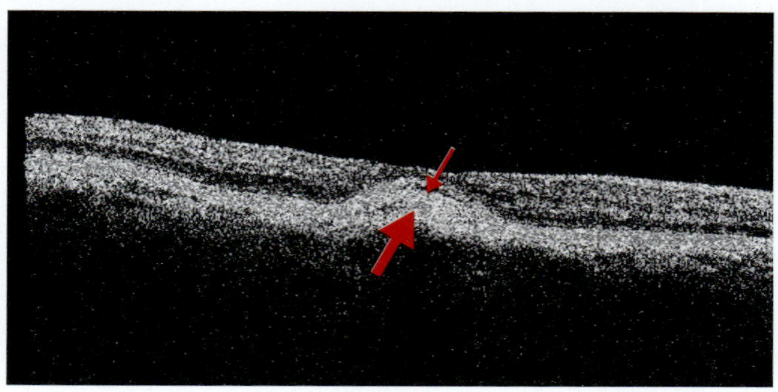

Male of 74 year old with right amblyopia and decreased visual acuity in the left eye of six months duration. Clinical examination reveals cataract of the left eye.

A. Right eye. There is a smooth elevation of high reflectivity in the retinal pigment epithelium and under it that causes elimination of the foveal depression (small arrow) due to the deposition of the vitelliform material (big arrow).

ADULT VITELLIFORM MACULAR DYSTROPHY

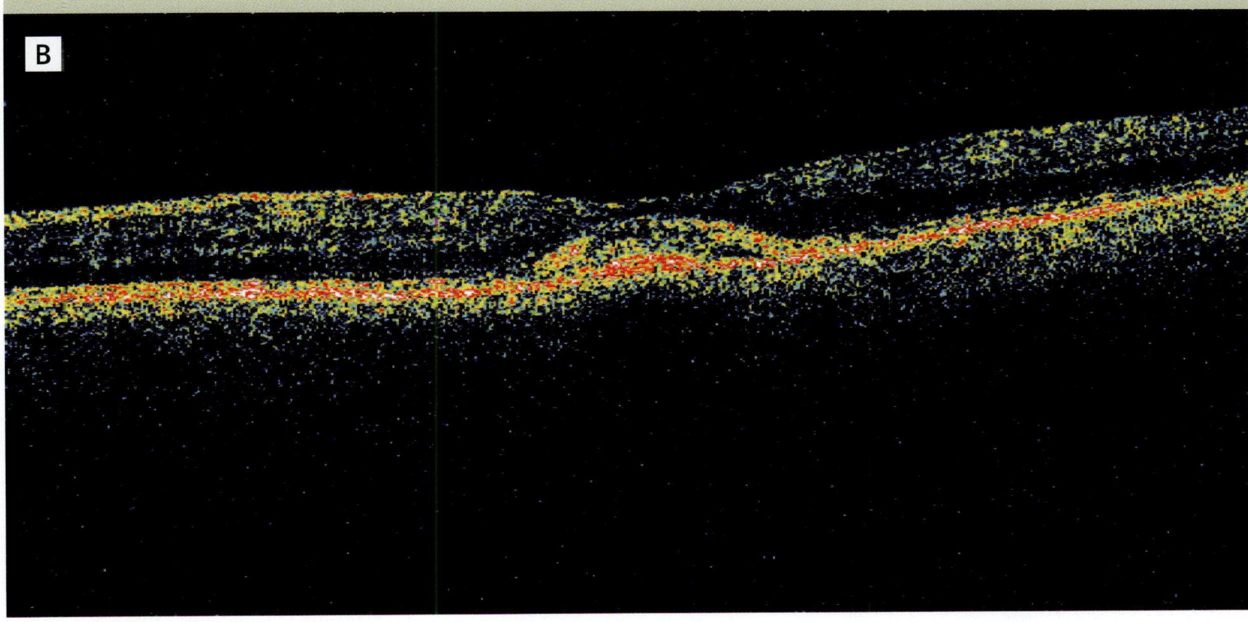

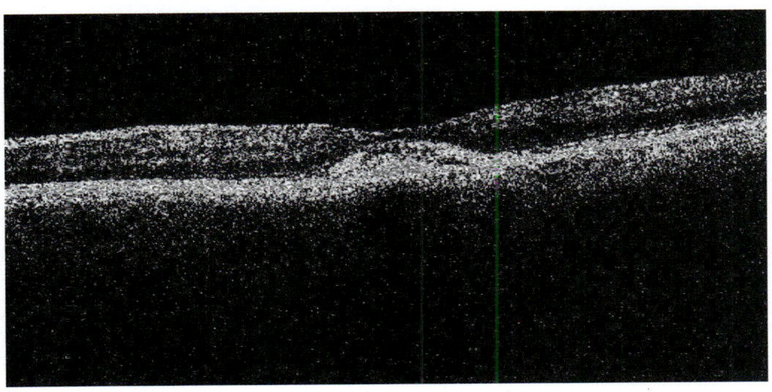

B. The left eye of the patient of page 266. A macular lesion similar to the one of the right eye but of smaller diameter is observed under the fovea.

ADULT VITELLIFORM MACULAR DYSTROPHY

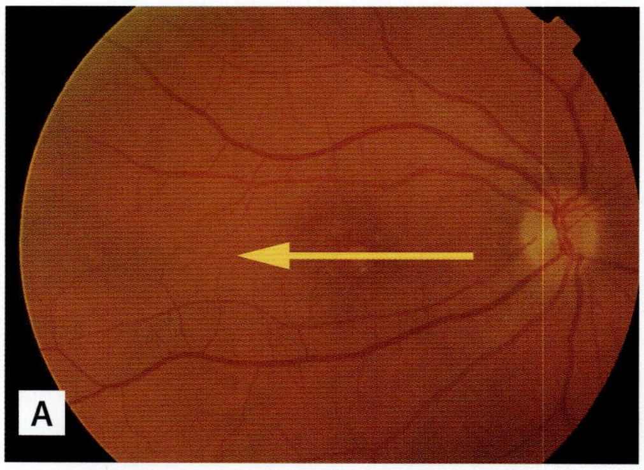

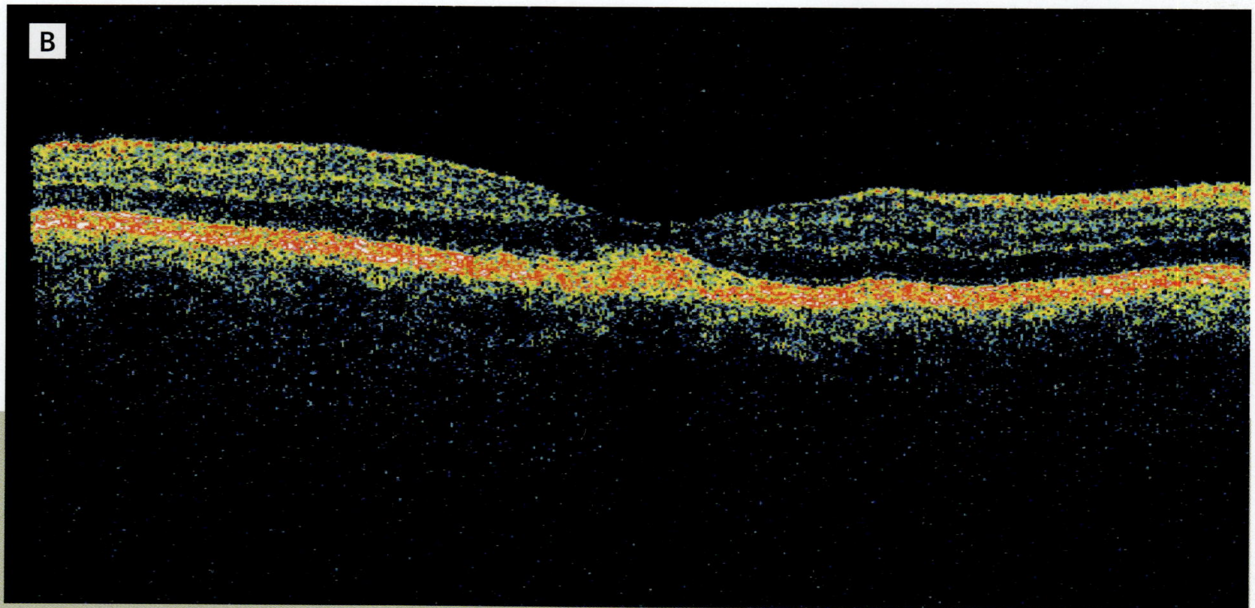

A. The right eye of a 55 year old patient with bilateral adult vitelliform macular dystrophy (the arrow shows the scan direction). B. There is a smooth elevation of high reflectivity in the retinal pigment epithelium due to the deposition of the vitelliform material (small arrow).

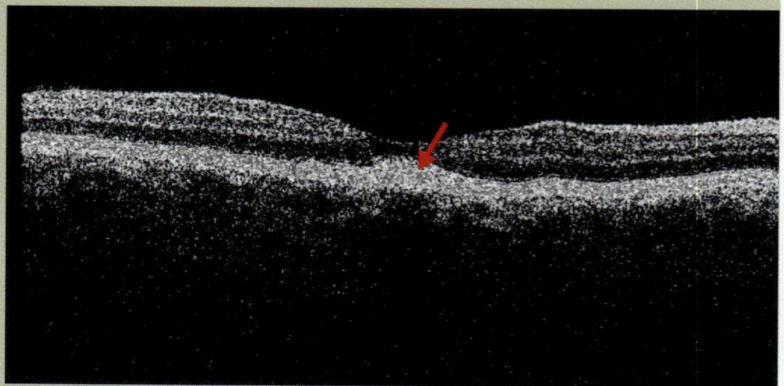

ADULT VITELLIFORM MACULAR DYSTROPHY

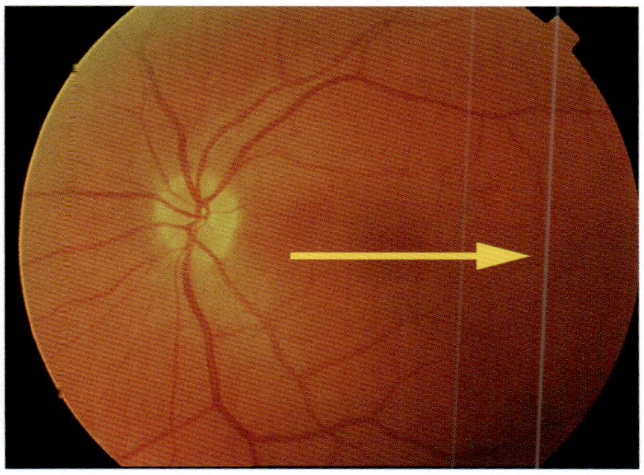

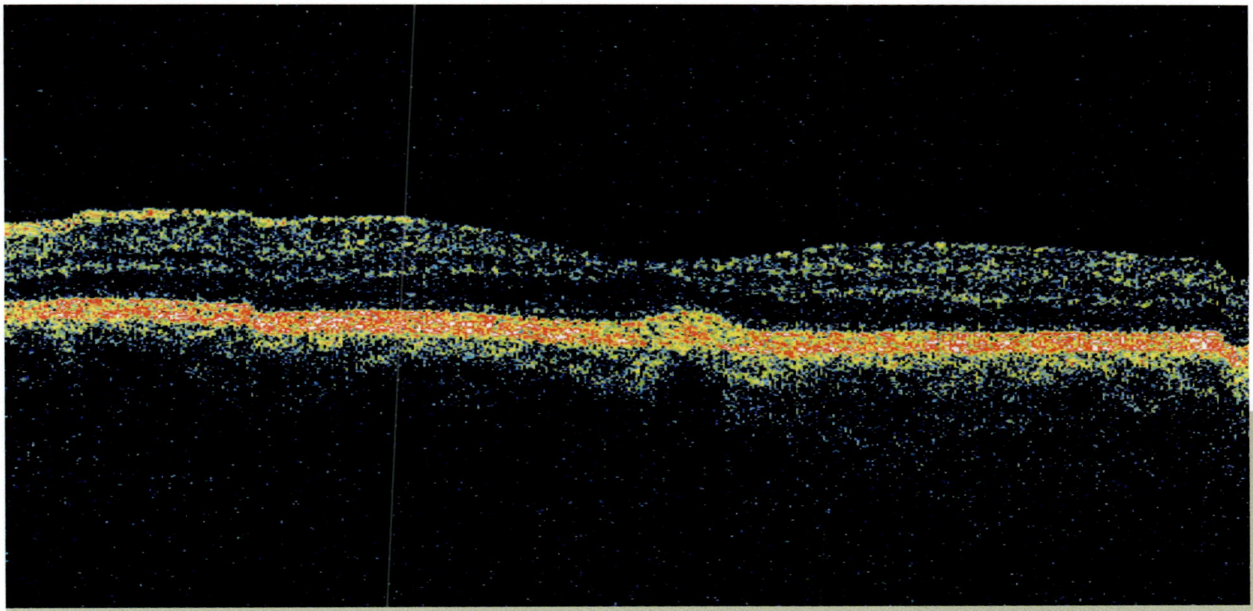

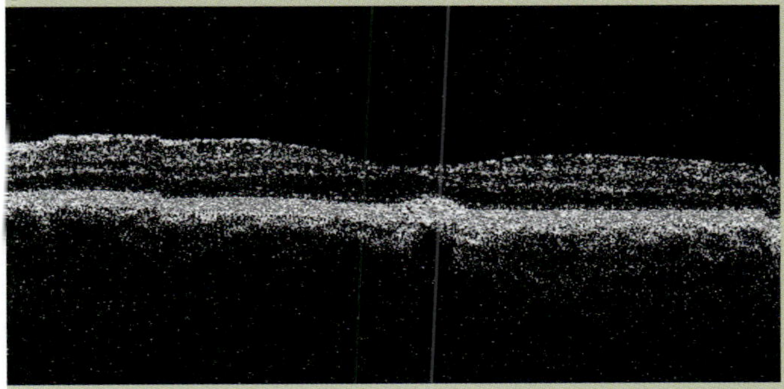

The left eye of the patient of page 268 (the arrow shows the scan direction). Vitelliform material in the macula is present.

STARGARDT - FLAVIMACULATUS DYSTROPHY

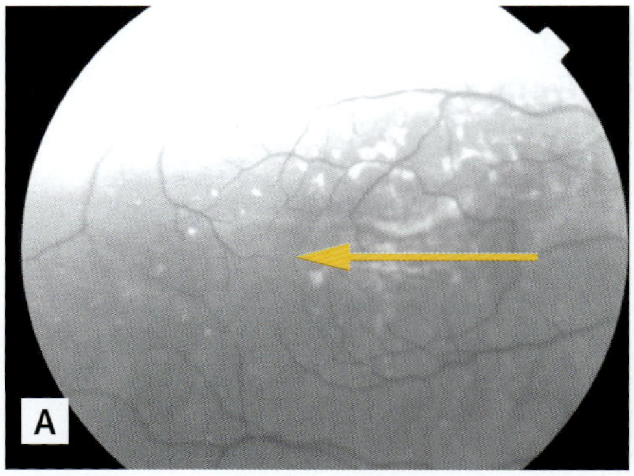

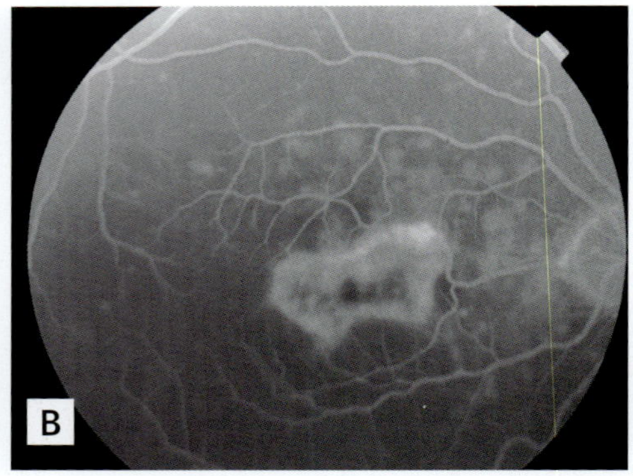

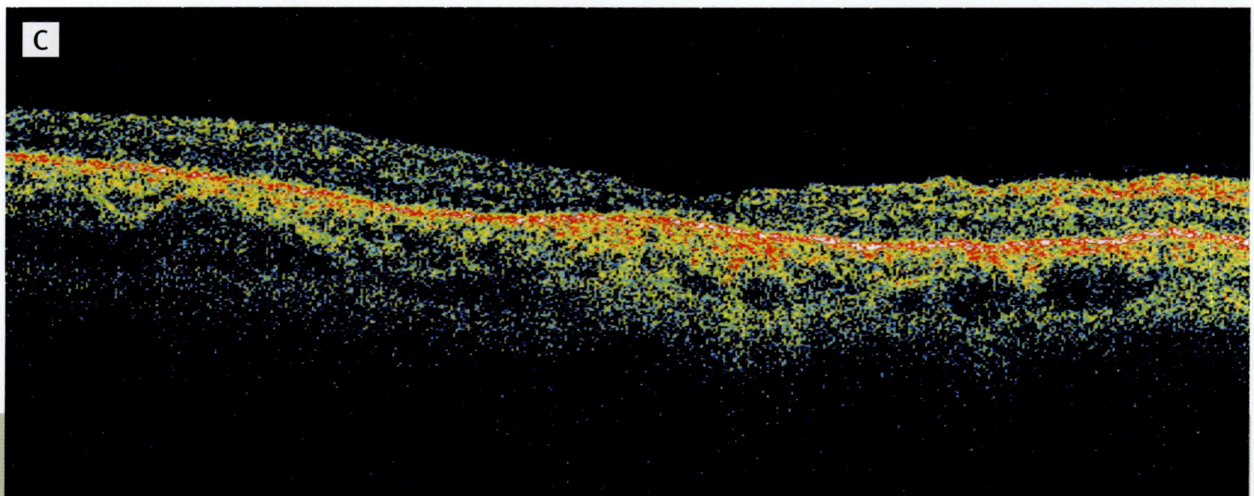

A. Patient with Stargardt-flavimaculatus dystrophy. There is macular atrophy and the characteristic flecks of the disease in the posterior pole and the periphery (the arrow shows the scan direction). B. Fluorescein angiography shows the typical choroidal silence and window defect type hyperfluorescence corresponding to the atrophic area and hyperfluorescence from the flecks' staining. C. Optical Coherence Tomography clearly shows thinning of the retinal layers (small arrow). That causes a higher degree of light penetration, resulting in higher choroidal reflectivity and delineation of the choroidal vessels (big arrow). The high choroidal reflectivity, which is observed is due to the thinning of the retinal layers.

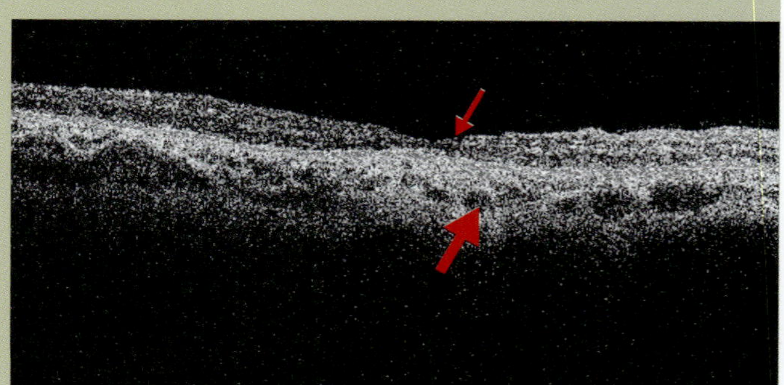

STARGARDT - FLAVIMACULATUS DYSTROPHY

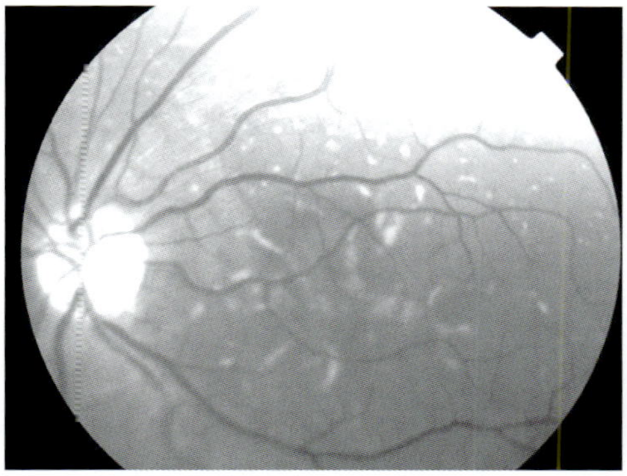

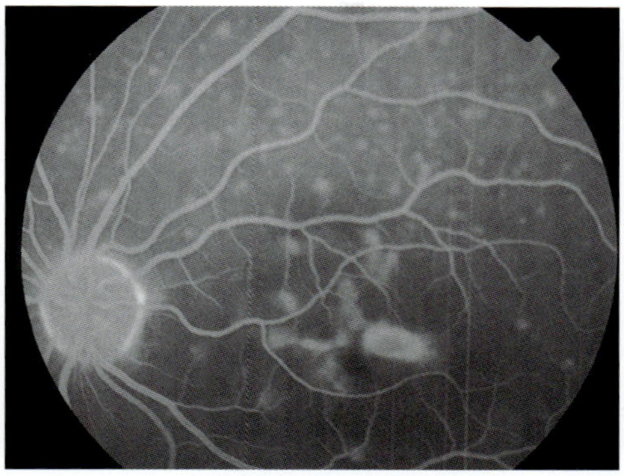

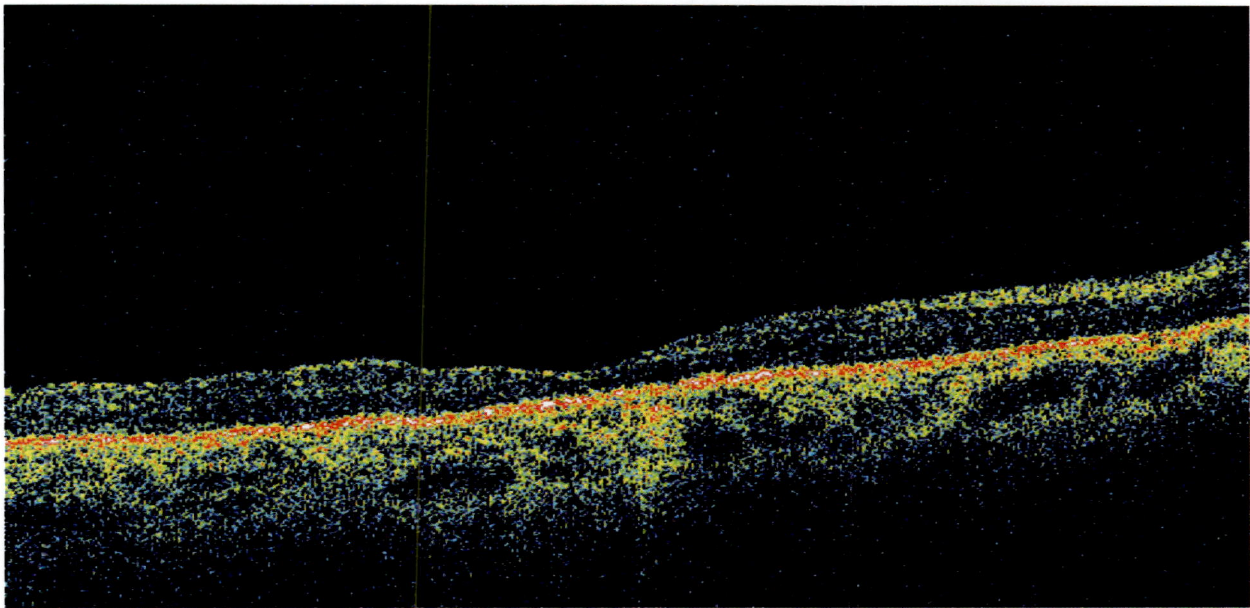

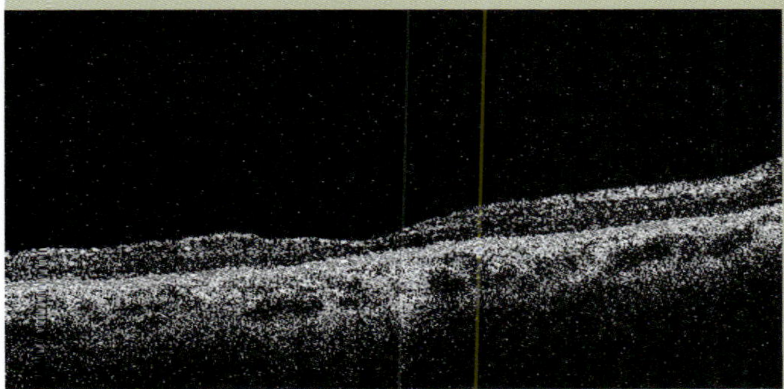

The other eye of the patient of page 270 with similar findings.

X-LINKED RETINOSCHISIS

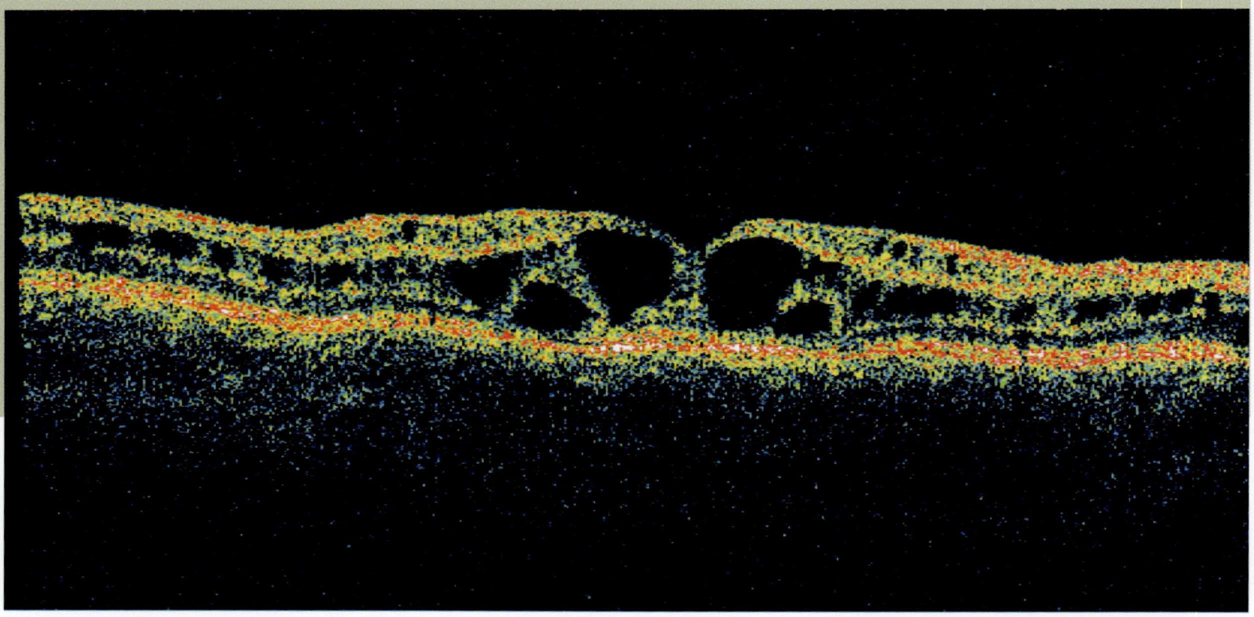

Patient with x-linked retinoschisis. Multiple intraretinal round areas of low reflectivity that correspond to retinal cysts are detected in the posterior pole within the retina (big arrow). There are also cysts of smaller dimension under the nerve fibre layer (small arrow).

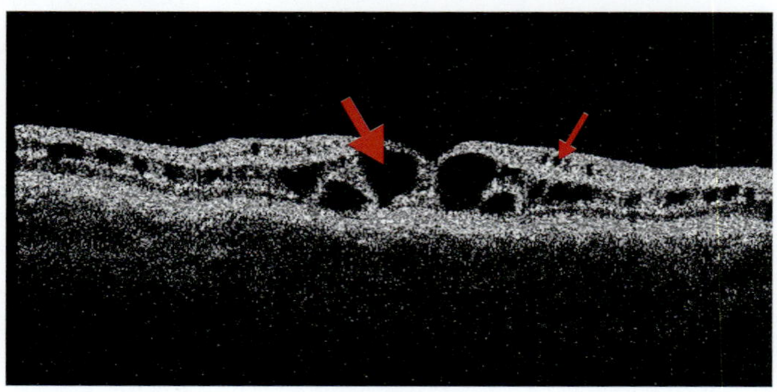

X-LINKED RETINOSCHISIS

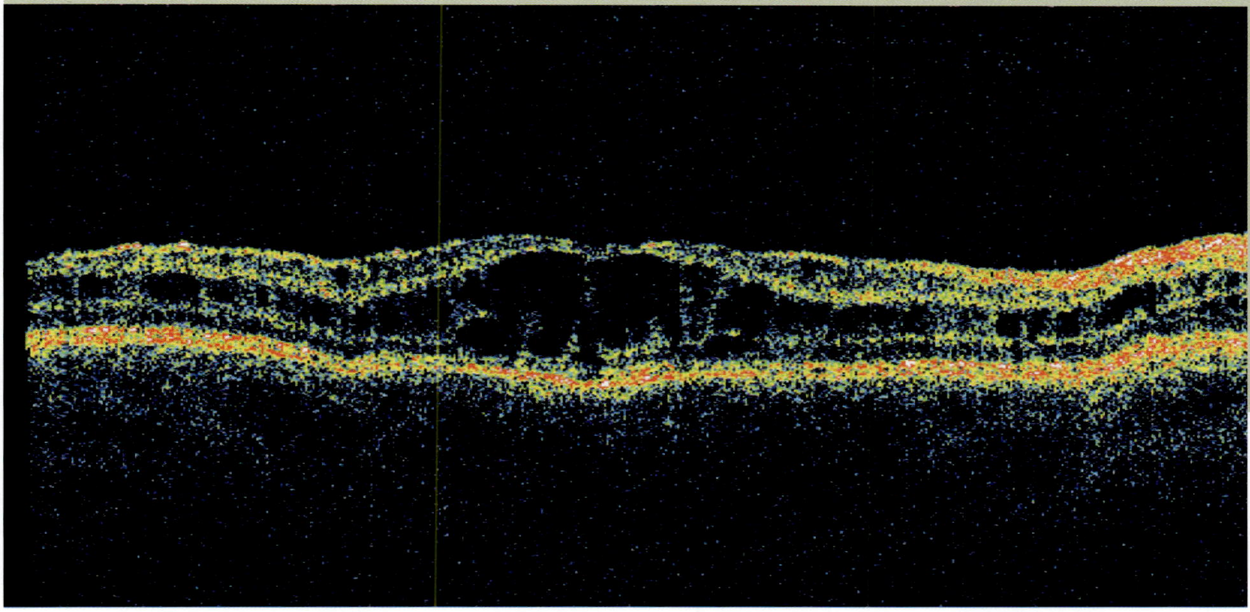

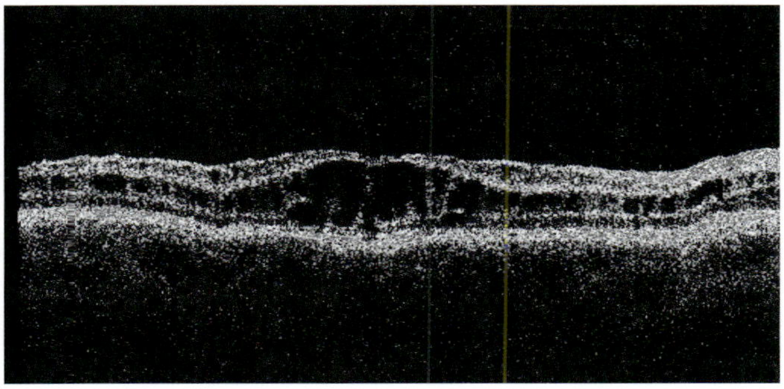

The other eye of the patient of page 272 with intraretinal cysts.

RETINITIS PIGMENTOSA

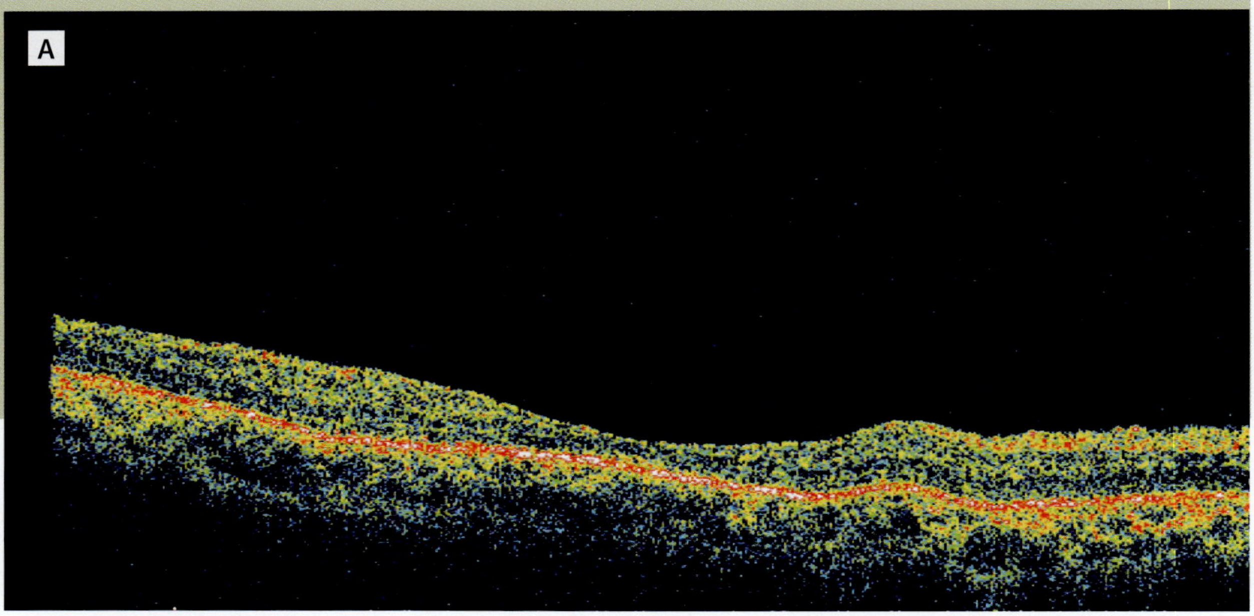

A. Right eye of a patient with retinitis pigmentosa. The thinning of the retinal layers, particularly in the left eye, is characteristic.

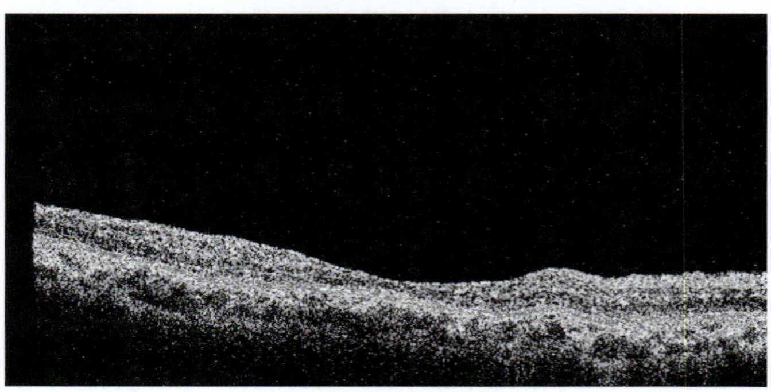

RETINITIS PIGMENTOSA

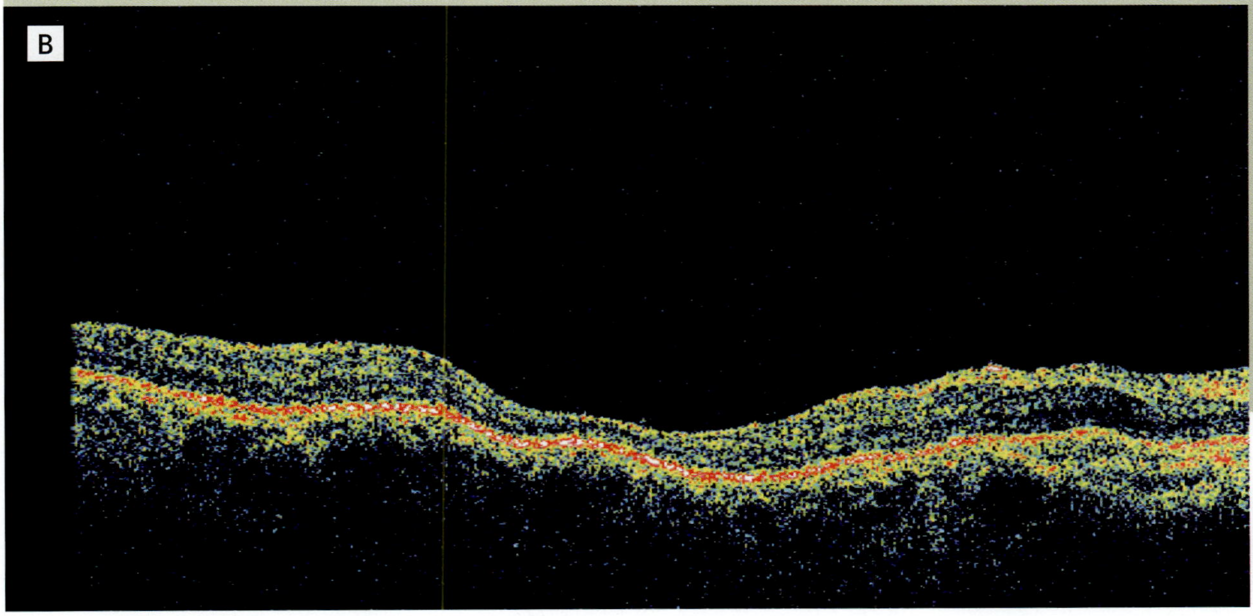

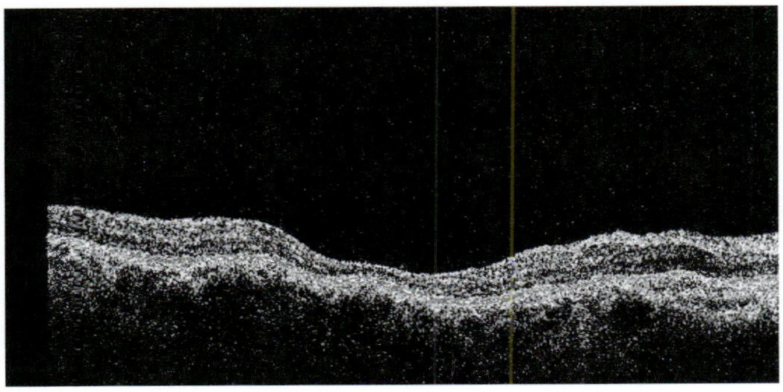

B. Left eye of patient of page 274. The thinning of the retinal layers is evident.

RETINITIS PIGMENTOSA

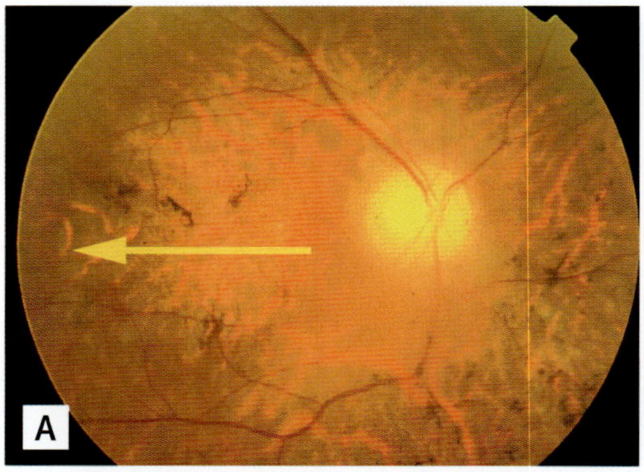

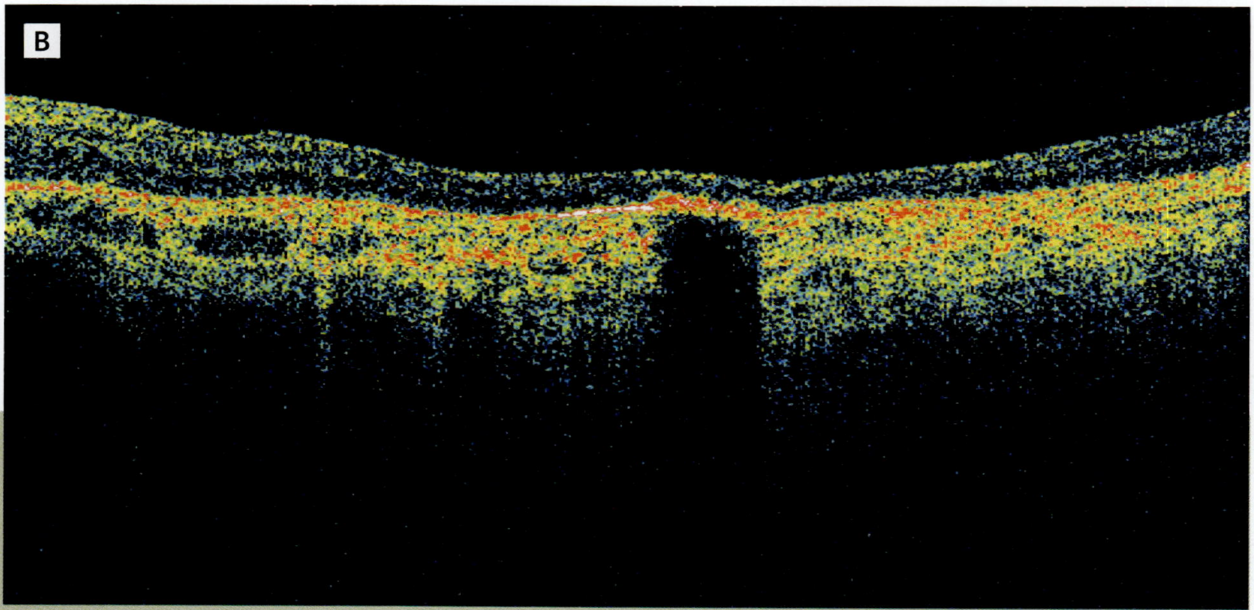

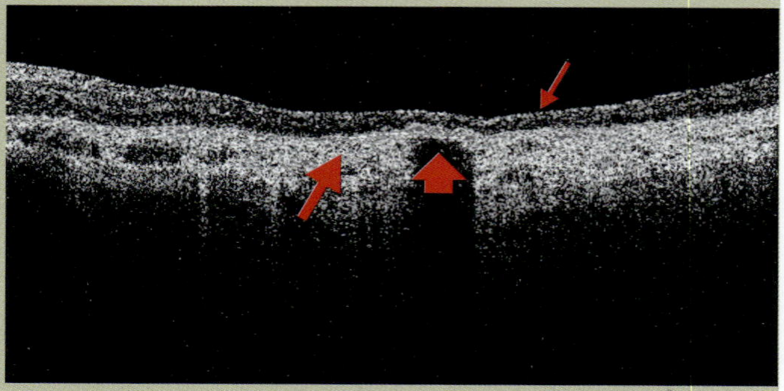

A. Patient with retinitis pigmentosa (the arrow shows the scan direction). B. Optical Coherence Tomography depicts diffuse thinning of all retinal layers due to their atrophy (small arrow). The apparent increase of the choroidal thickness is due to the retinal layers' thinning that reduces the light absorption by the retina, thus allowing for more light to reach the choroid (big arrow). Also note the well demarcated area of low reflectivity (shadowing) (thick arrow) that is due to the presence of pigment deposits at the retinal pigment epithelium and the subsequent absorption of light.

CONE DYSTROPHY

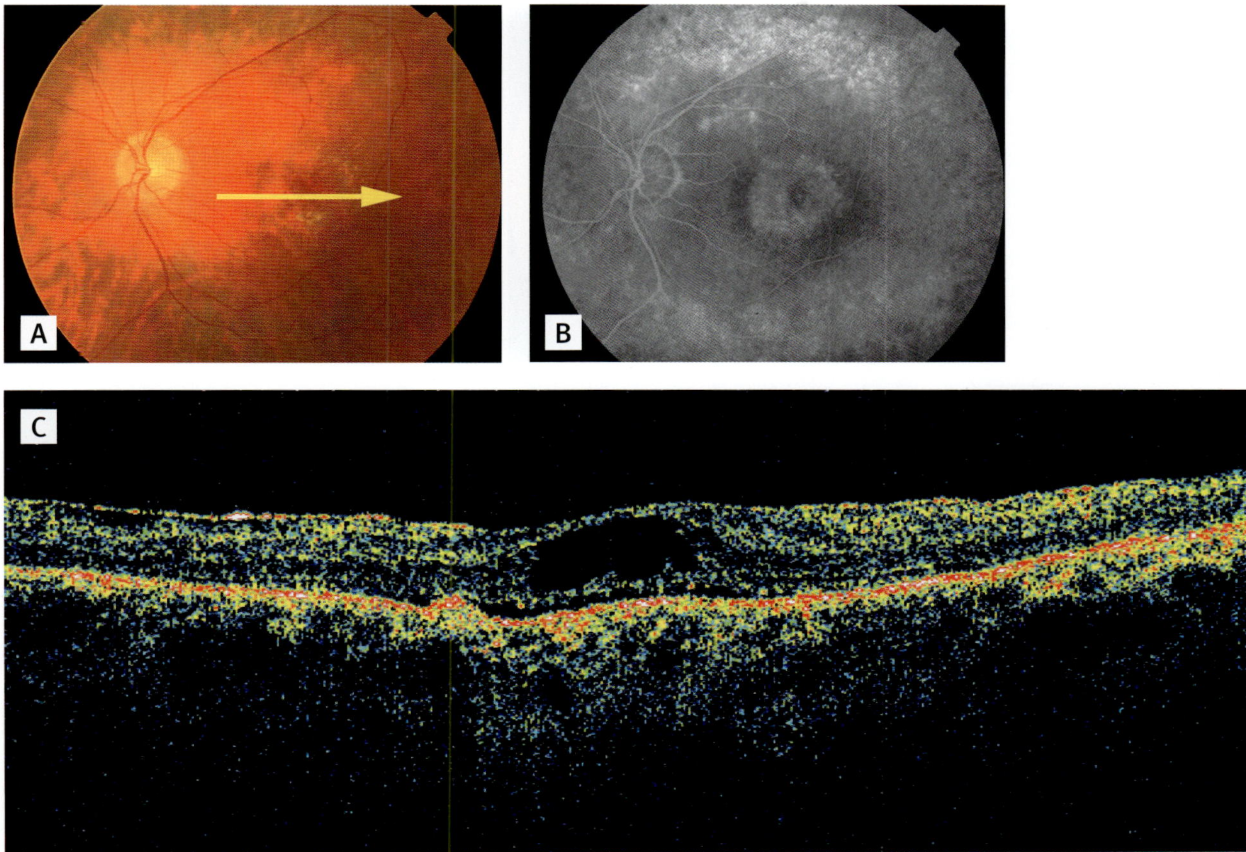

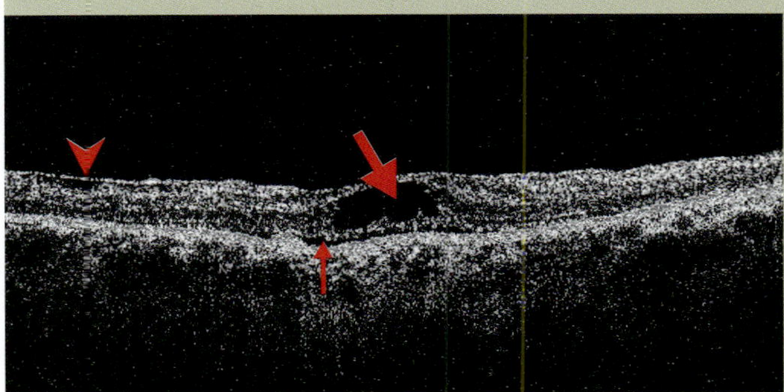

A. A 45 year old patient with cone dystrophy. Note the thinning of the retinal vessels and the bull's eye pattern in the macula (the arrow shows the scan direction). B. Fluorescein angiography shows a window defect type hyperfluorescence in the posterior pole without active dye leakage. C. Optical Coherence Tomography shows an area of low reflectivity between the retina and the retinal pigment epithelium that corresponds to subretinal fluid accumulation in the fovea (small arrow). There are also cystic intraretinal formations of low reflectivity corresponding to cystoid retinal edema (big arrow). Note the linear area of high reflectivity located on the retinal surface that represents an epiretinal membrane in the macula (arrow head).

CONE DYSTROPHY

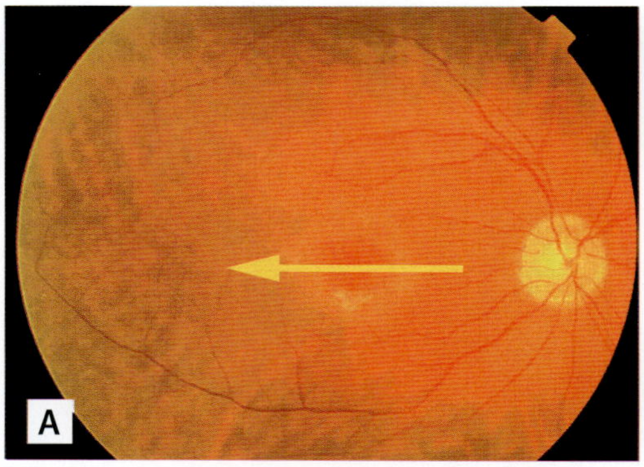

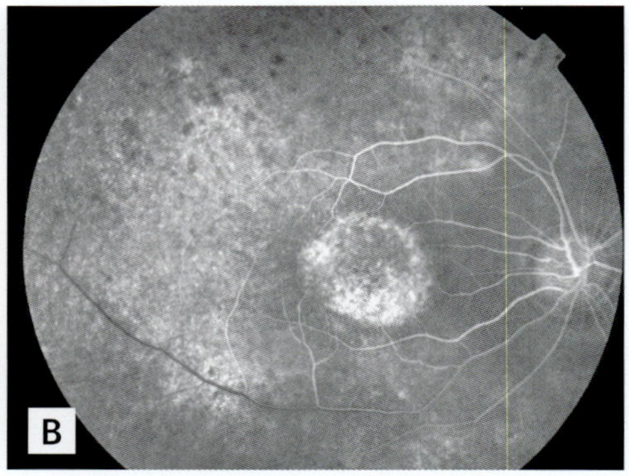

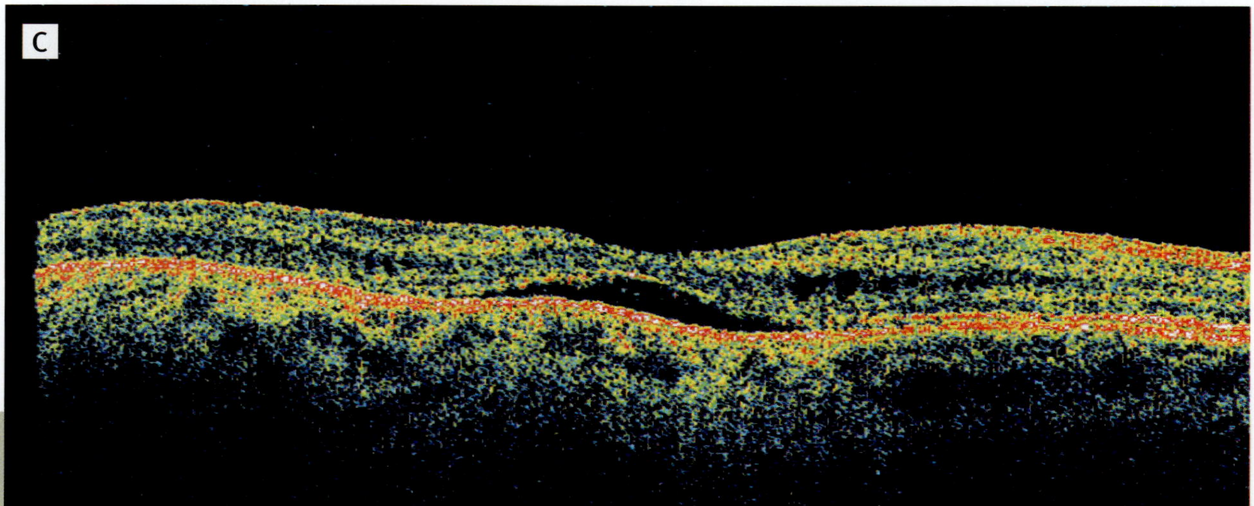

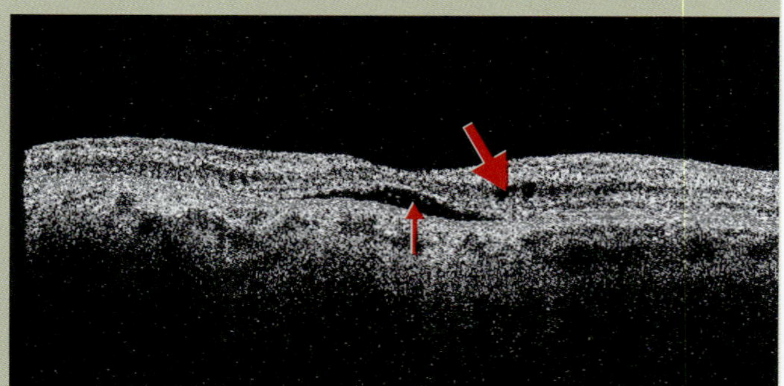

A. The right eye of the patient of page 277. The narrowing of the vessels and the appearance of the macula are similar to the fellow eye (the arrow shows the scan direction). B. Fluorescein angiography shows the same hyperfluorescence from window defect in the posterior pole without active dye leakage. C. Optical Coherence Tomography shows an area of low reflectivity between the retina and the retinal pigment epithelium that corresponds to subretinal fluid accumulation in the fovea (small arrow). There are also cystic intraretinal formations of low reflectivity corresponding to cystoid retinal edema, to a lesser extent compared to the left eye (big arrow).

CHAPTER 13

SELECTED DISEASES OF THE POSTERIOR SEGMENT

George Theodossiadis

ASTEROID HYALOSIS

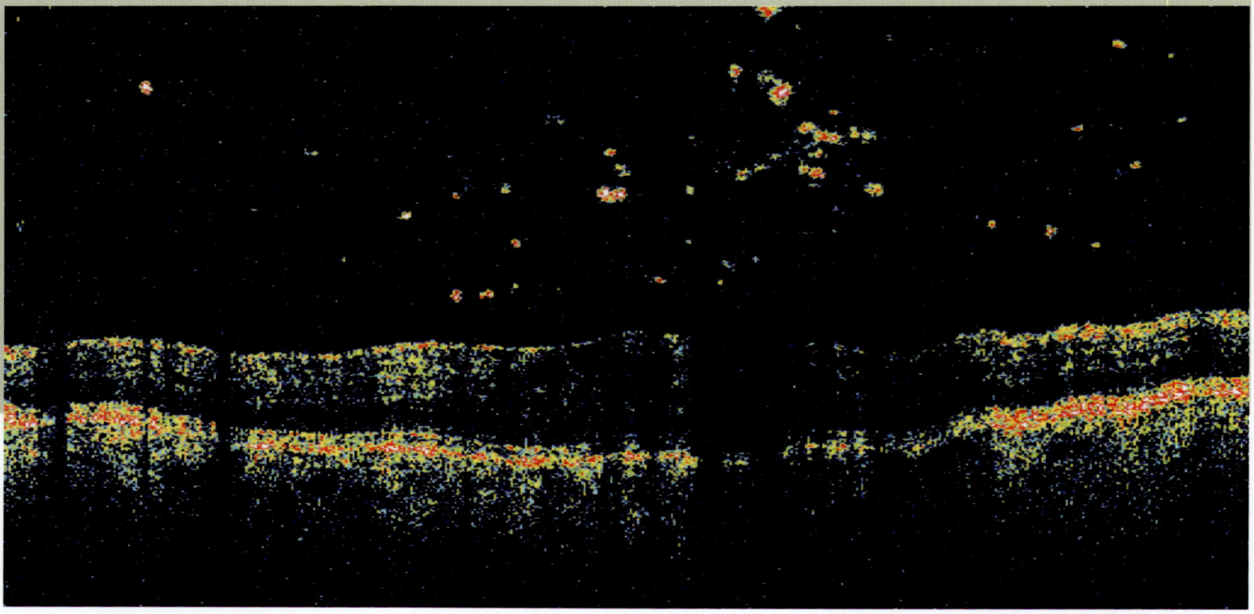

Diabetic patient with dense asteroid hyalosis that doesn't allow biomicroscopic macular examination. Multiple spheroidal areas of high reflectivity corresponding to the intravitreous crystals are detected inside the vitreous cavity, (small arrow). The appearance of the underlying retina is not of adequate quality because of the shadowing caused by the high reflectivity of the intravitreous crystals (big arrow). Nevertheless, retinal edema is clearly visible in the macular area in the form of thickened retina (arrow head).

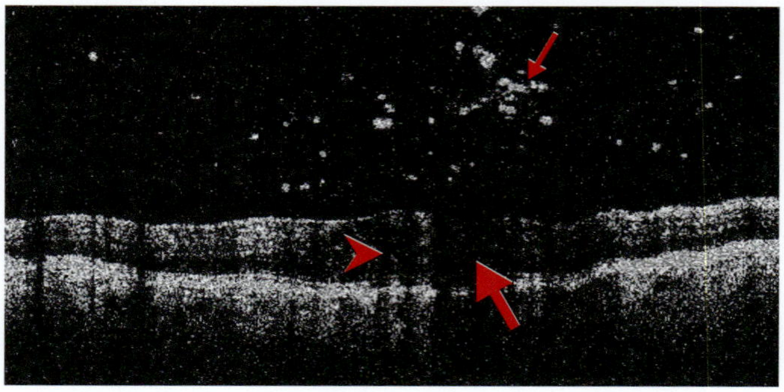

CHOROIDAL FOLDS

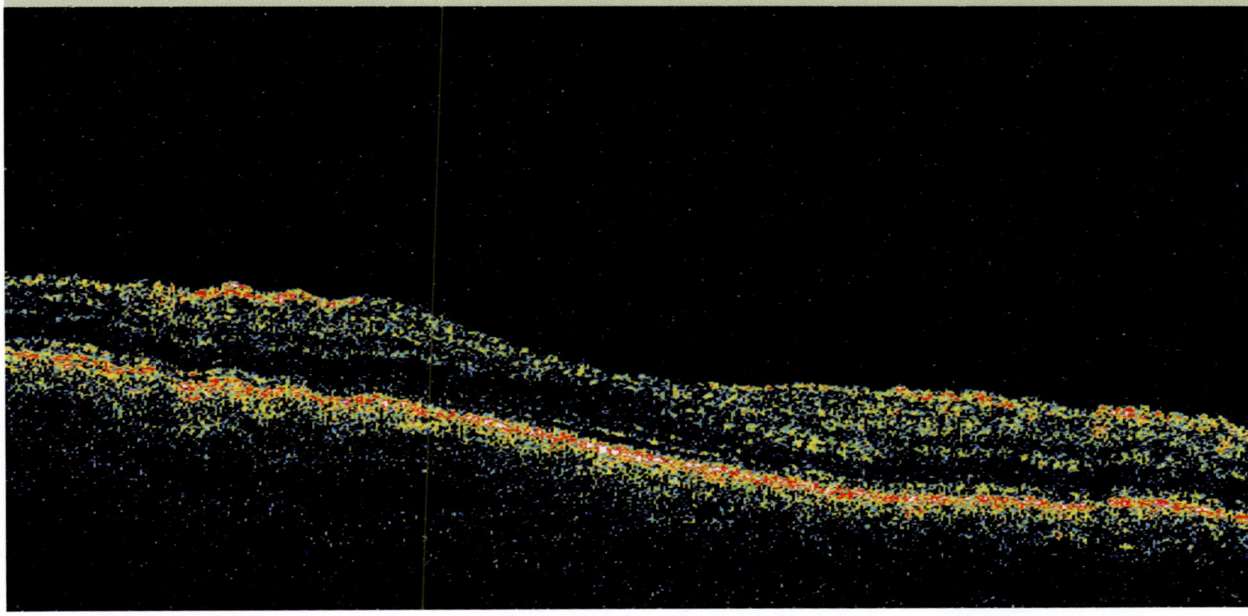

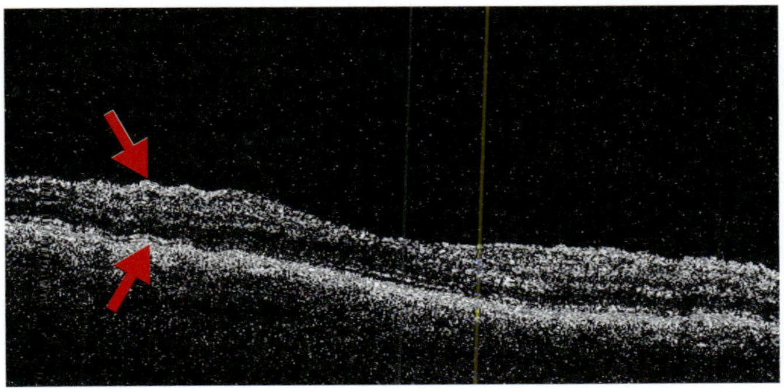

Patient having recently undergone a trabeculectomy with postoperative hypotony. The undulating appearance of the retinal surface and the retinal pigment epithelium-choriocapillaries complex (arrows) is due to the choroidal and retinal folds located nasally to the fovea.

CHOROIDAL FOLDS

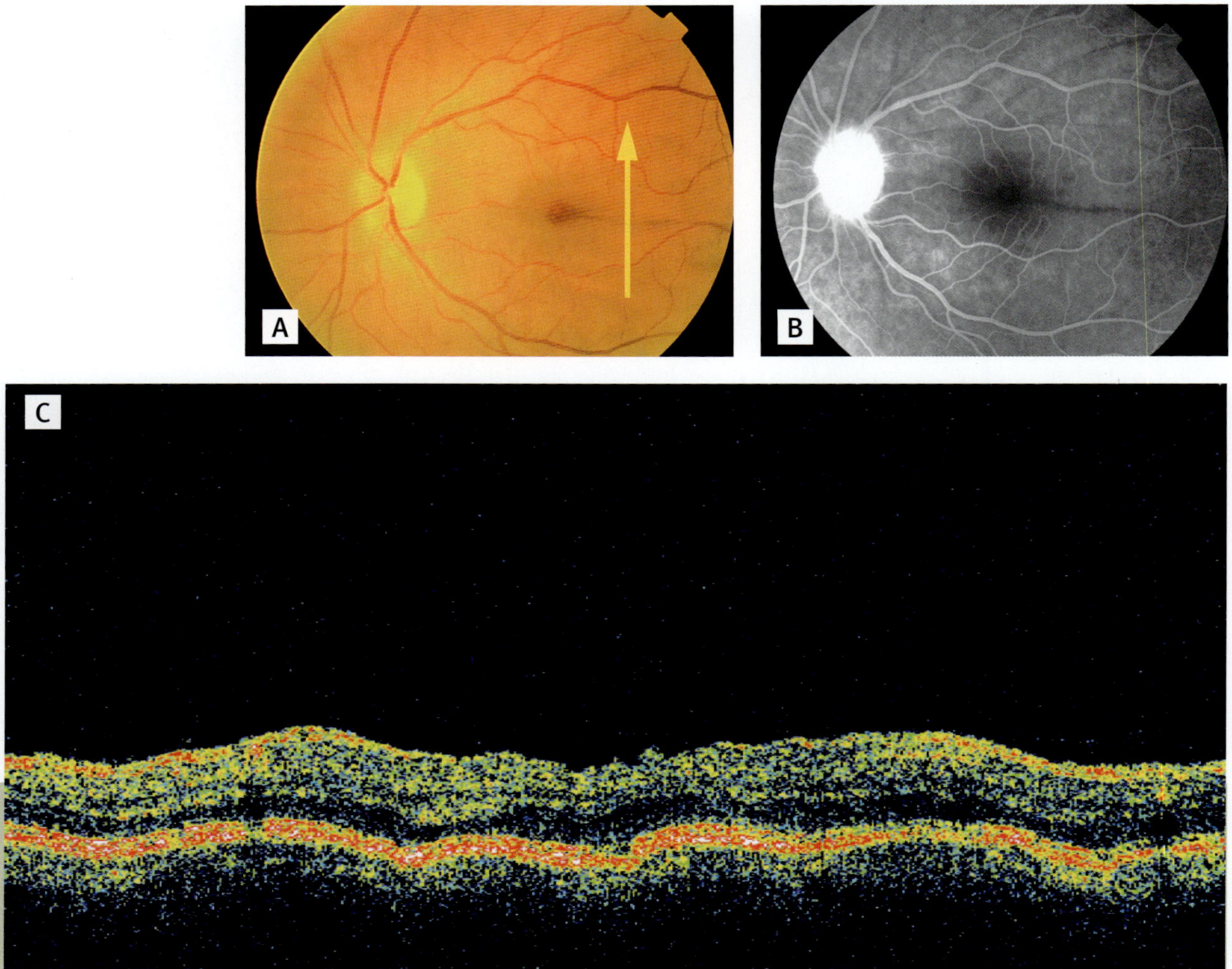

A. Patient with uveitis and choroidal folds with suspected posterior scleritis (the arrow shows the scan direction). B. Fluorescein angiography shows linear hypofluorescence corresponding to the choroidal folds and optic disc hyperfluorescence (hot disc). C. Optical Coherence Tomography shows an undulating retinal pigment epithelium-choriocapillaries complex (arrows) that is not accompanied by wrinkling of the overlying retina.

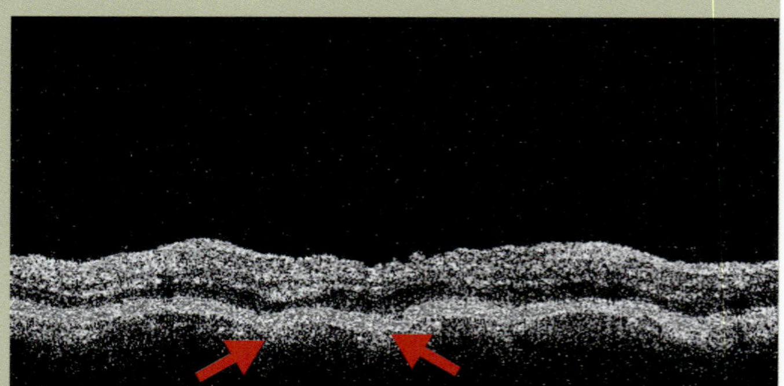

CENTRAL RETINAL ARTERY OCCLUSION

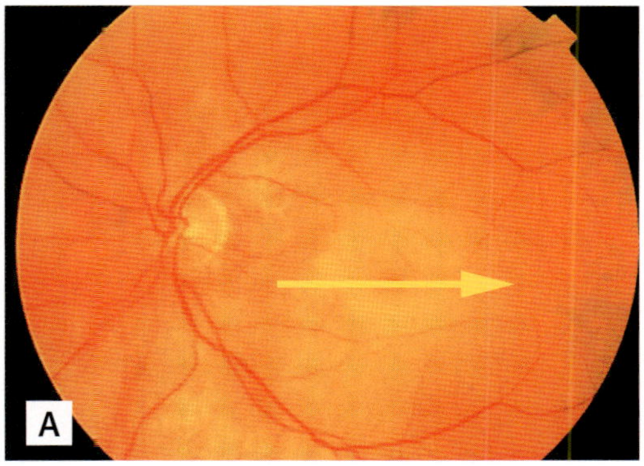

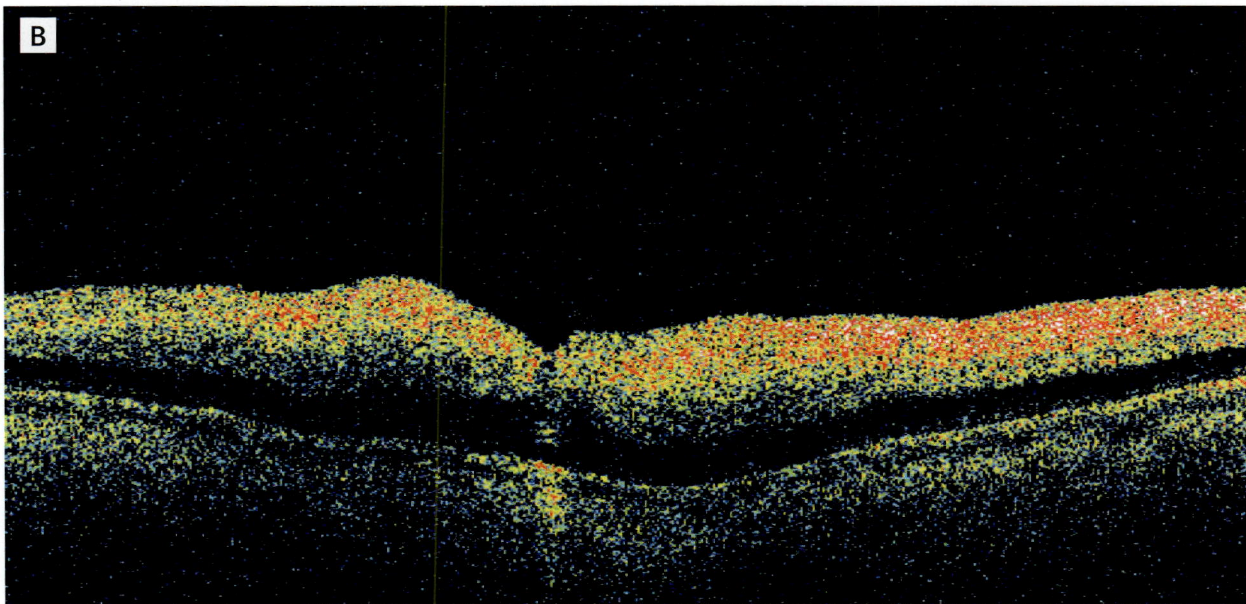

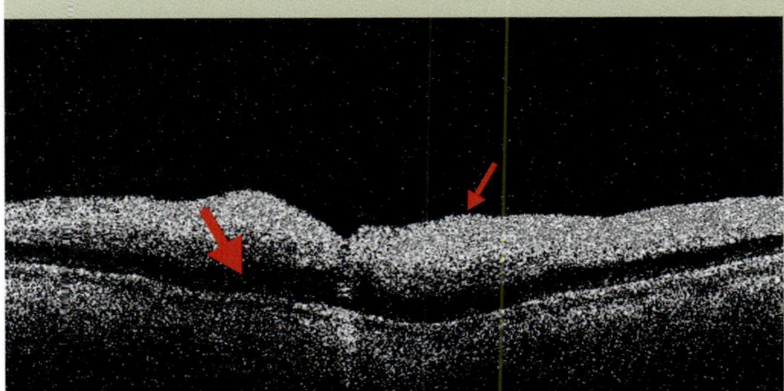

A. Patient with a 3 days old central retinal artery occlusion (the arrow shows the scan direction). B. Optical Coherence Tomography shows high reflectivity of the inner retinal layer due to ischemic intracellular retinal edema (small arrow). The decreased reflectivity of the outer retinal layers is a result of the overlying retinal edema (big arrow).

INTERFERON TREATMENT

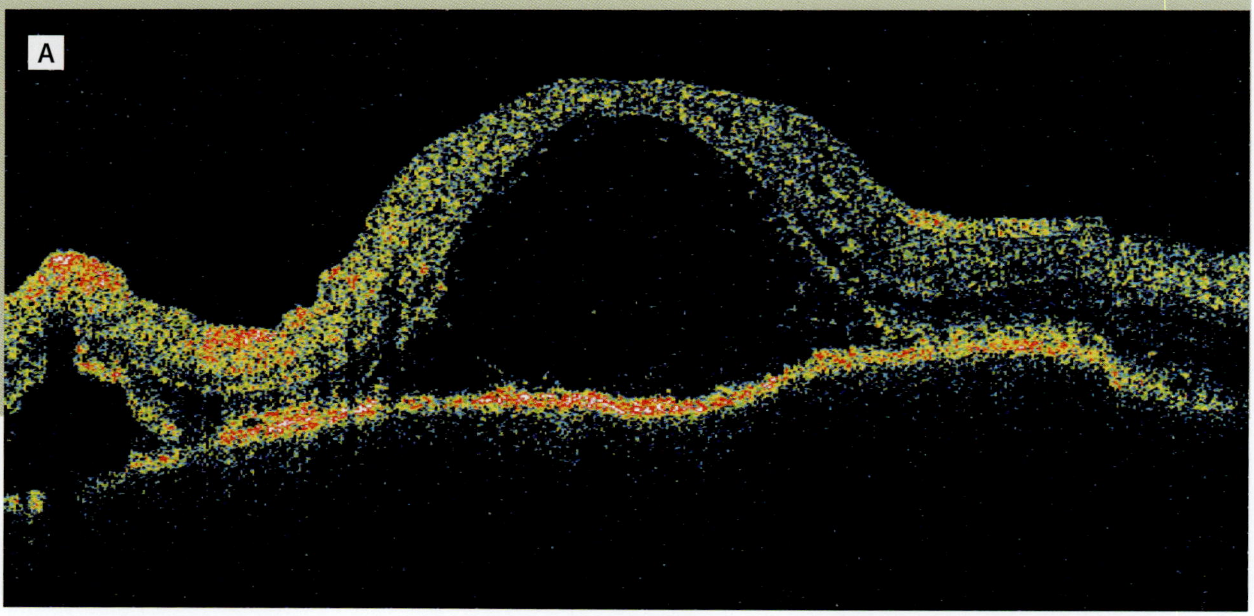

A. Right eye of a patient with hepatitis treated with interferon. Note the extensive area of low reflectivity between the retina and the retinal pigment epithelium that corresponds to a serous retinal detachment (small arrow). Areas of low reflectivity inside the retina are caused by diffuse and cystoid retinal edema (big arrow).

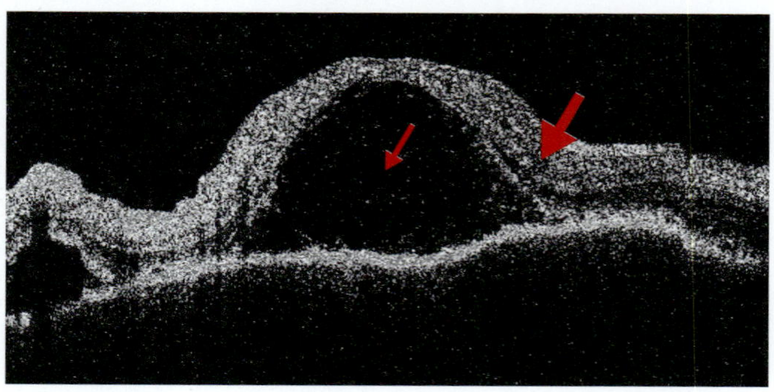

INTERFERON TREATMENT

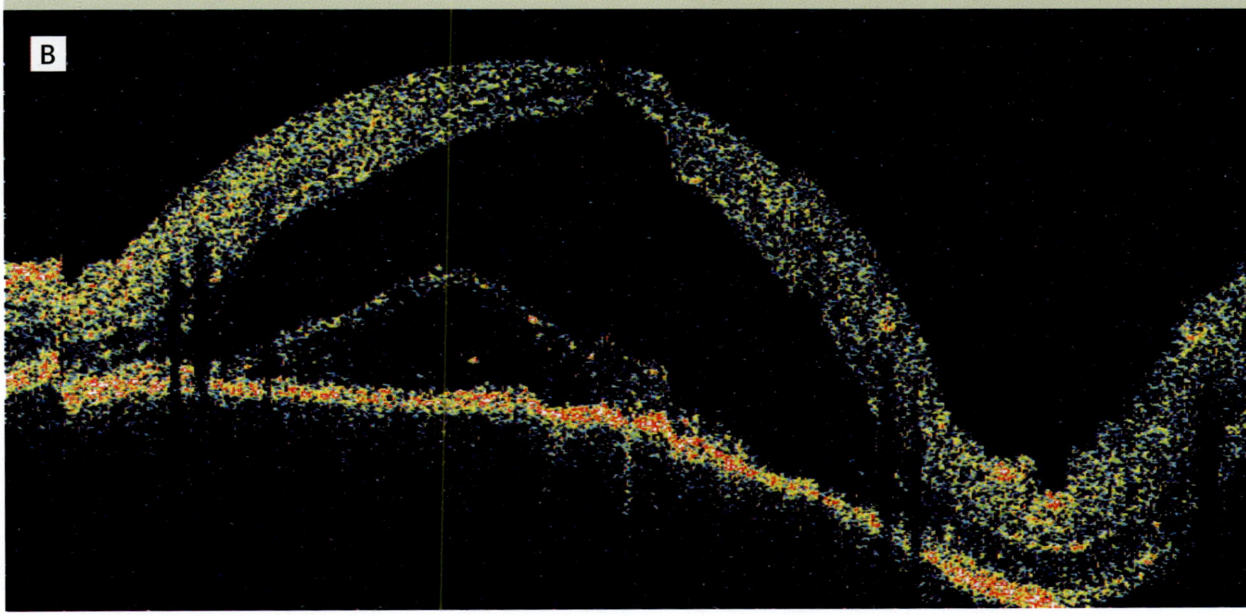

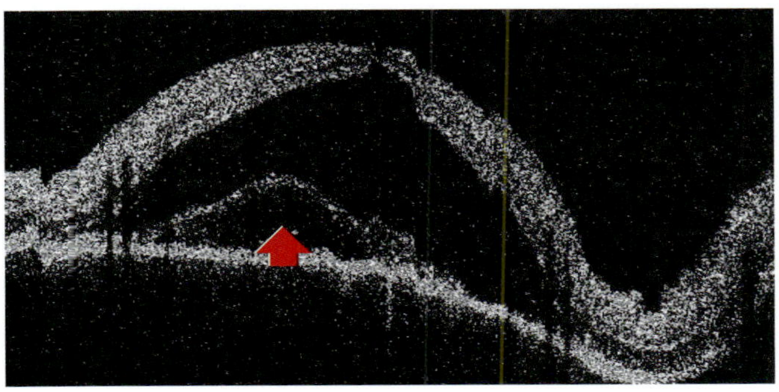

B. Left eye of the patient of page 286. The presence of a local detachment of the retinal pigment epithelium is also characteristic (arrow).

INTERFERON TREATMENT

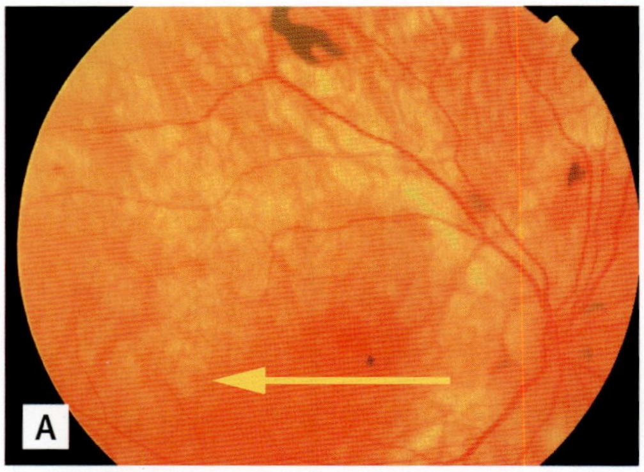

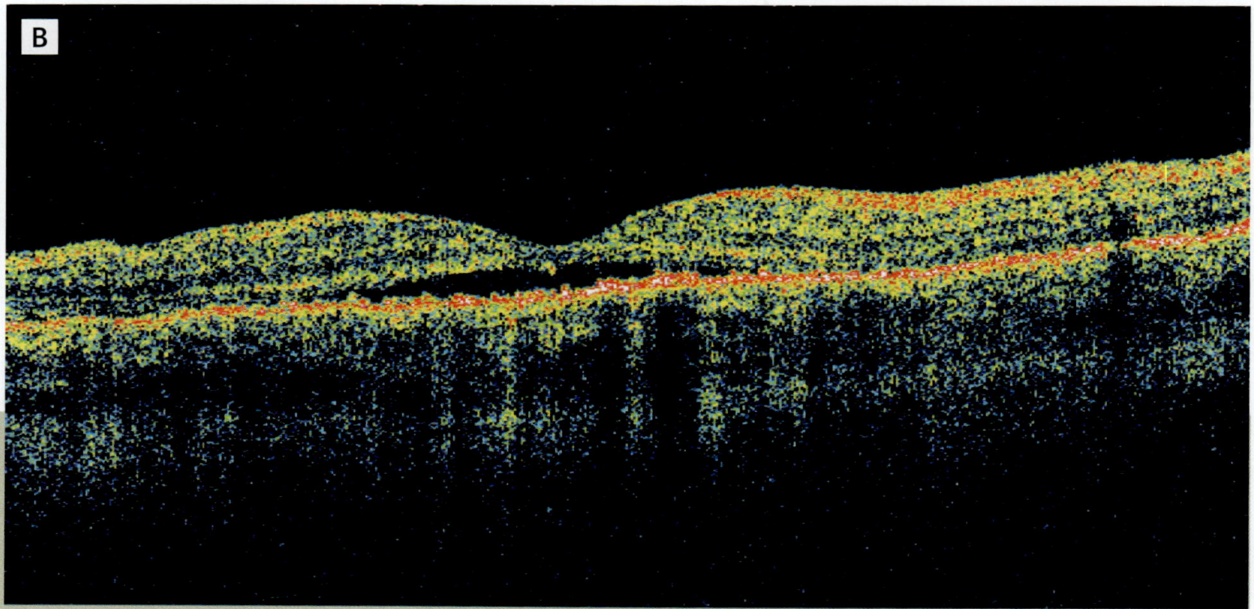

A. The right eye of the patient of page 286 four months after discontinuation of interferon (the arrow shows the scan direction). B. Optical Coherence Tomography shows a significant decrease of the subretinal fluid in the fovea (small arrow). The multiple shadows in the choroid correspond to the choroidal vessels (big arrows).

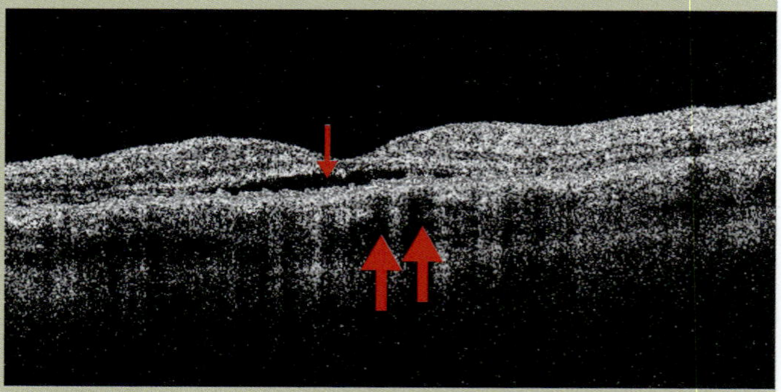

INTERFERON TREATMENT

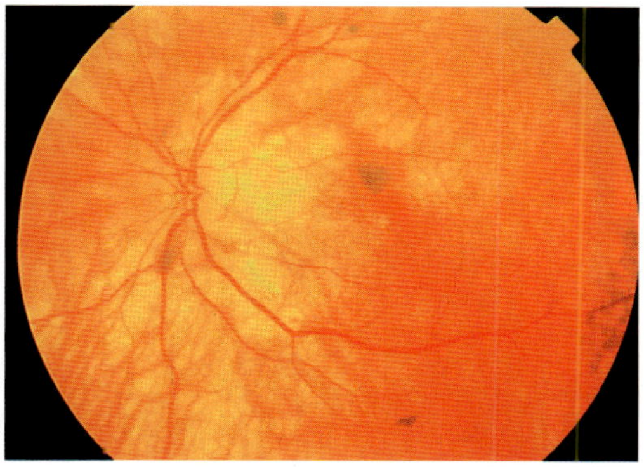

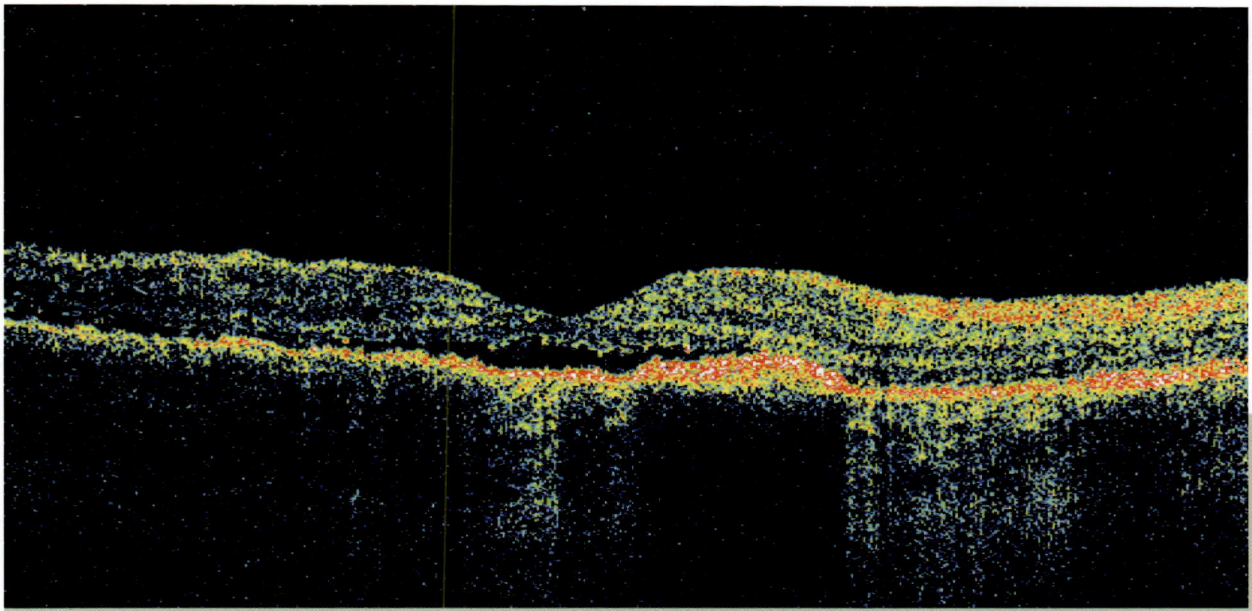

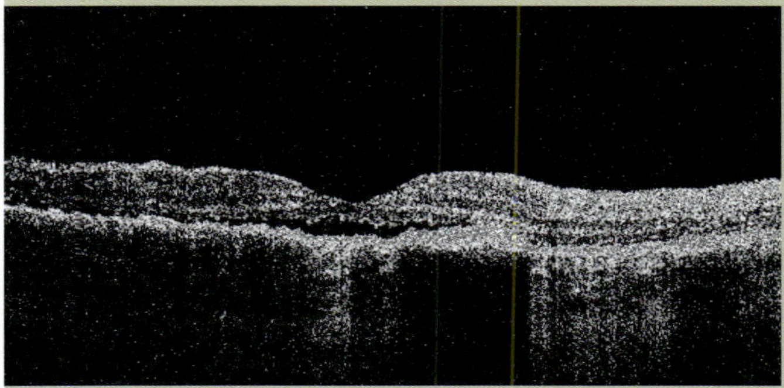

The left eye of the patient in page 288. Note the significant decrease of the macular detachment.

IDIOPATHIC PARAFOVEAL TELANGIECTASIS

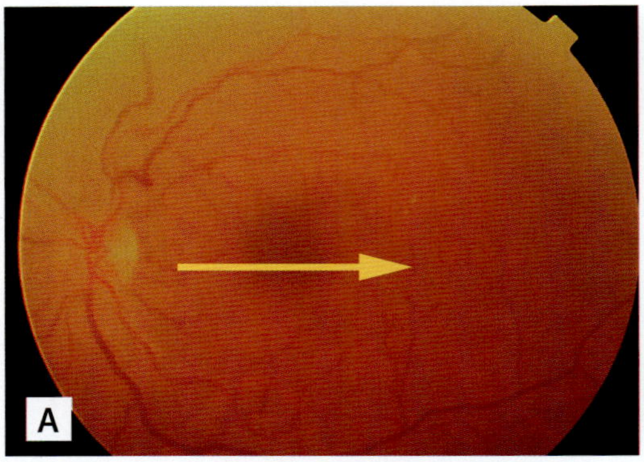

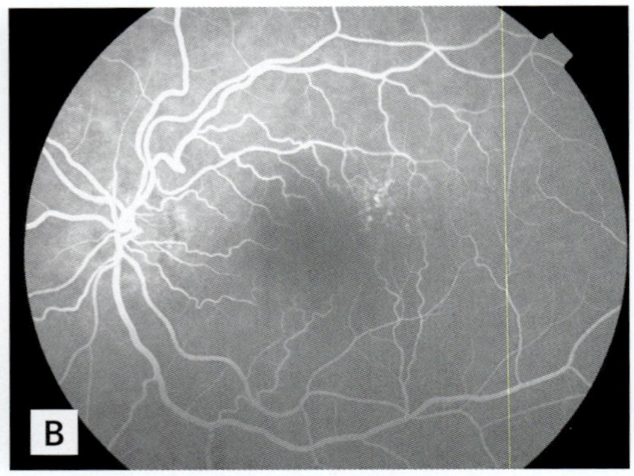

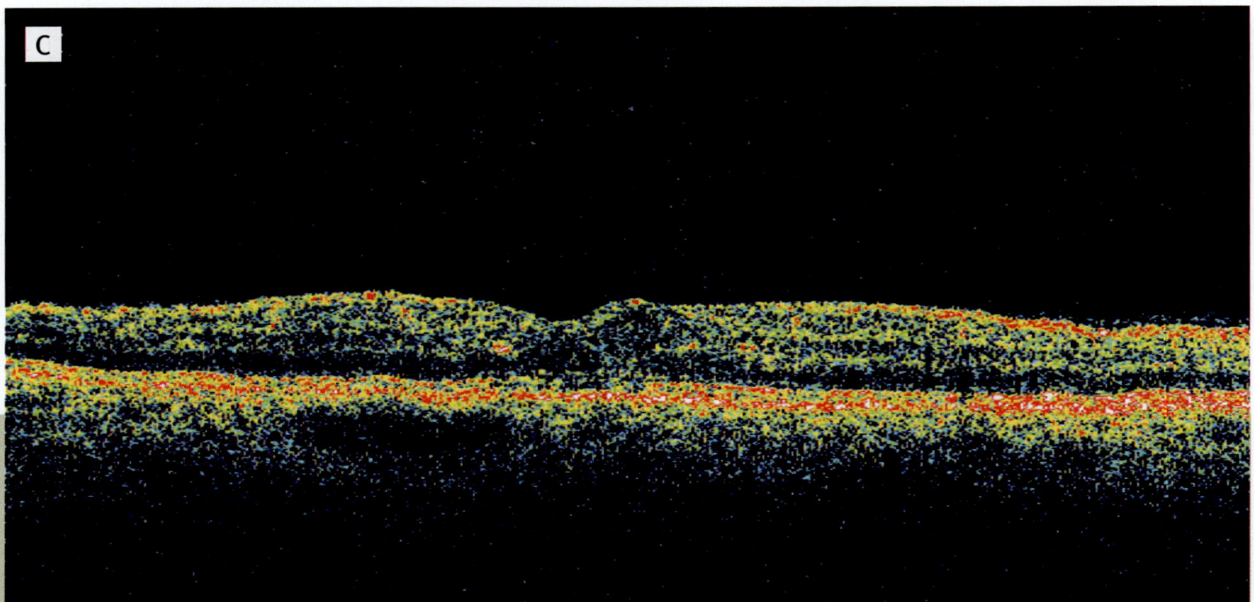

Patient with type I idiopathic parafoveal telangiectasis. A. Biomicroscopy shows the presence of perifoveal edema and focal exudates (the arrow shows the scan direction). B. Fluorescein angiography reveals the presence of telangiectasis superotemporally to the fovea. C. Note the localized increase of the retinal thickness temporally to the fovea due to the edema (small arrow). A small area of high intraretinal reflectivity is detected corresponding to a hard exudate (big arrow).

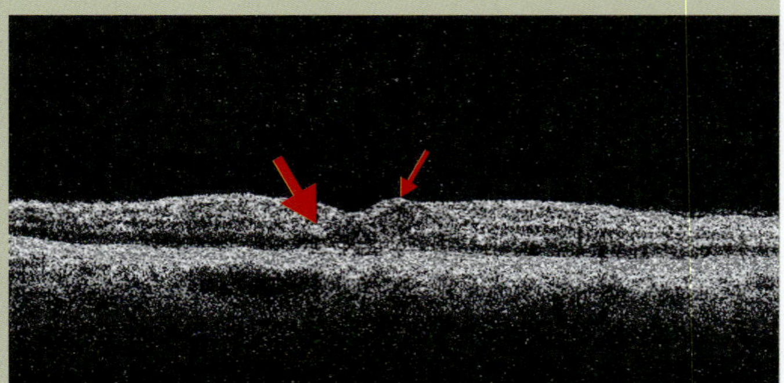

VALSALVA RETINOPATHY

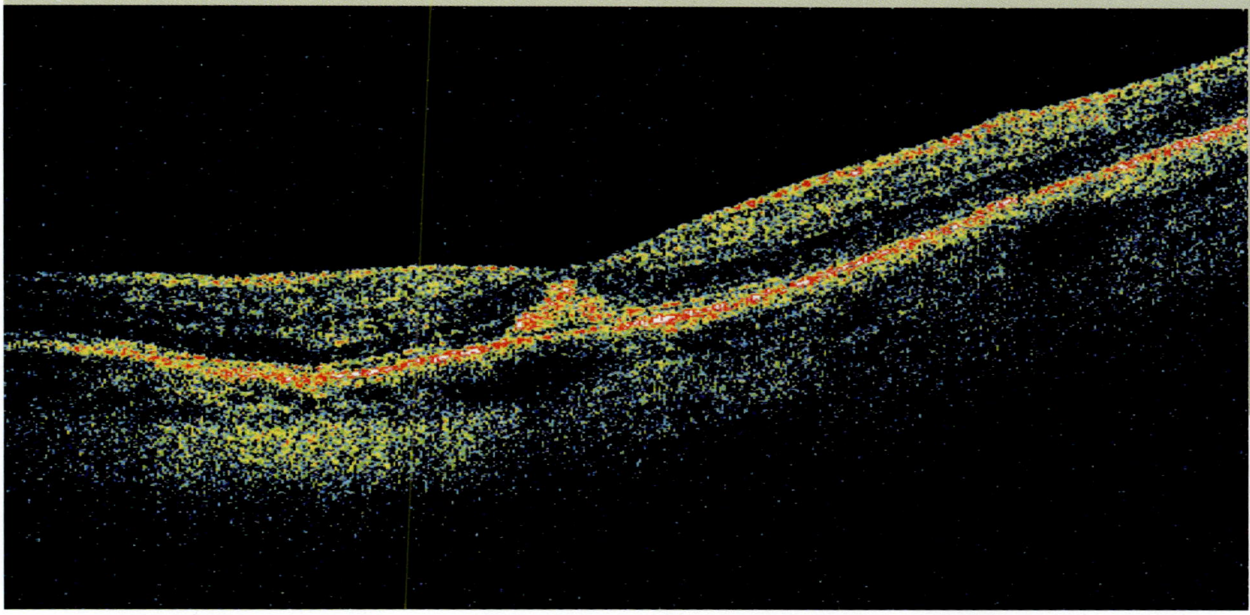

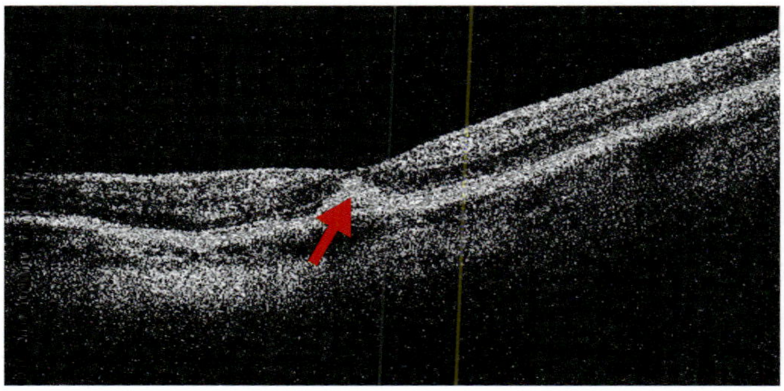

Patient with Valsalva retinopathy. The patient suffered a decrease in his visual acuity after an episode of vomit. Note the area of high reflectivity in the fovea that corresponds to an intraretinal haemorrhage (arrow).

TRAUMATIC CHOROIDAL RUPTURE

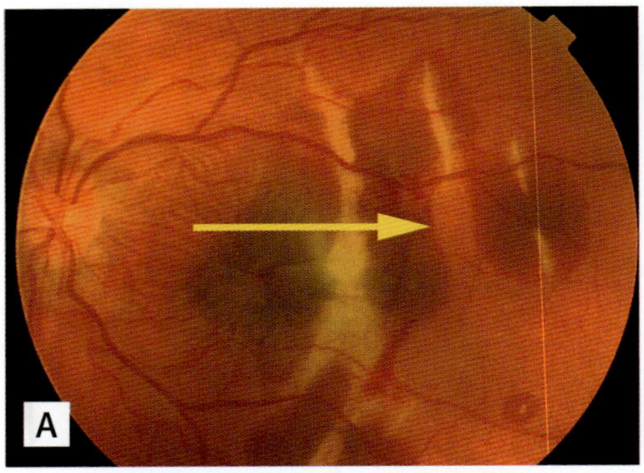

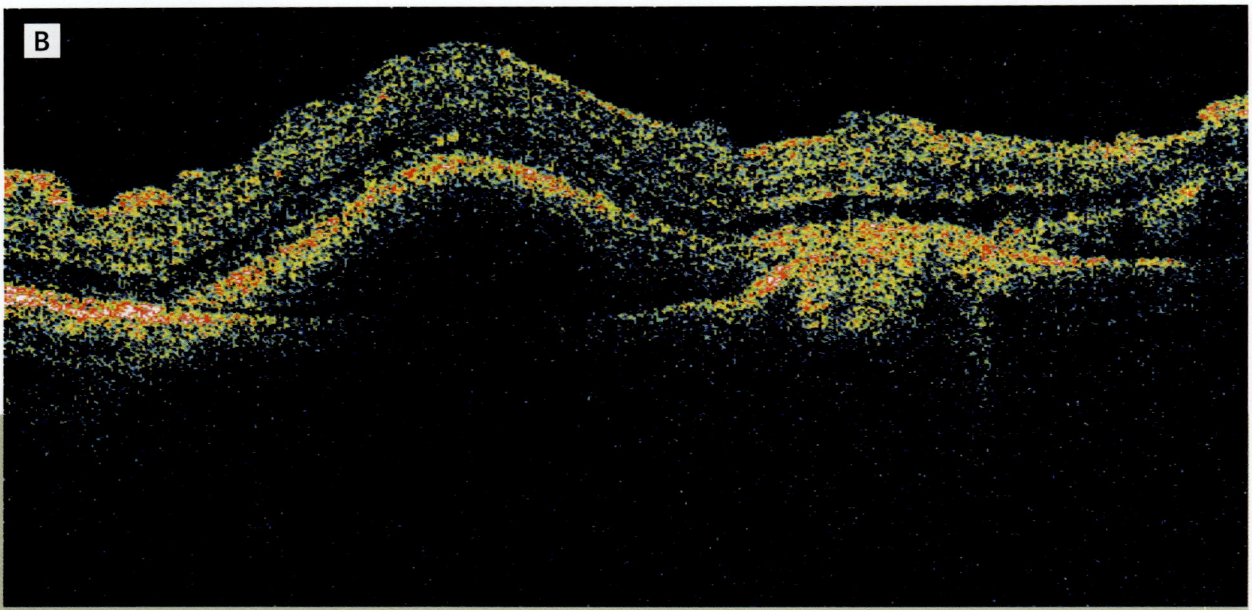

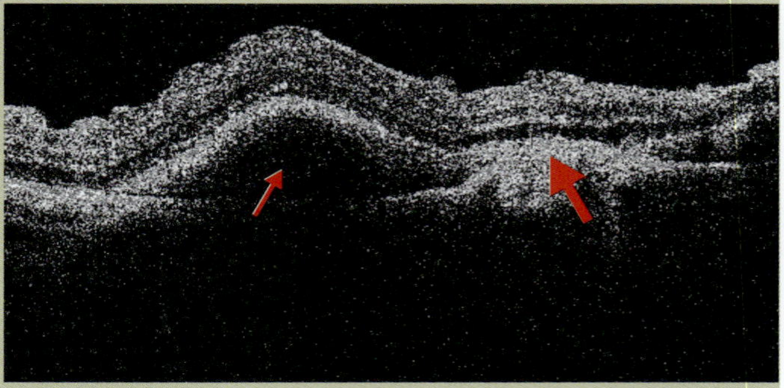

A. Patient with choroidal rupture and subretinal hemorrhage after an injury (the arrow shows the scan direction). B. Optical Coherence Tomography shows a dome-shaped area of high reflectivity deriving from the choroid that causes retinal elevation and corresponds to the choroidal rupture (big arrow). An area of low reflectivity which corresponds to the haemorrhage is also detected under the retinal pigment epithelium (small arrow). The haemorrhage causes an elevation of the retinal pigment epithelium and shadowing underneath.

CHOROIDAL HEMANGIOMA

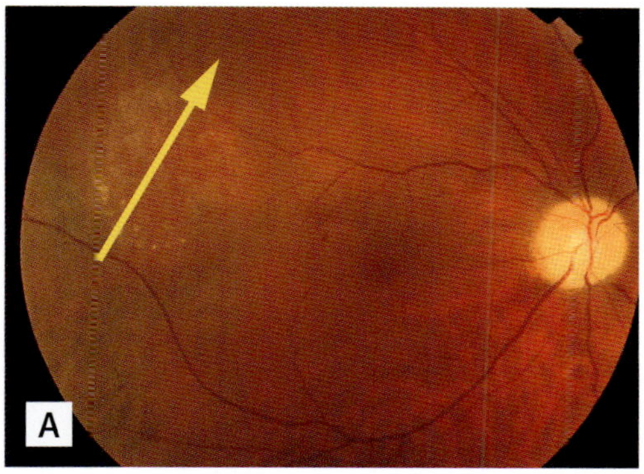

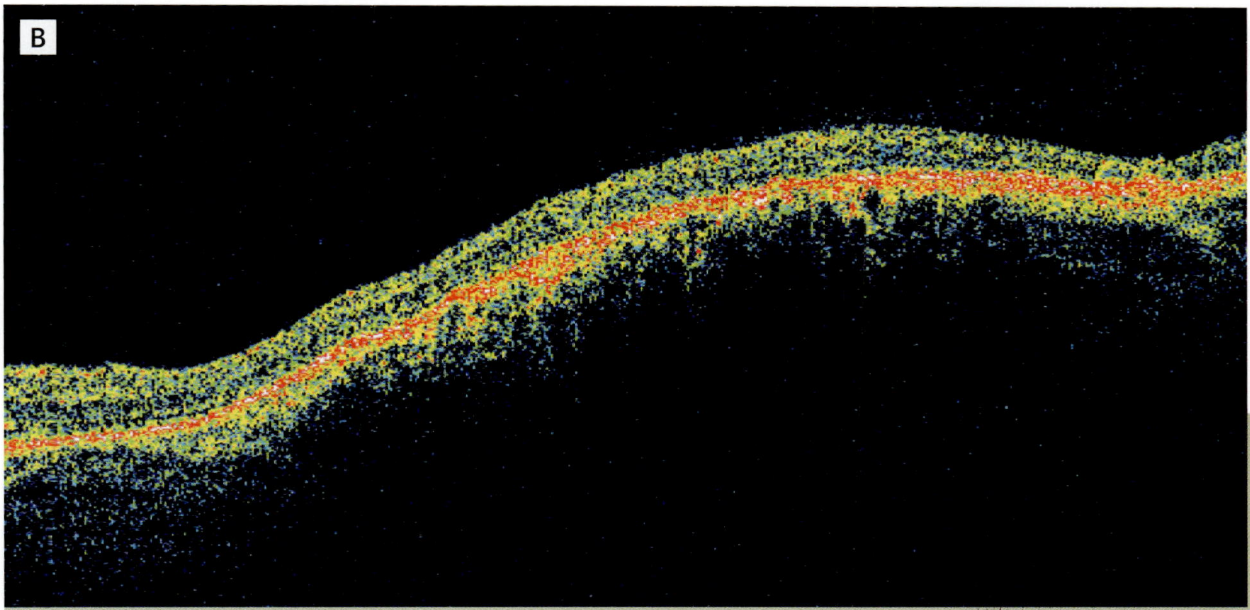

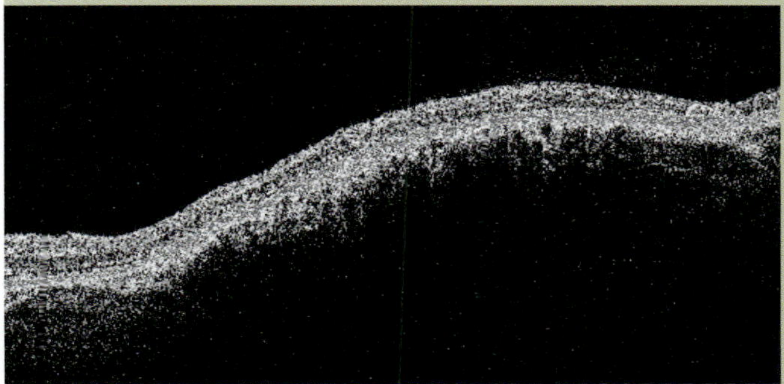

A. Patient with choroidal hemangioma superotemporally to the macula (the arrow shows the scan direction). B. Optical Coherence Tomography shows a smooth elevation of the retina and the retinal pigment epithelium-choriocapillaries complex due to the underlying choroidal tumor. Optical Coherence Tomography cannot determine the nature of the tumor.

ANGIOID STREAKS

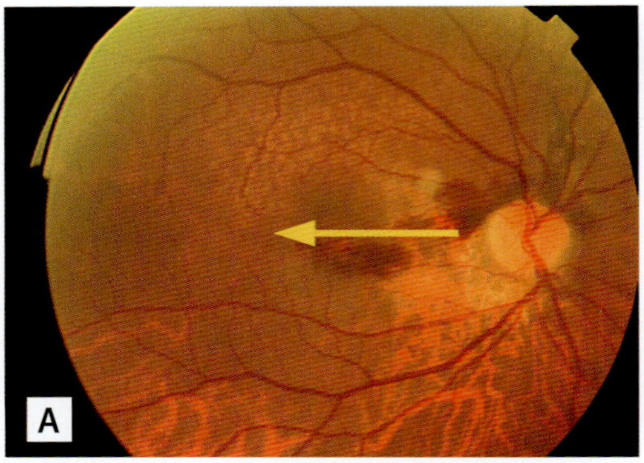

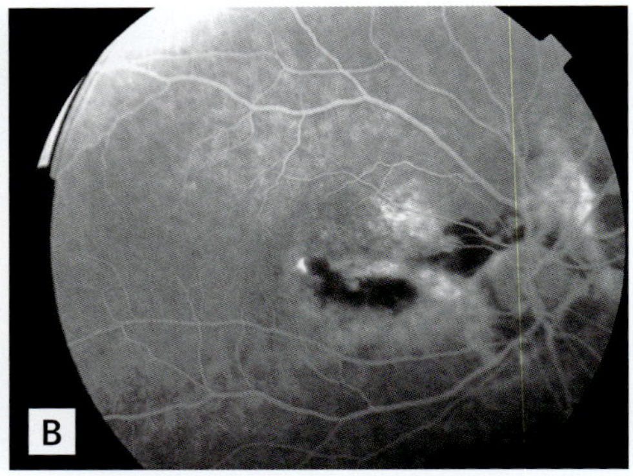

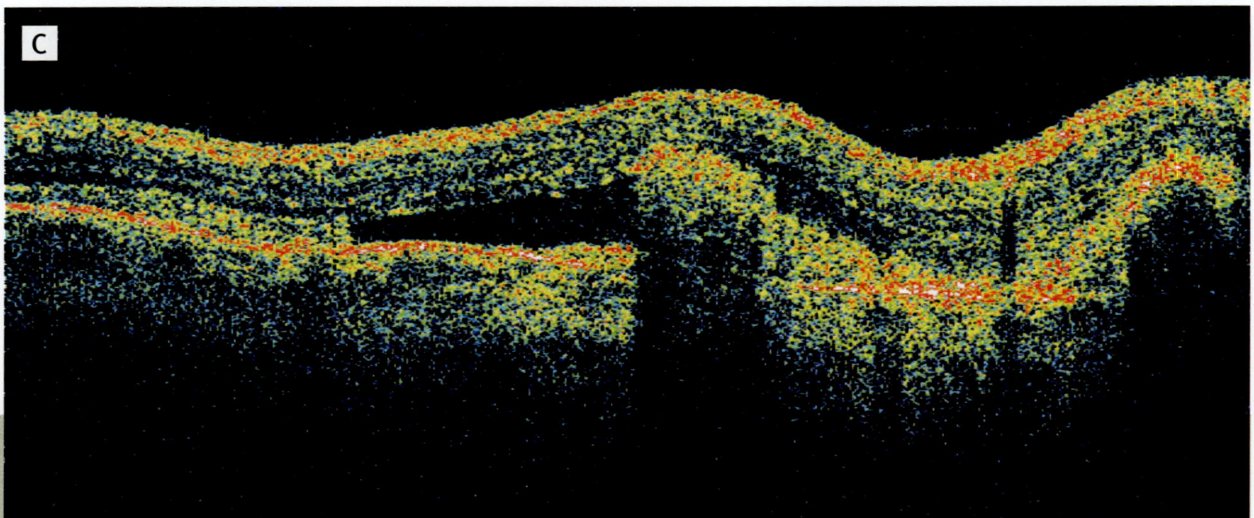

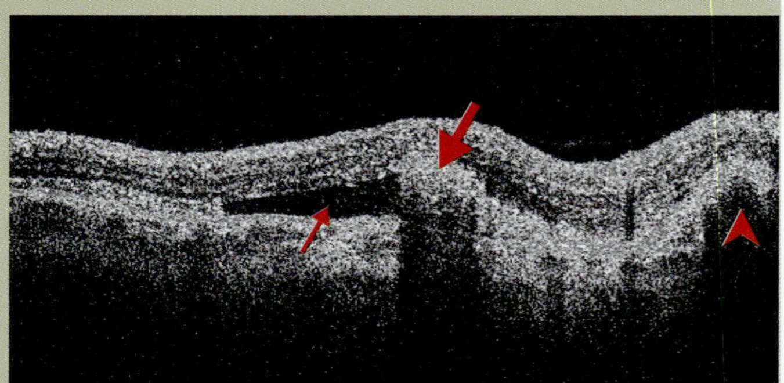

A. Patient with angioid streaks and active choroidal neovascularization (the arrow shows the scan direction). B. Fluorescein angiography shows dye leakage in the posterior pole and hypofluorescence corresponding to the haemorrhages. Angioid streaks are also detected. C. Optical Coherence Tomography depicts an area of low reflectivity between the retina and the retinal pigment epithelium that corresponds to the subretinal fluid accumulation in the fovea (small arrow). The area of high reflectivity located inside the subretinal space corresponds to the choroidal neovascularization (big arrow). Subretinal haemorrhage is detected as an elevated area of low reflectivity under the retinal pigment epithelium and the choriocapillaries (arrow head).

ANGIOID STREAKS

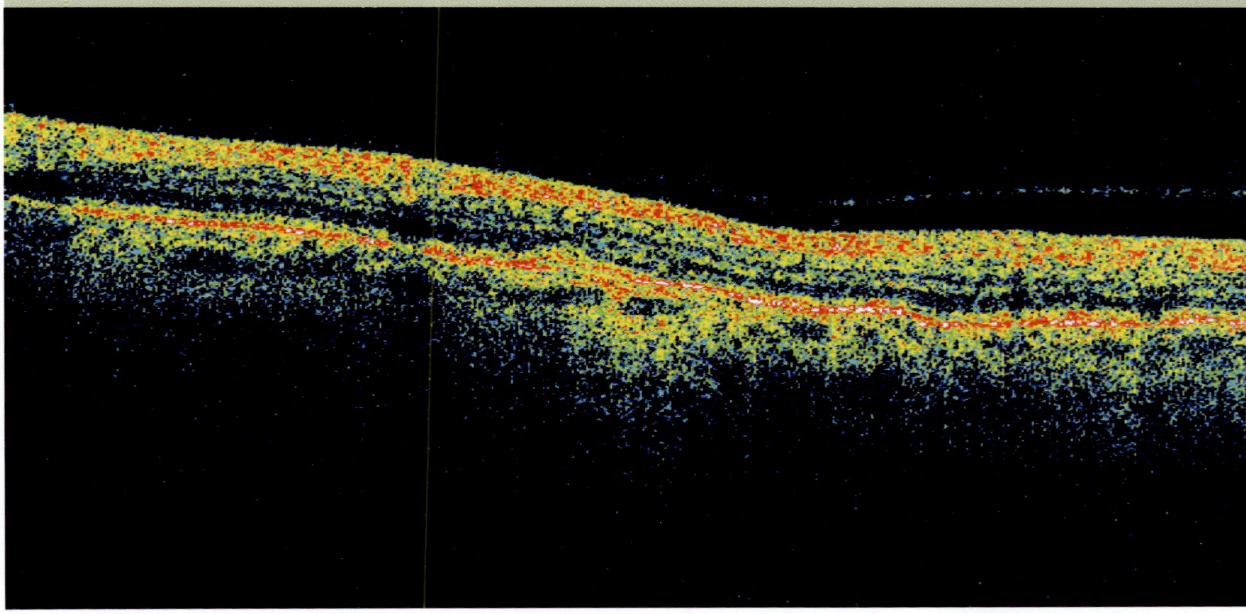

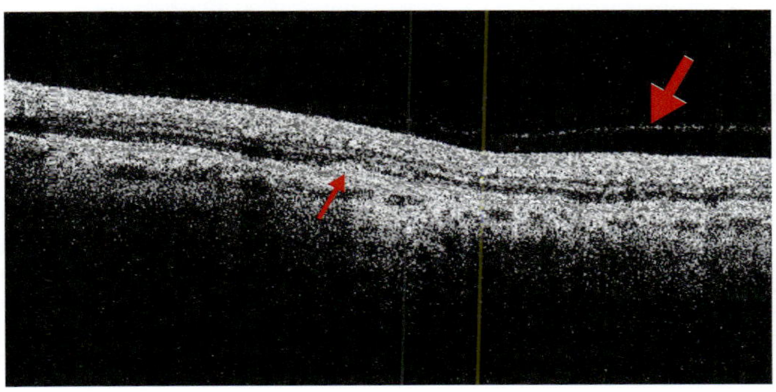

Another scan of the patient of page 294. The area of angioid streaks is detected as a separation of the retinal pigment epithelium-choriocapillaries layers (small arrow). The vitreous appears partially attached to the retina (big arrow).

ACUTE MYELOGENOUS LEUKEMIA

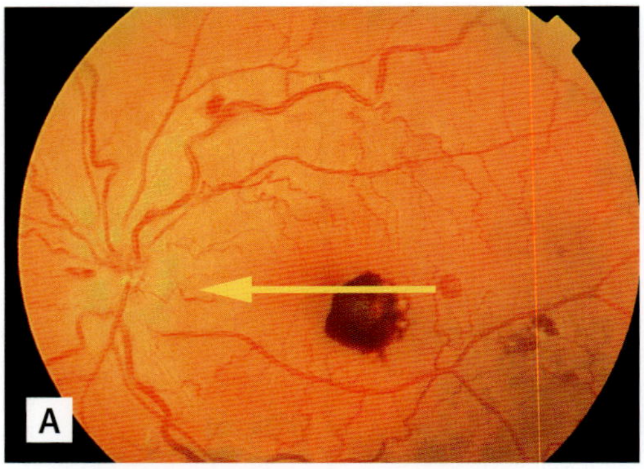

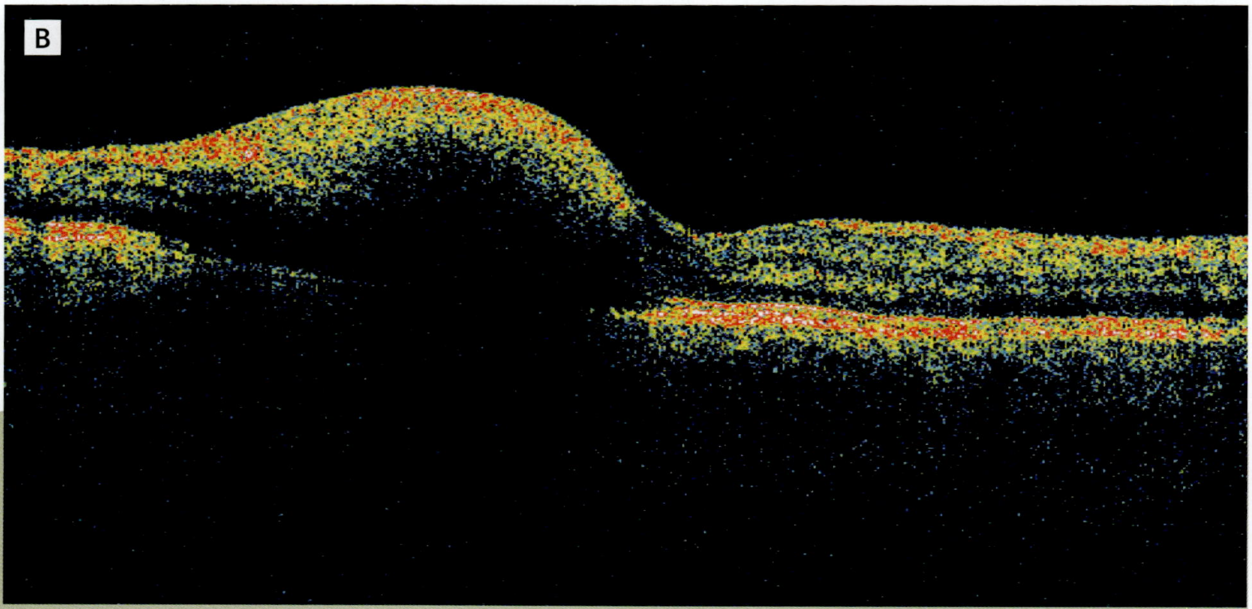

A. Patient with acute myelogenous leukemia and macular haemorrhage (the arrow shows the scan direction). B. Optical Coherence Tomography depicts a thick area of high reflectivity on the retinal surface in the central fovea that corresponds to the retinal haemorrhage (small arrow). Note the almost complete shadowing of the underlying tissue caused by the high reflectivity of the haemorrhage (big arrow).

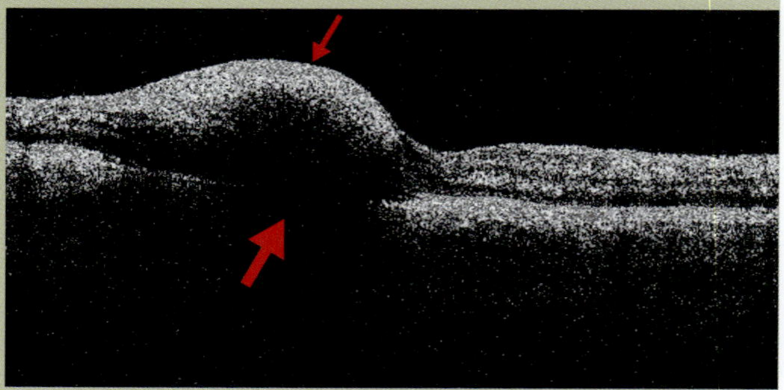

ACUTE MYELOGENOUS LEUKEMIA

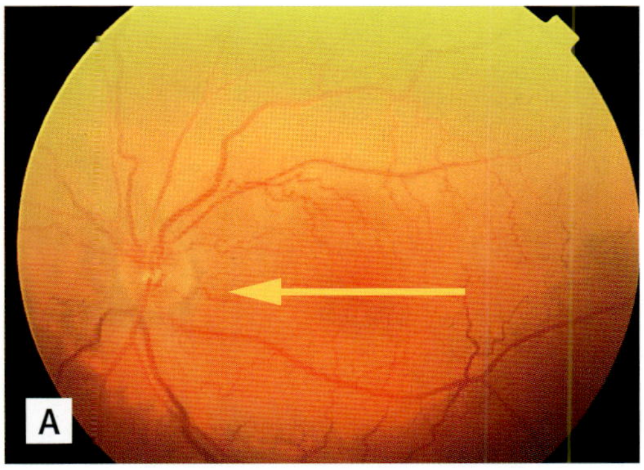

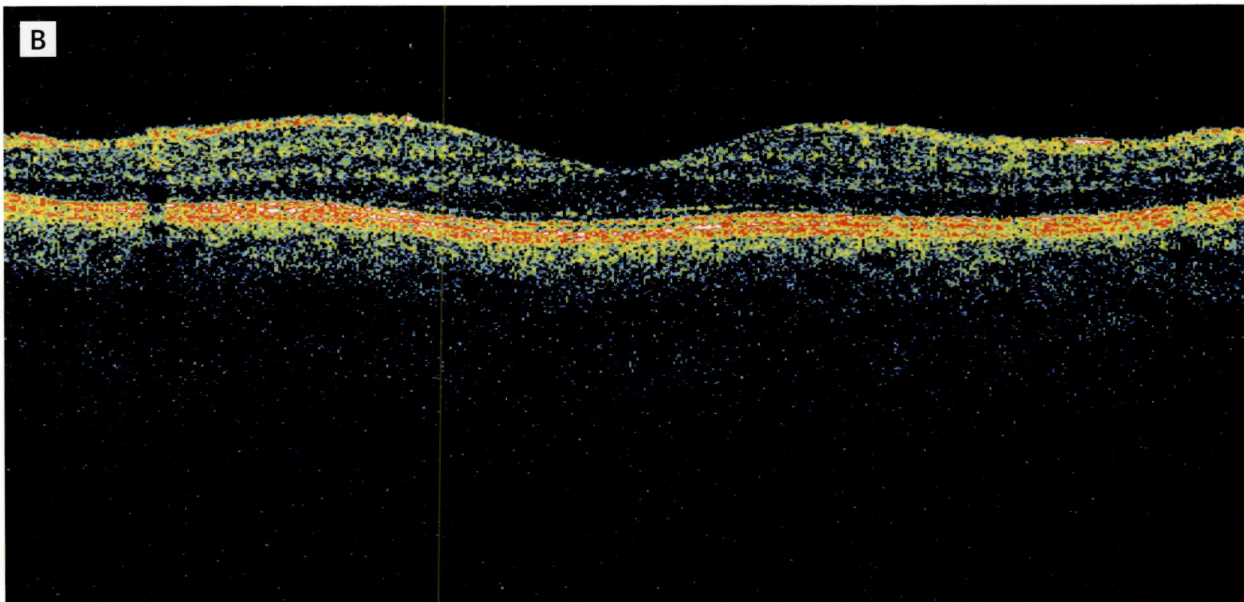

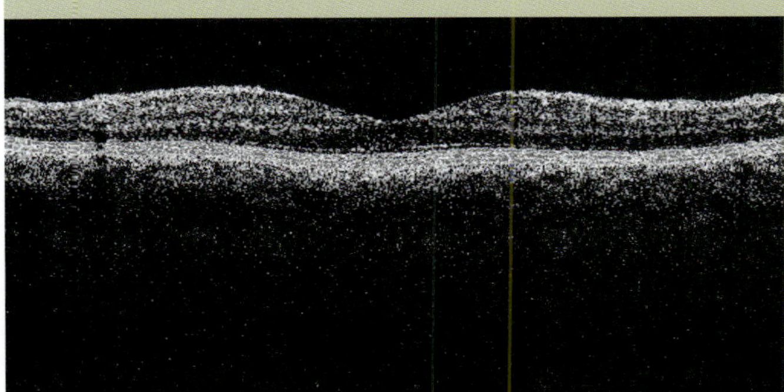

A. The patient of page 296 ten months after systemic treatment (the arrow shows the scan direction). B. Note the complete recovery of the physiologic macular anatomy and the disappearance of the haemorrhages.

METASTATIC CHOROIDAL TUMOR

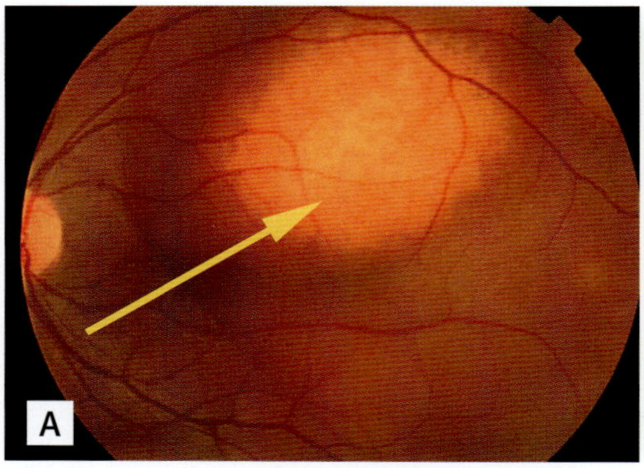

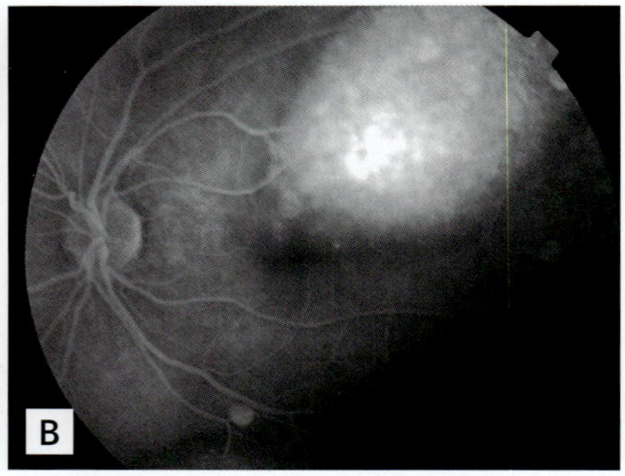

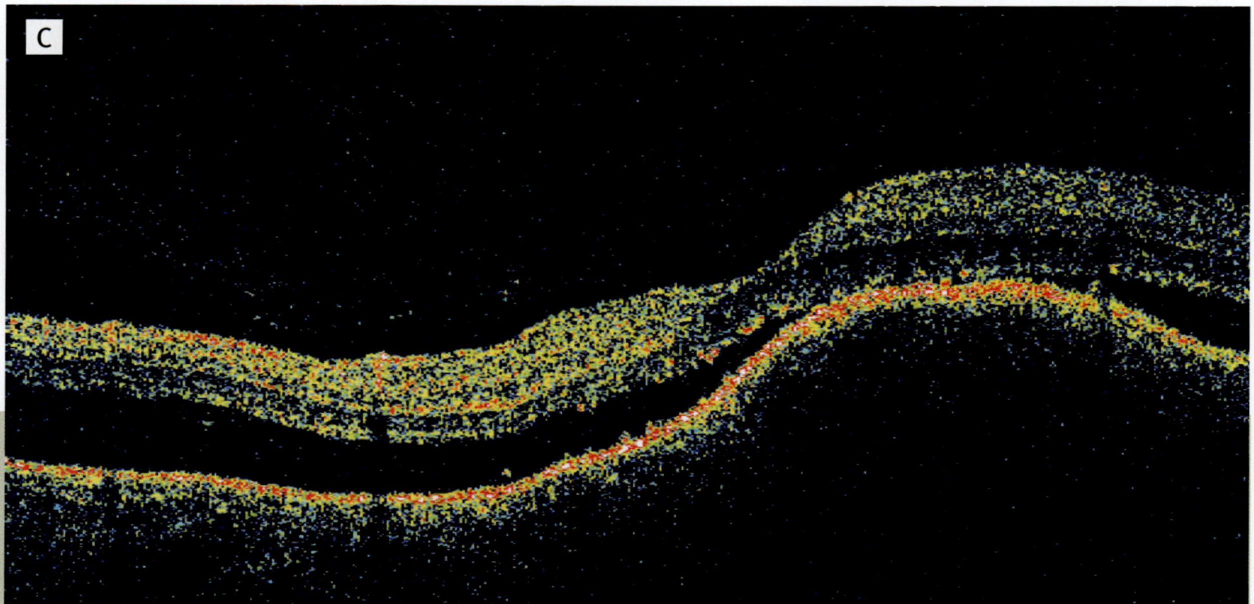

A. Patient with metastatic choroidal tumor (the arrow shows the scan direction). B. Fluorescein angiography shows hyperfluorescence corresponding to the tumor. C. Optical Coherence Tomography demonstrates a smooth elevation of the retina and the retinal pigment epithelium-choriocapillaries complex due to the underlying choroidal tumor (small arrow). An area of low reflectivity, located between the retina and the retinal pigment epithelium around the tumor (big arrows) due to a secondary retinal detachment also exists. Note the appearance of the fovea (thick arrow).

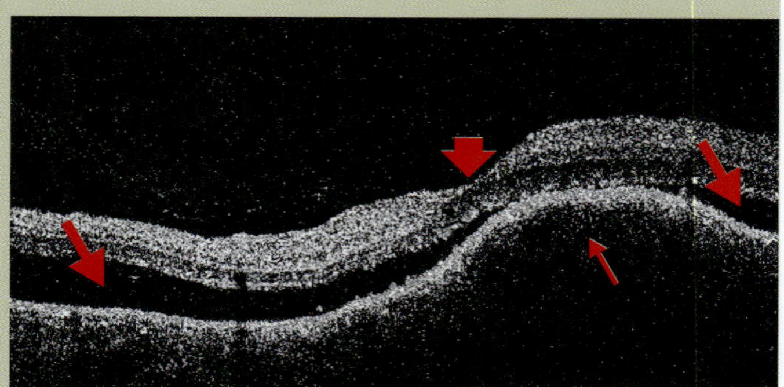

CHOROIDAL NEVUS

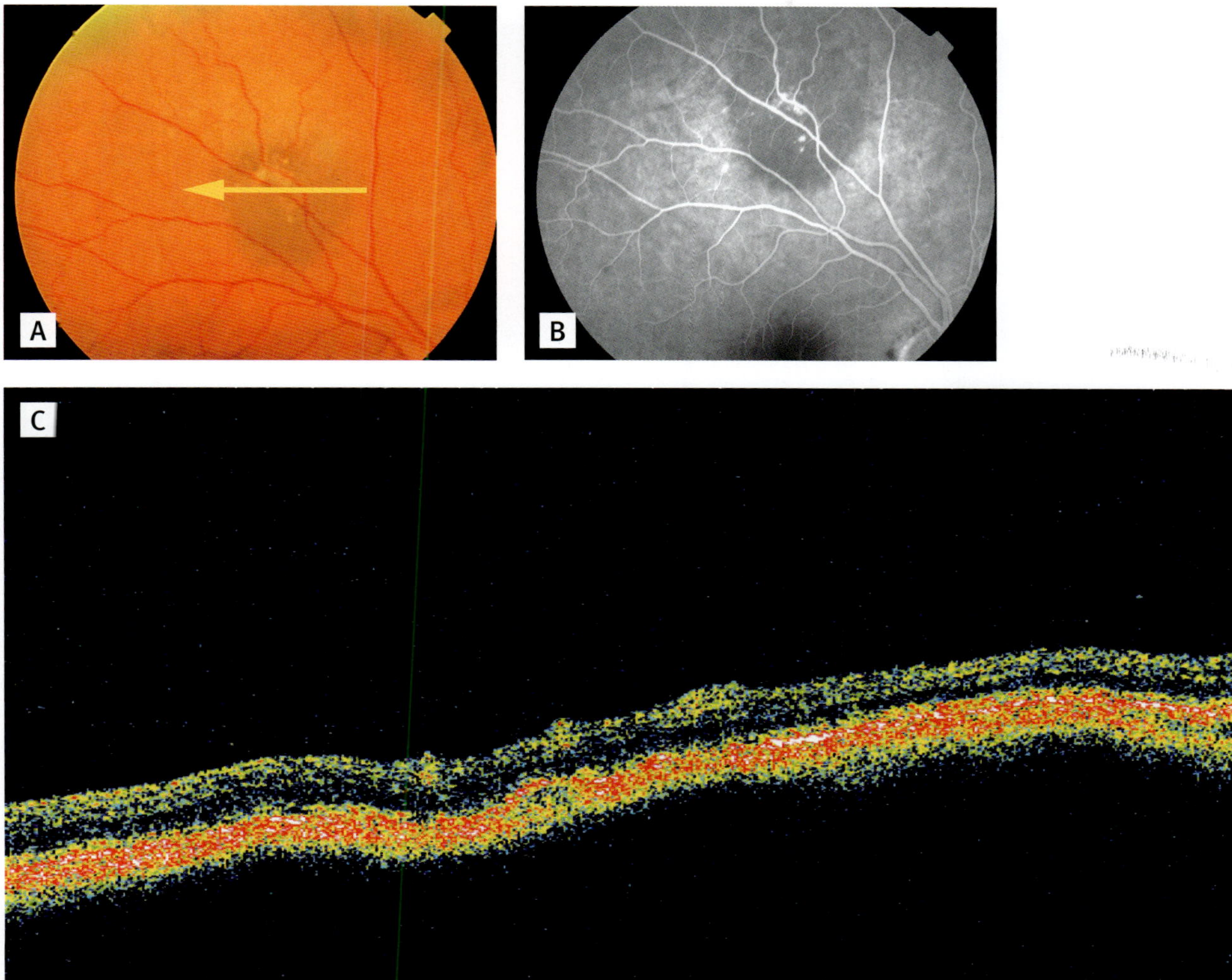

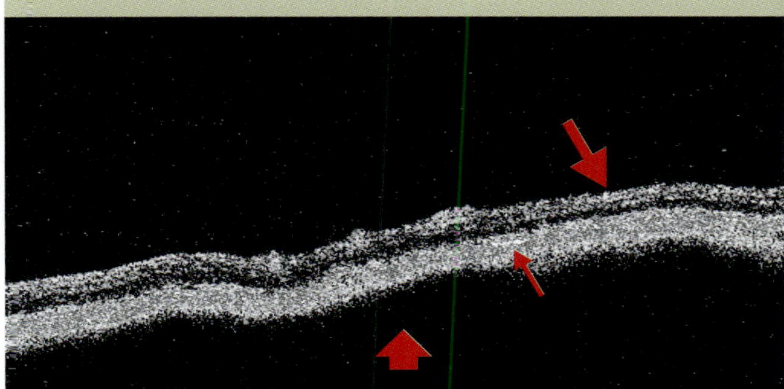

Patient with choroidal nevus outside the superotemporal vascular arcade. B. Fluorescein angiography shows hypofluorescence corresponding to the tumor and staining of the drusen located within its area. C. Optical Coherence Tomography shows an increase of thickness and reflectivity of the retinal pigment epithelium–choriocapillaries complex (small arrow) with retinal thinning (big arrow). The choroid is not detected by Optical Coherence Tomography (thick arrow).

CONGENITAL HYPERTROPHY OF THE RETINAL PIGMENT EPITHELIUM

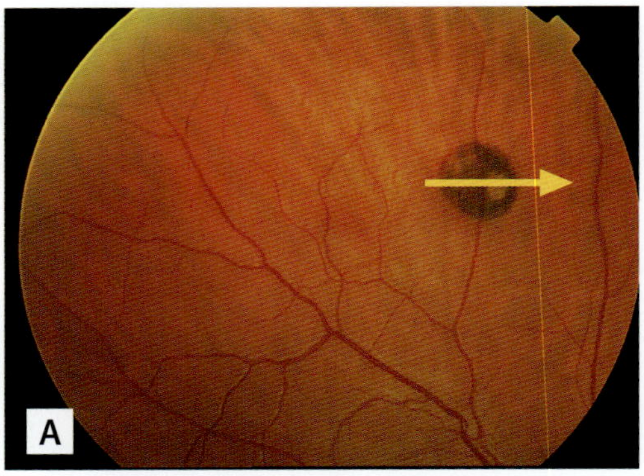

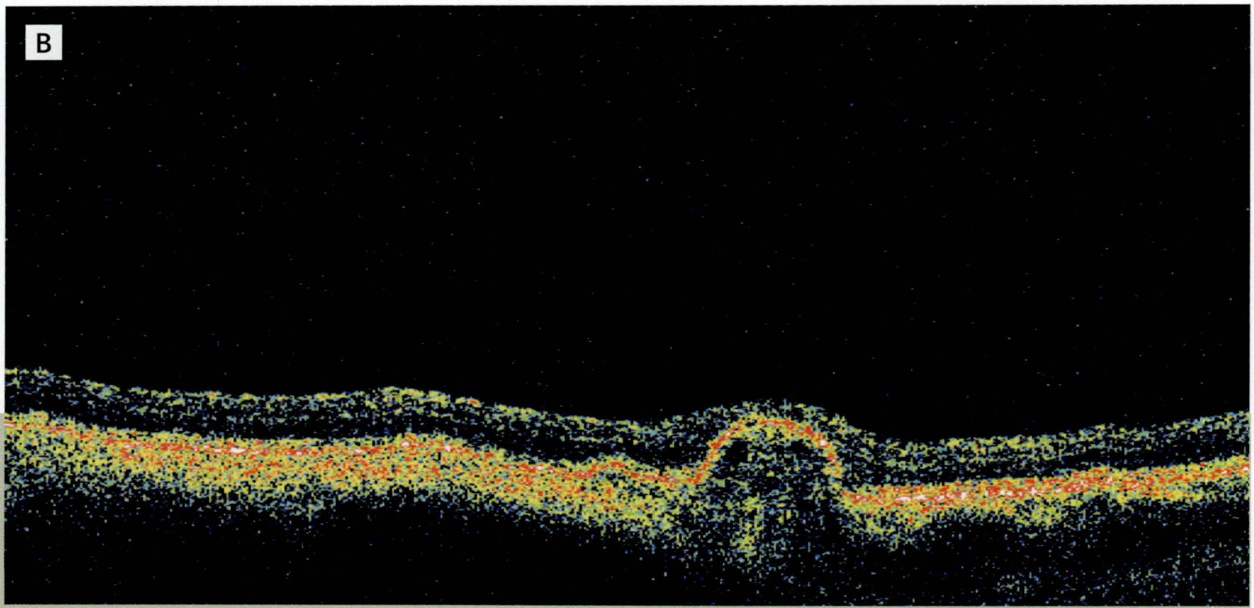

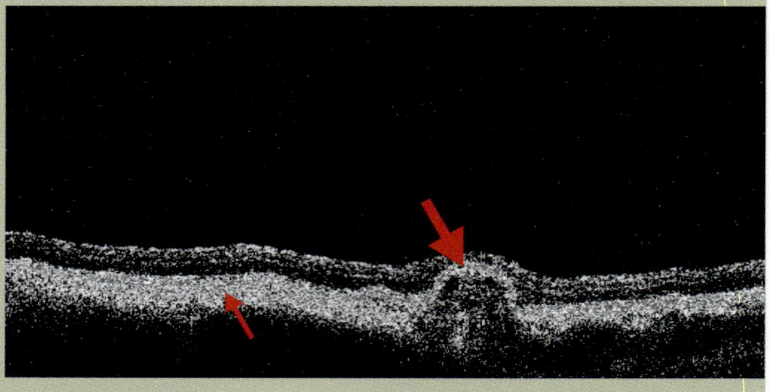

A. Patient with congenital hypertrophy of the retinal pigment epithelium (the arrow shows the scan direction). B. Optical Coherence Tomography shows an increased thickness of the retinal pigment epithelium-choriocapillaries complex (small arrow). The smooth elevation that is detected at the hypertrophy margins is due to the presence of large drusen (big arrow).

CHOROIDAL OSTEOMA

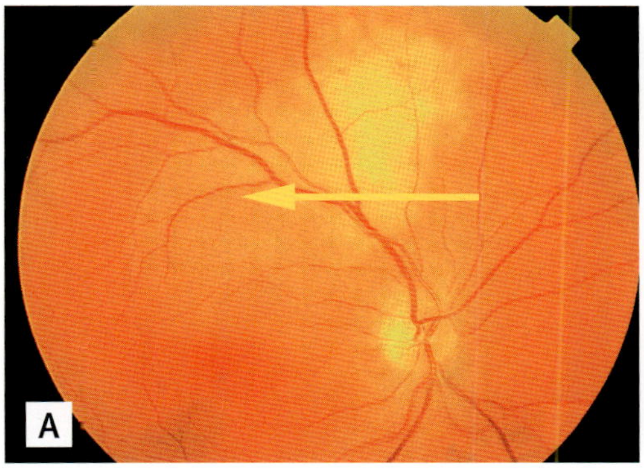

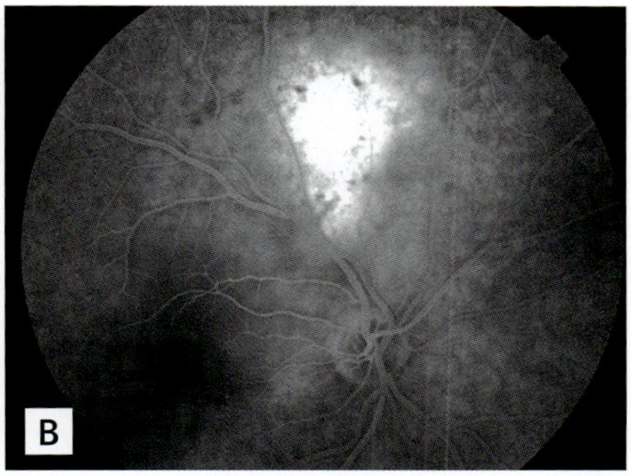

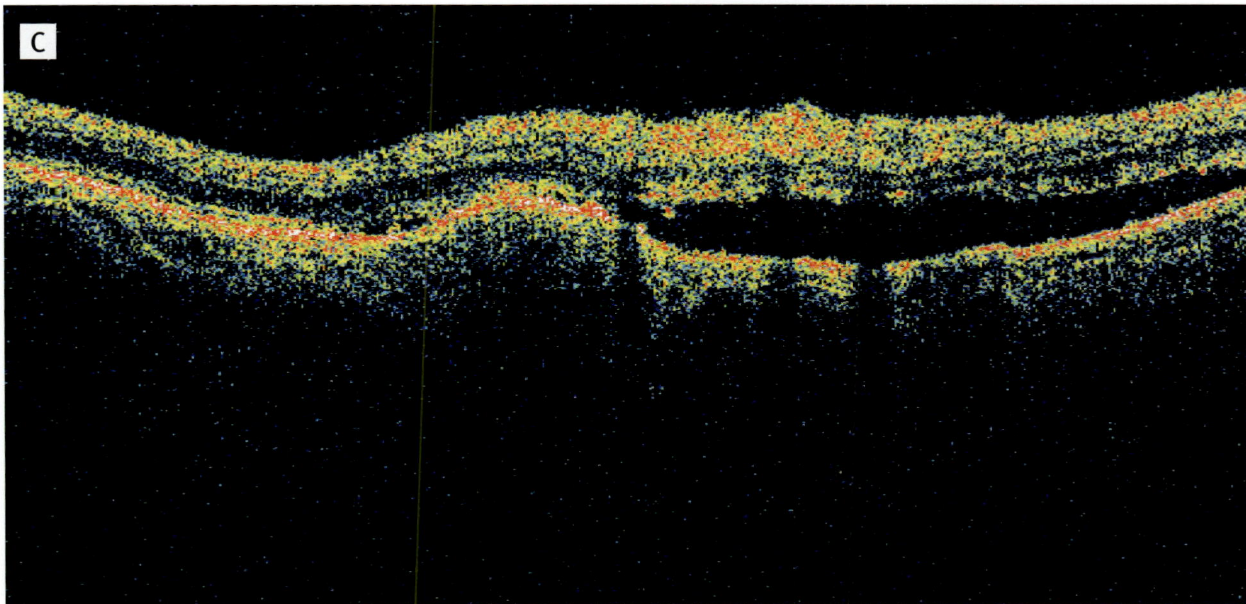

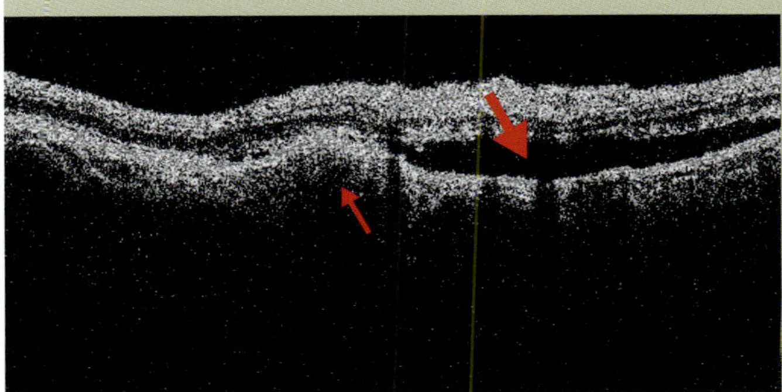

A. A 55 year old woman with suspected choroidal osteoma above the optic disc (the arrow shows the scan direction). B. Fluorescein angiography shows hyperfluorescence with staining of the tumor. C. Optical Coherence Tomography depicts a smooth elevation of the retina and the retinal pigment epithelium-choriocapillaries complex due to the underlying choroidal tumor (small arrow). Next to the tumor there also exists an area of low reflectivity, located between the retina and the retinal pigment epithelium (big arrow) corresponding to a secondary retinal detachment.

IDIOPATHIC RETINAL EDEMA

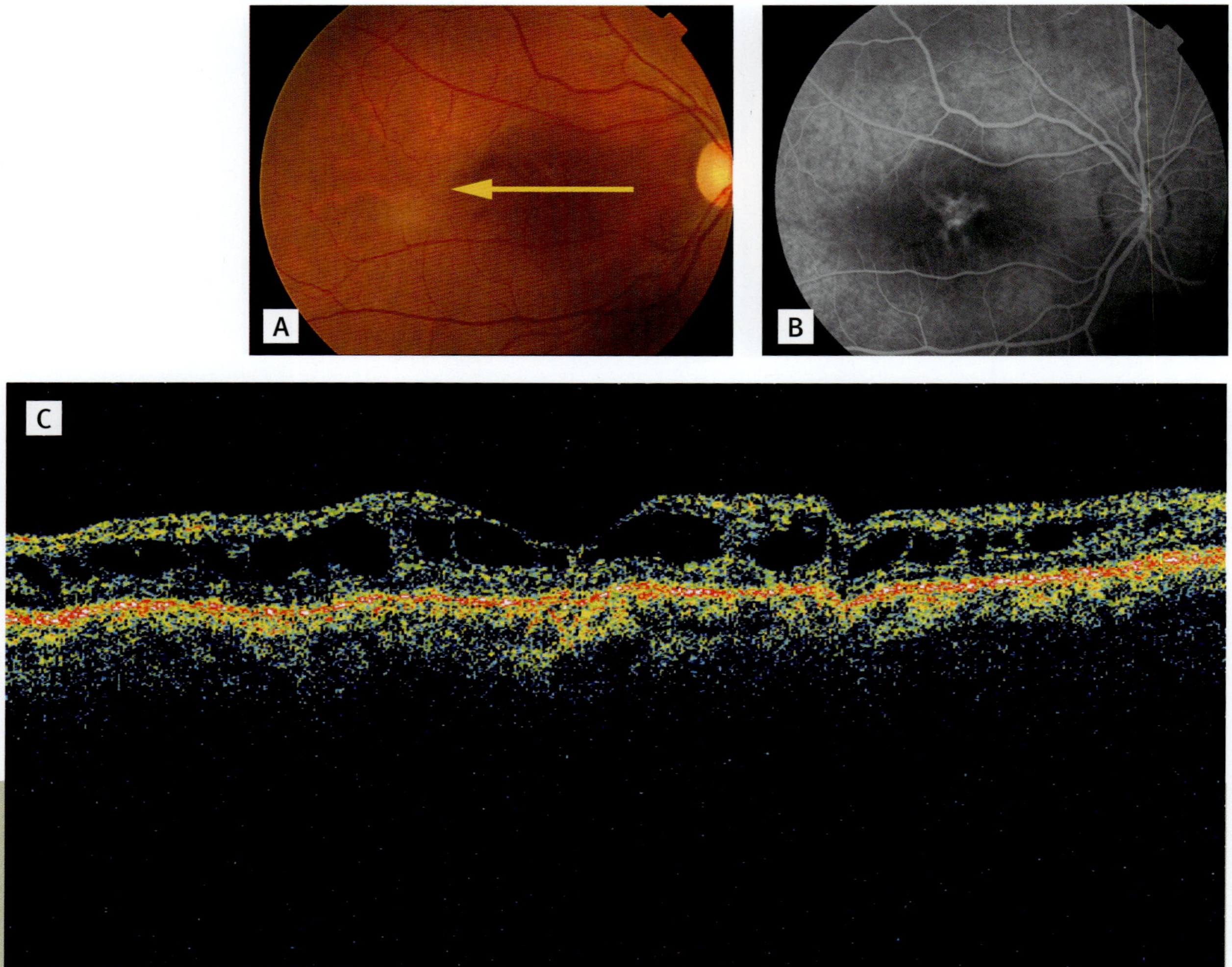

A. A 38-year-old patient with idiopathic cystoid macular edema (the arrow shows the scan direction). B. Fluorescein angiography shows macular hyperfluorescence. C. Optical Coherence Tomography demonstrates diffuse and multiple cystic areas of low reflectivity corresponding to the cystoid retinal edema (small arrows).

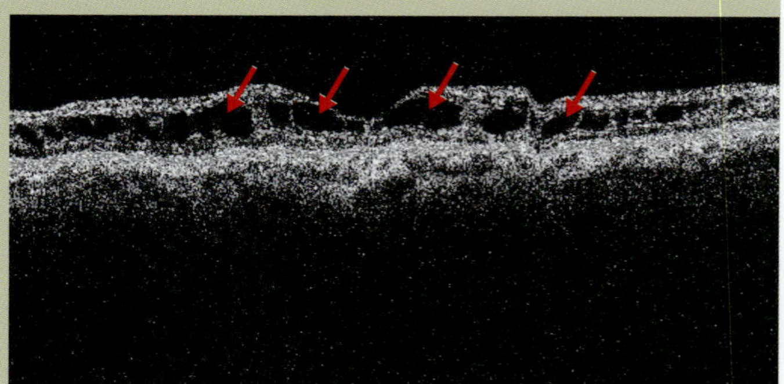

IDIOPATHIC RETINAL EDEMA

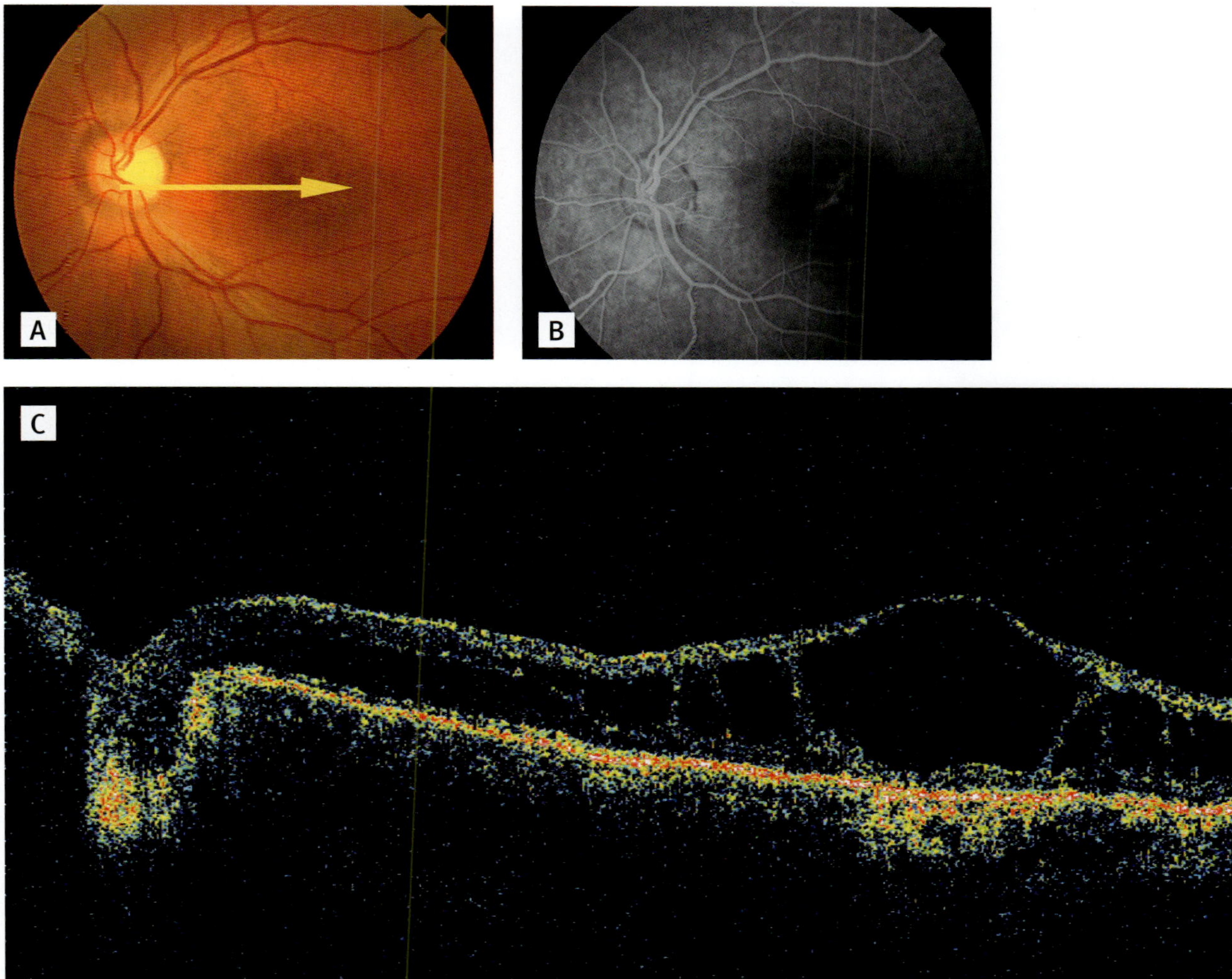

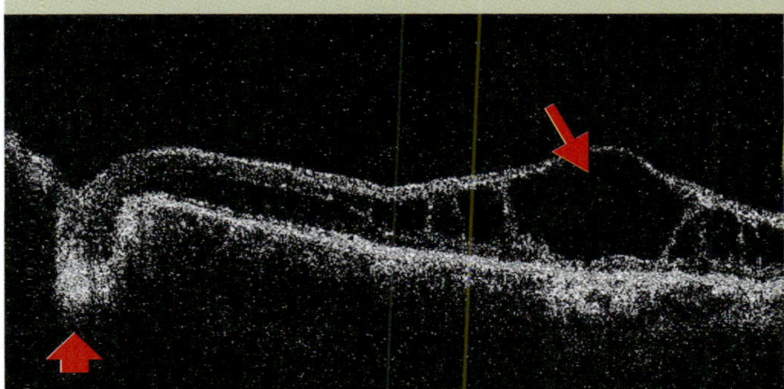

A, B. The other eye of the patient of page 302 (the arrow shows the scan direction). C. Optical Coherence Tomography shows multiple diffuse cystic areas of low reflectivity corresponding to the so called cystoid retinal edema (big arrow). Thick arrow: optic disc.

LEBER CONGENITAL AMAUROSIS

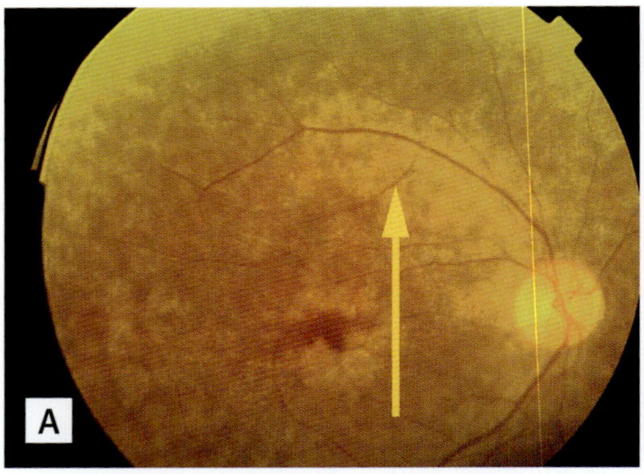

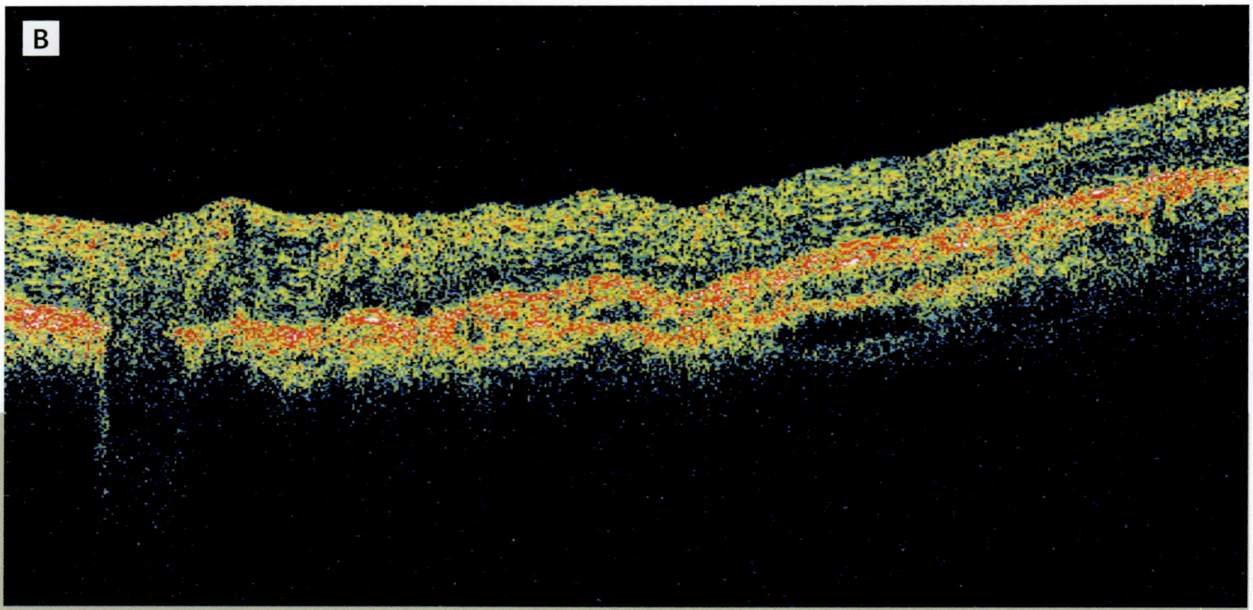

A. Patient with Leber congenital amaurosis. There is a paleness of the optic disc, thinning of the blood vessels and perifoveal atrophy (the arrow shows the scan direction). B. Optical Coherence Tomography reveals a thickening of the retinal pigment epithelium-choriocapillaries complex in the parafoveal area (thick arrow), a local interruption of it (small arrow) and disorganization of the retinal architecture.

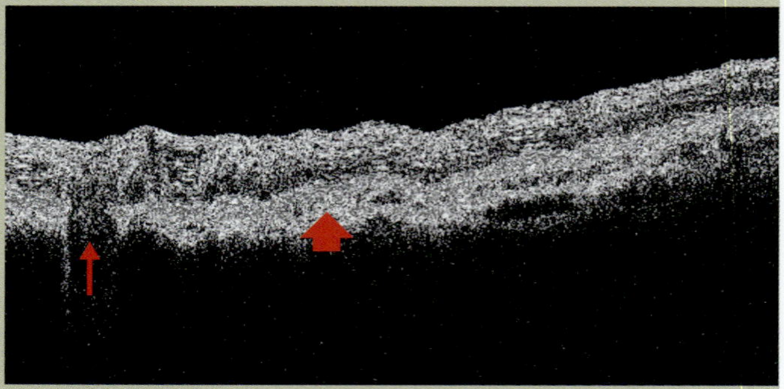

CHAPTER 14

GLAUCOMA

George Theodossiadis, Pantelis Nikolaidis

Primary open angle glaucoma is the most common type of glaucoma in adults. It affects both eyes asymmetrically and it is characterized by the presence of: 1) Open angle of the anterior chamber and normal gonioscopy. 2) Optic neuropathy due to a progressive ganglion cells and neural fiber damage. 3) Characteristic visual field defects.

The disease is often caused by an increase of the intraocular pressure. Primary open angle glaucoma differs from ocular hypertension since in the latter there are no visual fields and optic disc alterations. Five percent of patients with ocular hypertension may develop glaucoma in 10 years. Loss of ganglion cells and of the nerve fibers in primary open angle glaucoma is assessed mainly by visual fields testing. However, according to the findings so far, visual fields defects are detected when there is a nerve fiber loss of at least 30-40%. Additionally, the visual fields examination is subjective requiring the patient's cooperation. Therefore, the necessity for early diagnosis (in order to initiate prompt treatment) or for exclusion of the disease cannot be underestimated. Early diagnosis or exclusion of the disease is achieved in most cases by new technology with the following examinations:

1. Confocal Scanning Laser Ophthalmoscopy (Heidelberg): This examination scans the optic disc giving a three-dimensional image of the scanning area. Confocal Scanning Laser Ophthalmoscopy can only scan the optic disc and therefore,

because of the physiologic anatomical optic disc variations, the possibility for detection of glaucomatous lesions is very limited[5]. In addition, the examiner should delineate himself the optic disc borders manually, a fact that limits the examination's repeatability. The transverse resolution of the examination is 10μm and the axial is 300μm.

2. Scanning Laser Polarimetry (GDX): This is a useful examination that evaluates retinal nerve fiber layer thickness around the optic disc and the final result is independent of other parameters like the corneal thickness . It is an accurate method that helps in detecting early stage glaucoma. The resolution of this method is 13μm[10]. For a better understanding of the examination, a Scanning Laser Polarimetry map is presented (figure C, page 317), that shows the following:

a. Color image of the optic disc and peripapillary area.

b. Topographic analysis of the nerve fiber layer coded in false colors. In particular, hot colors (red, orange, and yellow) represent an increase of the nerve fiber layer thickness, while cold colors (blue, azure, and green) represent a decrease of the nerve fiber layer thickness. Normally the nerve fiber layer is thicker in the superior temporal and inferior temporal peripapillary quadrants and progressively becomes thinner towards the periphery assuming the appearance of a vertical bow-tie. In glaucomatous areas the hot colors are replaced by colder ones.
c. Red-free image of the optic disc and the peripapillary area.

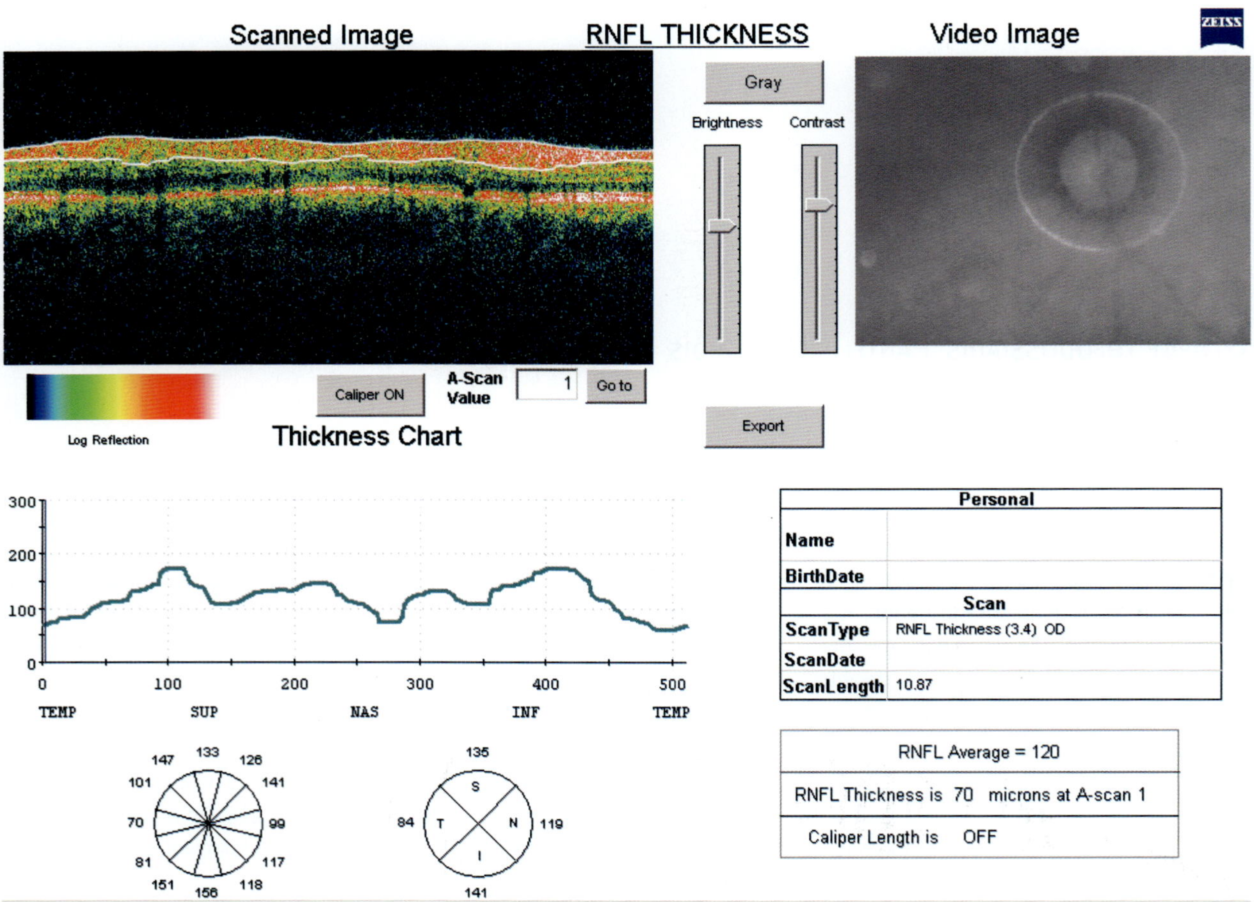

Fig. 1: The retinal nerve fiber layer thickness analysis protocol as obtained by Optical Coherence Tomography. It is based on circular scans centered on the optic disc with diameter 2.3mm or 3.4mm. The resulting image is presented "unfolded". The software of Optical Coherence Tomography identifies automatically the inner and outer limits of the nerve fiber layer and calculates its thickness in all quadrants.

RNFL THICKNESS AVERAGE ANALYSIS

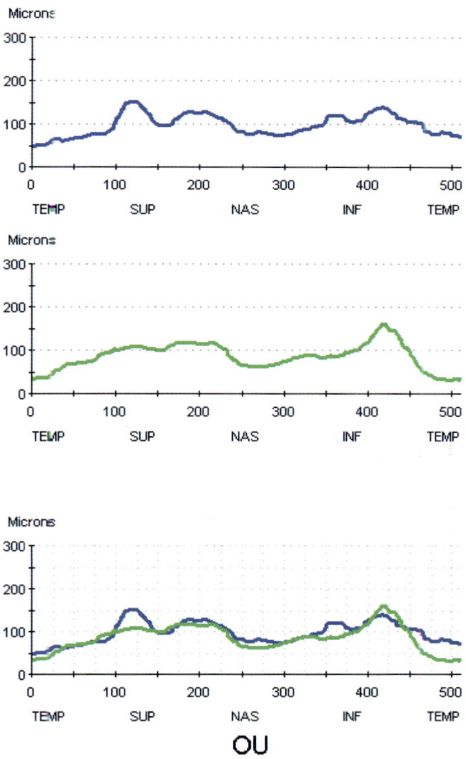

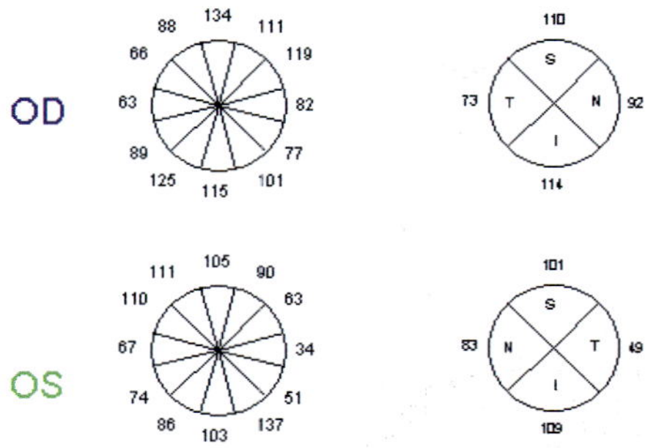

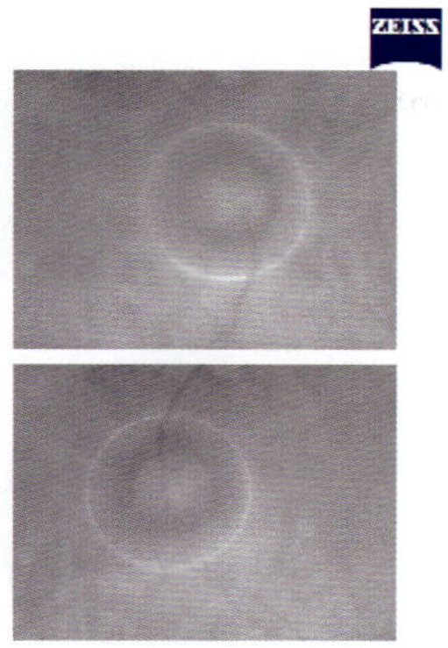

Personal	
Name	
BirthDate	
Scan	
ScanType	RNFL Thickness (3.4)
ScanDate	
ScanLength	10.87

	OD (N=3)	OS (N=3)	Diff(OD-OS)
Smax/Imax	1.086	0.727	0.36
Smax/Tavg	2.068	2.388	-0.319
Imax/Tavg	1.904	3.286	-1.382
Smax/Navg	1.641	1.41	0.232
Max-Min	102	129	-27
Smax	151	117	34
Imax	139	161	-22
Savg	110	101	9
Iavg	114	109	5
Avg.Thickness	97.25	85.75	11.5

Fig. 2

The color squares represent points where the nerve fiber layer thickness has a high probability to be pathologically reduced due to corresponding nerve fiber loss. The difference emerges from the comparison between the nerve fiber layer thickness detected and a normative database for persons of the same age. The probability of nerve fiber loss is bigger when hot color squares are shown (red 99.5%) and progressively decreases as the colors become colder (blue 95%).

d. Linear representation of the nerve fiber layer across a circle positioned around the optic disc. This line is normally double-humped with the humps corresponding to the superior and the inferior quadrants, where the nerve fiber layer is thicker. In normal subjects this line is confined within a physiologic range of values for all four quadrants of the same color. In cases where there is a thinning of the nerve fiber layer the line goes beyond the lower physiologic limits in the area corresponding to the nerve fiber loss. The greater the distance of the line from the lower normal limits the bigger the nerve fiber loss.

3. Optical Coherence Tomography: It is a quantitative, objective method of high resolution that studies the optic disc and the peripapillary area[1,2,6,7,8,17,18]. Optical Coherence Tomography resolution varies from 8μm to 10μm and therefore it enables the detection of early changes of the nerve fiber layer that cannot be found with visual fields testing[3,4]. Optical Coherence Tomography offers 18 linear or circular scanning protocols and 6 analysis protocols that are used for the quantitative analysis for the optic disc[9,11,12]. Each of these 6 analysis protocols have the following use:

I. RNFL Thickness (retinal nerve fiber layer thickness in the peripapillary area) evaluates the nerve fiber layer thickness by performing circular scans around the optic disc. The physiologic values of the four quadrants are: superior 122.8μm

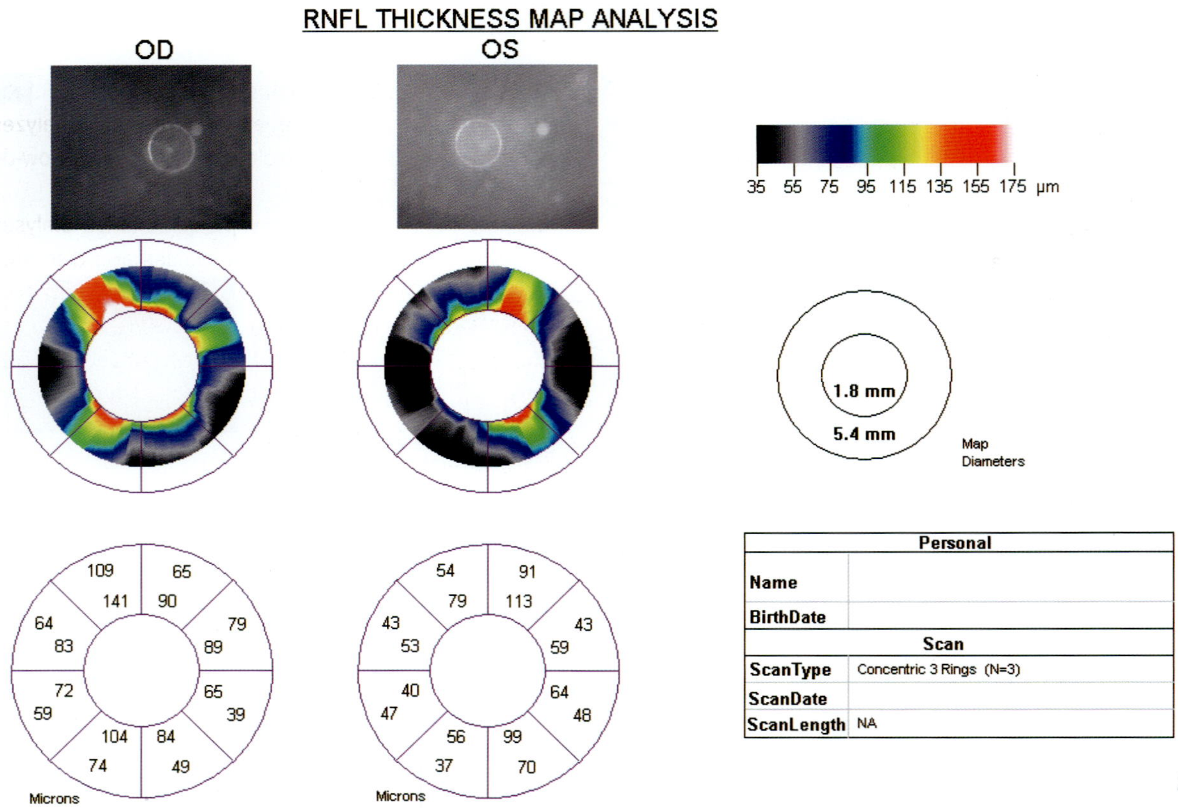
RNFL THICKNESS MAP ANALYSIS
OD
OS
35 55 75 95 115 135 155 175 µm
1.8 mm
5.4 mm
Map Diameters
109 65 141 90 64 79 83 89 72 65 59 39 104 84 74 49
Microns
54 91 79 113 43 43 53 59 40 64 47 48 56 99 37 70
Microns
Personal
Name
BirthDate
Scan
ScanType Concentric 3 Rings (N=3)
ScanDate
ScanLength NA

Fig. 3

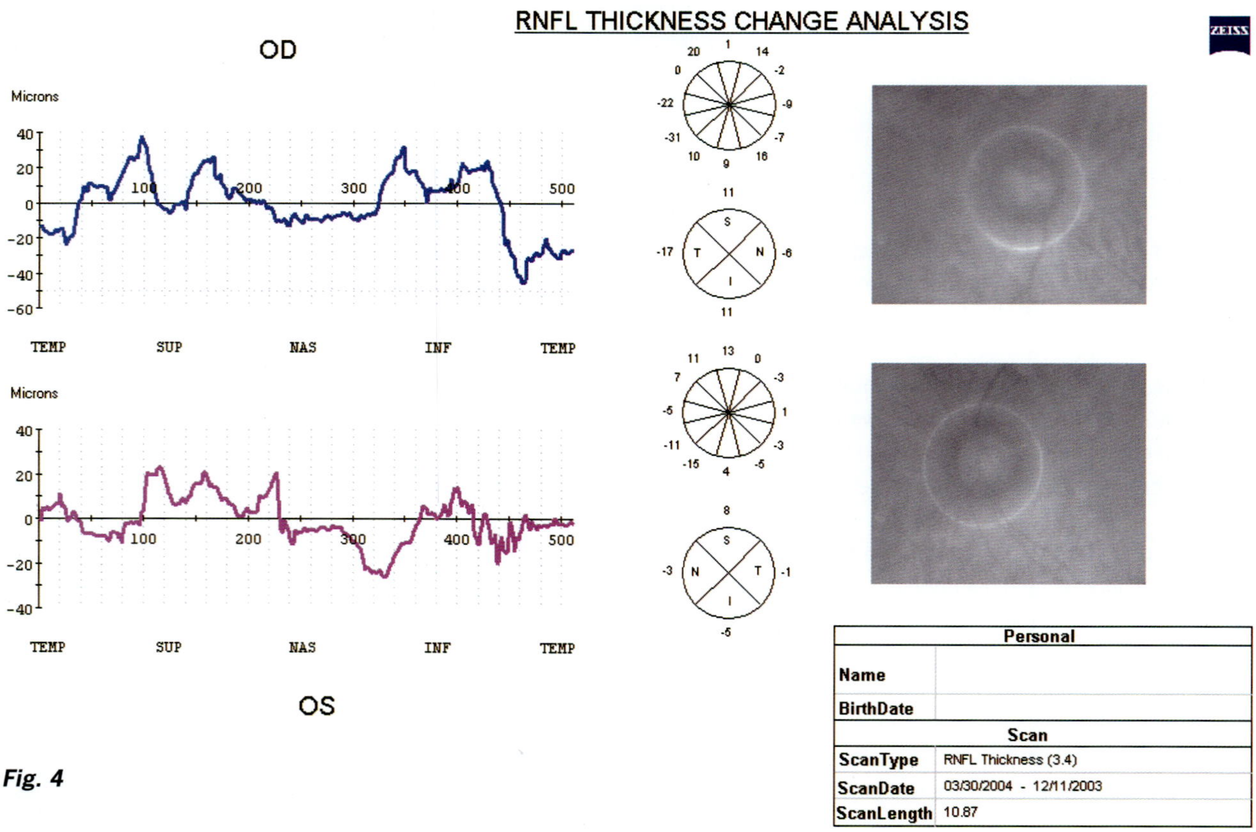
RNFL THICKNESS CHANGE ANALYSIS
OD
Microns
TEMP SUP NAS INF TEMP
Microns
TEMP SUP NAS INF TEMP
OS
Personal
Name
BirthDate
Scan
ScanType RNFL Thickness (3.4)
ScanDate 03/30/2004 - 12/11/2003
ScanLength 10.87

Fig. 4

(± 2.9), inferior 127.4μm (± 2.7), temporal 69.4μm (± 2.7) and nasal 73.6μm (± 2.1) *(figure 1)*[12a].

II. RNFL Thickness Average (mean value of the retinal nerve fiber layer thickness in the peripapillary area). It shows a graphic representation of the thickness of both eyes with the possibility of comparison *(figure 2)*.

III. RNFL Thickness Map (map of the peripapillary retinal nerve fiber layer thickness). It presents a map of the peripapillary nerve fiber layer thickness *(figure 3)*.

IV. RNFL Thickness Change (changes of the peripapillary retinal nerve fiber layer thickness). It compares the changes in the retinal nerve fiber layer thickness between two examinations of the same patient *(figure 4)*.

V. RNFL Serial Analysis (serial comparison and analysis of the peripapillary retinal nerve fiber layer thickness). It analyzes the retinal nerve fiber layer thickness during the follow-up period *(figure 5)*.

VI. Optic Nerve Head. It offers multiple quantitative analyses of the optic nerve head. Physiologic values are: disc area 2.27mm^2 (± 0.07), cup area 0.67mm^2 (± 0.07), rim area 1.60mm^2 (± 0.07), cup/disc area ratio 0.29 (± 0.02), cup/disc horizontal ratio 0.55 (± 0.02), cup/disc vertical ratio 0.48 (± 0.02), vertical integrated rim area (vol.) 0.43mm^3 (± 0.04), horizontal integrated rim width (area) 1.60mm^2 (± 0.07) *(figure 6)* [1a,12a,13-16].

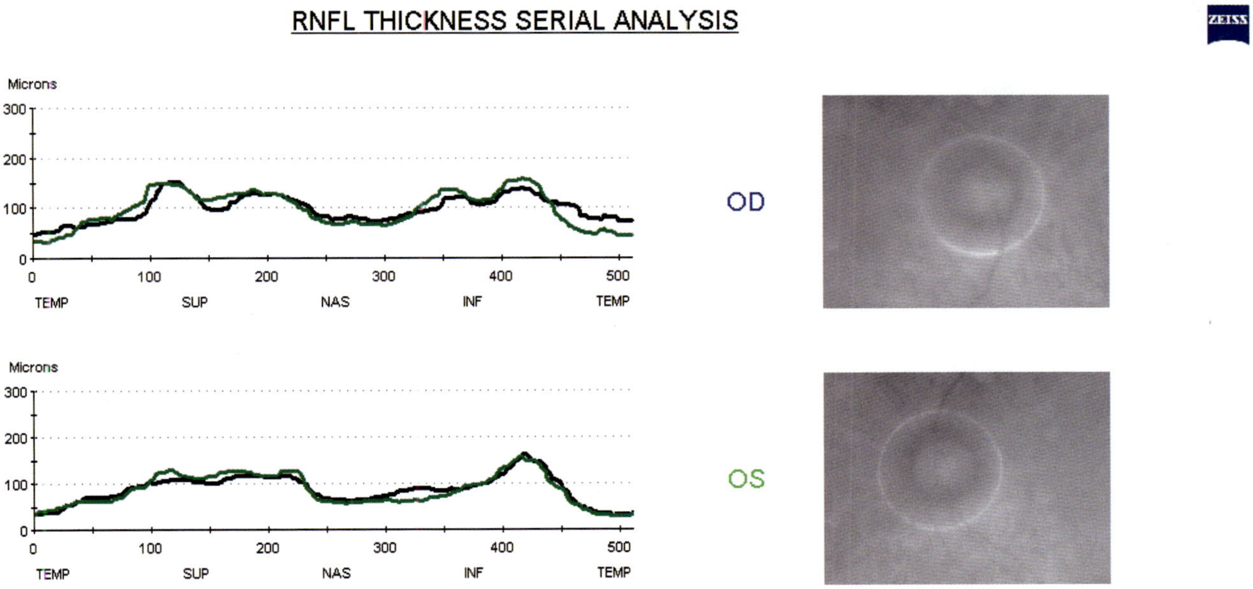

Color Legend and Exam Dates

	OD	OS
First Exam	12/11/2003	12/11/2003
Second Exam	03/30/2004	03/30/2004
Third Exam	NA	NA
Fourth Exam	NA	NA

Personal	
Name	
BirthDate	
Scan	
ScanType	RNFL Thickness (3.4)
ScanDate	Multiple, See Table
ScanLength	10.87

Fig. 5

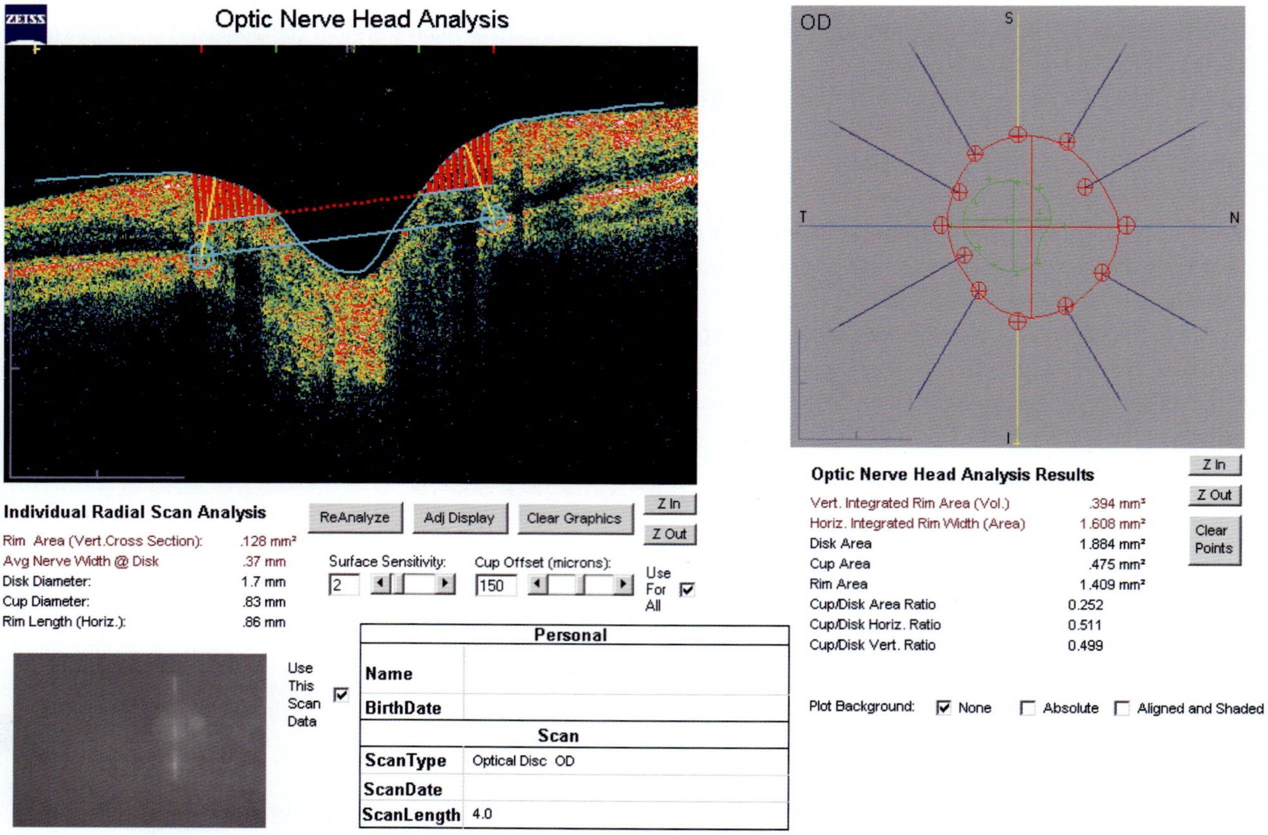

Fig. 6: The borders of the optic nerve head are defined by an area of high reflectivity that represents the neuroretinal rim and is located at the point of separation between the shadowing caused by the optic disc tissue and the high reflectivity band of the retinal pigment epithelium-choriocapillaris complex. Analysis of the data by the software of Optical Coherence Tomography offers parameters such as the optic disc diameter, the area, volume and length of the neuroretinal rim, the diameter and area of the optic disc and cupping, the horizontal and vertical cup to disc ratio.

GLAUCOMA

1. Bagga H, Greenfield DS, Knighton RW. Macular symmetry testing for glaucoma detection. J Glaucoma 2005; 14:358-363.

1a. Brancato R, Lumbroso B. Guide to optical coherence tomography interpretation. Part III. Glaucoma. Page 71.

2. Bourne RR, Medeiros FA, Bowd C, Jahanbakhsh K, Zangwill LM, Weinreb RN. Comparability of retinal nerve fiber layer thickness measurements of optical coherence tomography instruments. Invest Ophthalmol Vis Sci 2005; 46:1280-1285.

3. Burgansky-Eliash Z, Wollstein G, Chu T, Ramsey JD, Glymour C, Noecker RJ, Ishikawa H, Schuman JS. Optical coherence tomography machine learning classifiers for glaucoma detection: a preliminary study. Invest Ophthalomol Vis Sci 2005;46:4147-4152.

4. Chen HY, Huang ML. Discrimination between normal and glaucomatous eyes using Stratus optical coherence tomography in Taiwan Chinese subjects. Graefes Arch Clin Exp Ophthalmol 2005;243:894-902.

5. Greenfield DS, Bagga H. Clinical variables associated with glaucomatous injury in eyes with large optic disc cupping. Ophthalmic Surg Lasers Imaging 2005; 36:401-409.

6. Hess DB, Asrani SG, Bhide MG, Enyedi LB, Stinnett SS, Freedman SF. Macular and retinal nerve fiber layer analysis of normal and glaucomatous eyes in children using optical coherence tomography. Am J Ophthalmol 2005;139:509-517.

7. Huang ML, Chen HY. Development and comparison of automated classifiers for glaucoma diagnosis using Stratus optical coherence tomography. Invest Ophthalmol Vis Sci 2005; 46:4121-4129.

8. Jeoung JW, Park KH, Kim TW, Khwarg SI, Kim DM. Diagnostic ability of optical coherence tomography with a normative database localized retinal nerve fiber layer defects. Ophthalmology 2005;112:2157-2163.

9. Iliev ME, Meyenberg A, Garweg JG. Morphometric assessment of normal, suspect and glaucomatous optic discs with Stratus OCT and HRT II. Eye 2005;23.

10. Kanamori A, Nagai-Kusuhara A, Escano MF, MaedA h, Nakamura M, Negi A. Comparison of confocal scanning laser ophthalmoscopy, scanning laser polarimetry and optical coherence tomography to discriminate ocular hypertension and glaucoma at an early stage. Graefes Arch Clin Exp Ophthalmol 2006;244:58-68.

11. Leung CK, Chan WM, Yung WH, Ng AC, Woo J, Tsang MK, Yse RK. Comparison of macular and peripapillary measurements for the detection of glaucoma: an optical coherence tomography study. Ophthalmology 2005;112:391-400.

12. Leung CK, Chan WM, Hui YL, Yung WH, Woo J, Tsang MK, Tse KK. Analysis of retinal nerve fiber layer and optic nerve head in glaucoma with different reference plane offsets, using optical coherence tomography. Invest Ophthalmol Vis Sci 2005;46:891-899.

12a. Manassakorn A, Nouri-Mahdavi K, Caprioli J. Comparison of retinal nerve fiber layer thickness and optic disk algorithms with optical coherence tomography to detect glaucoma. Am J Ophthalmol 2006;141:105-115.

13. Medeiros FA, Zangwill LM, Bowd C, Vessani Rm, Susanna R Jr, Weinreb RN. Evaluation of retinal nerve fiber layer, optic nerve head, and macular thickness measurements for glaucoma detection using optical coherence tomography. Am J Ophthalmol 2005;139:44-55.

14. Sellem E. Practical assessment. Early-stage or advanced glaucoma. Fr J Ophthalmol 2005;28:17-24.

15. Sihota R, Sony P, Gupta V, Dada T, Singh R. Comparing glaucomatous optic neuropathy in primary open angle and chronic primary angle closure glaucoma eyes by optical coherence tomography. Ophthalmic Physiol Opt 2005;25:408-415.

16. Wollstein G, Paunescu LA, Ko TH, Fujimoto JG, Kowaleviez A, Hart I, Beaton S, Ishihawa H, Mattox C, Singh O, Duker J, Drexler W, Schuman JS. Ultrahigh-resolution optical coherence tomography in glaucoma. Ophthalmology 2005;112:229-237.

17. Wollstein G, Ishikawa H, Wang J, Beaton SA, Schuman JS. Comparison of three optical coherence tomography scanning areas for detection of glaucomatous damage. Am J Ophthalmol 2005;139:39-43.

18. Wollstein G, Schuman JS, Price LL, Aydin A, Stark PC, Hertzmark E, Lai E, Ishikawa H, Mattox C, Fujimoto JG, Paunescu LA. Optical coherence tomography longitudinal evaluation of retinal nerve fiber layer thickness in glaucoma. Arch Ophthalmol 2005;123:464-470.

FAST RETINAL NERVE FIBER LAYER SCANNING PROTOCOL

Fast retinal nerve fiber layer scan (RNFL) is the only peripapillary Retinal Nerve Fiber Layer scan type available in the Stratus Optical Coherence Tomography software that has normative database analysis. The normative data used in the software were collected by studying approximately 350 normal individuals equally distributed into decades between the ages of 20 and 80 years.

With this scan type, during a single scan the Retinal Nerve Fiber Layer thickness is determined at 256 points at a set

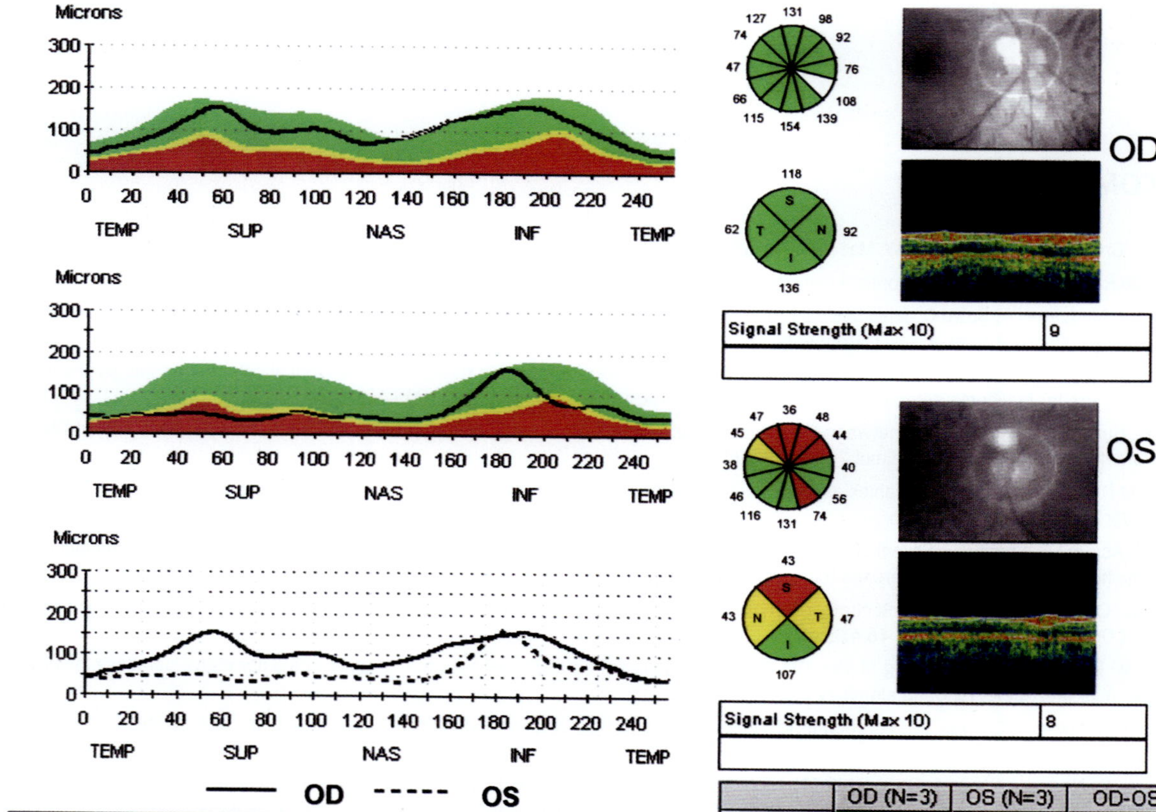

OD	Scans used	1, 2, 3
OS	Scans used	1, 2, 3

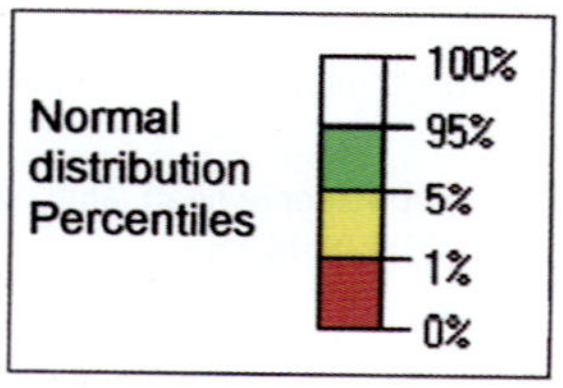

	OD (N=3)	OS (N=3)	OD-OS
Imax/Smax	1.02	2.98	-1.97
Smax/Imax	0.98	0.34	0.65
Smax/Tavg	2.48	1.15	1.33
Imax/Tavg	2.52	3.43	-0.91
Smax/Navg	1.68	1.25	0.43
Max-Min	117.00	129.00	-12.00
Smax	155.00	54.00	101.00
Imax	157.00	161.00	-4.00
Savg	118.00	43.00	75.00
Iavg	136.00	107.00	29.00
Avg.Thick	102.21	60.11	42.10

Figure 7. StratusOCT Fast retinal nerve fiber layer (RNFL) scan from a patient with glaucoma in the left eye only. Areas that are colored in white and green indicate normal RNFL thickness. Areas with RNFL thicknesses expected in <5% of age-matched controls are colored in yellow and areas with RNFL thicknesses expected in <1% of age-matched controls are colored in red. In addition many summary parameters are outside normal, including superior average (Savg) and average thickness (Avg Thick)

diameter (3.4mm) around the center of the optic disc 3 times. These values are averaged to yield 12 clock-hour thicknesses, 4 quadrant thicknesses and a single overall Retinal Nerve Fiber Layer thickness measurement. Summary parameters are also provided including ratios and maximum Retinal Nerve Fiber Layer thickness values in the superior and inferior quadrants. These values are then compared against a normative database of age-matched controls to derive percentile values. Parameters for a given eye are noted on the Stratus Optical Coherence Tomography printout as to whether they fall outside of the 99% confidence interval (CI) (pathological), between the 95% and 99% (borderline), or within the 95% CI.

Several investigators have reported that Retinal Nerve Fiber Layer inferior thickness and average thickness have the best diagnostic accuracy of Stratus Optical Coherence Tomography Retinal Nerve Fiber Layer measurements.[1,2]

When full circle mean Retinal Nerve Fiber Layer thickness and the mean thickness values of one or more quadrants or clock hours, were evaluated at the P<5% limit, sensitivities were 84%, 89% and 89%, respectively, in patients with visual field loss and the corresponding specificities were 98%, 95% and 92%.[3]

Figure 7 shows an example of the printout from the Stratus Optical Coherence Tomography fast Retinal Nerve Fiber Layer analysis.

BIBLIOGRAPHY

1. Shah NN, Bowd C, Medeiros FA, Weinreb RN, Samble PA, Hoffmann EM, Zangwill LM. Combining structural and functional testing for detection of glaucoma. Ophthalmology. 2006; 113:1593-602.

2. Kanamori A, Nagai-Kusuhara A, Escano MF, Maeda H, N, Nakamura M, Negi A. Comparison of confocal scanning laser ophthalmoscopy, scanning laser polarimetry and optical coherence tomography to discriminate ocular hypertension and glaucomaat an early stage. Graefes Arch Clin Exp Ophthalmol. 2006;244:58-68.

3. Budenz DL, Michael A, Chang RT, McSoley J, Katz J. Sensitivity and specificity of the StratusOCT for perimetric glaucoma. Ophthalmology. 2005;112(1):3-9

EARLY UNILATERAL PIGMENTARY GLAUCOMA

A

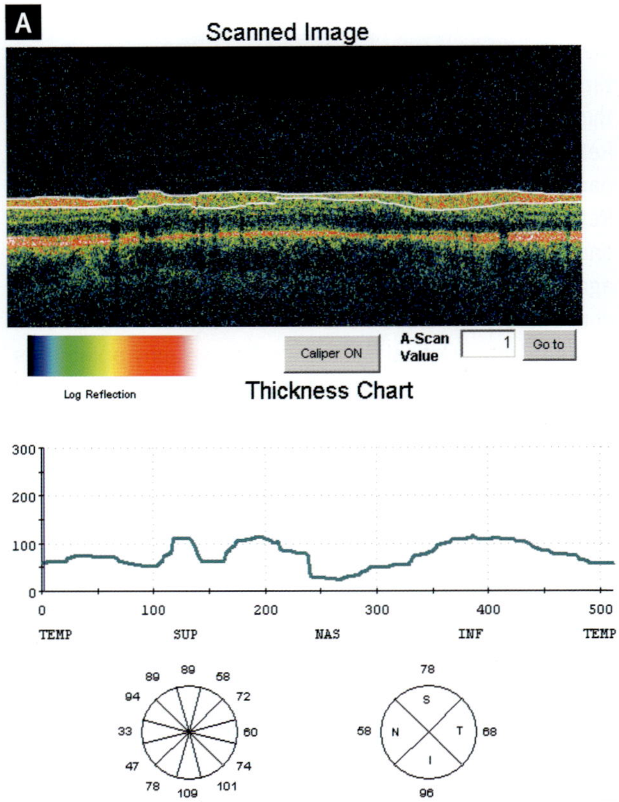

B

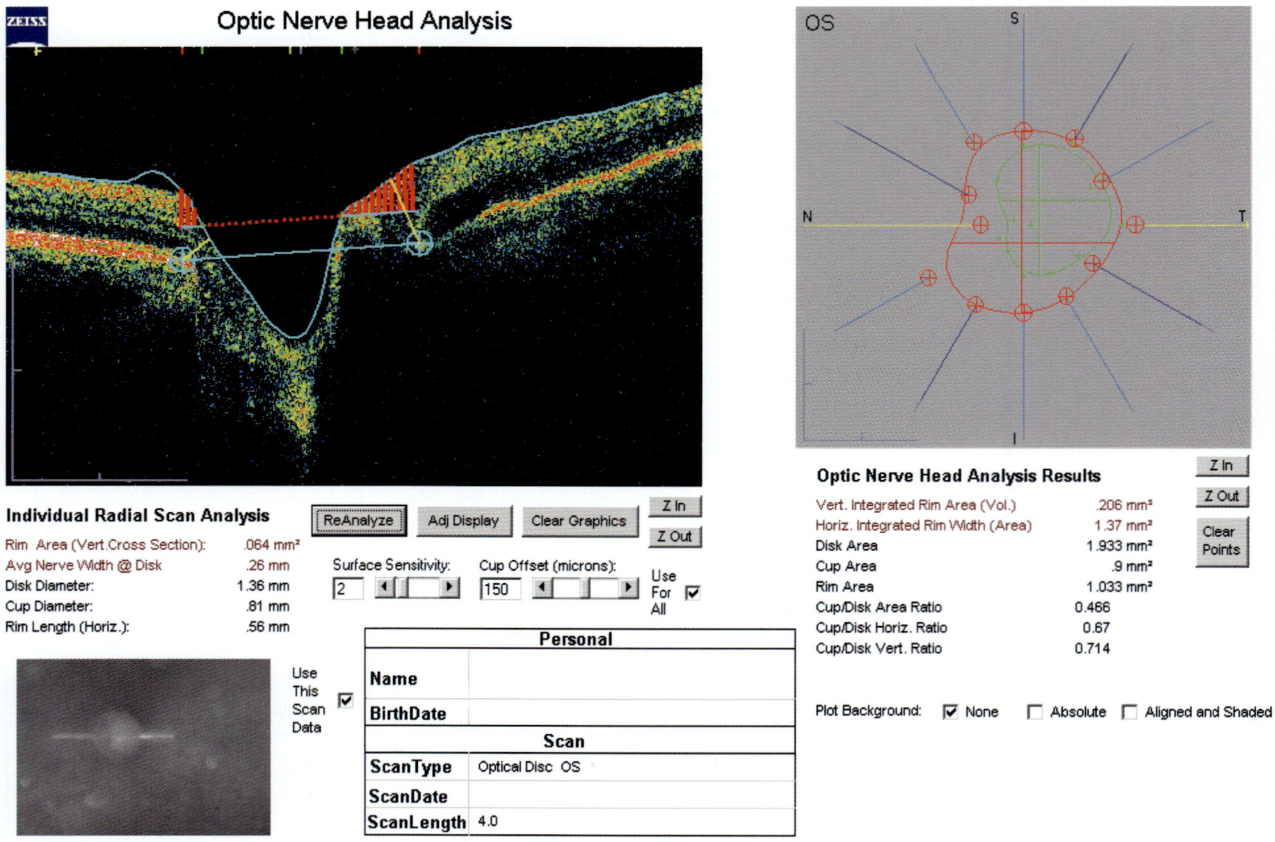

C

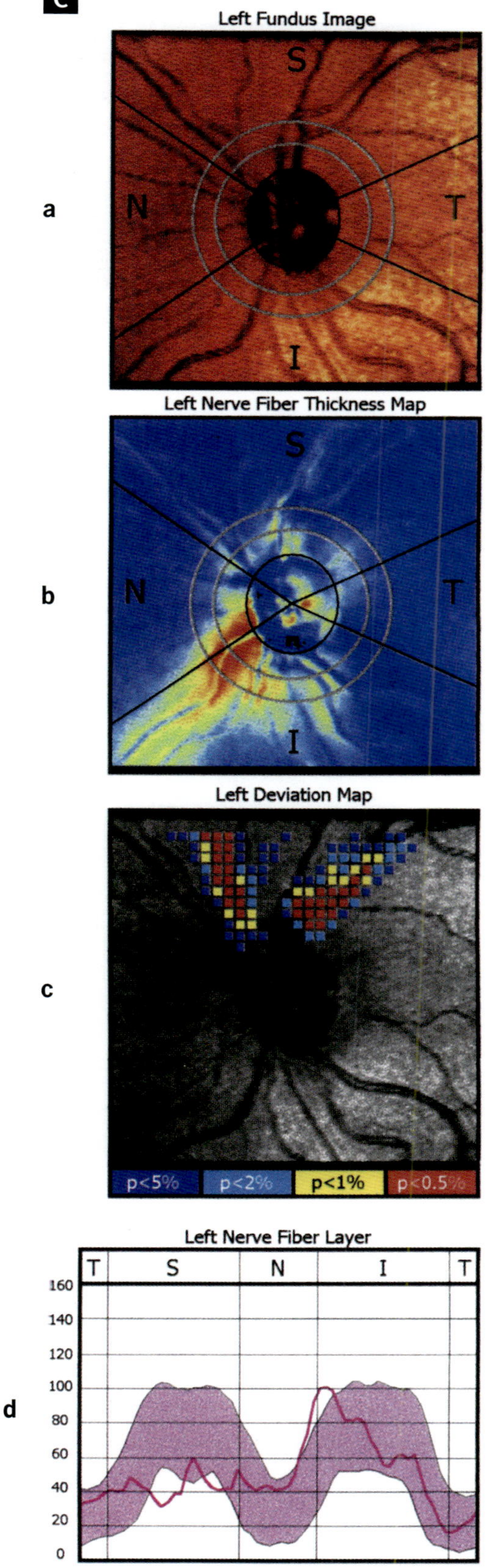

D

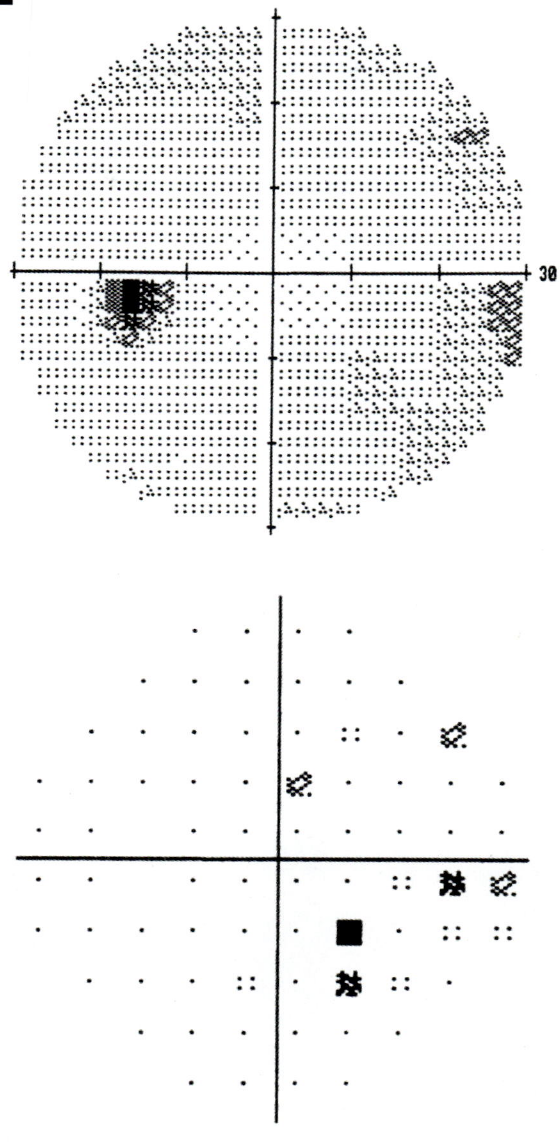

Patient 44-year-old with early pigmentary glaucoma in one eye. A. Optical Coherence Tomography shows a significant decrease of the mean thickness of the nerve fiber layer (73.75μm) with a bigger decrease of the thickness at the superior quadrant (78μm). B. Optic disc C/D ratio in the horizontal axis is 0.67 and in the vertical is 0.71. C. Scanning Laser Polarimetry shows decrease of the nerve fiber layer thickness in the superior quadrant corresponding to the inferior defect in the visual field test. D. Visual fields reveal early paracentral inferior lesions.

EARLY UNILATERAL PIGMENTARY GLAUCOMA

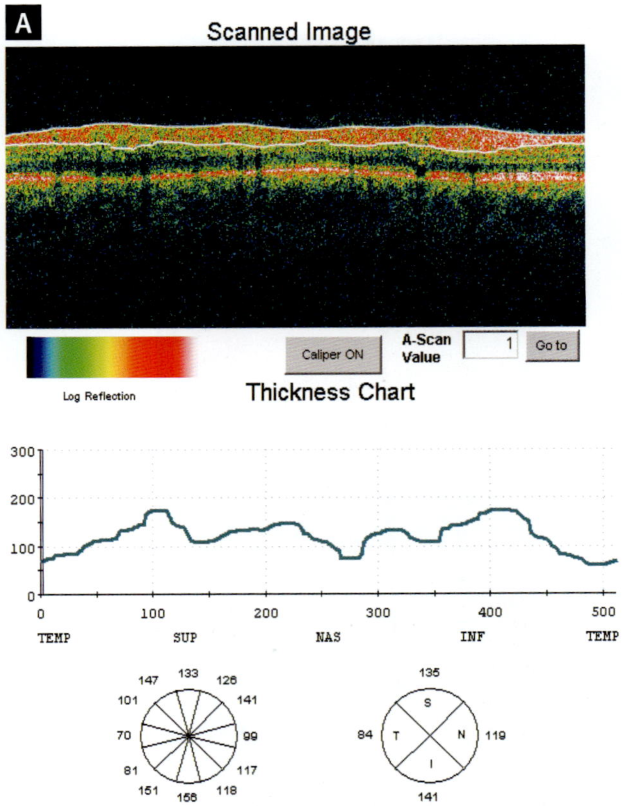

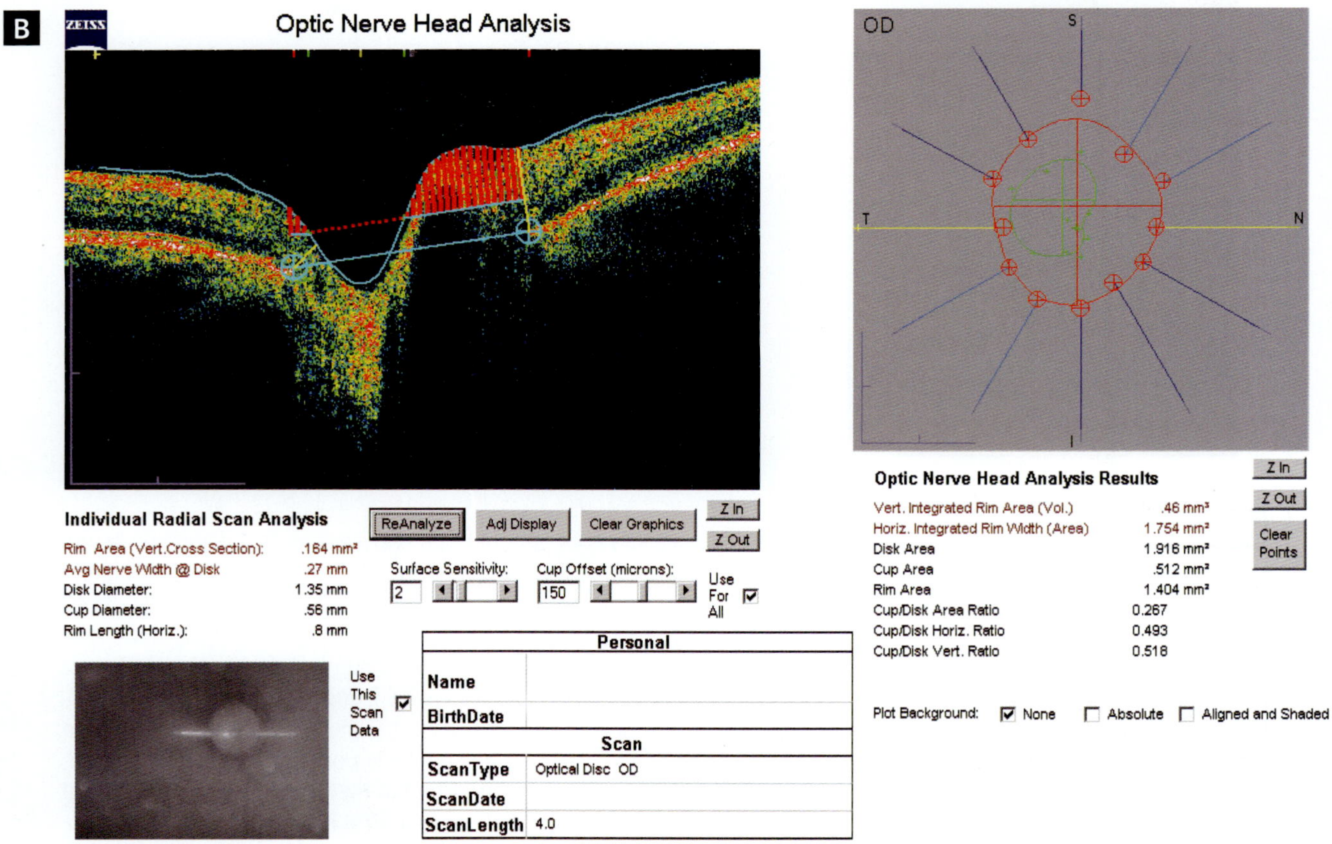

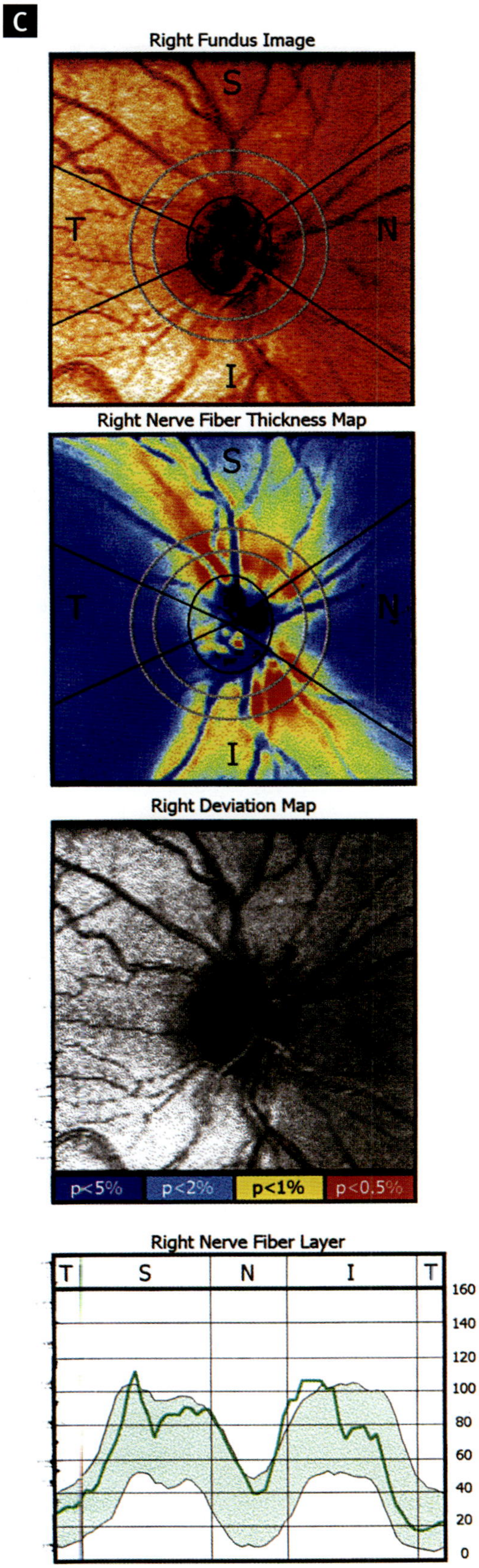

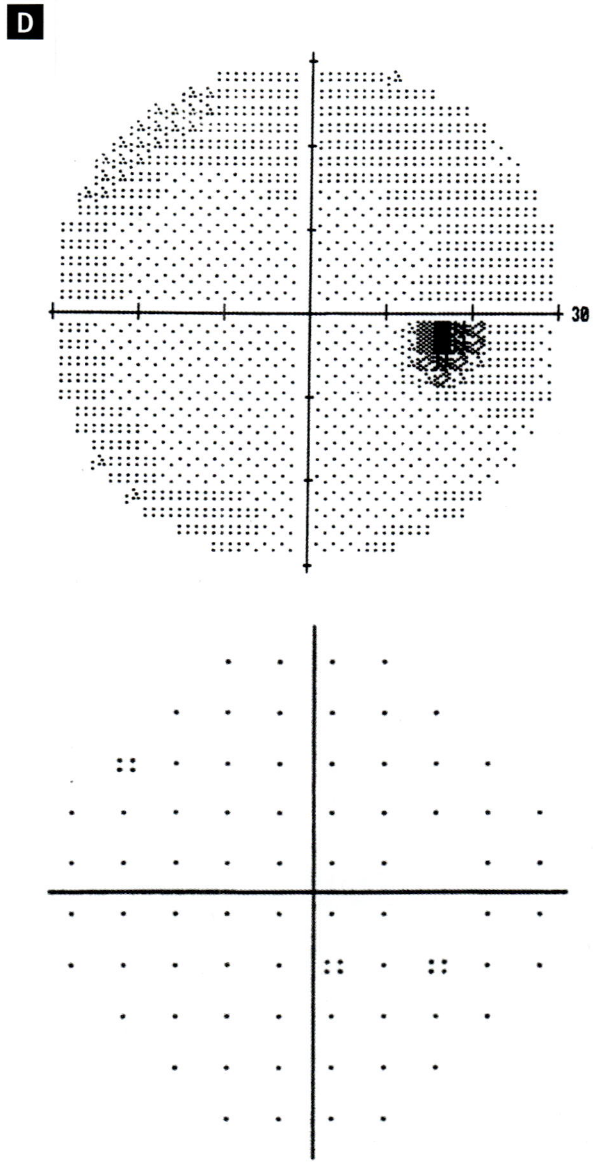

The other eye of the same patient (page 316).
A. Optical Coherence Tomography shows a normal mean nerve fiber layer thickness (117.7μm). B. Optic disc C/D ratio in the horizontal axis is 0.5 and in the vertical is 0.51. There is asymmetry observed between the two eyes. C, D. Visual fields and Scanning Laser Polarimetry are normal.

UNILATERAL GLAUCOMA

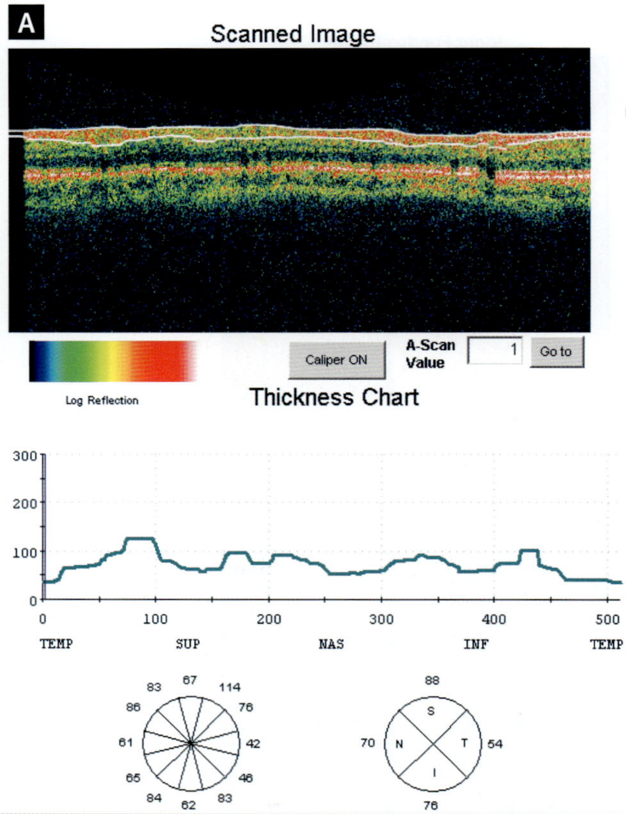

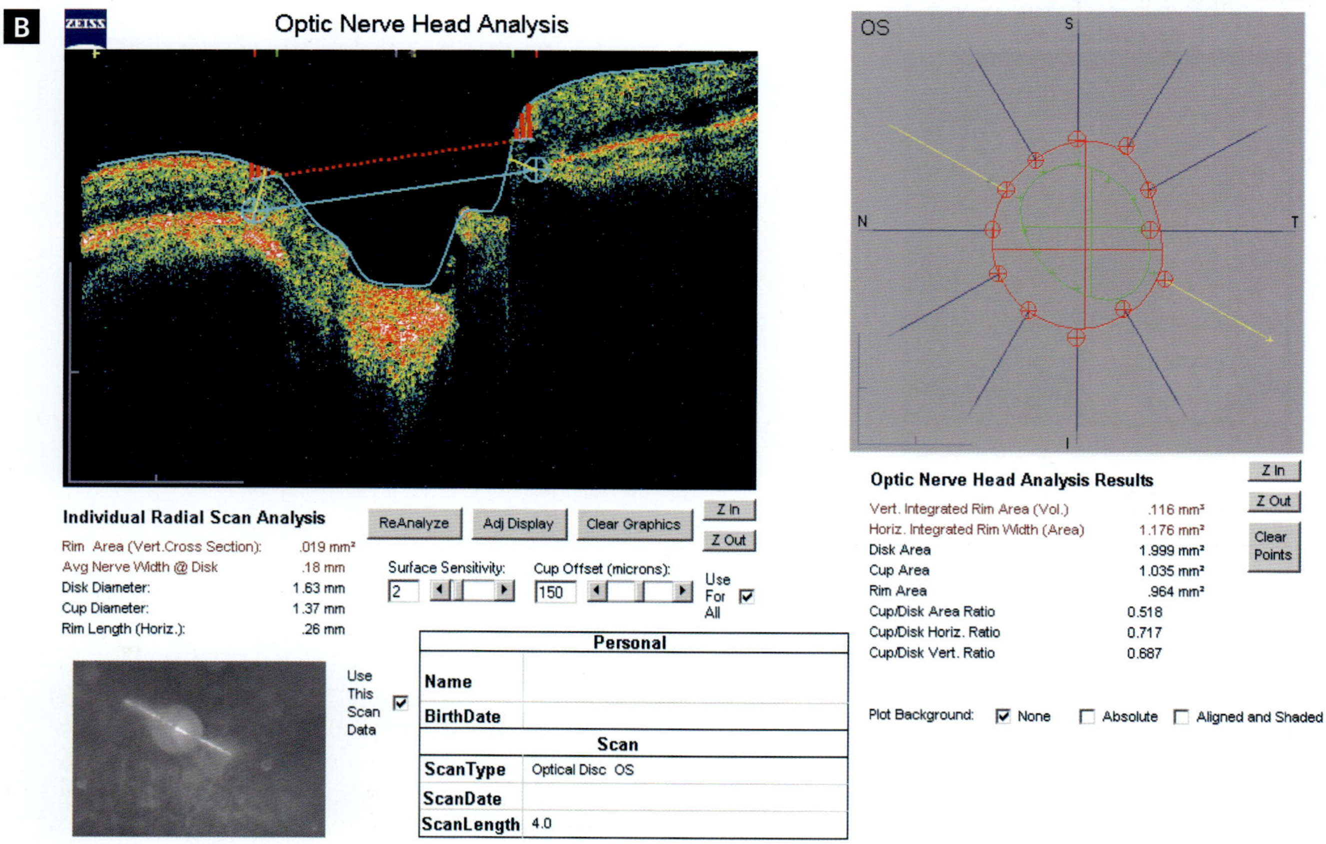

C

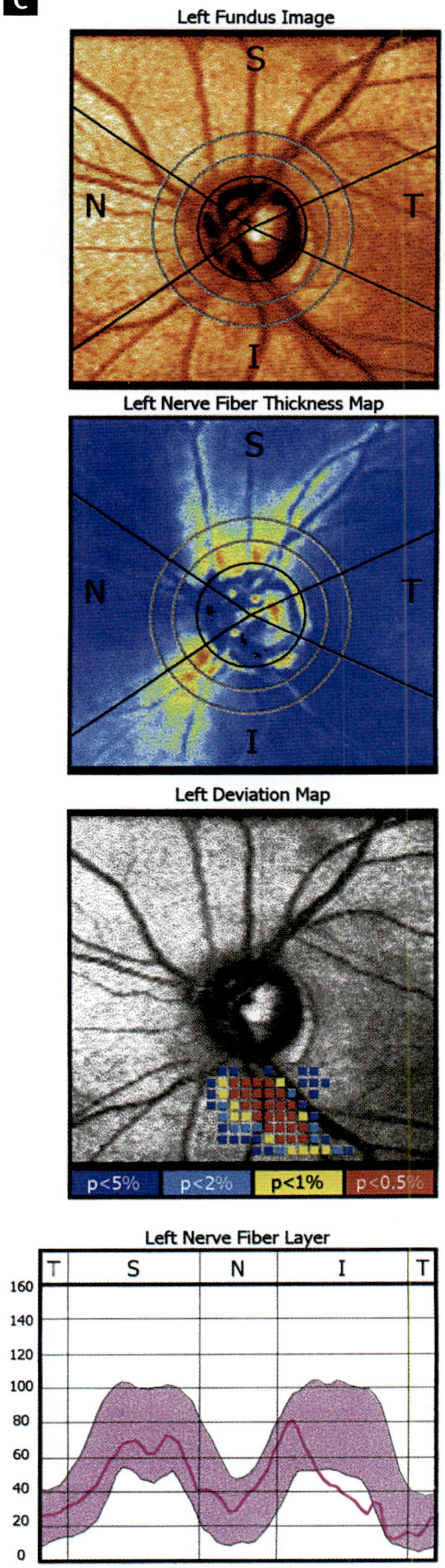

D

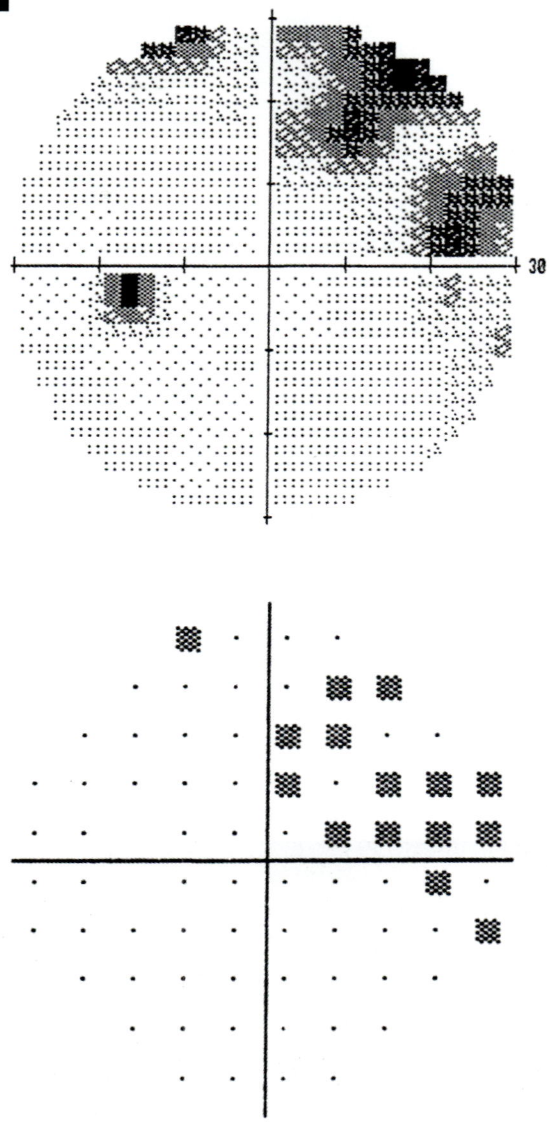

Patient 50-year-old with unilateral glaucoma. A. Optical Coherence Tomography shows a significant decrease of mean thickness of the nerve fiber layer (70.6μm) with bigger decrease of the thickness in the inferior quadrant (76μm). B. Optic disc C/D ratio in the horizontal axis is 0.71 and in the vertical is 0.68 with a notching located inferotemporally. C. Scanning Laser Polarimetry shows a decrease of the nerve fiber layer thickness in the inferior quadrant, a finding that corresponds to the superior lesion found in the visual field testing. D. Visual fields reveal significantly reduced sensitivity in the superior nasal quadrant.

UNILATERAL GLAUCOMA

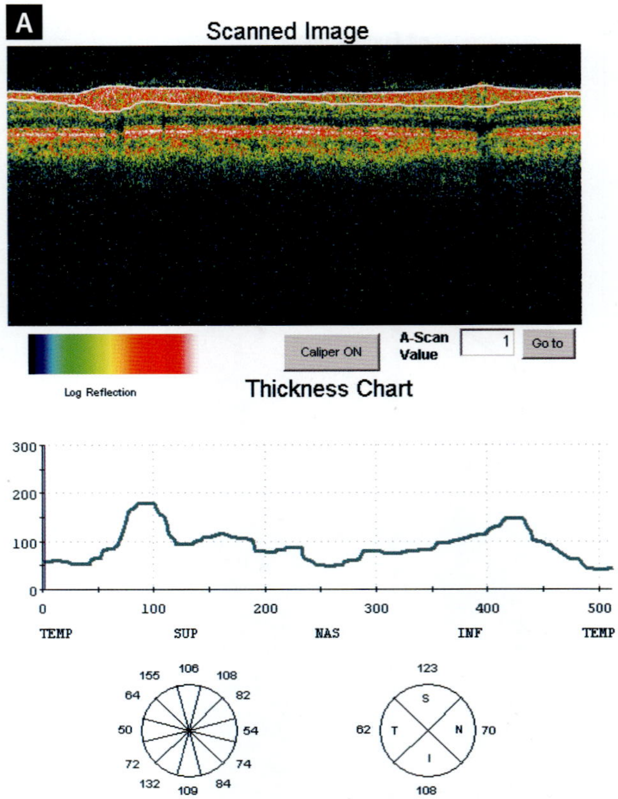

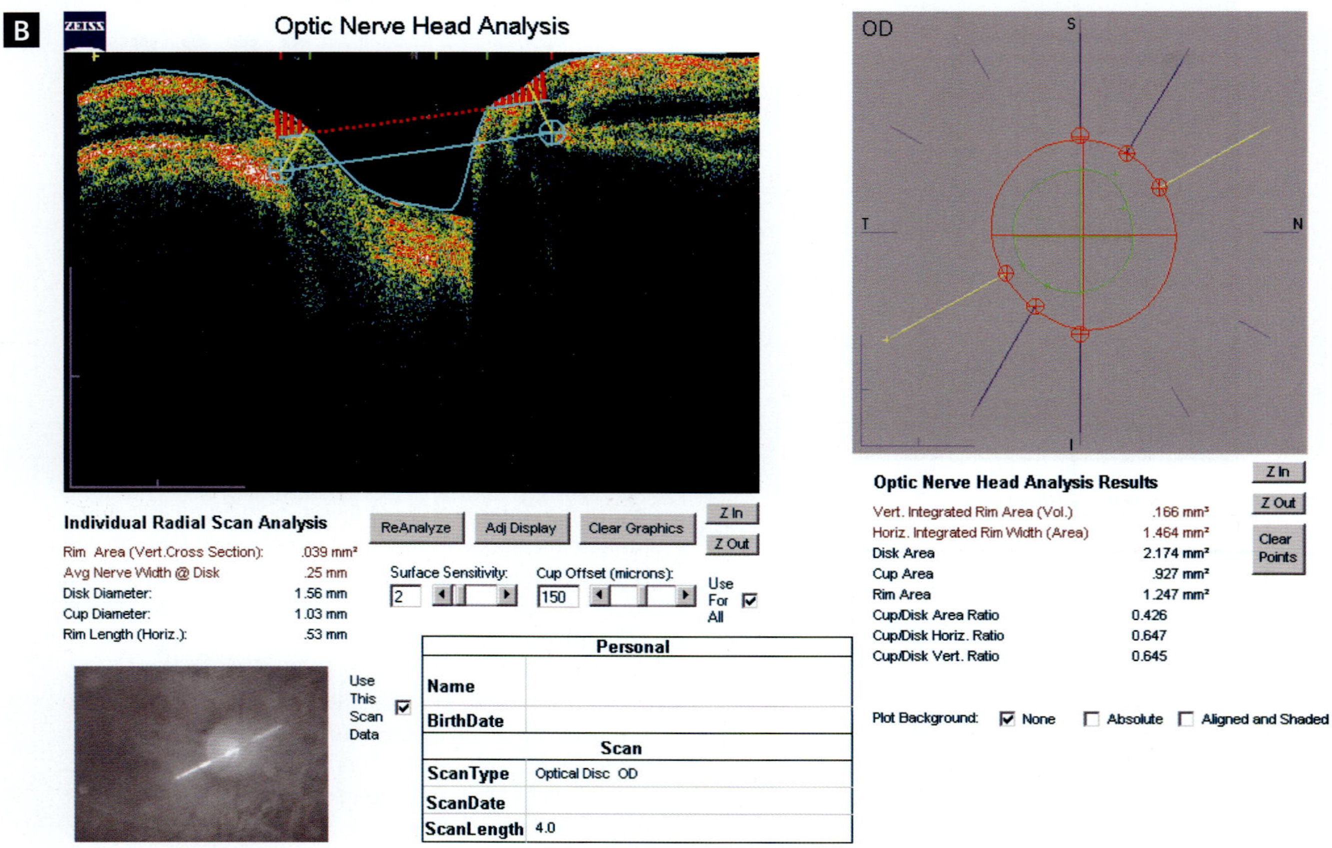

C

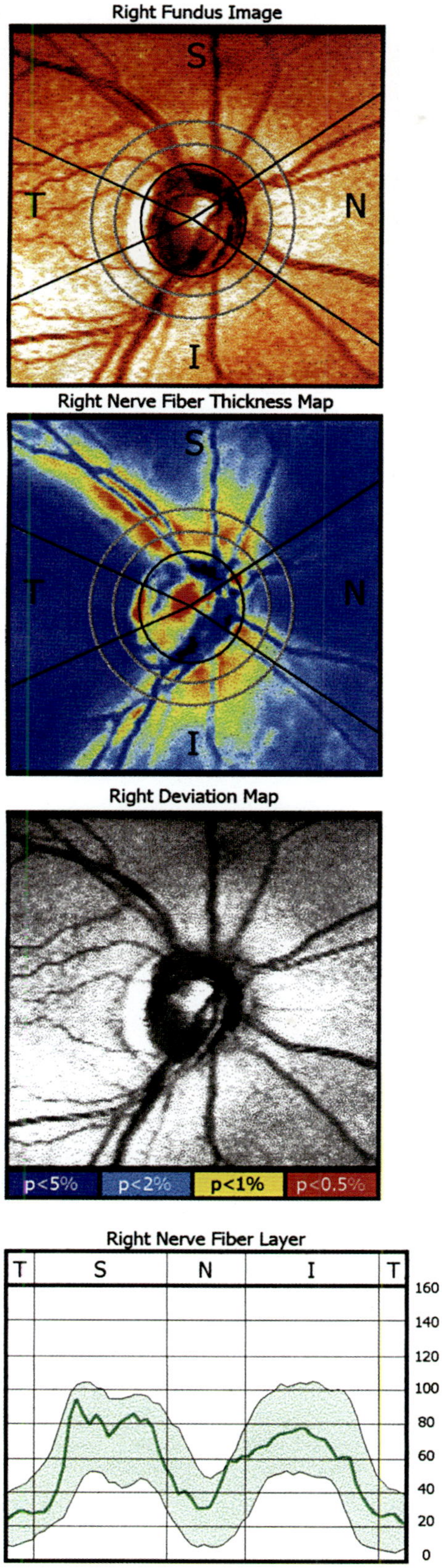

D

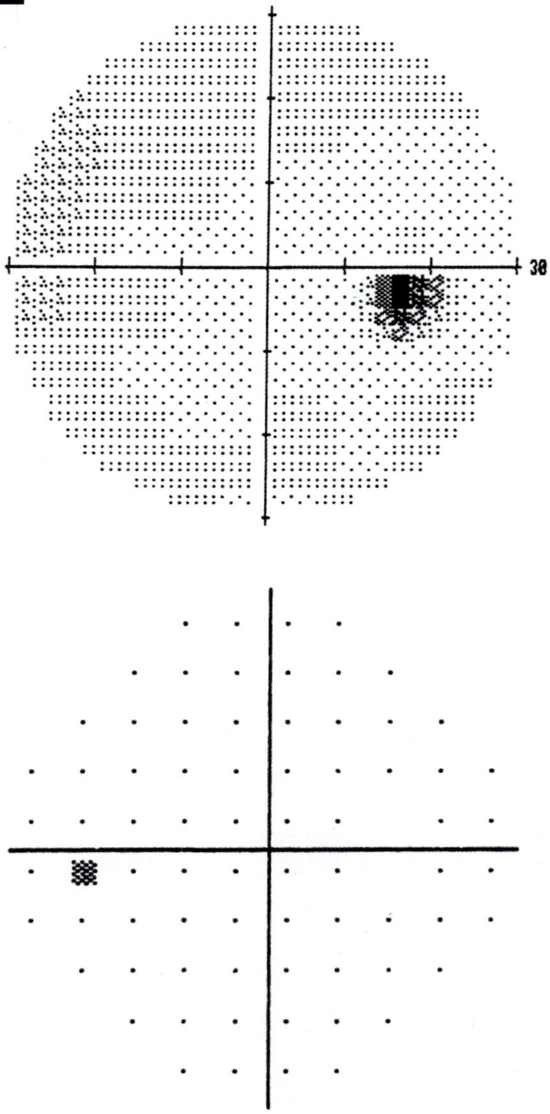

The other eye of the same patient (page 320).
A. Optical Coherence Tomography shows normal mean nerve fiber layer thickness (93.17μm). B. Optic disc C/D ratio in the horizontal and vertical axis is 0.64 with symmetrical cupping. C, D. Visual fields and Scanning Laser Polarimetry are normal.

EARLY GLAUCOMA

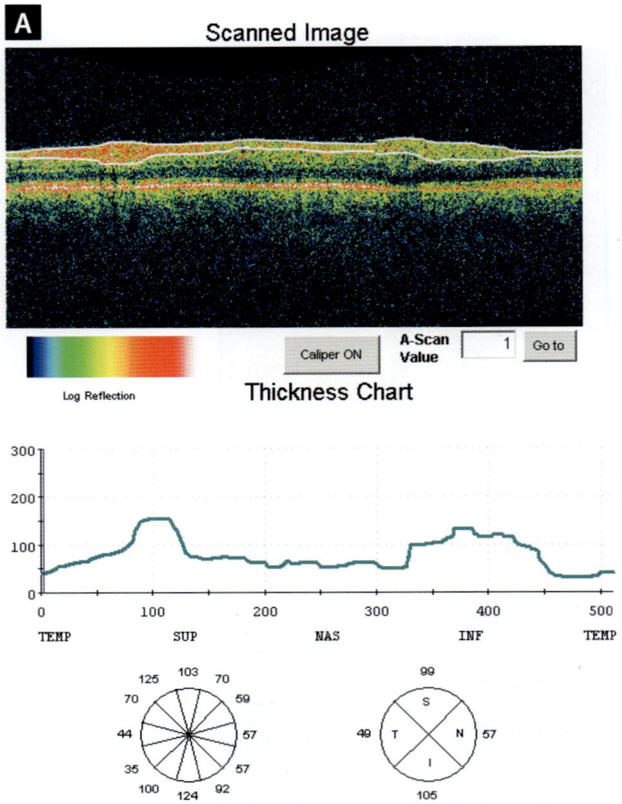

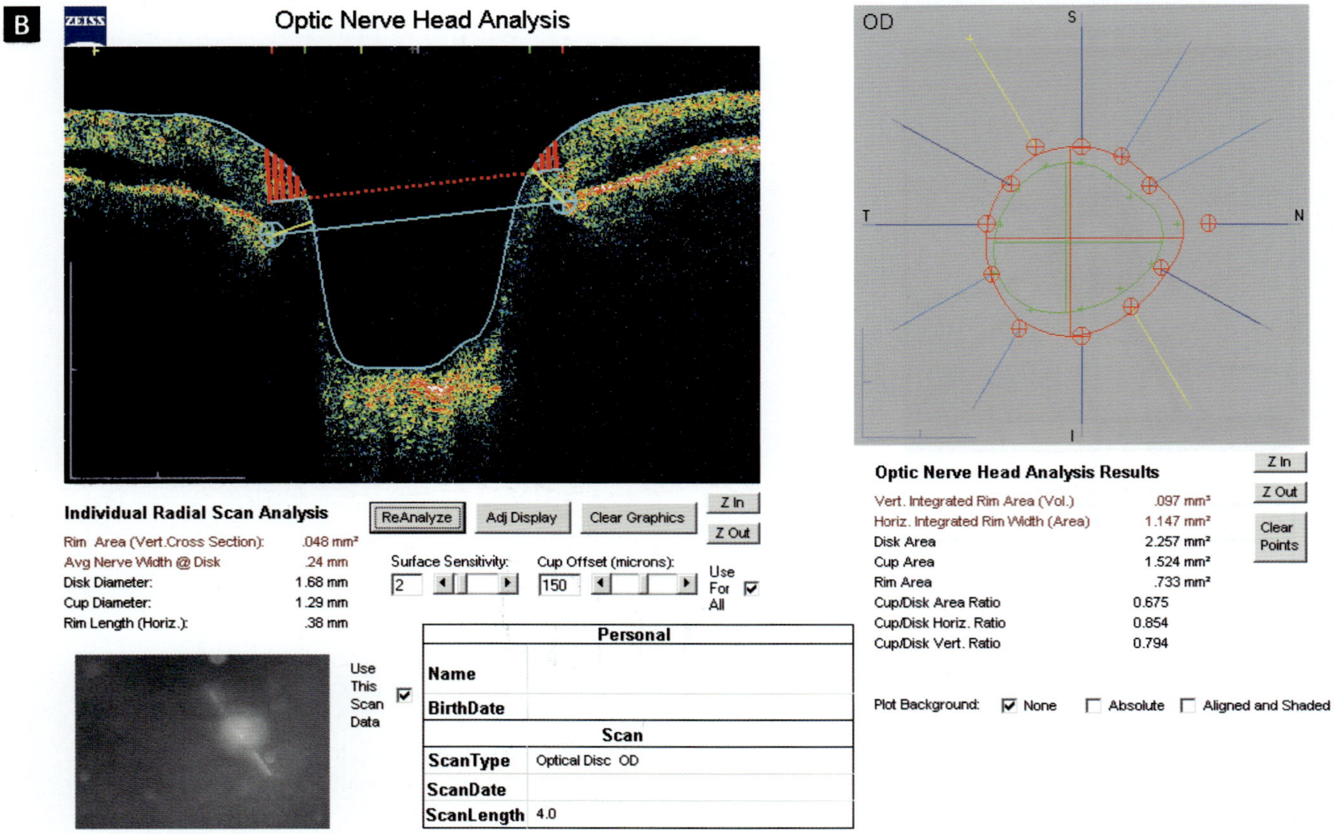

C

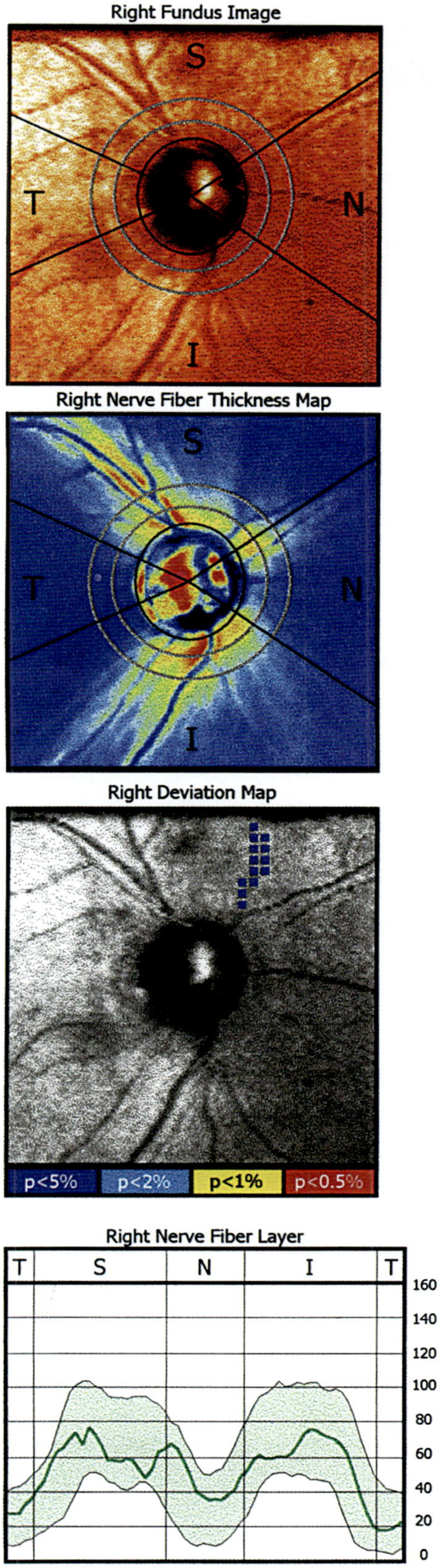

D

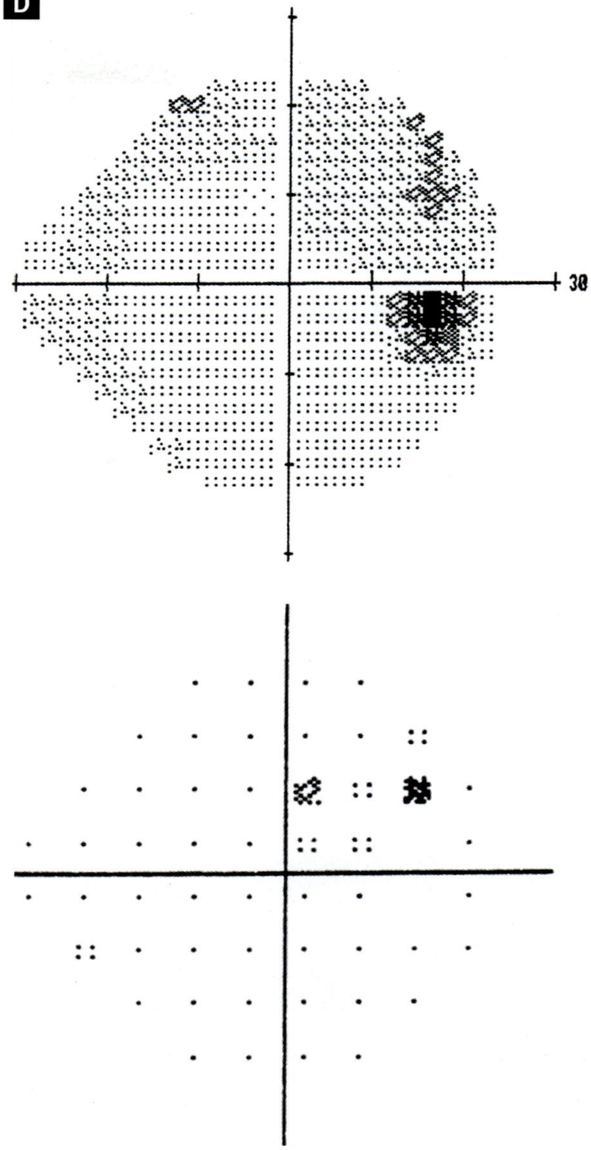

Patient 58-year-old with increased intraocular pressures and cupping of the optic discs. A. Optical Coherence Tomography shows a decrease of the mean nerve fibre layer thickness (79.5μm). B. Optic disc C/D ratio in the horizontal axis is 0.85 and in the vertical 0.80. C, D. Visual fields and Scanning Laser Polarimetry don't detect any particular changes.

EARLY GLAUCOMA

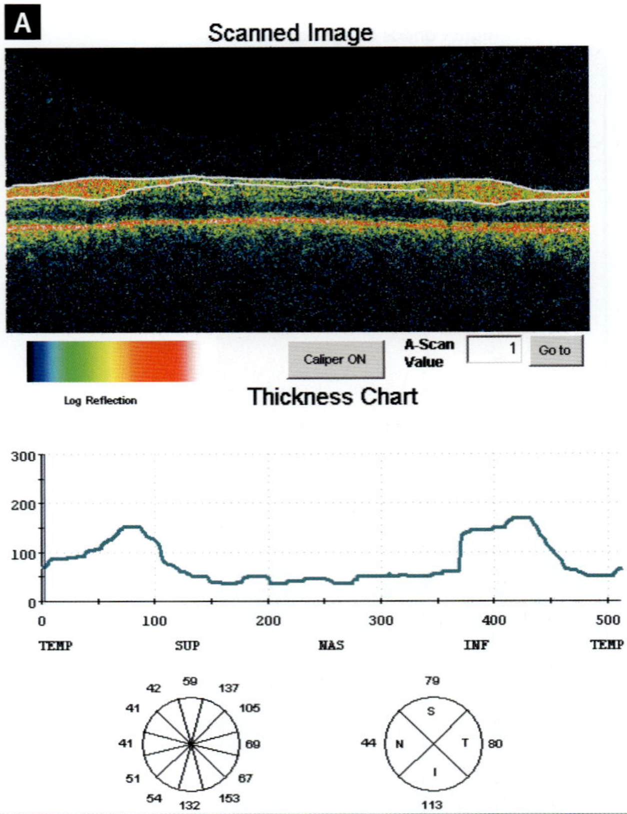

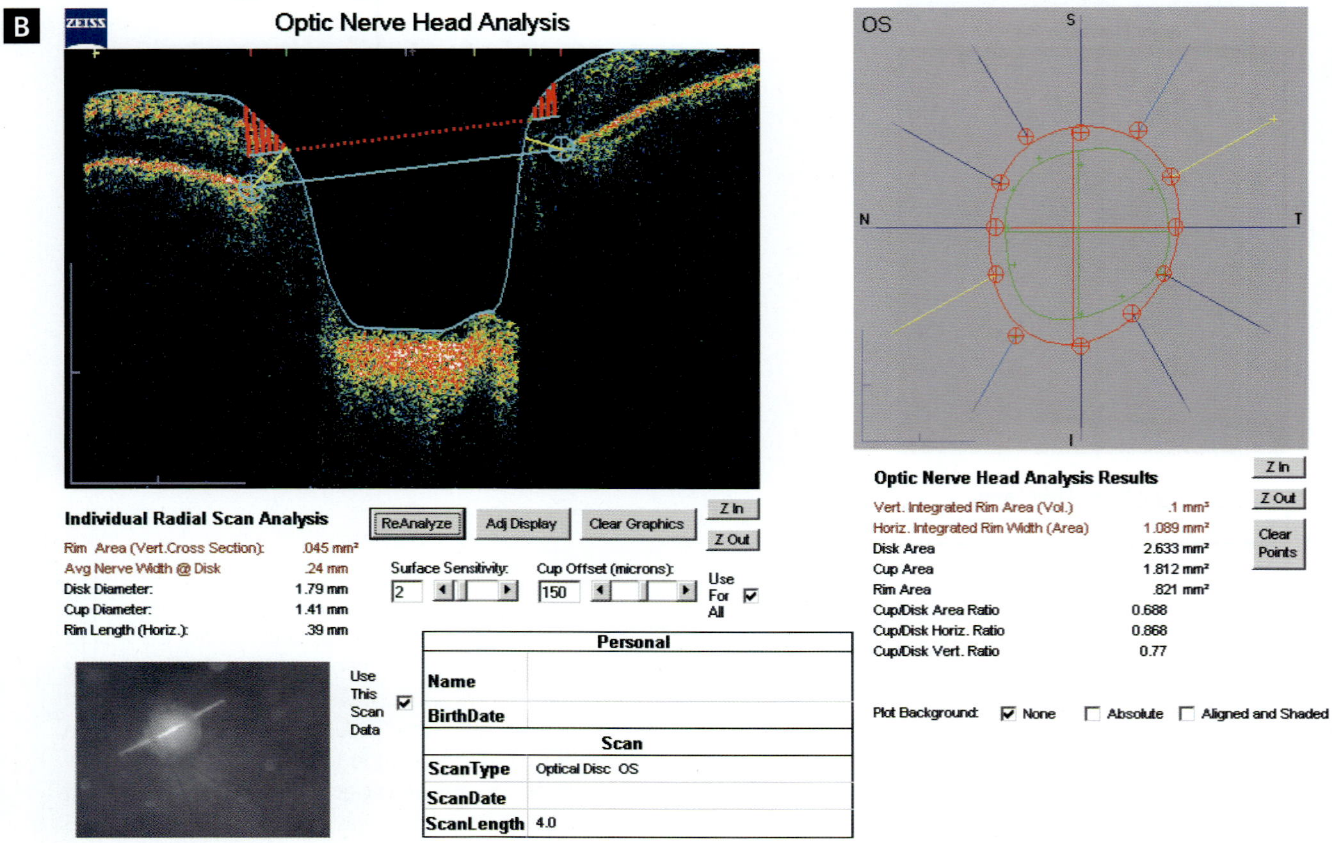

C

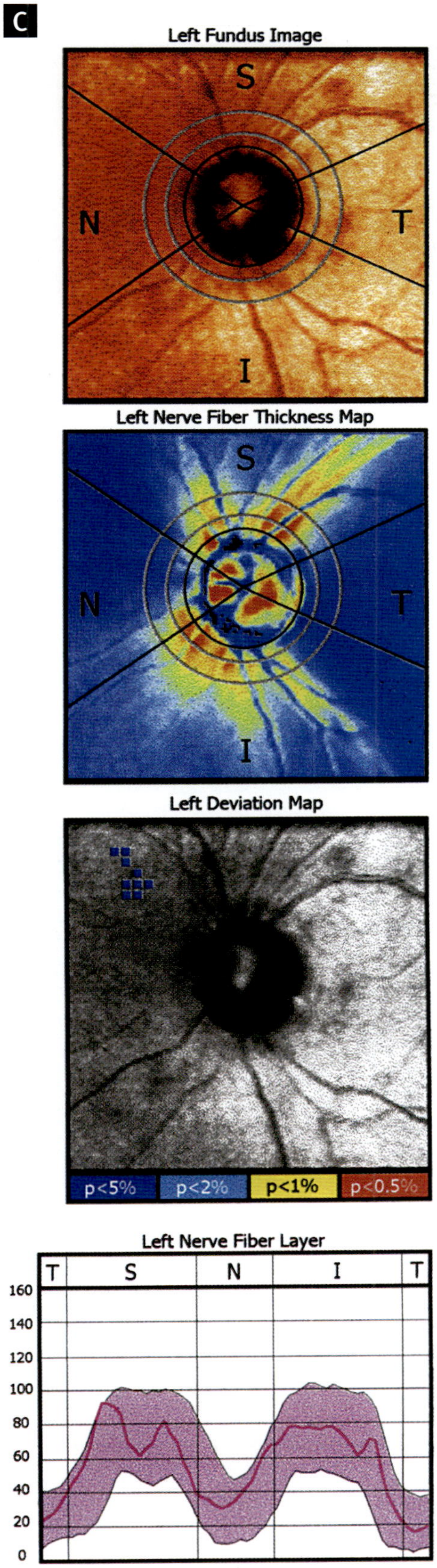

D

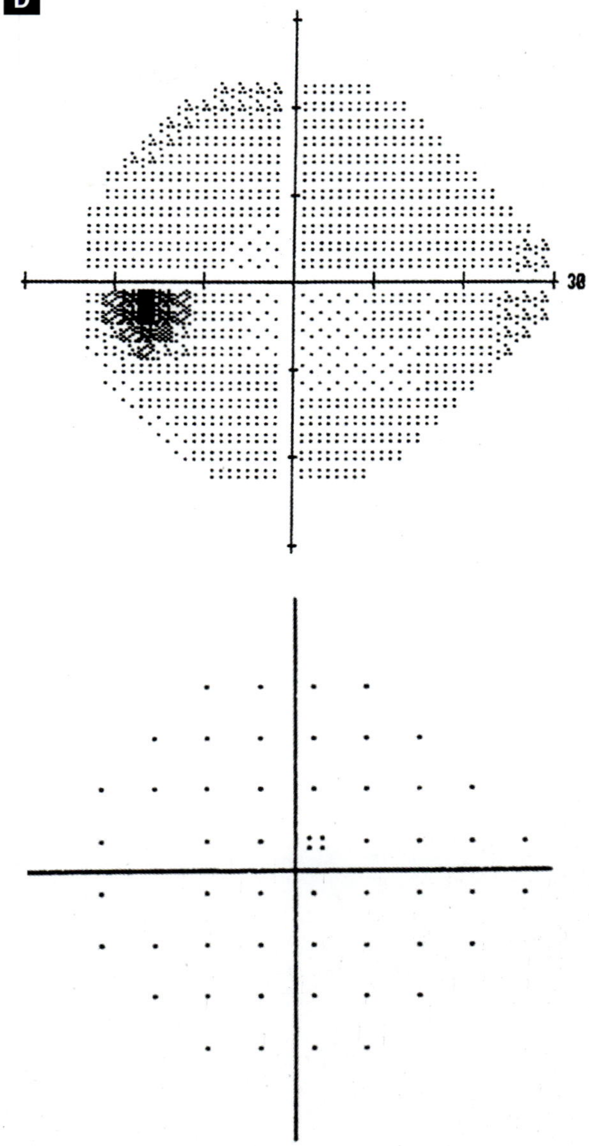

The other eye of the same patient (page 324). A. Optical Coherence Tomography shows a decrease of the mean nerve fibre layer thickness (79μm). B. Optic disc C/D ratio in the horizontal axis is 0.87 and in the vertical 0.77. Although Scanning Laser Polarimetry and visual fields are not outside the normal limits, the detection of decreased nerve fiber layer thickness in both eyes underlines early glaucomatous damage (preperimetric glaucoma). C, D. Visual fields and Scanning Laser Polarimetry are normal.

BILATERAL GLAUCOMA

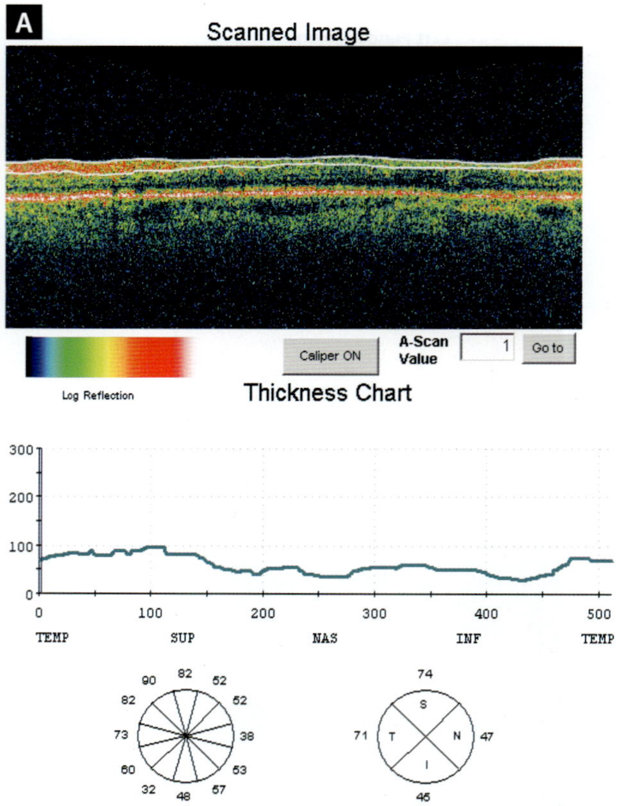

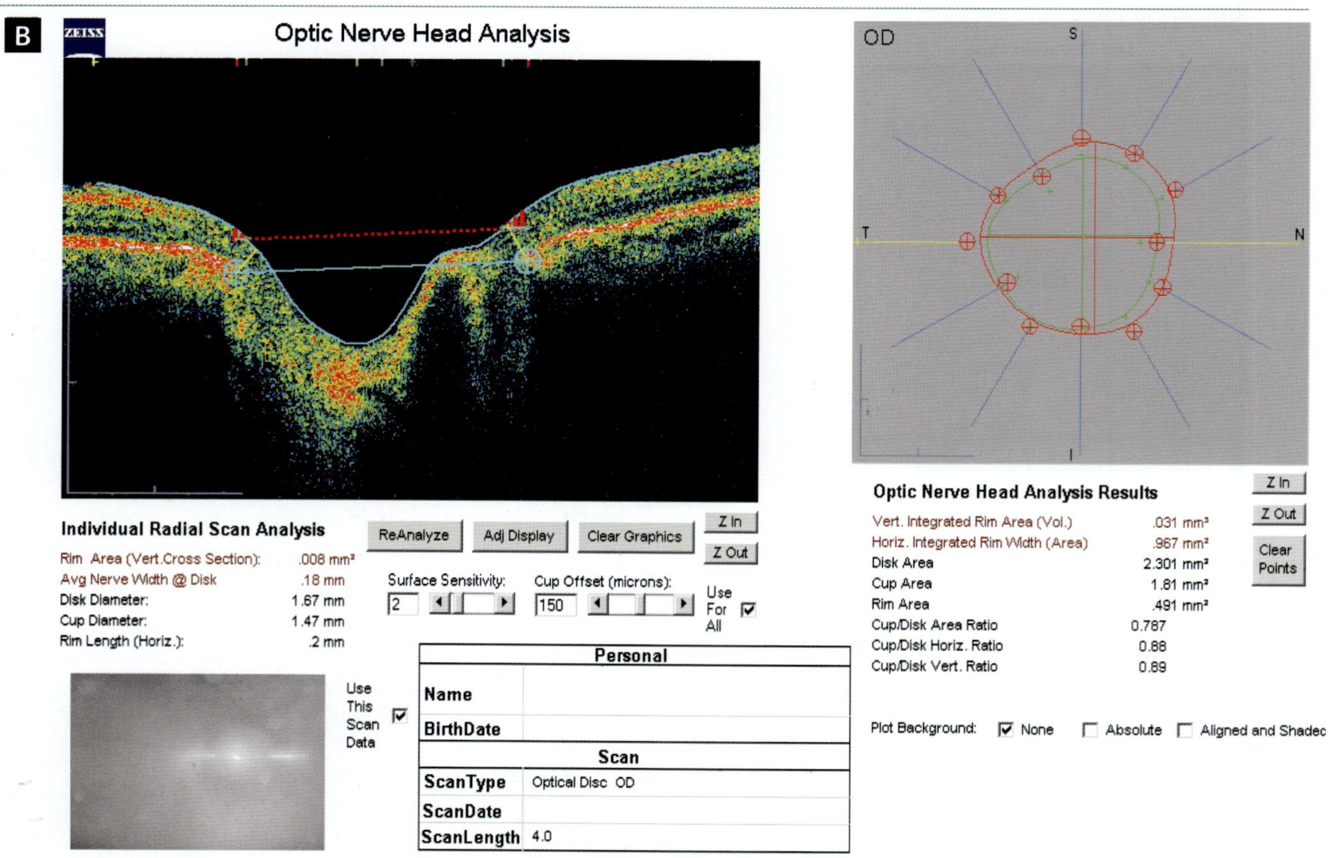

C

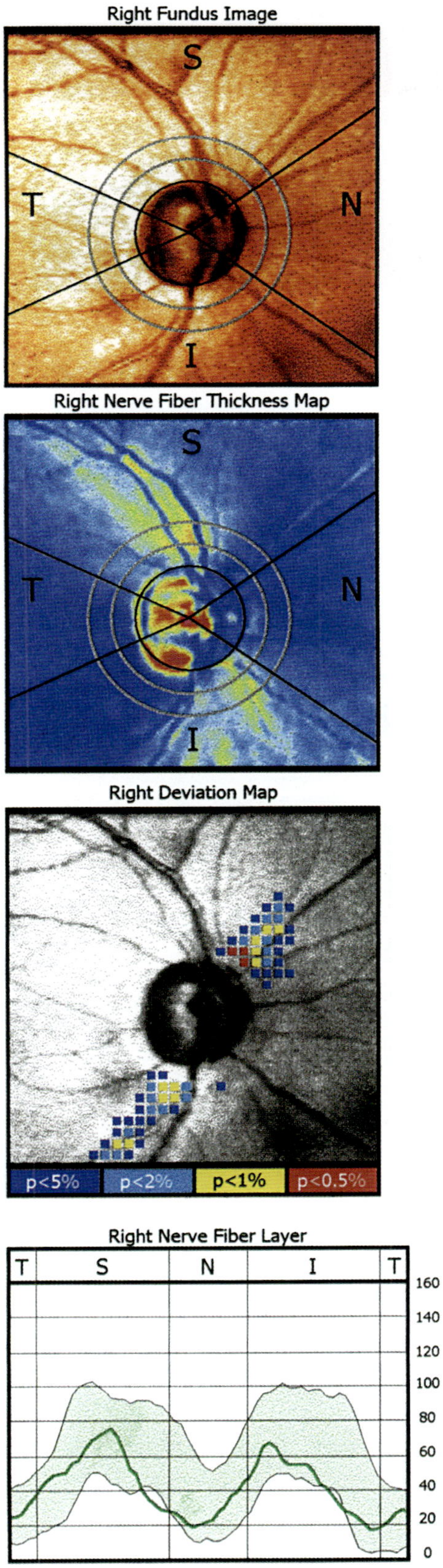

D

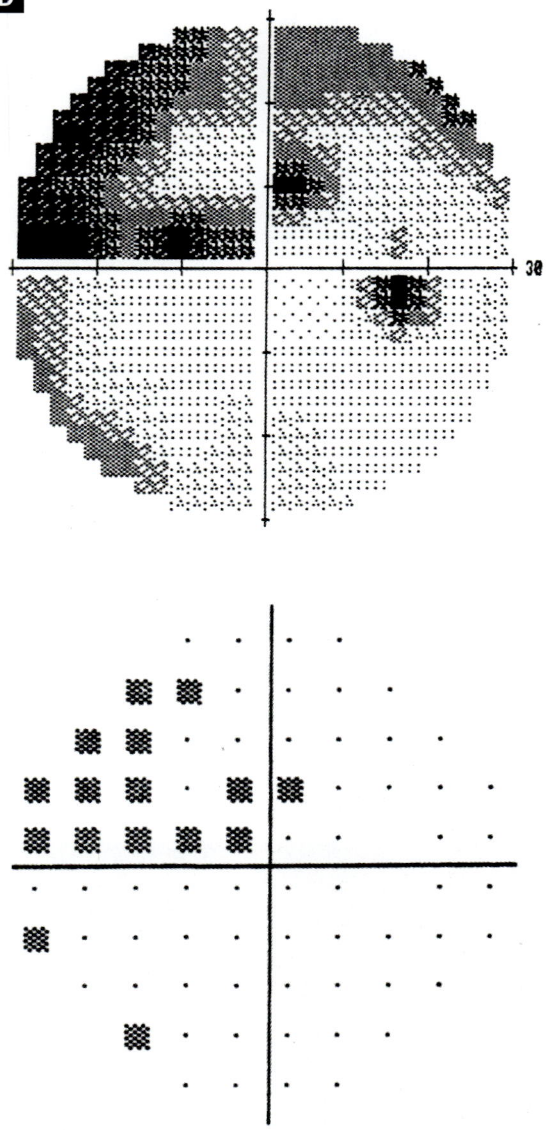

Patient 84-year-old with bilateral glaucoma. A. Optical Coherence Tomography shows a significant decrease of the mean thickness of the nerve fiber layer (60.25μm) with a bigger decrease of thickness in the inferior quadrant (45μm). B. Optic disc C/D ratio in the horizontal axis is 0.88 and in the vertical 0.89. C. Scanning Laser Polarimetry shows a relative decrease of nerve fiber layer thickness in the superior nasal and inferior temporal quadrants, findings that correspond partly to the changes of the visual field testing. D. Visual fields reveal a significant decrease of sensitivity in the superior nasal quadrant with central involvement.

BILATERAL GLAUCOMA

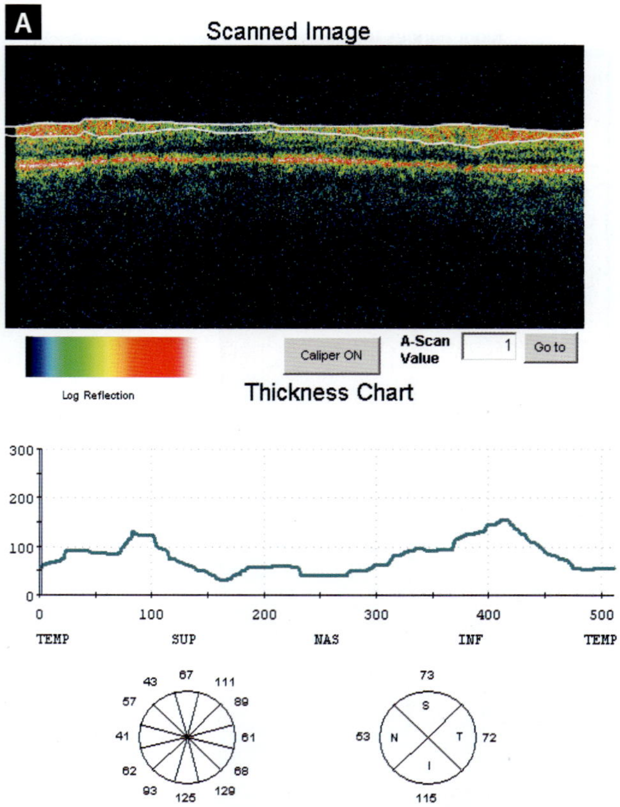

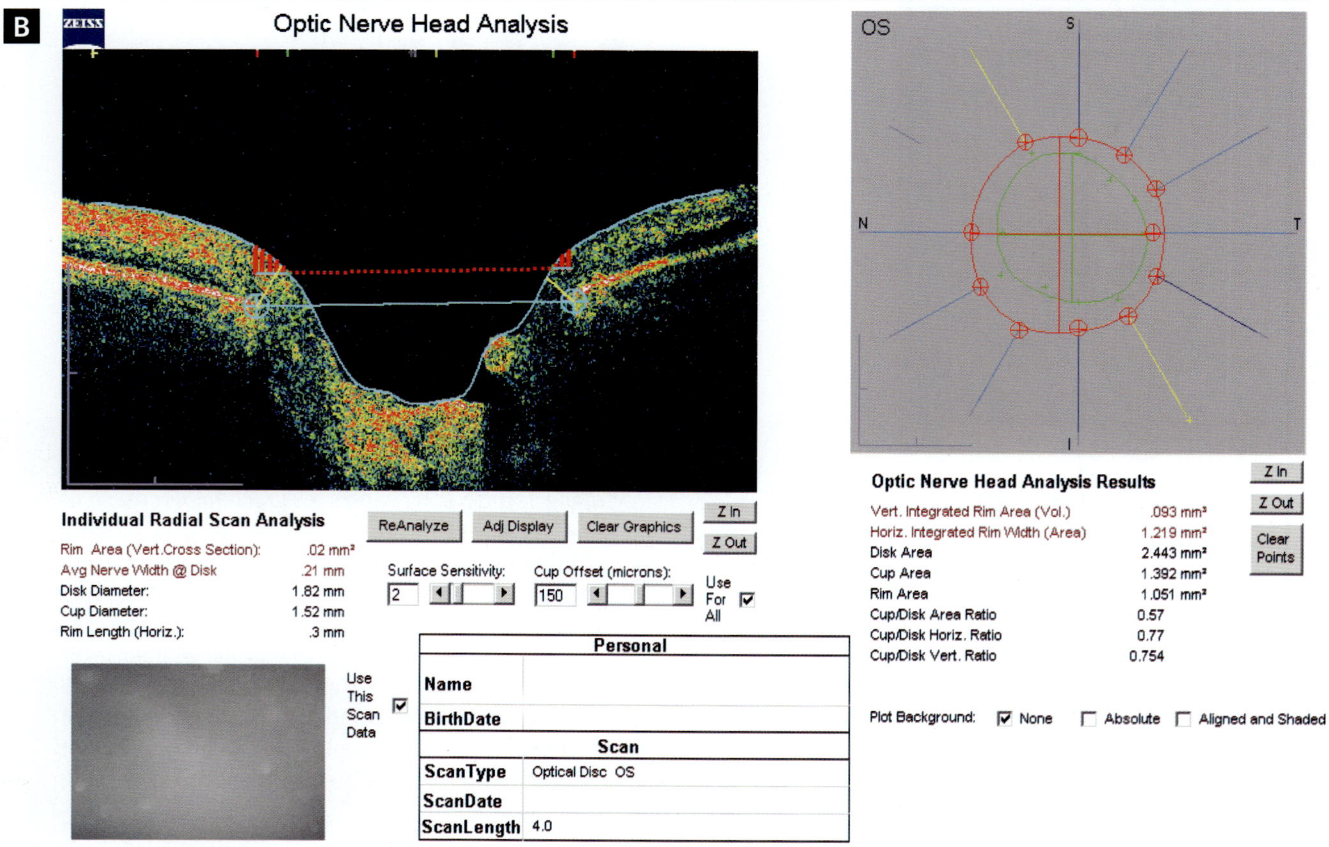

C

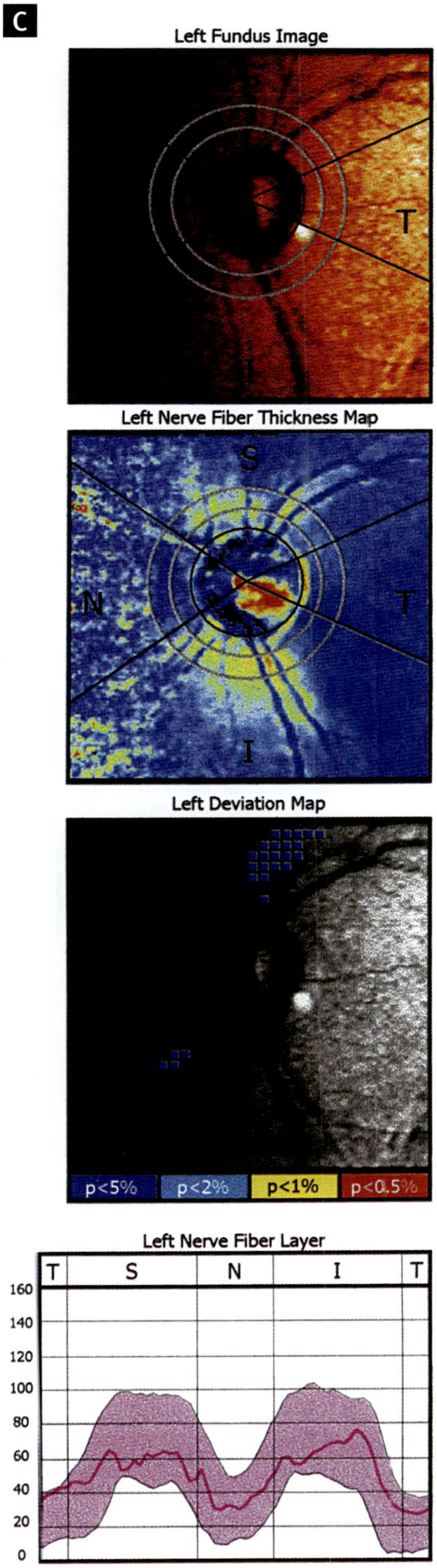

D

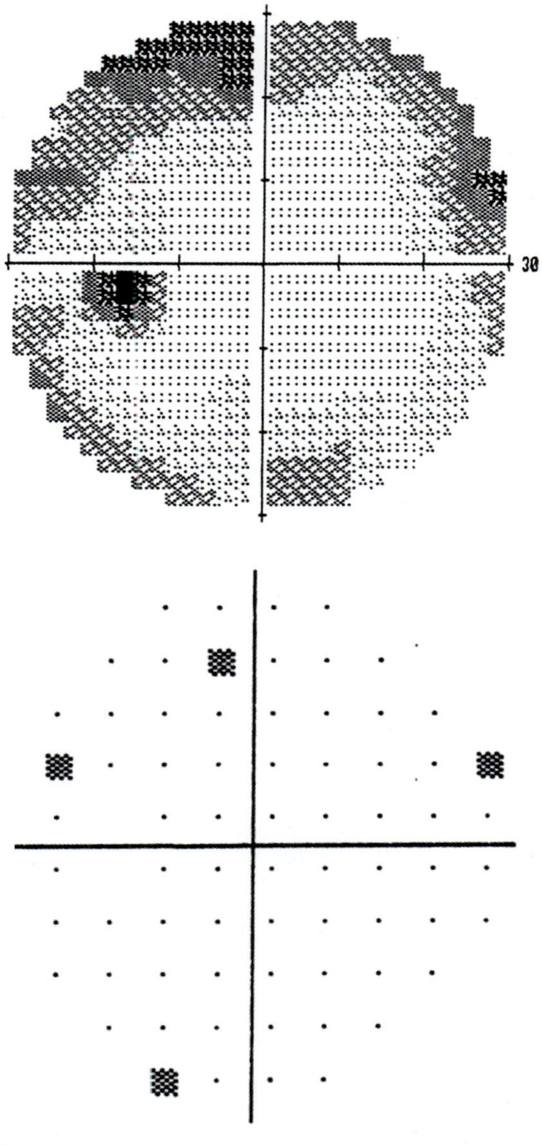

The other eye of the same patient (page 328). A. Optical Coherence Tomography shows a considerable decrease of the mean nerve fibre layer thickness (73.8μm) with a bigger decrease of the thickness in the superior quadrant (73 μm). B. Optic disc C/D ratio in the horizontal axis is 0.77 and in the vertical 0.75. C, D. Because of cataract, visual fields show a general reduction of sensitivity while Scanning Laser Polarimetry is of bad quality.

ADVANCED UNILATERAL GLAUCOMA

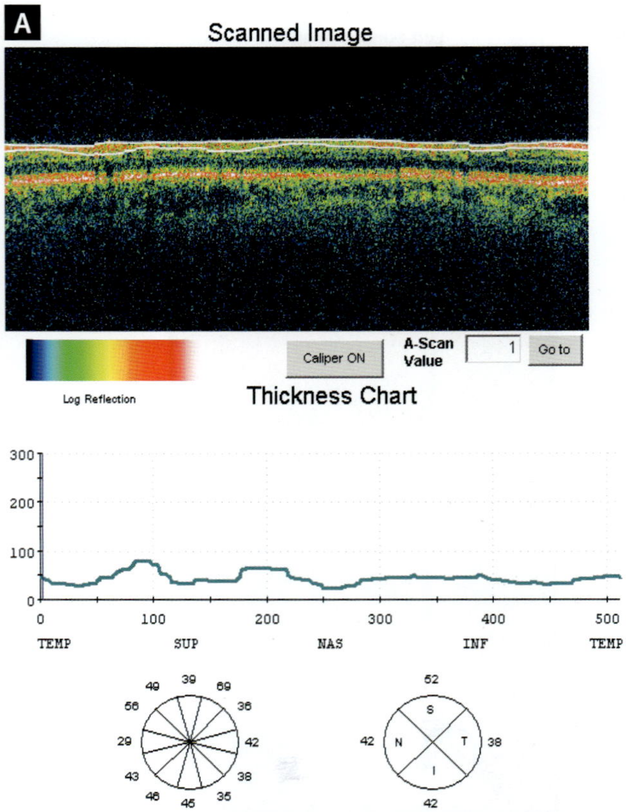

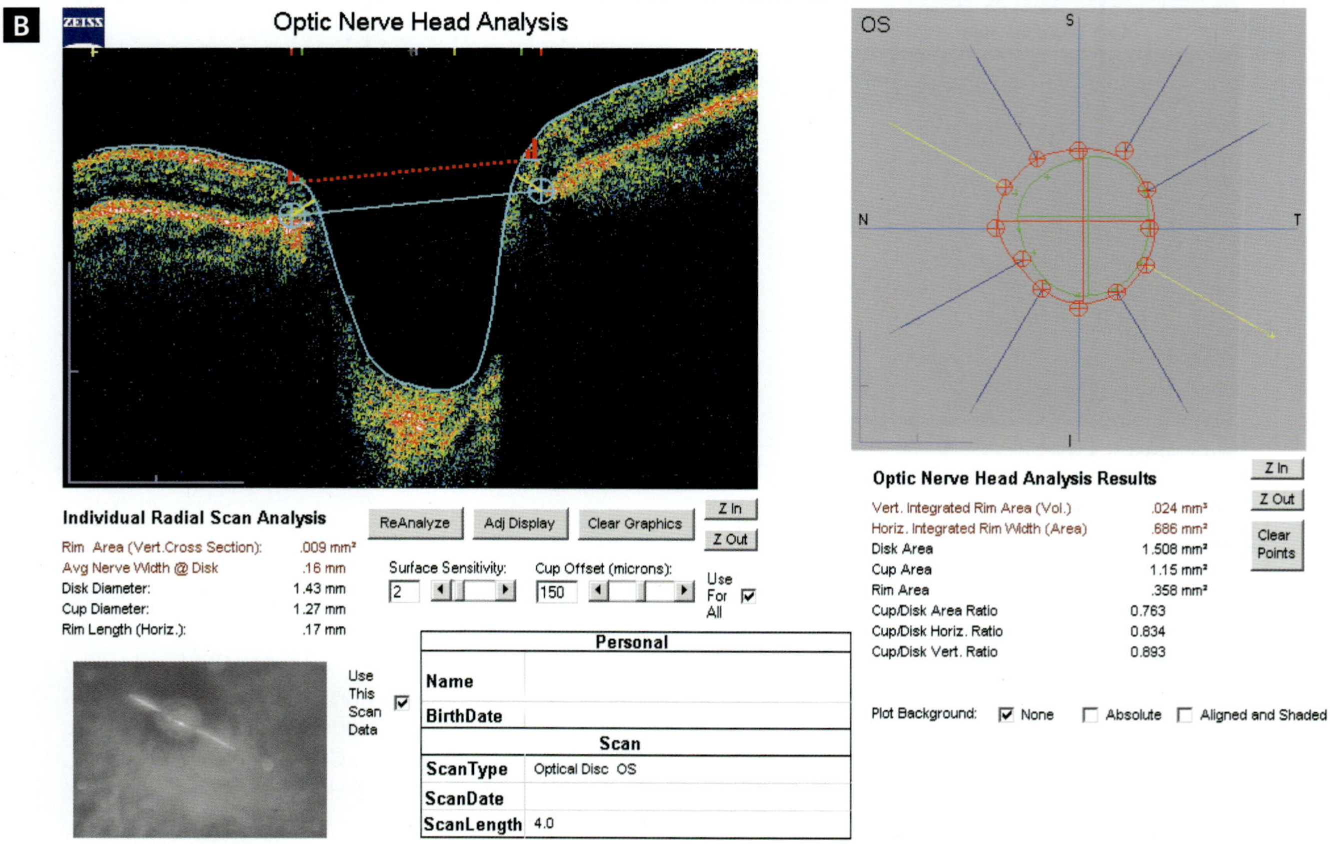

C

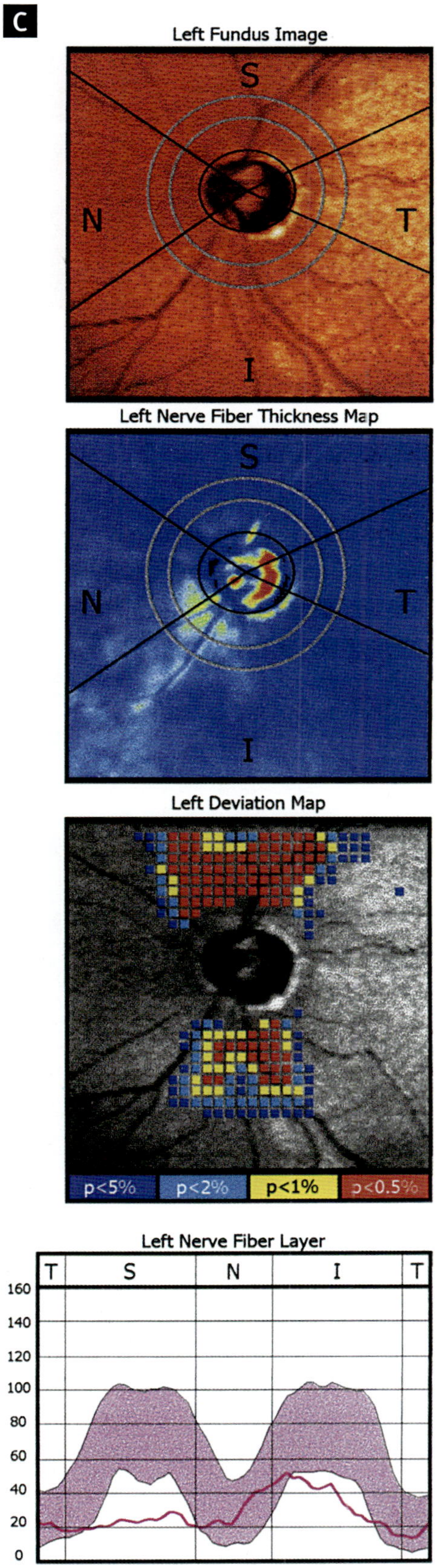

D

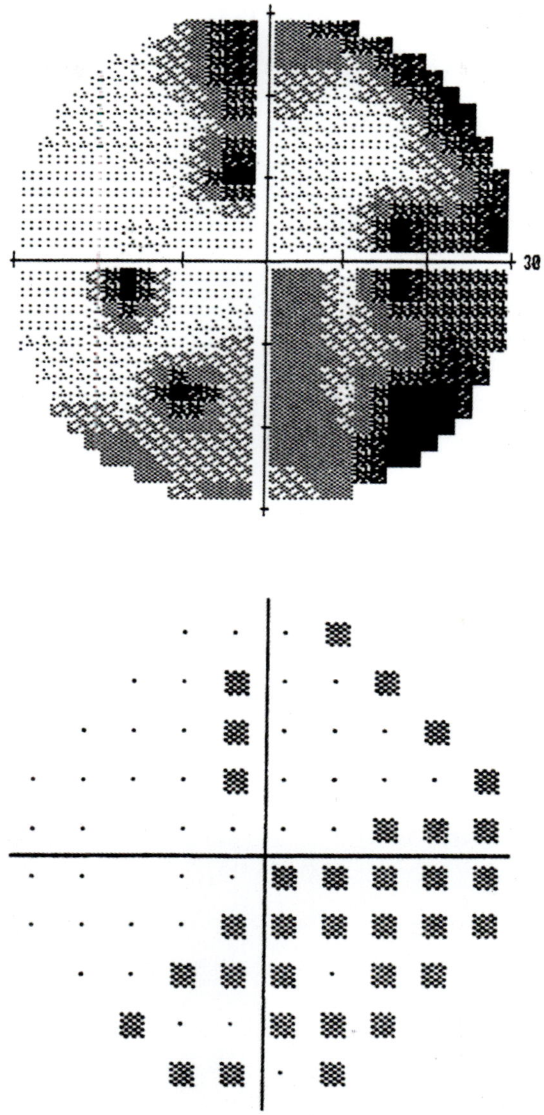

Patient 45-year-old with advanced glaucoma in one eye. A. Optical Coherence Tomography shows a substantial decrease of the mean thickness of the nerve fiber layer (38.9μm) with a bigger decrease in the inferior and superior quadrants. B. Optic disc C/D ratio in the horizontal axis is 0.83 and in the vertical 0.89. Note the great depth of the disc cupping. C. Scanning Laser Polarimetry shows a big decrease of the nerve fiber layer thickness in the superior and inferior quadrants. D. Visual fields reveal extensive changes in the nasal hemifield.

ADVANCED UNILATERAL GLAUCOMA

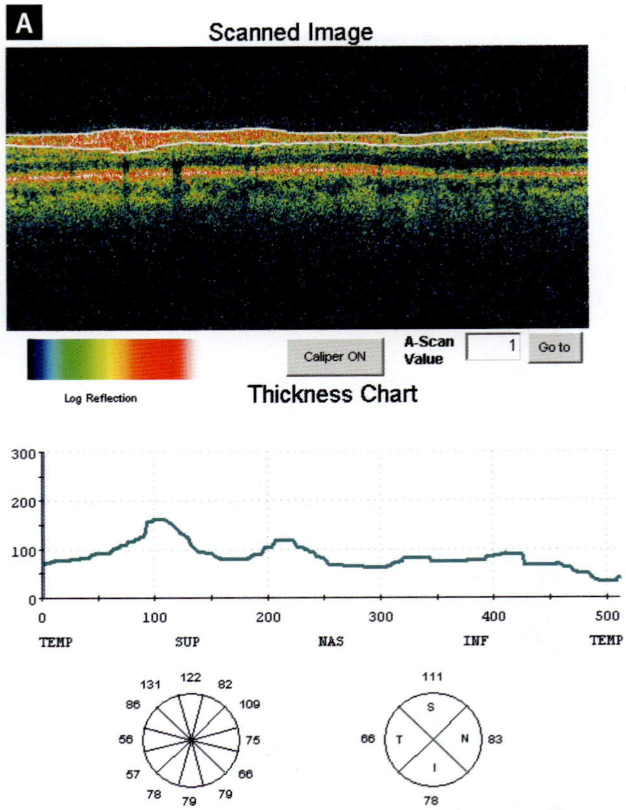

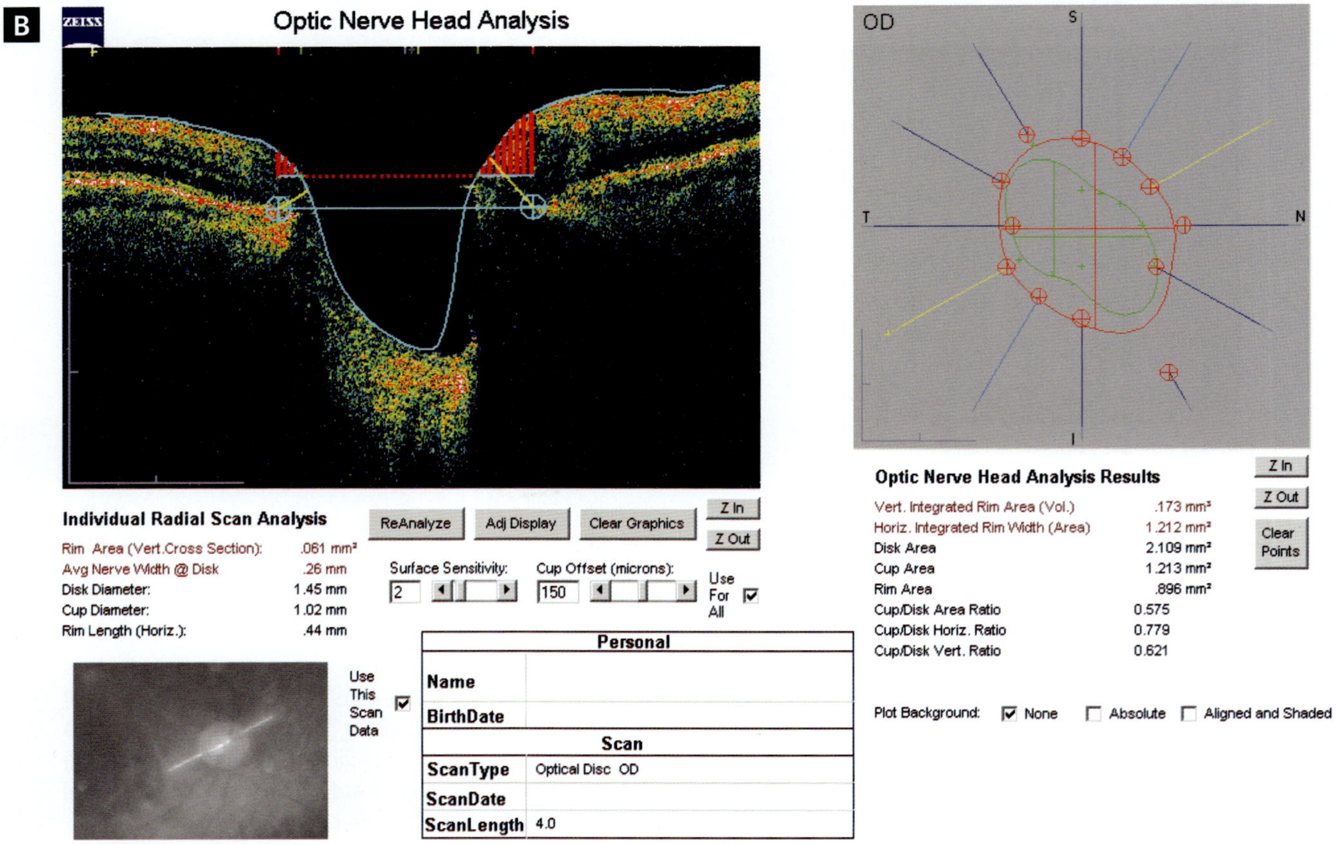

C

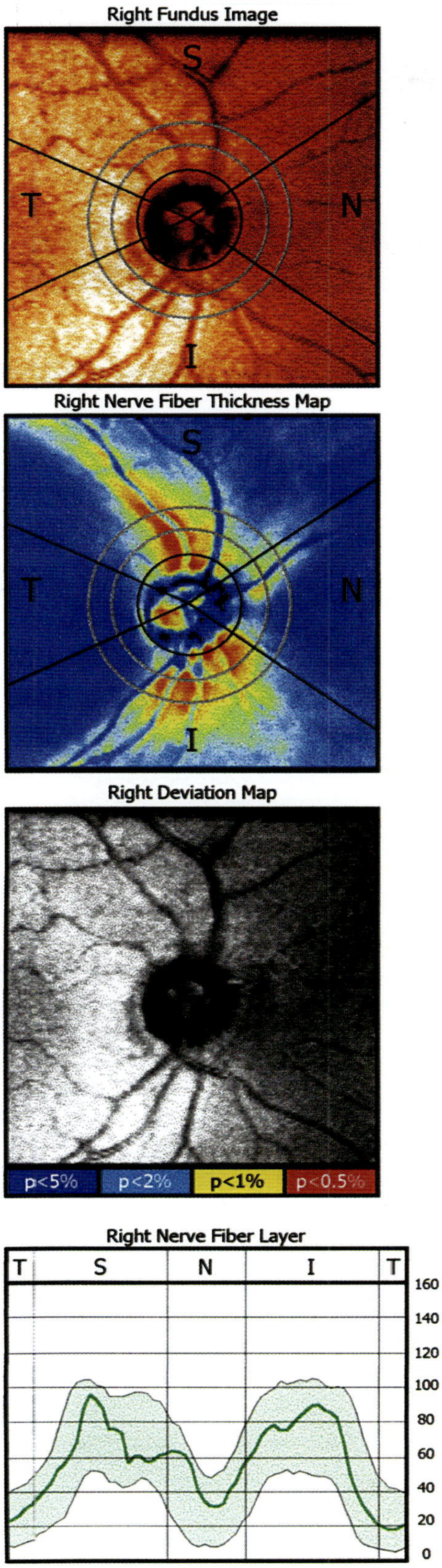

D

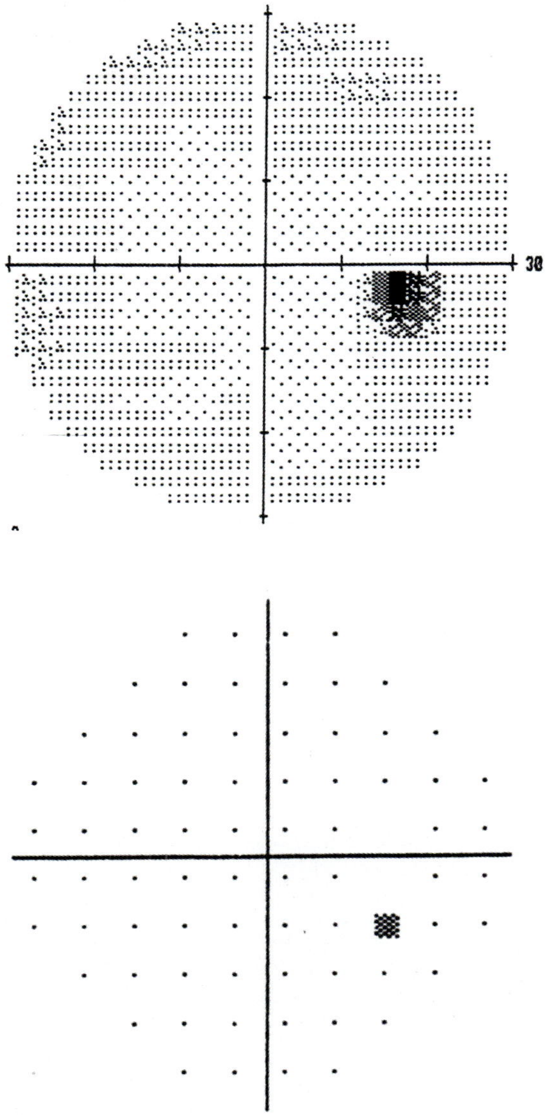

The other eye of the same patient (page 332). A. Optical Coherence Tomography shows a mild decrease of the mean nerve fibre layer thickness (84.75μm). B. Optic disc C/D ratio in the horizontal axis is 0.77 and in the vertical 0.62. The mild decrease of nerve fiber layer thickness, combined with the glaucomatous findings of the other eye, makes the regular control of this patient necessary. C, D. Visual fields and Scanning Laser Polarimetry are normal.

BILATERAL ADVANCED GLAUCOMA

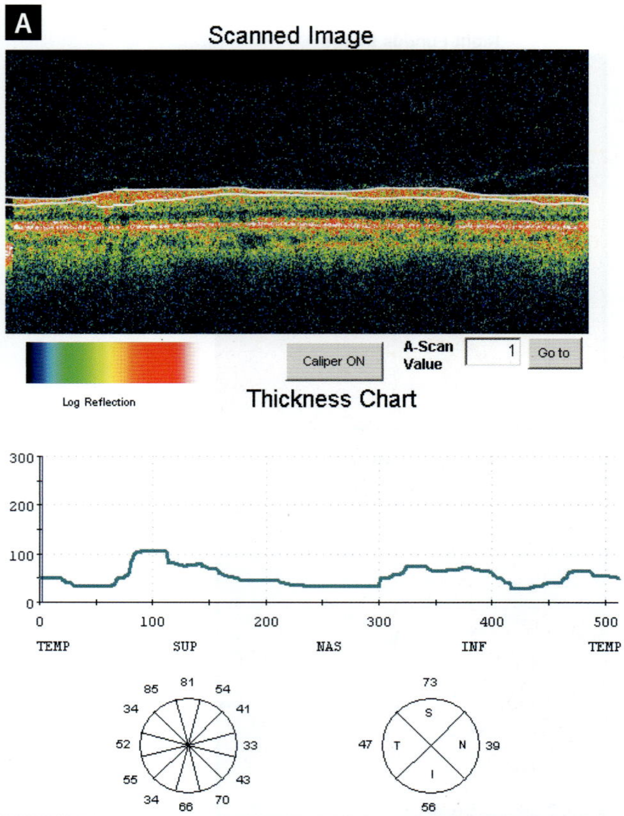

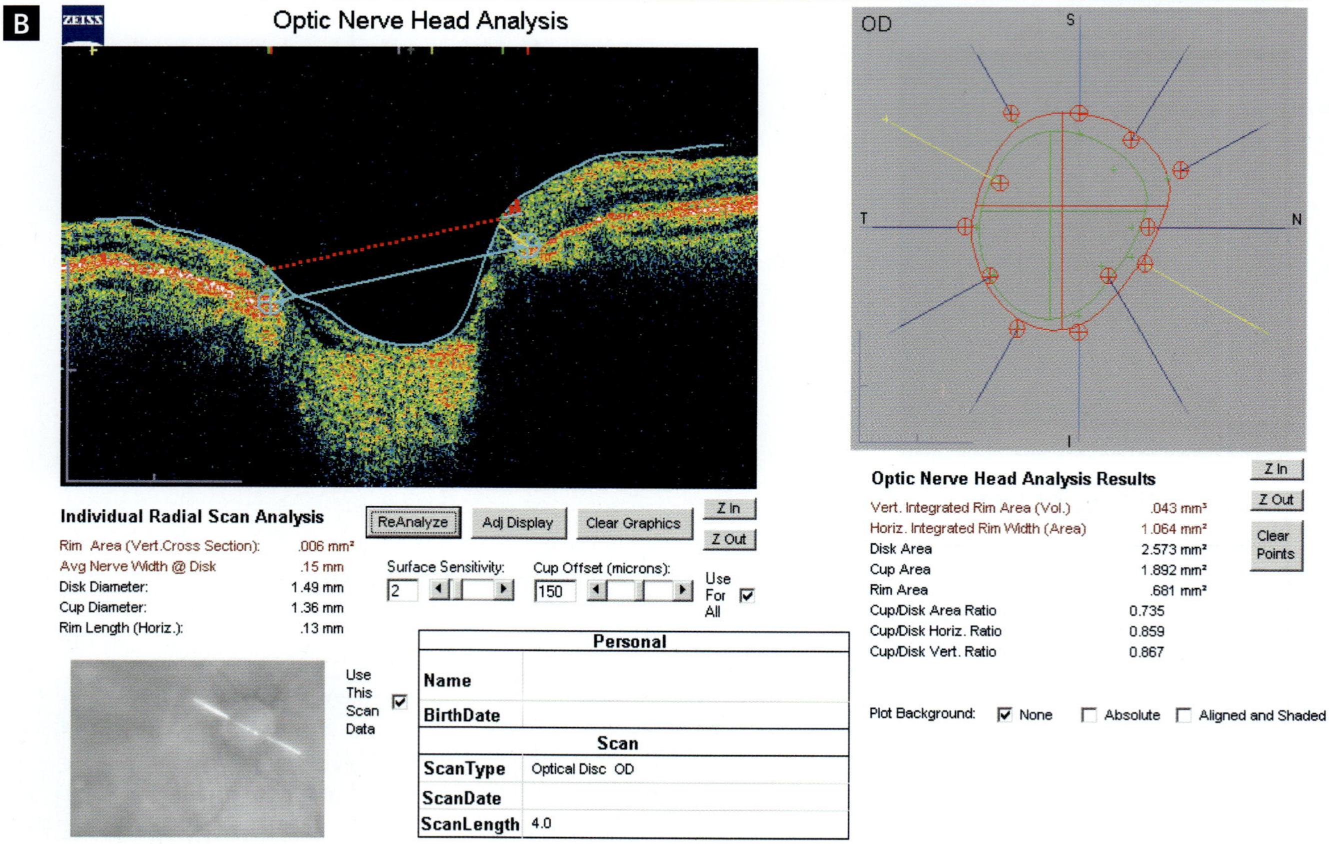

C

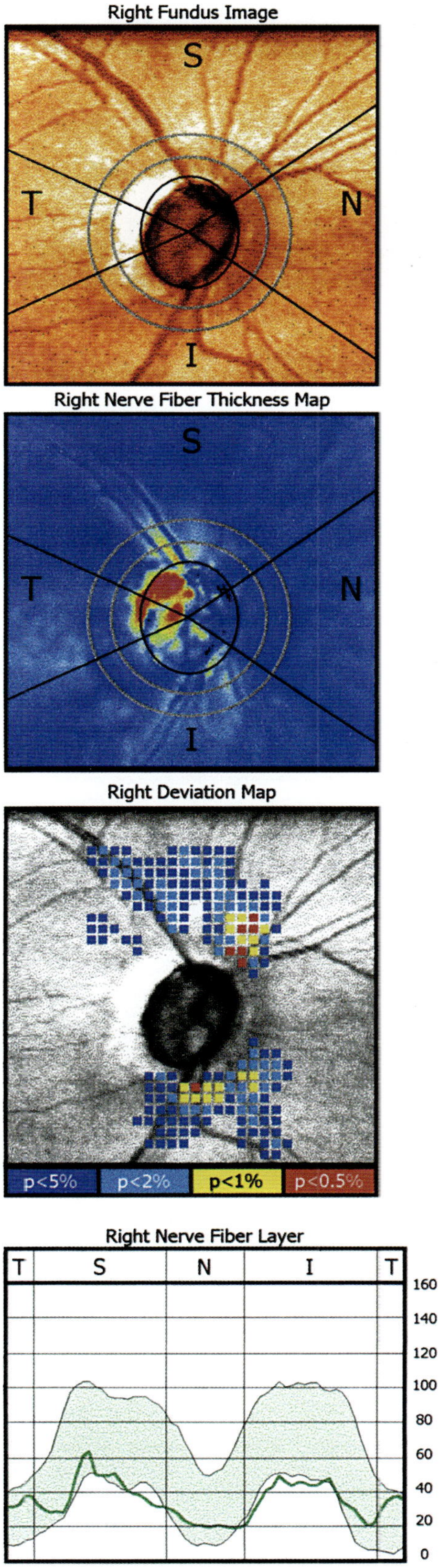

D

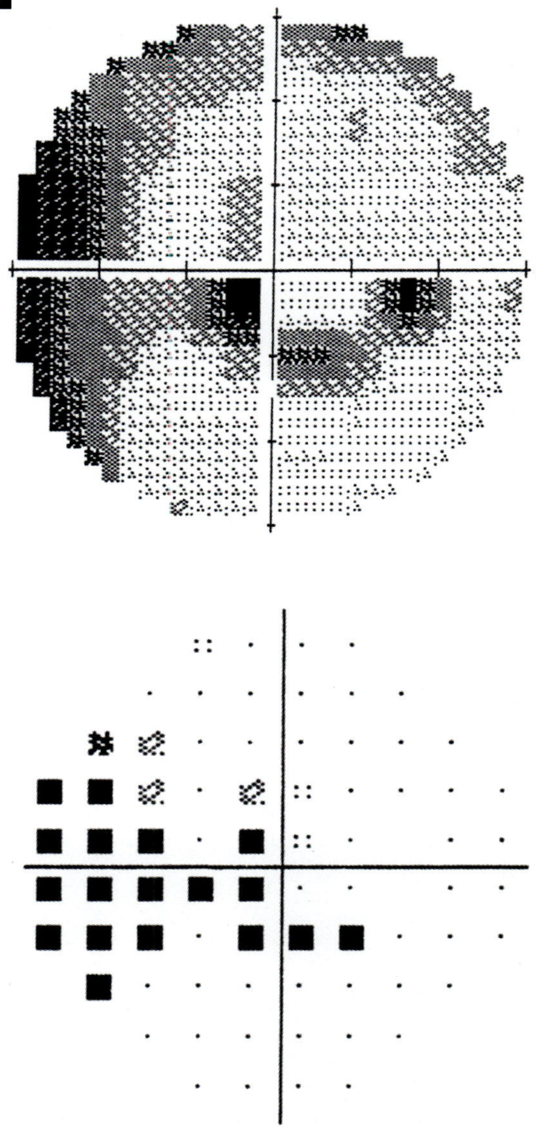

Patient 45-year-old with bilateral advanced glaucoma. A. Optical Coherence Tomography shows a significant decrease of the mean thickness of the nerve fiber layer (52.25μm) with a bigger decrease in the inferior quadrant (56μm). B. Optic disc C/D ratio in the horizontal and vertical axis is 0.86. C Scanning Laser Polarimetry shows a big decrease of nerve fiber layer thickness in the superior and inferior quadrants. D. Visual fields reveal a big decrease of sensitivity nasally with an inferior arcuate scotoma involving the center of fixation.

BILATERAL ADVANCED GLAUCOMA

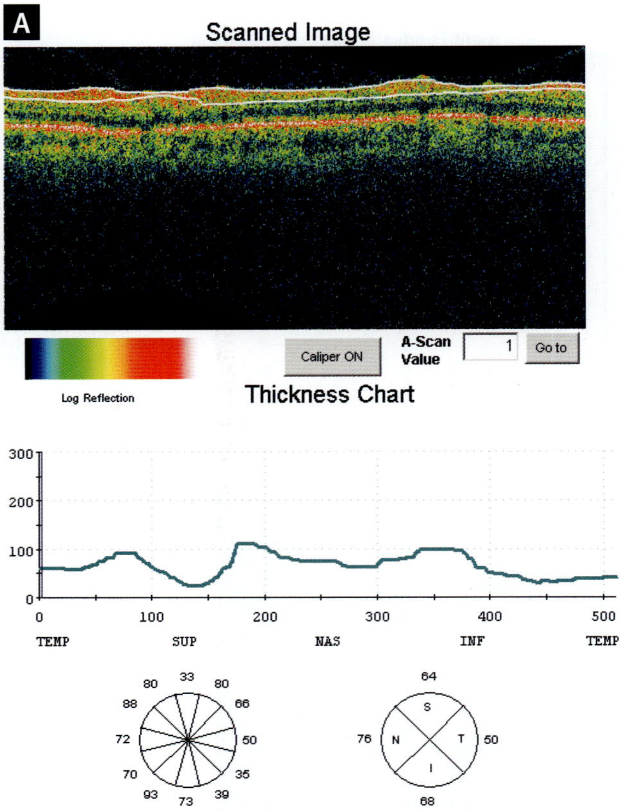

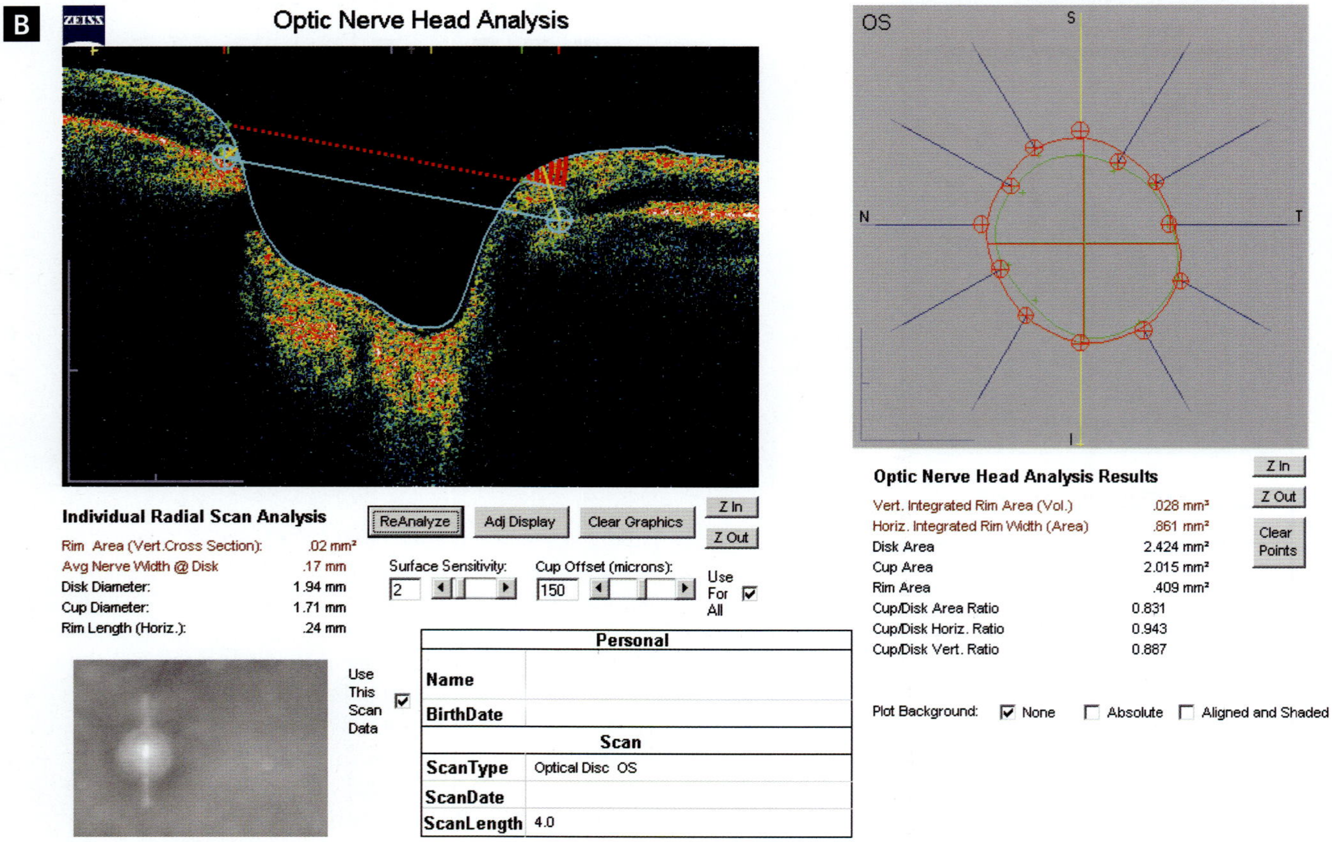

C

D

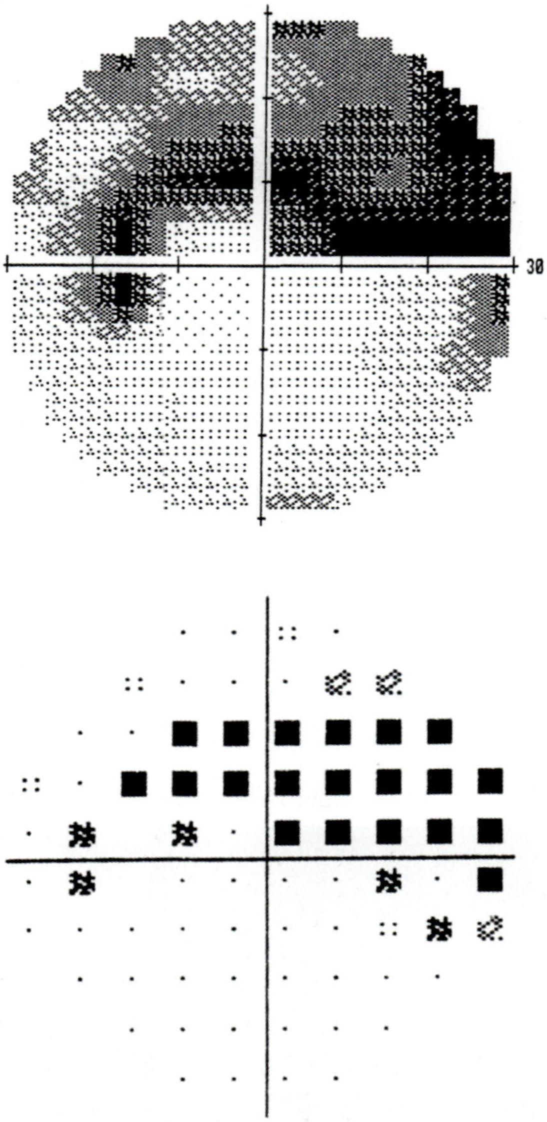

The other eye of the same patient (page 336). A. Optical Coherence Tomography shows a considerable decrease of the mean nerve fibre layer thickness (43.9μm). B. Optic disc C/D ratio in the horizontal axis is 0.94 and in the vertical 0.88. C. Scanning Laser Polarimetry was impossible to perform because of the patient's inability to fixate. D. Visual fields show a big decrease of sensitivity in the superior hemifield involving the fixation point.

LARGE OPTIC DISC CUPPING

A

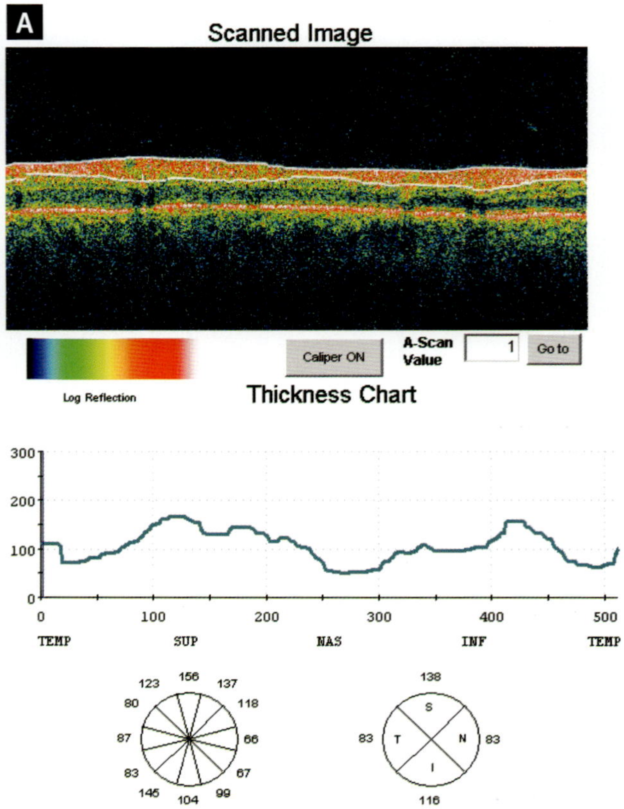

B

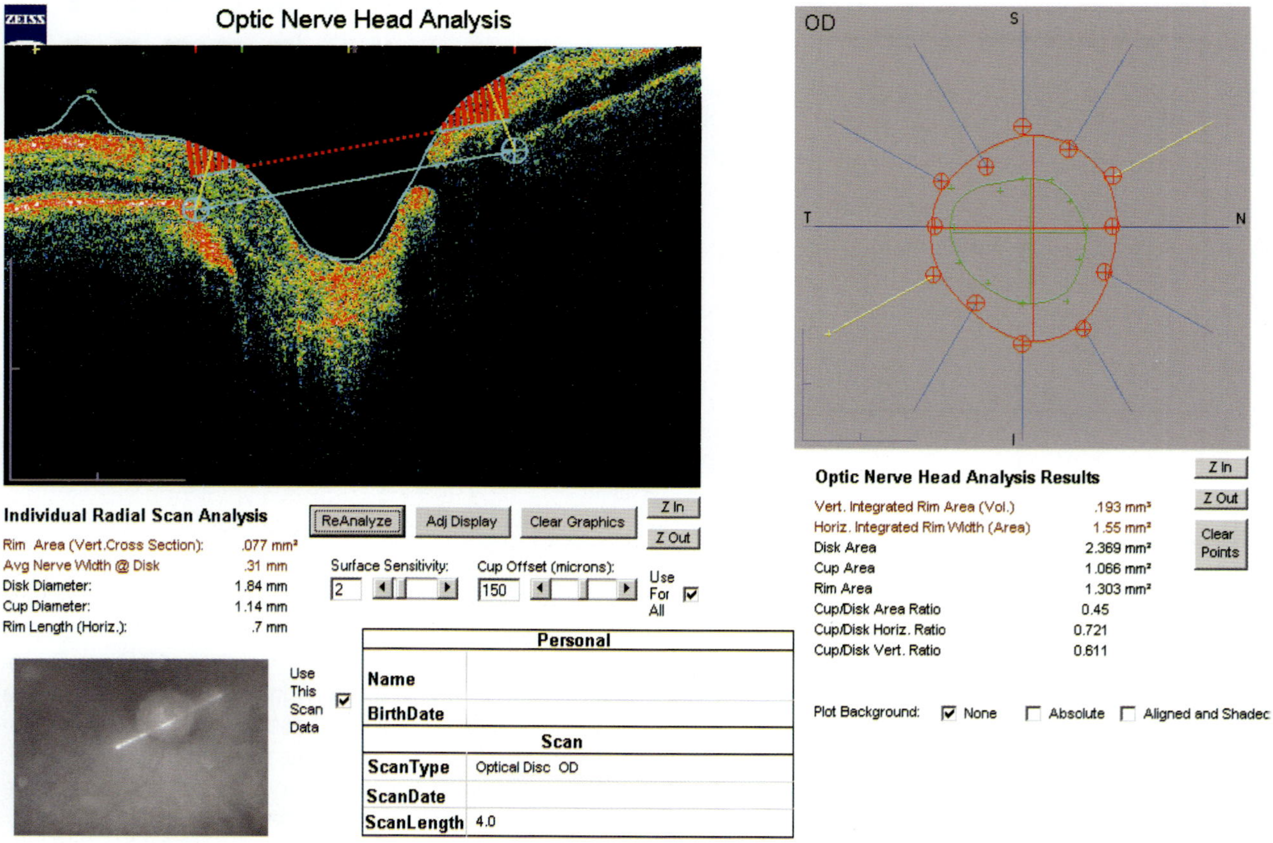

C

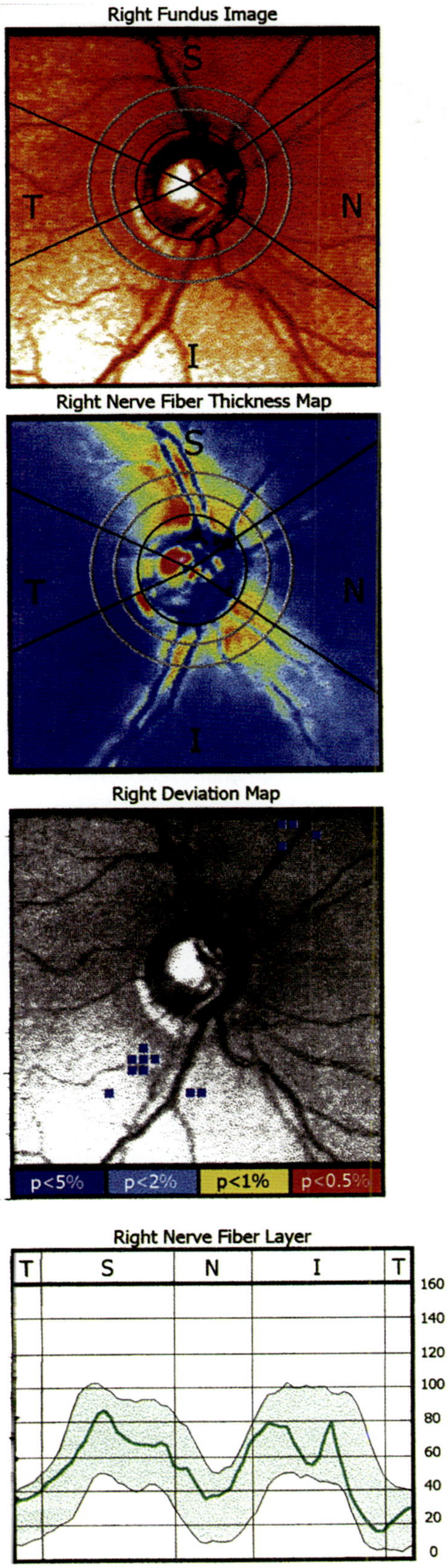

D

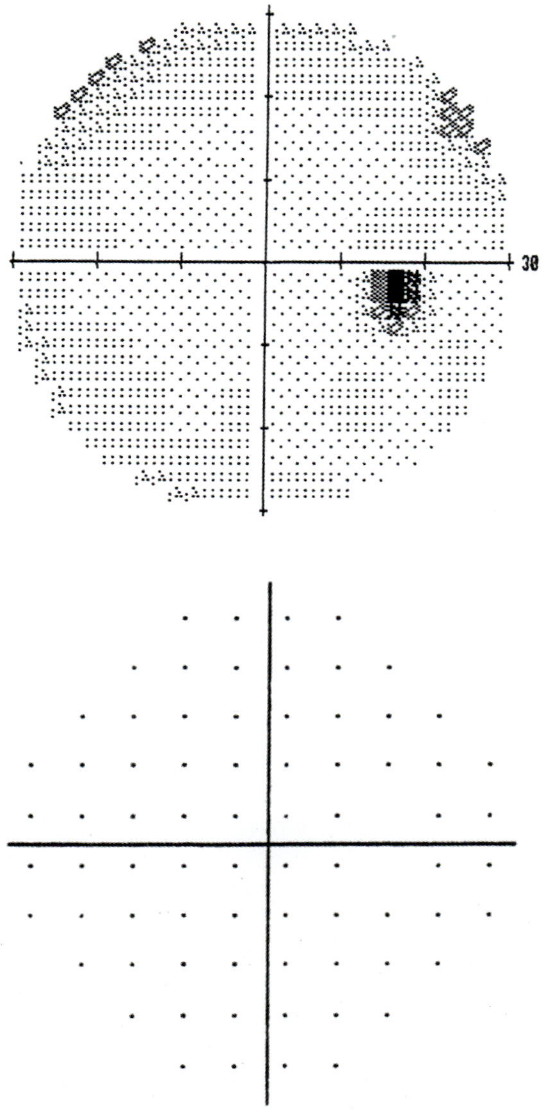

Patient 62-year-old with normal intraocular pressures. Biomicroscopically an asymmetrical increase of optic disc cupping is observed. A. Optical Coherence Tomography shows the mean thickness of nerve fiber layer (106μm) to be within normal limits. B. Optic disc C/D ratio in the horizontal axis is 0.71 and in the vertical 0.59. C, D. Visual fields and Scanning Laser Polarimetry don't reveal any particular alteration.

LARGE OPTIC DISC CUPPING

A

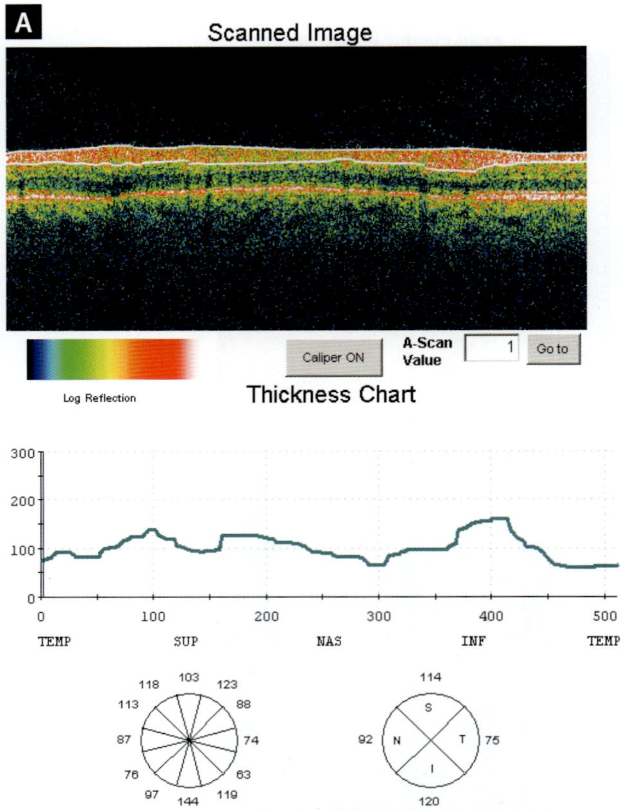

B

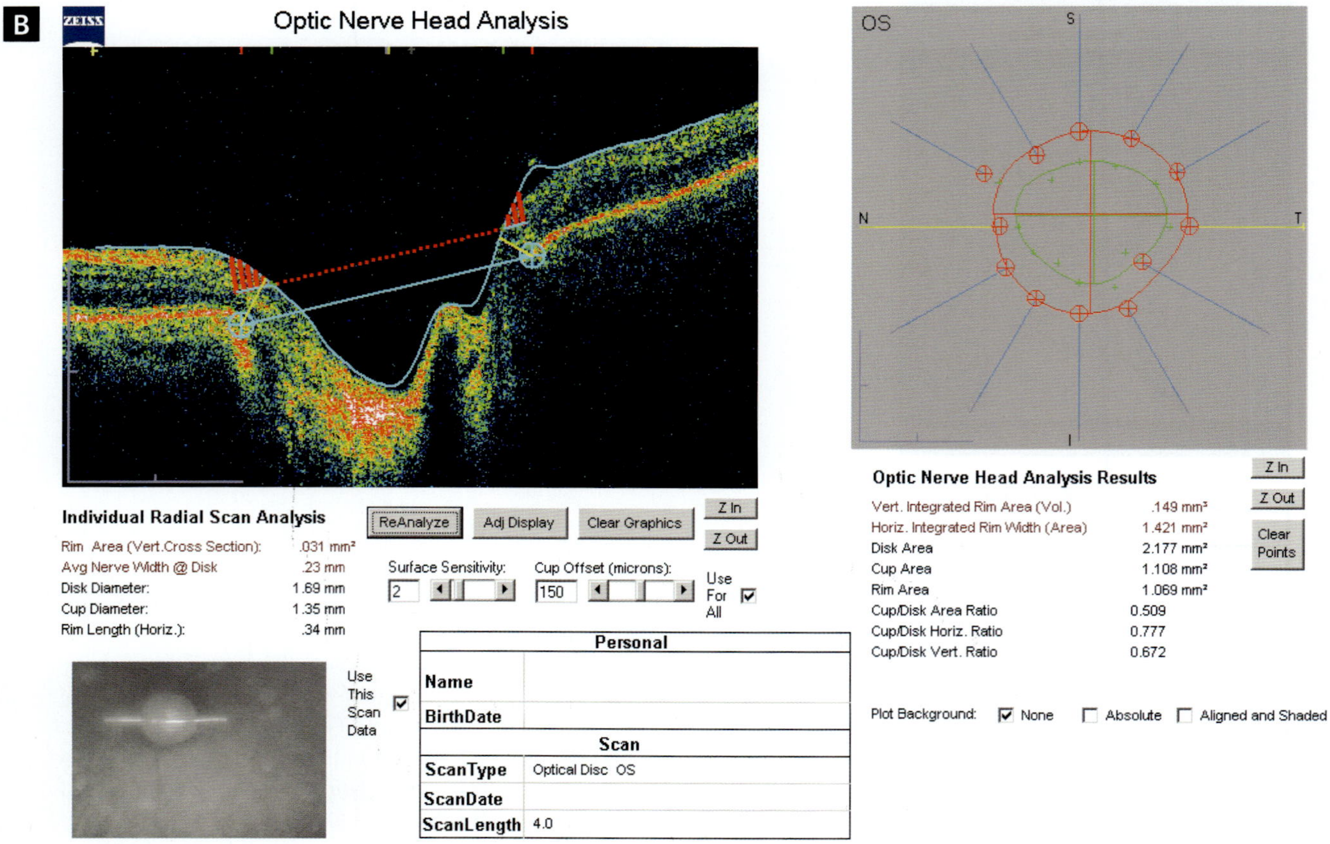

C

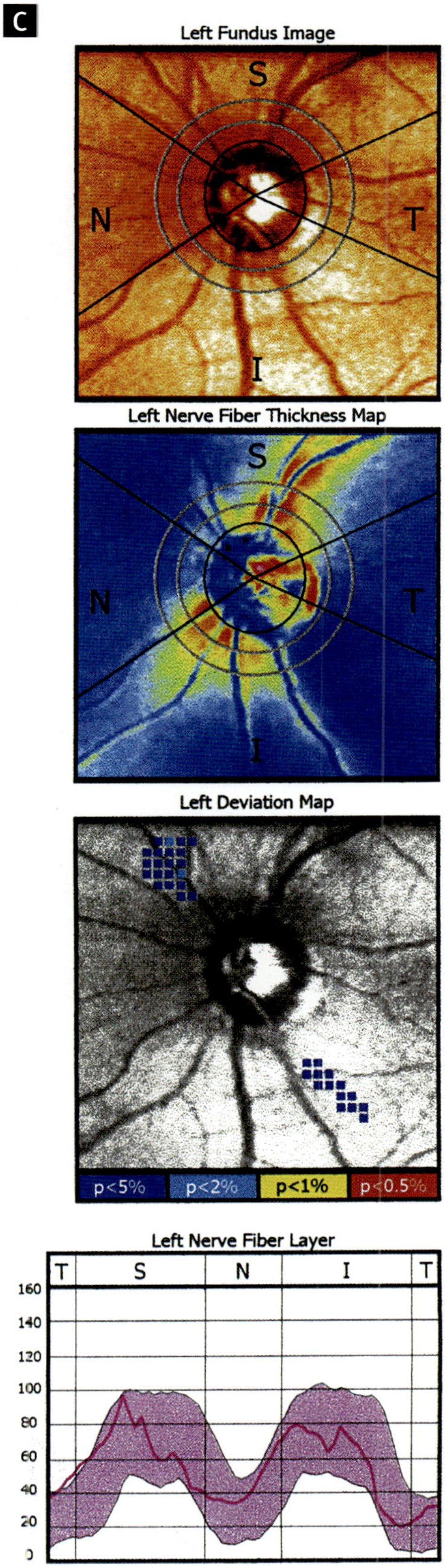

D

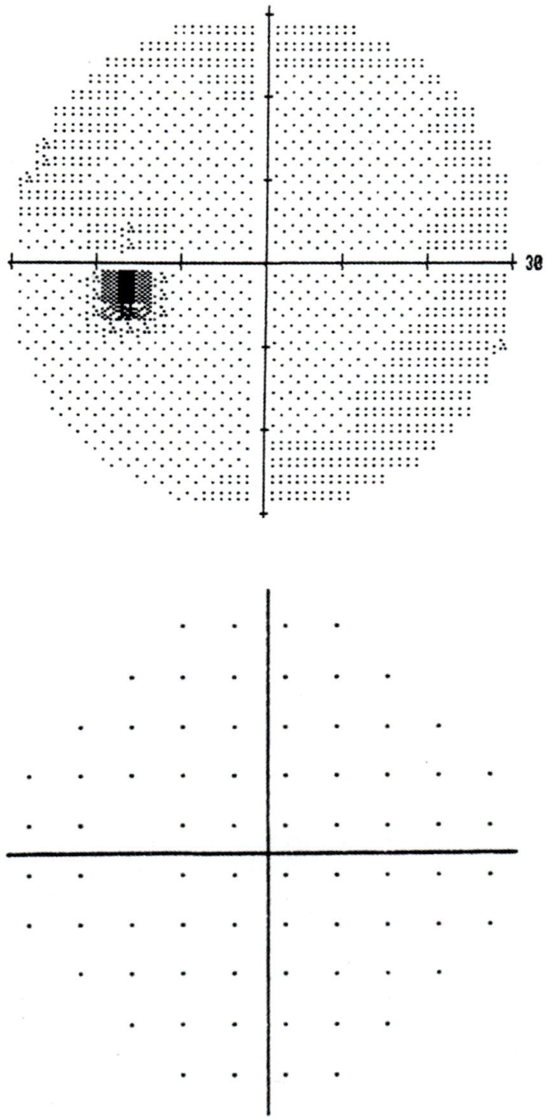

The other eye of the same patient (page 340). A. Optical Coherence Tomography shows that the mean nerve fibre layer thickness (100μm) is within normal limits. B. Optic disc C/D ratio in the horizontal axis is 0.71 and in the vertical 0.61. The normal nerve fiber layer thickness found with Optical Coherence Tomography confirms the normal findings from the visual fields and Scanning Laser Polarimetry in this patient with suspicious optic discs. C, D. Visual field and Scanning Laser Polarimetry are normal.

BIG OPTIC DISC WITH LARGE CUPPING

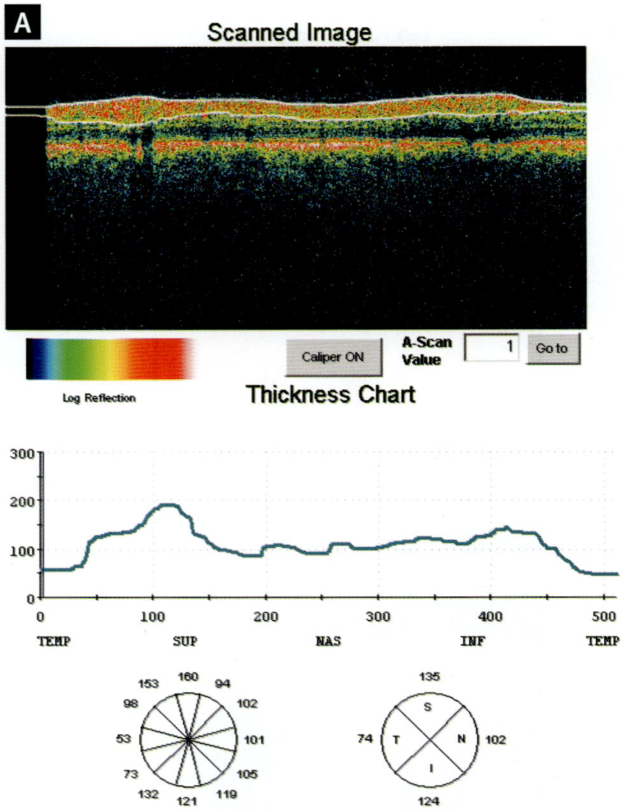

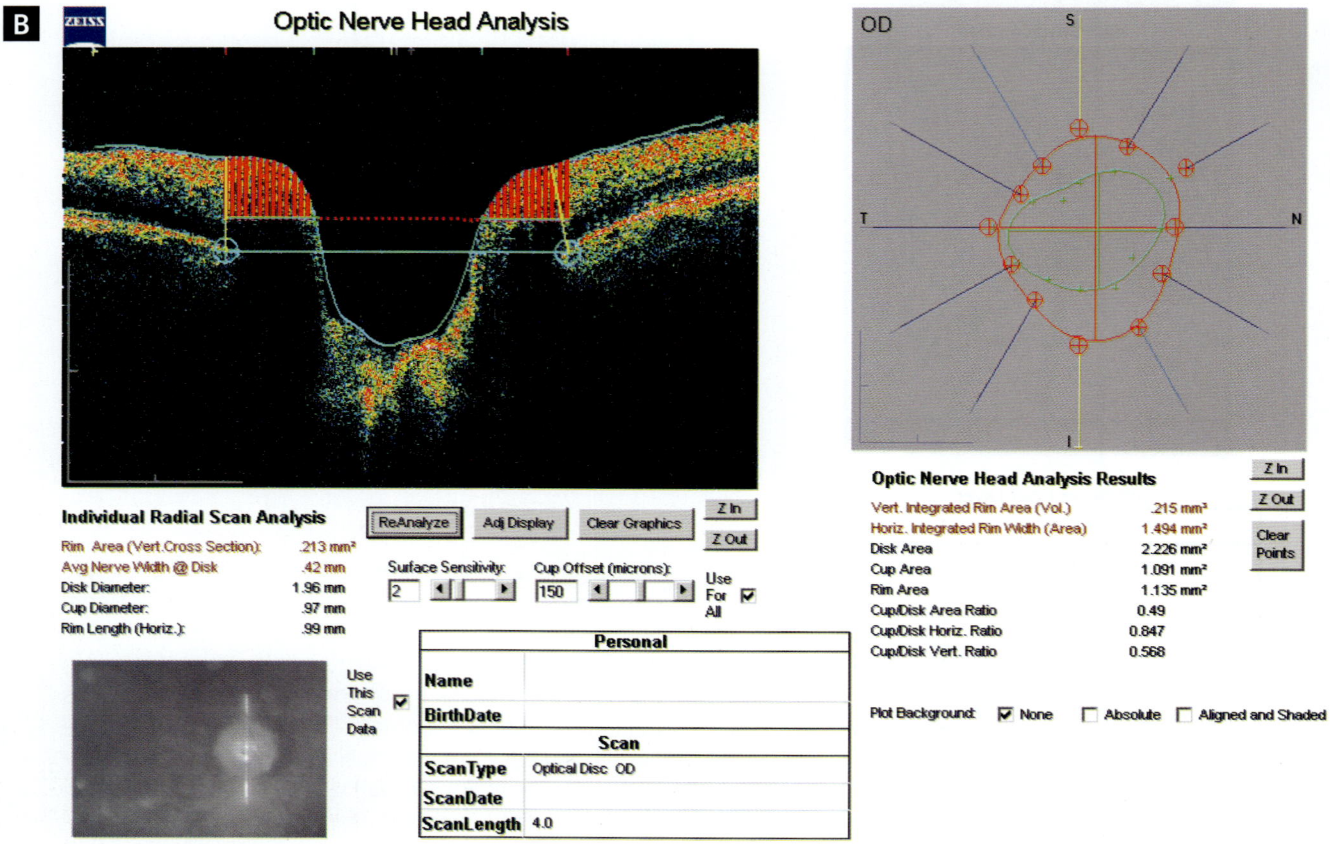

C

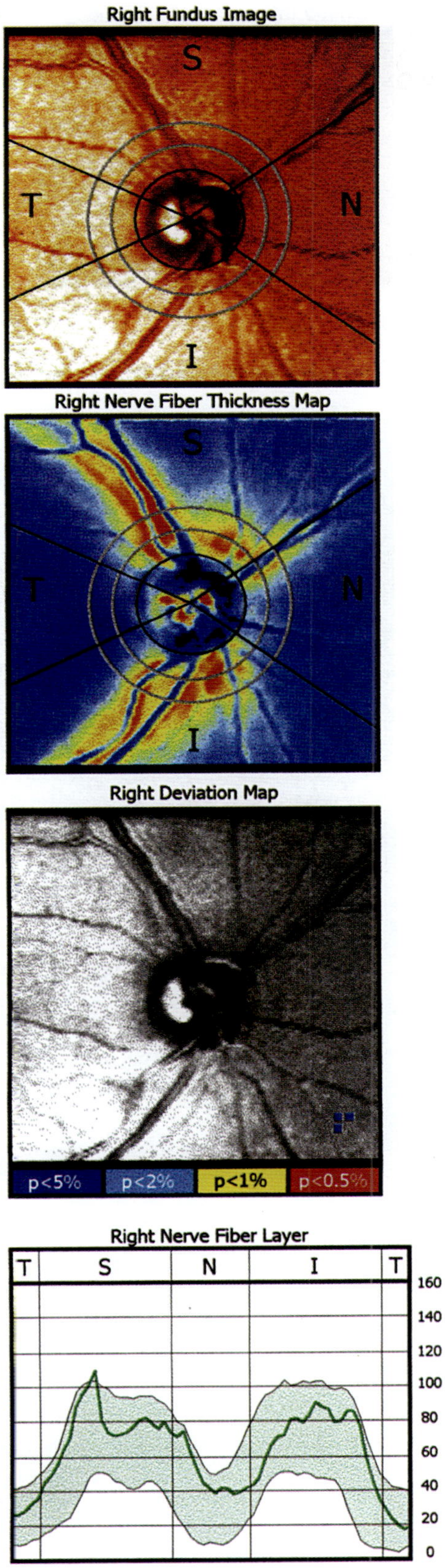

D

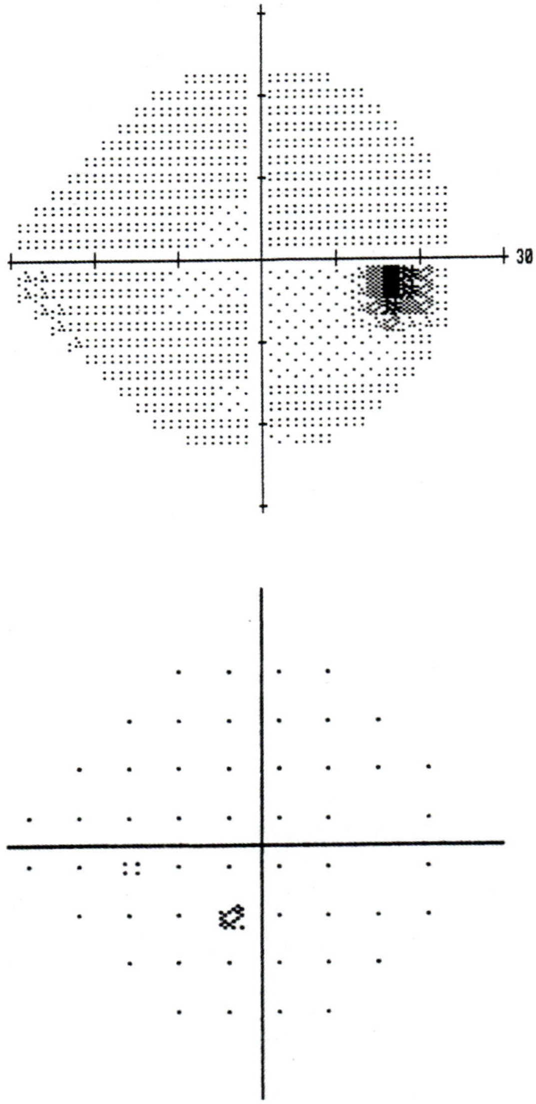

Patient 60-year-old with large optic discs and large cuppings without corresponding increase of intraocular pressure. A. Optical Coherence Tomography shows a normal mean thickness of the nerve fiber layer (115μm). B. Optic disc C/D ratio in the horizontal axis is 0.85 and in the vertical 0.57 and the vertical optic disc diameter is 1.96mm. C, D. Visual fields and Scanning Laser Polarimetry don't reveal any particular alteration.

BIG OPTIC DISC WITH LARGE CUPPING

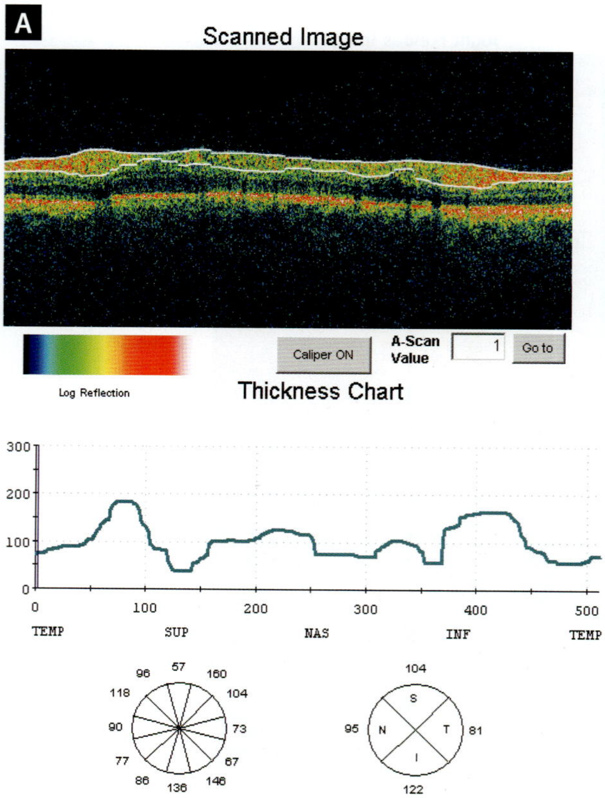

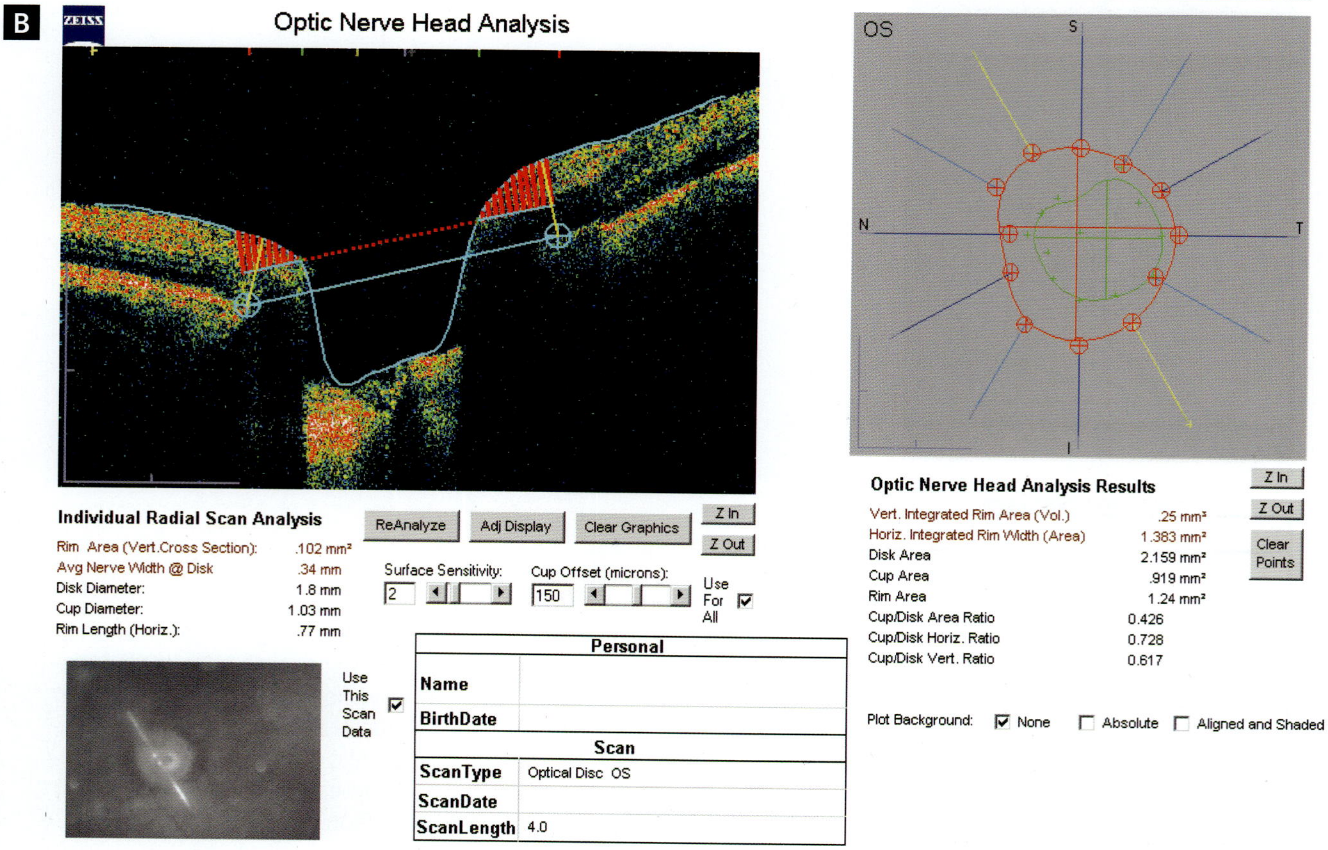

C

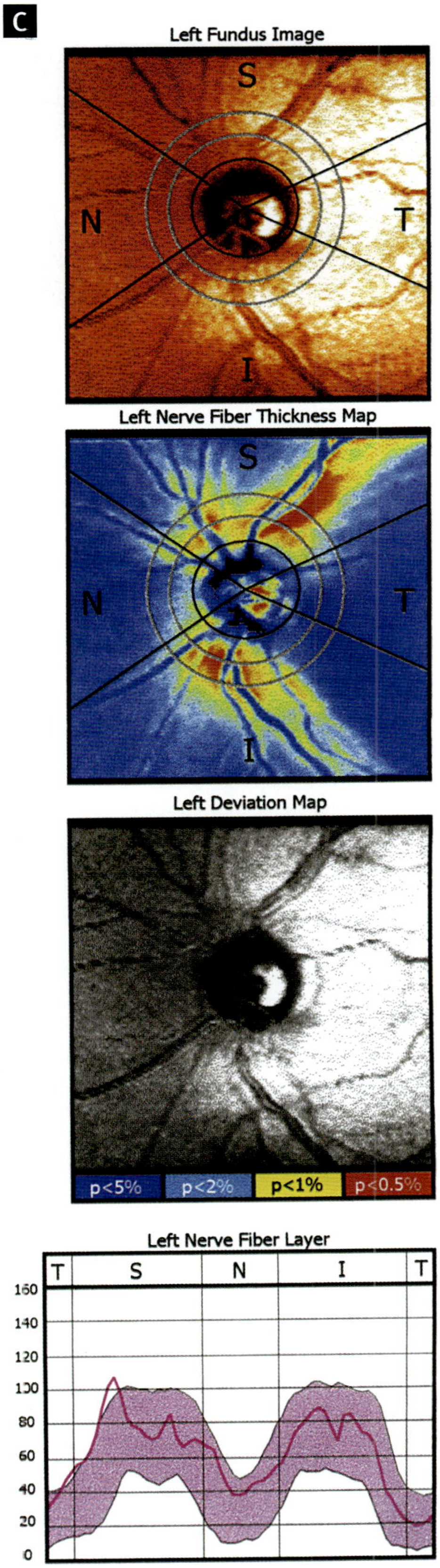

D

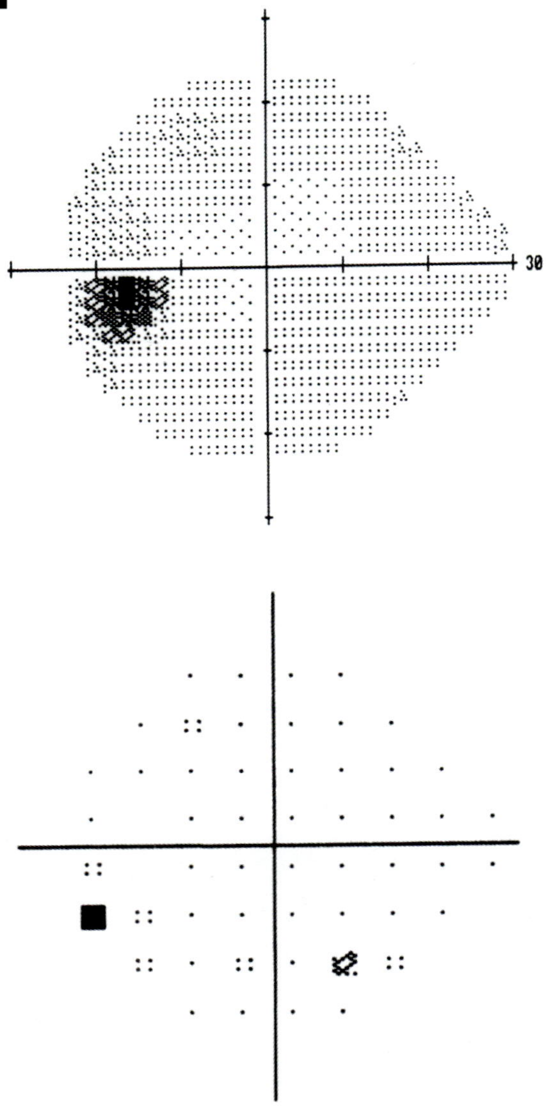

The other eye of the same patient (page 344). A. Optical Coherence Tomography shows a normal mean nerve fibre layer thickness (105μm). B. Optic disc C/D ratio in the horizontal axis is 0.73 and in the vertical 0.62 with optic disc diameter of 1.80mm. In this patient with large optic discs and increased cuppings, Optical Coherence Tomography findings are in agreement with those of visual fields and Scanning Laser Polarimetry. C, D. Visual fields and Scanning Laser Polarimetry don't show any particular alteration.

OCULAR HYPERTENSION

A

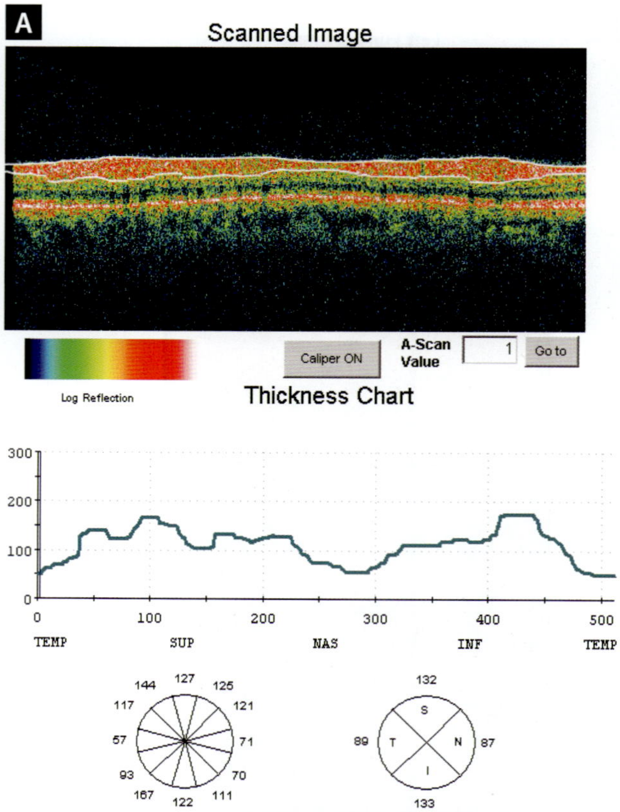

B

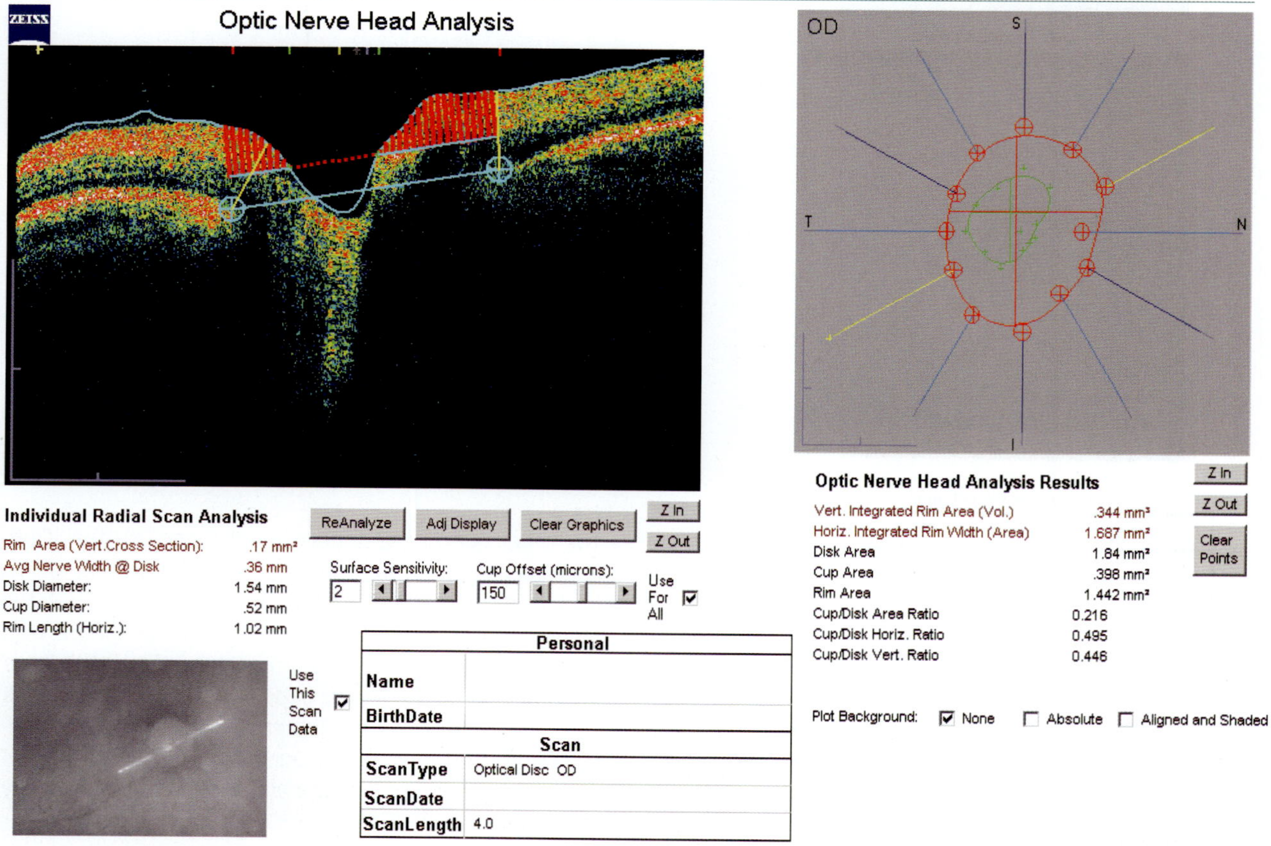

C

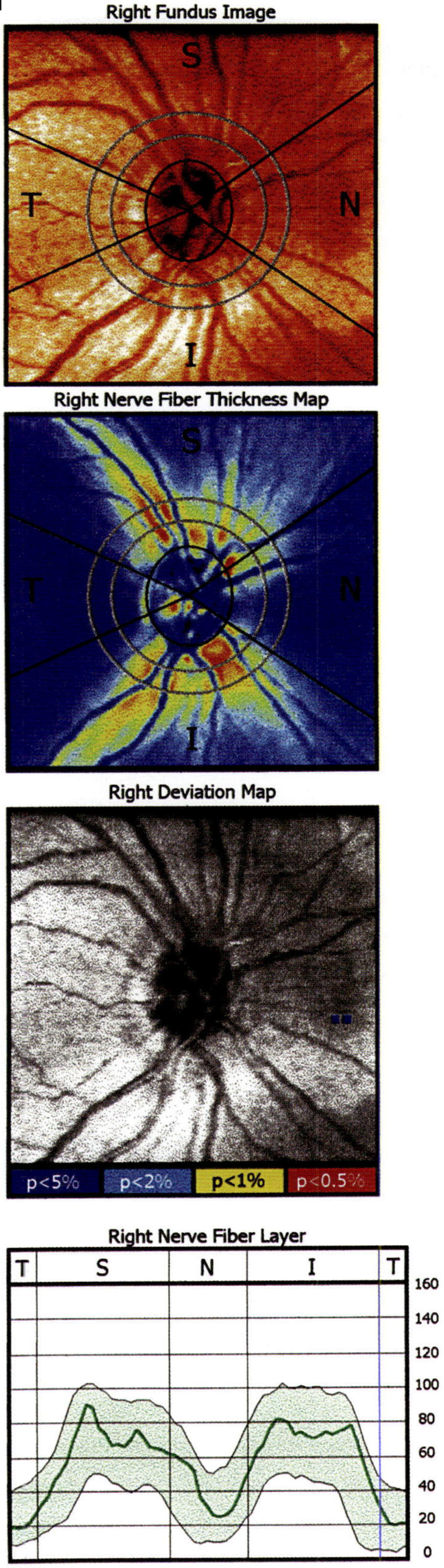

D

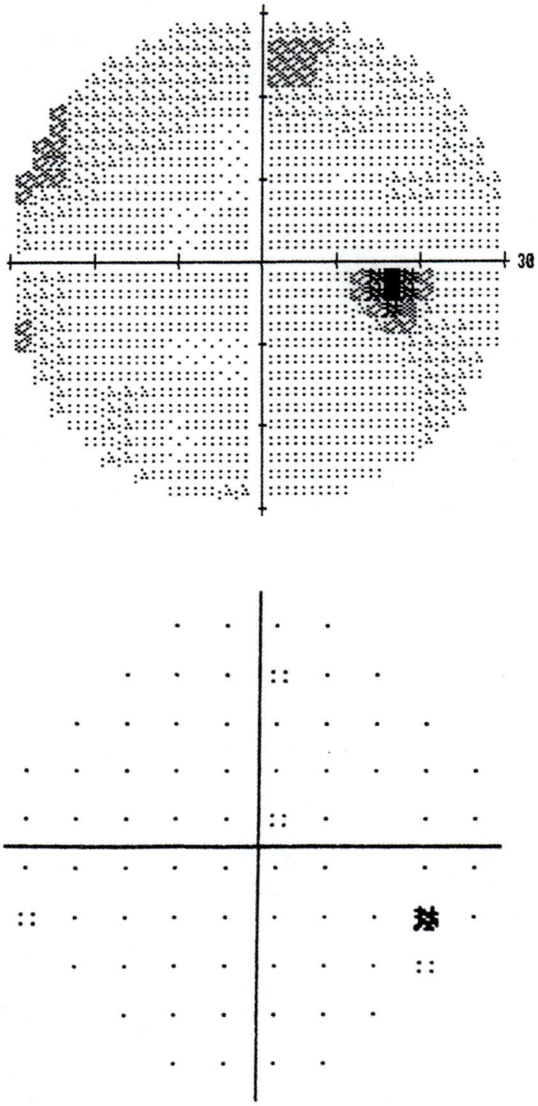

Patient 71-year-old with ocular hypertension. A. Optical Coherence Tomography shows a mean thickness of nerve fiber layer (112μm) within normal limits. B. Optic disc C/D ratio in the horizontal axis is 0.5 and in the vertical 0.45. C, D. Visual fields and Scanning Laser Polarimetry don't reveal any particular alteration.

OCULAR HYPERTENSION

A

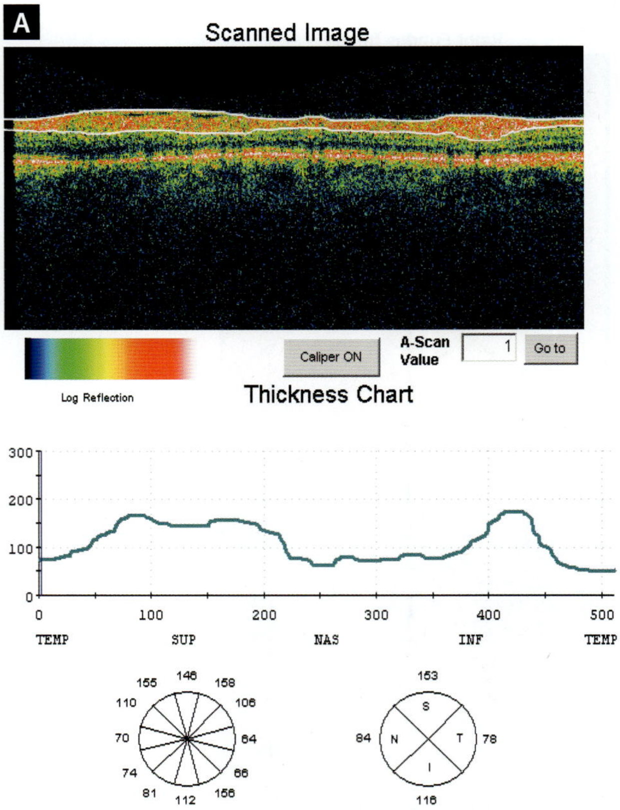

B

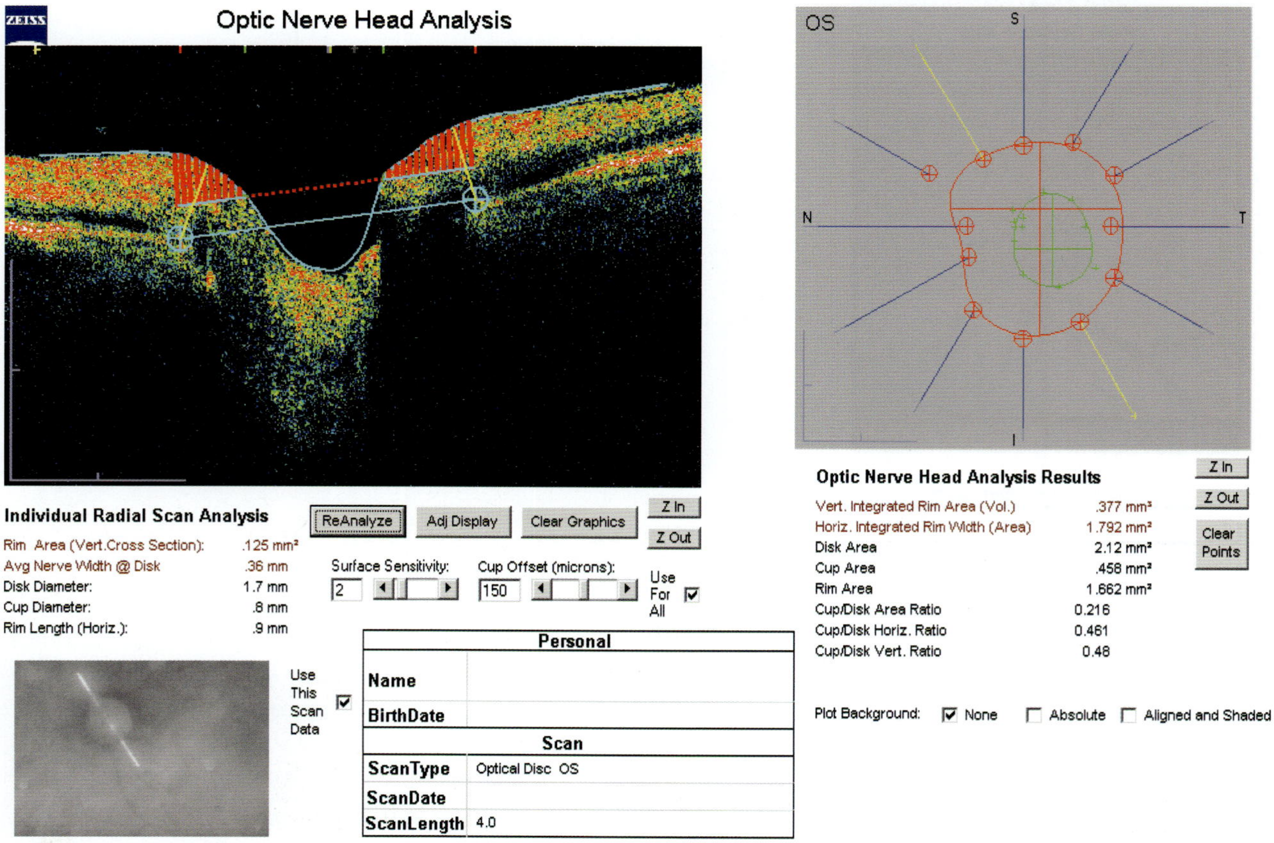

C

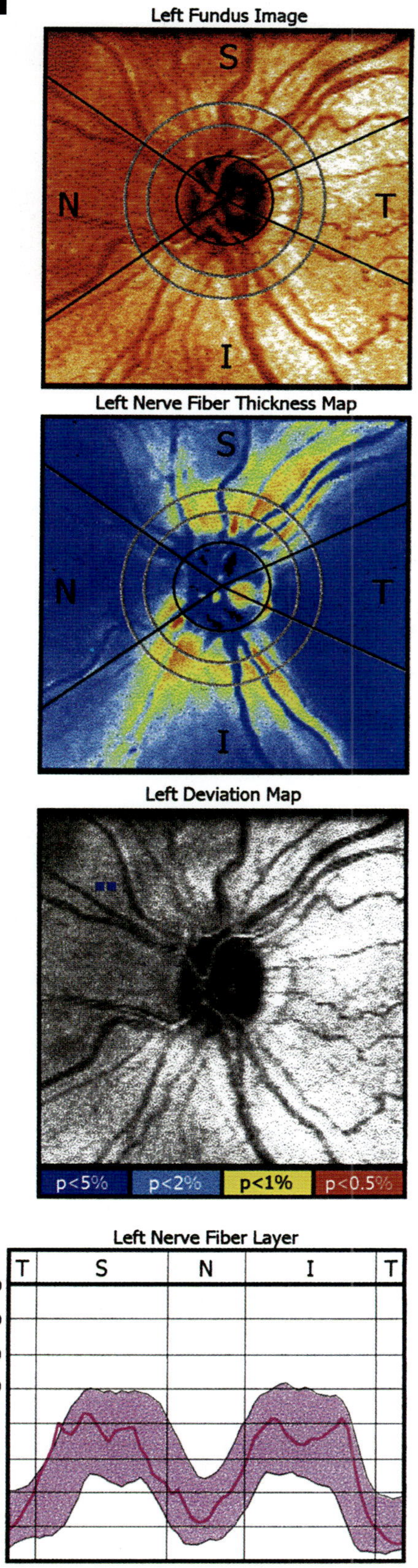

D

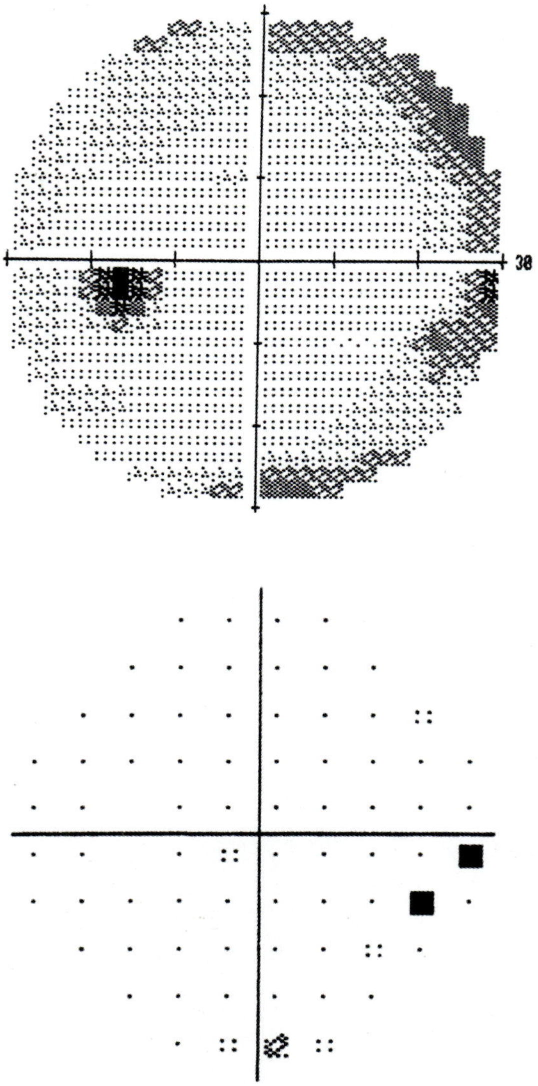

The other eye of the same patient (page 348). A. Optical Coherence Tomography shows a mean nerve fibre layer thickness (108μm) within normal limits. B. Optic disc C/D ratio in the horizontal axis is 0.46 and in the vertical 0.48. Optical Coherence Tomography shows that this patient doesn't have any early glaucoma changes. C, D. Visual fields and Scanning Laser Polarimetry are normal.

OCULAR HYPERTENSION

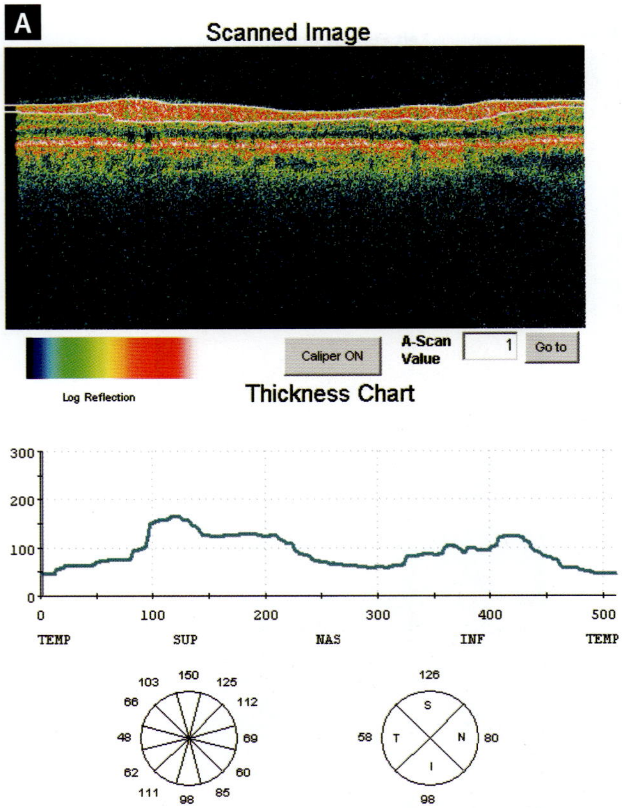

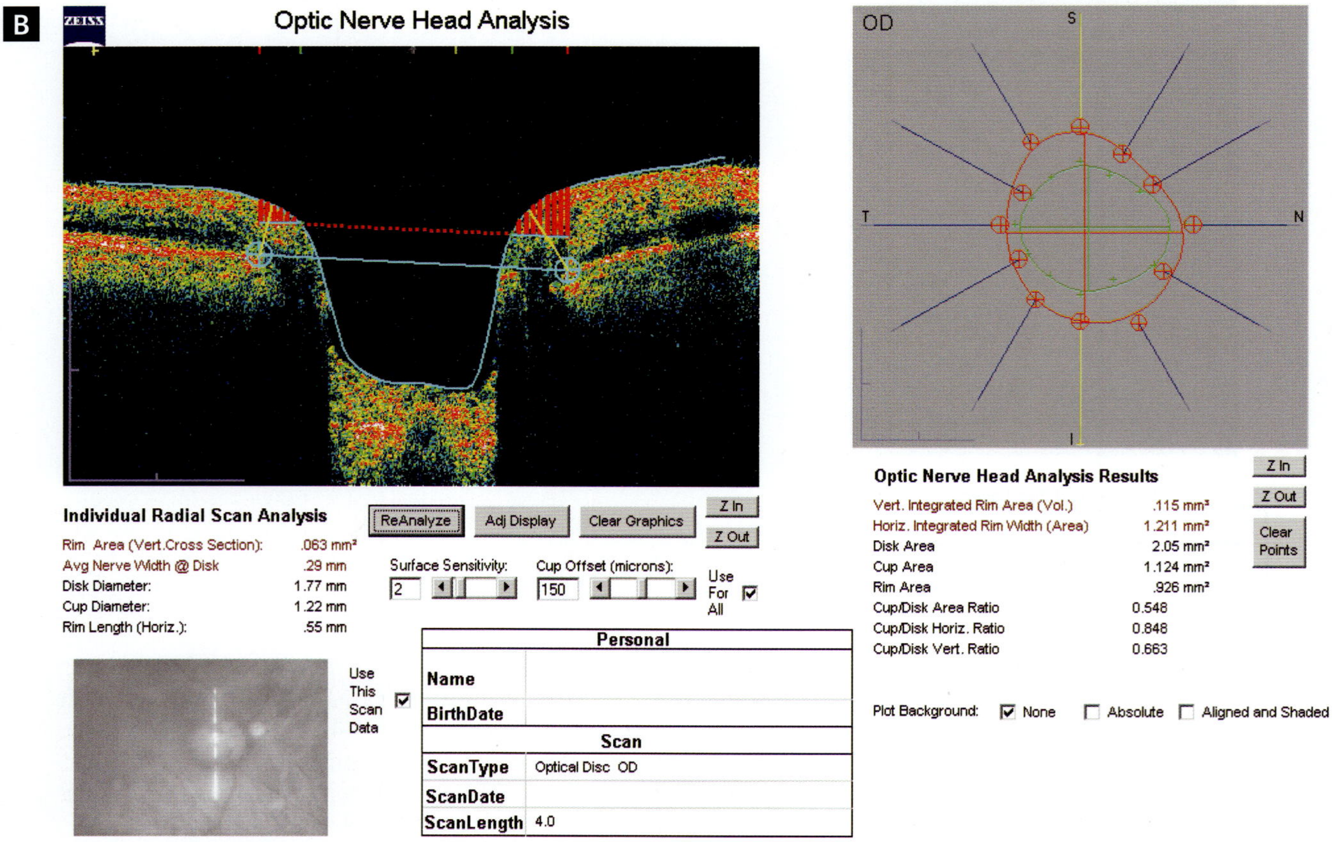

C

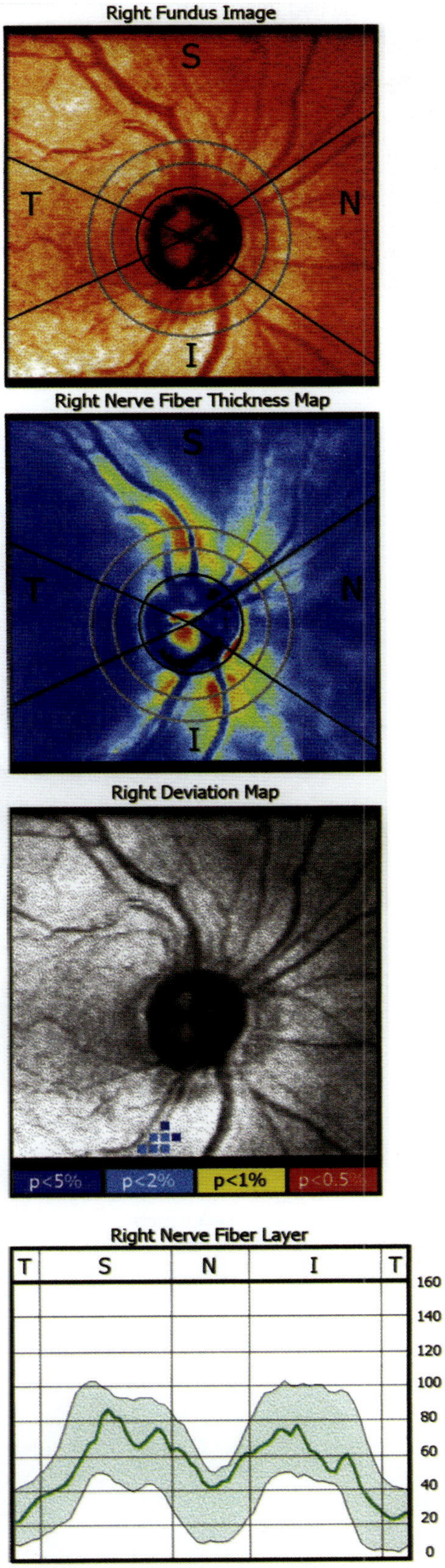

D

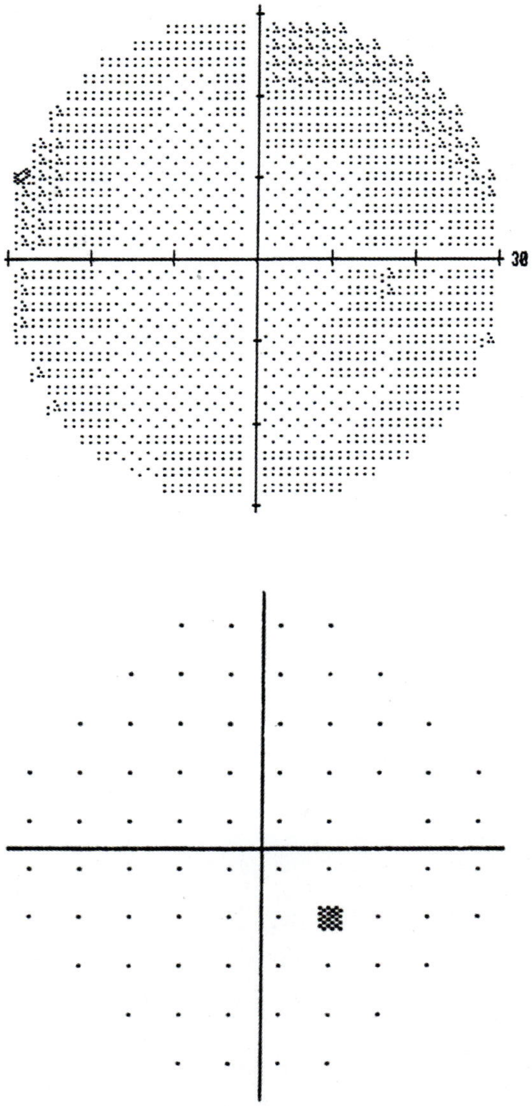

Patient 67-year-old with ocular hypertension and increased optic disc cupping. A. Optical Coherence Tomography shows a mean thickness of nerve fiber layer 90μm. B. Optic disc C/D ratio in the horizontal axis is 0.85 and in the vertical 0.65. C, D. Visual fields and Scanning Laser Polarimetry don't reveal any particular alteration.

OCULAR HYPERTENSION

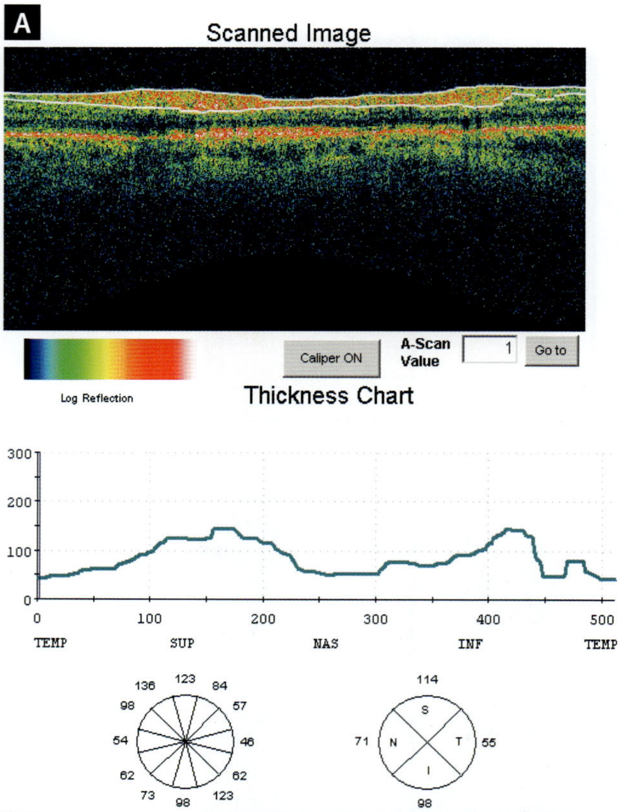

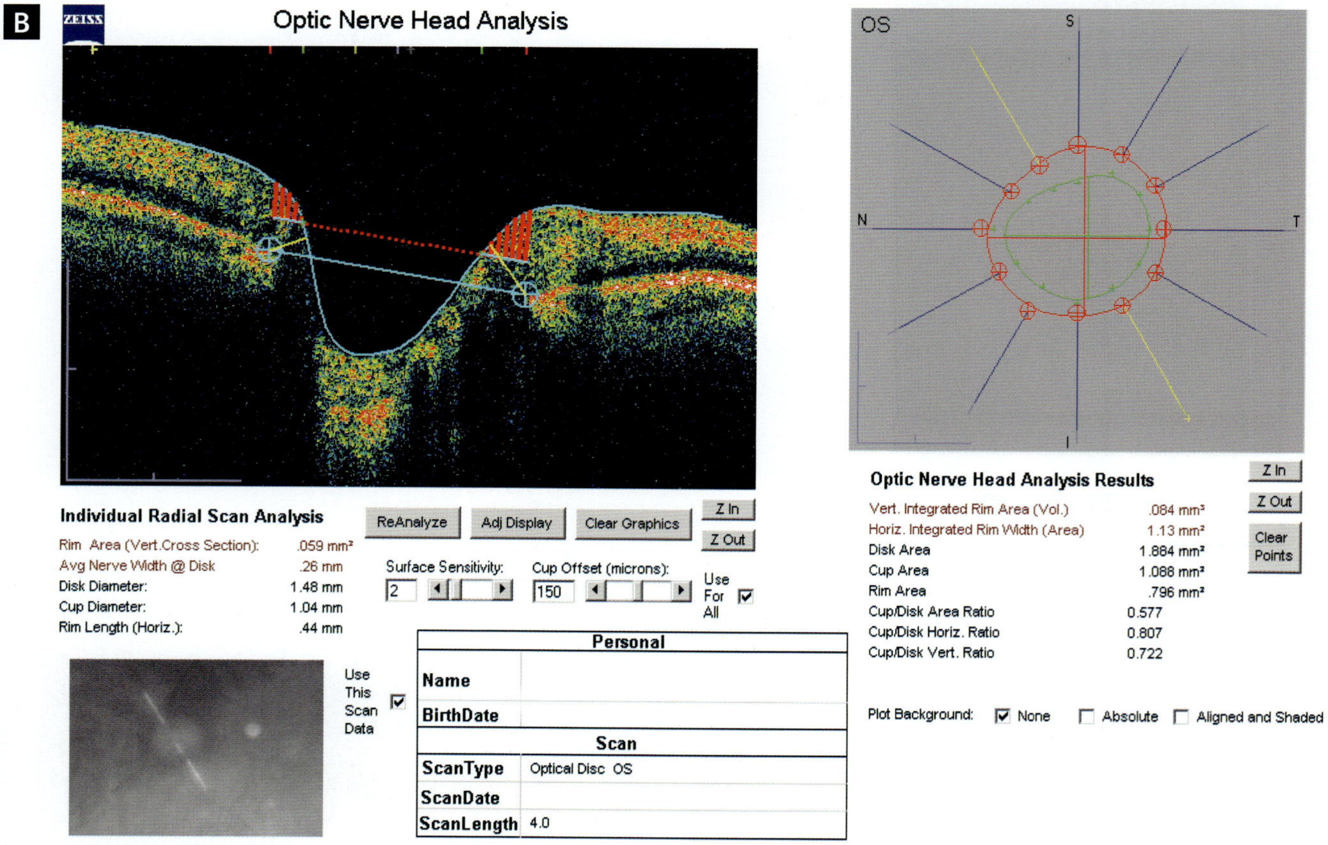

C

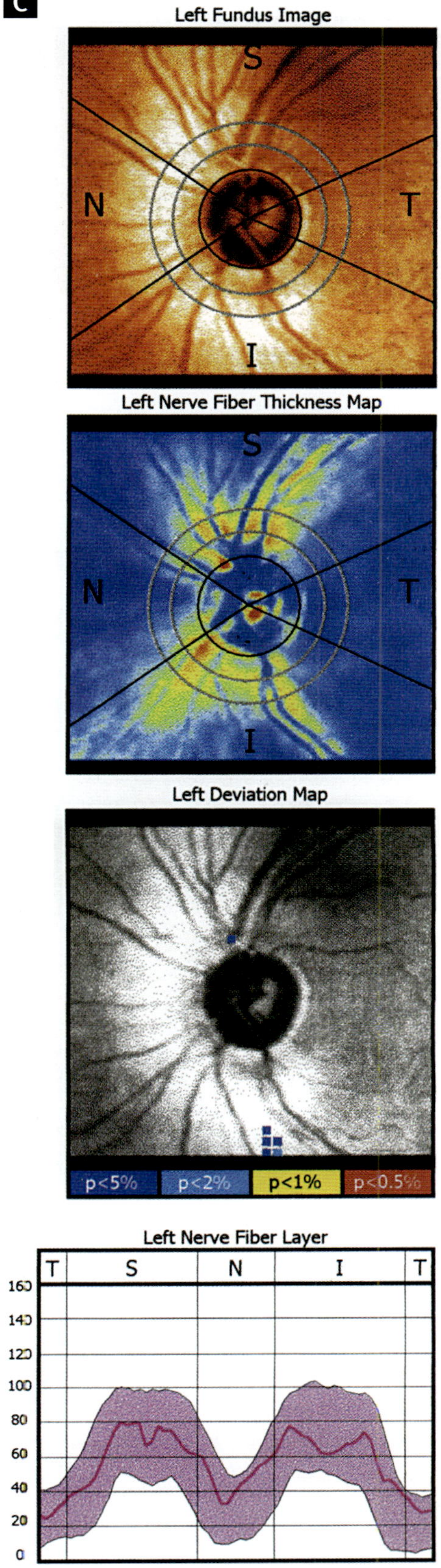

D

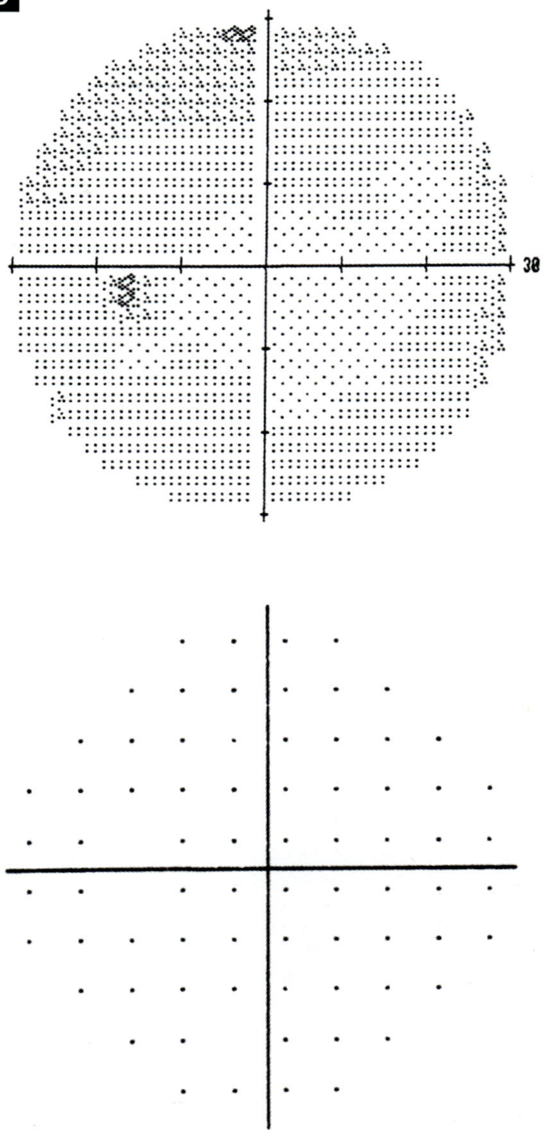

The other eye of the same patient (page 352). A. Optical Coherence Tomography shows a borderline mean nerve fibre layer thickness (84μm). B. Optic disc C/D ratio in the horizontal axis is 0.80 and in the vertical 0.72. Contrary to the previous patient, detection of a decreased nerve fiber layer thickness in the left eye renders necessary the regular control of this patient and possibly the initiation of treatment. C, D. Visual fields and Scanning Laser Polarimetry are normal.

TILTED OPTIC DISC

A

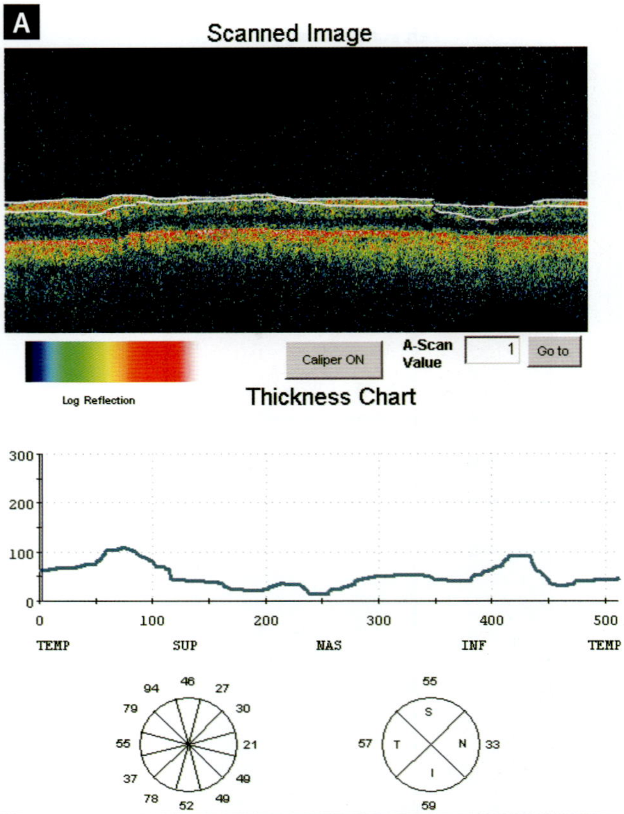

B

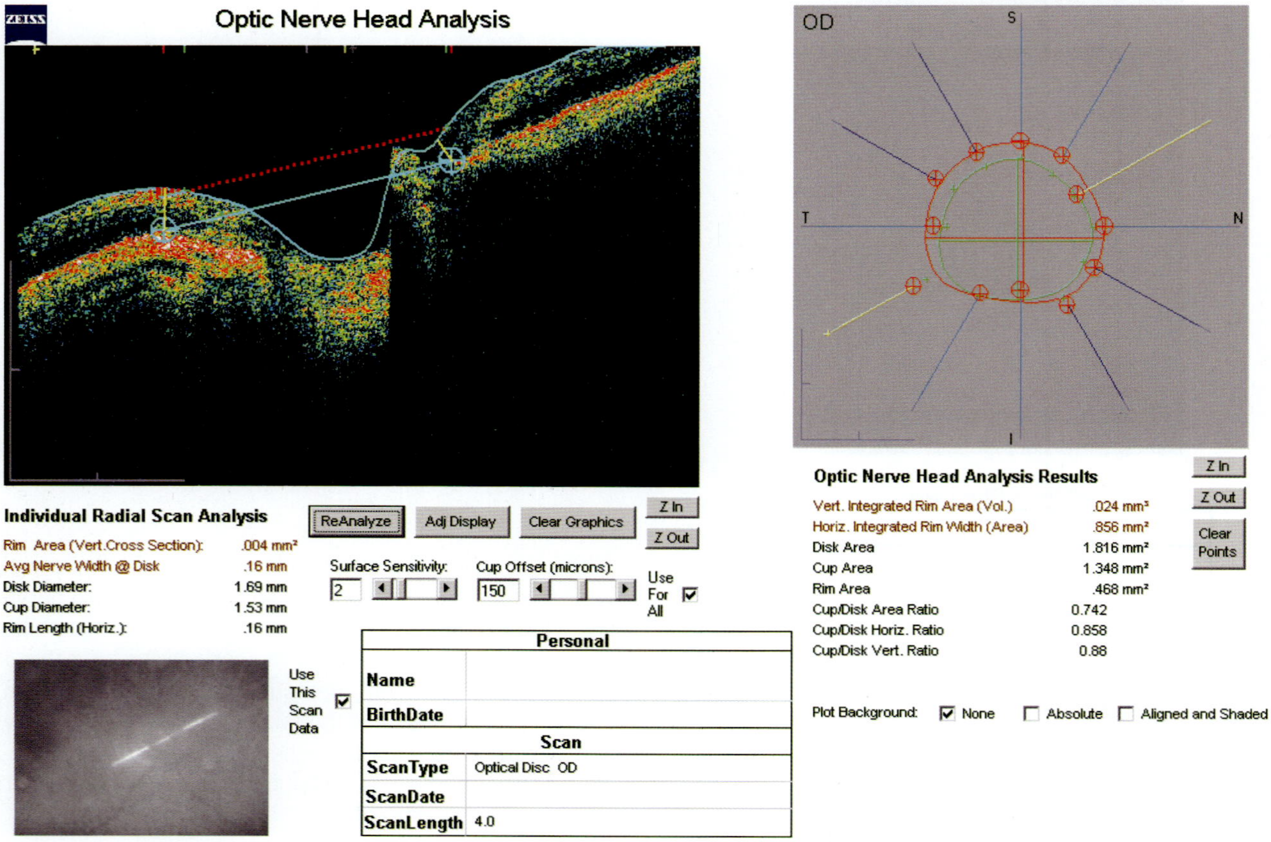

C

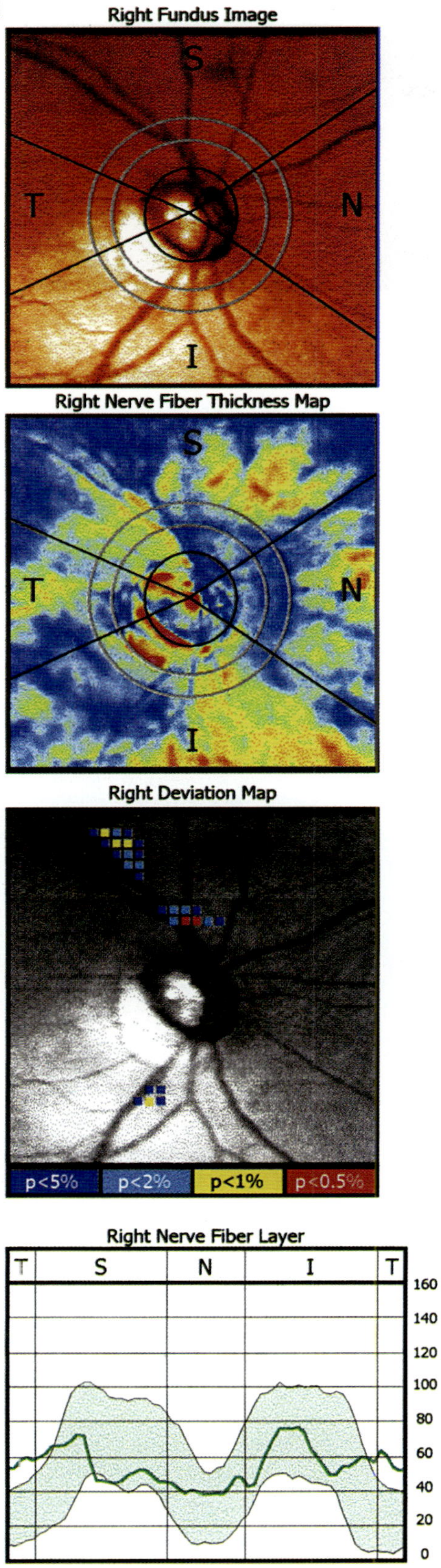

D

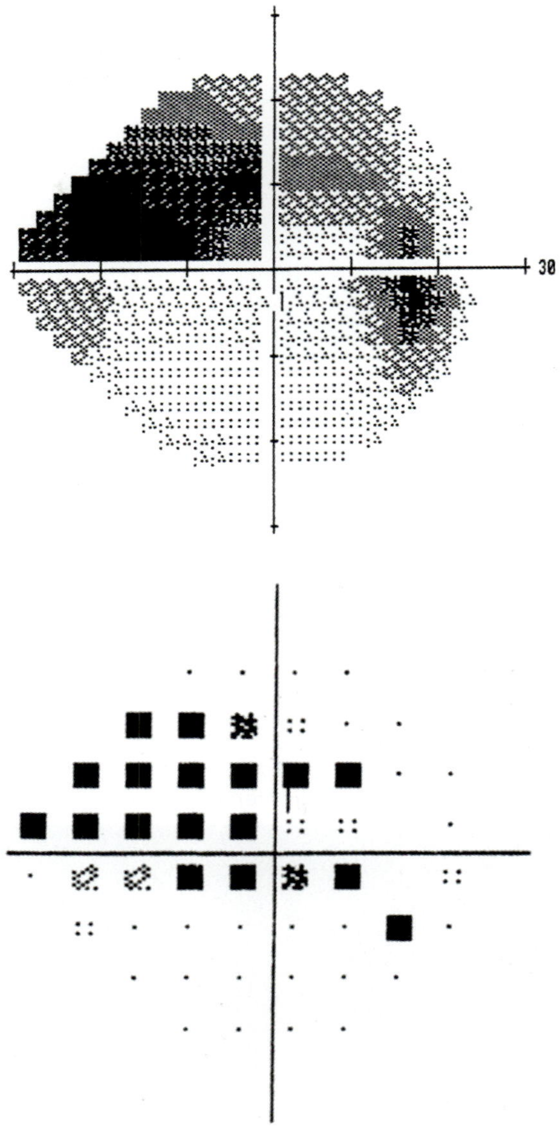

Patient 69-year-old with tilted optic discs and increased intraocular pressures. A. Optical Coherence Tomography shows a decrease of the mean thickness of the nerve fiber layer (48μm). B. Optic disc C/D ratio in the horizontal axis is 0.86 and in the vertical 0.88. C. Scanning Laser Polarimetry shows a mild decrease of nerve fiber layer in the superior quadrant. D. Visual fields show a large scotoma in the superior nasal quadrant.

TILTED OPTIC DISC

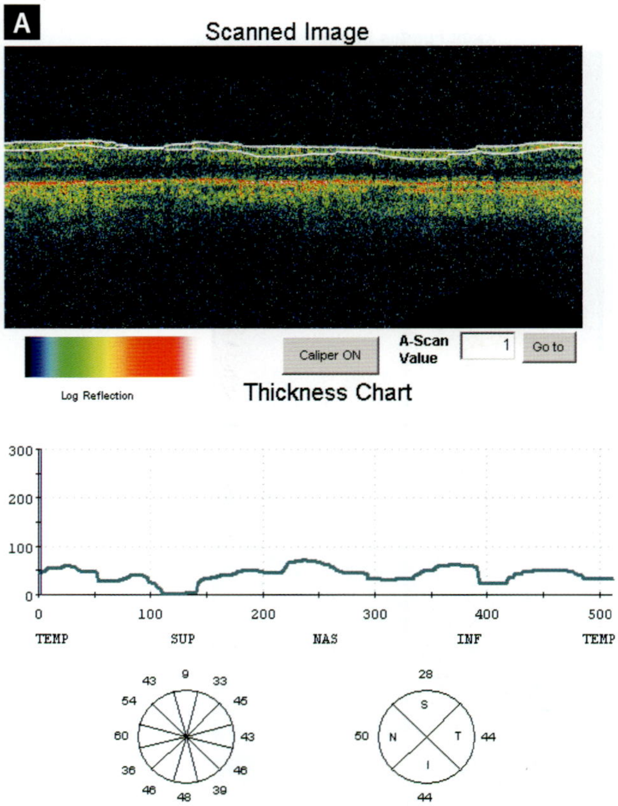

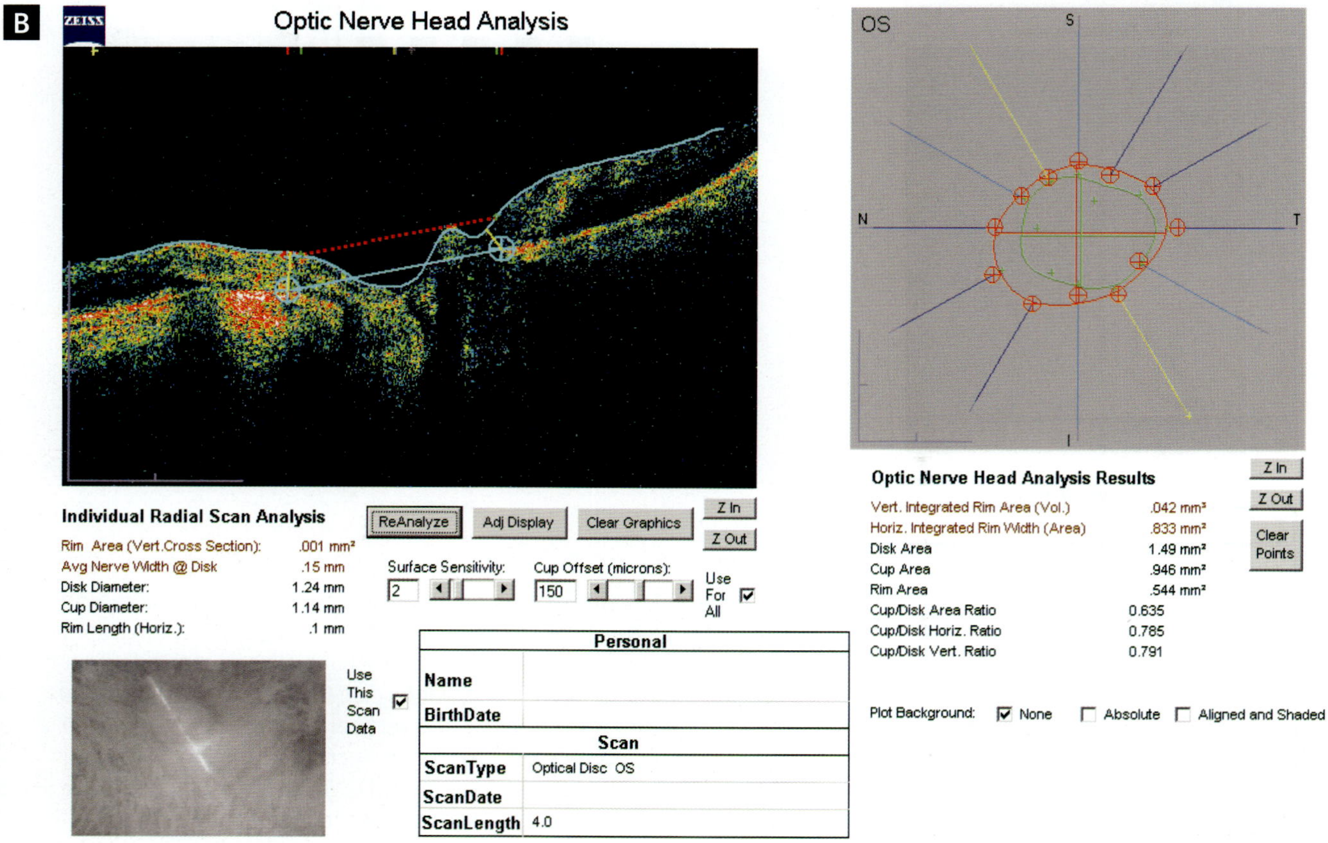

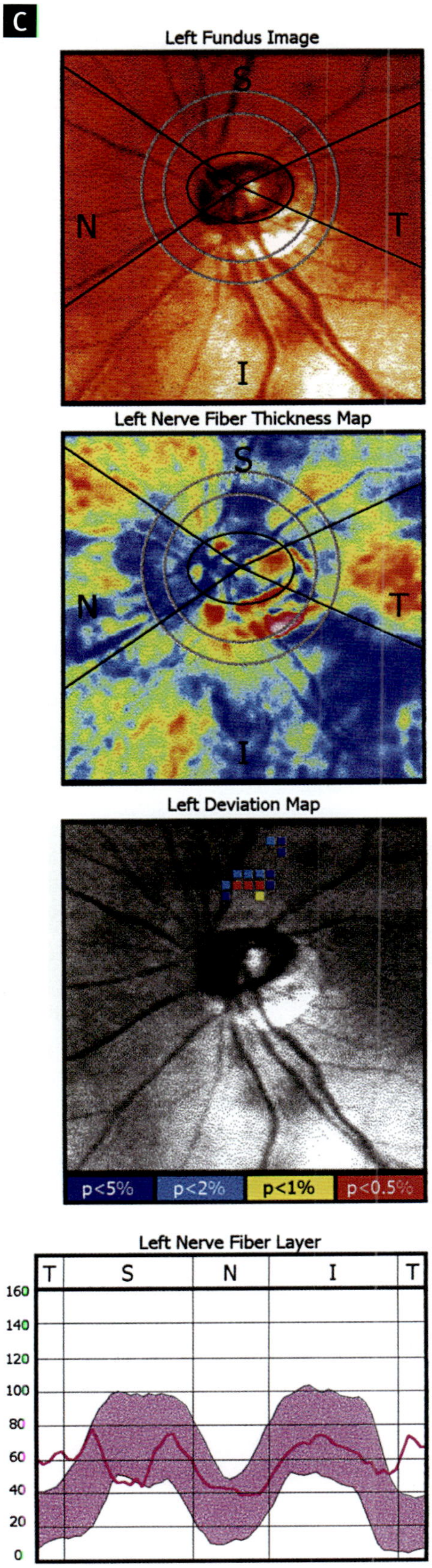

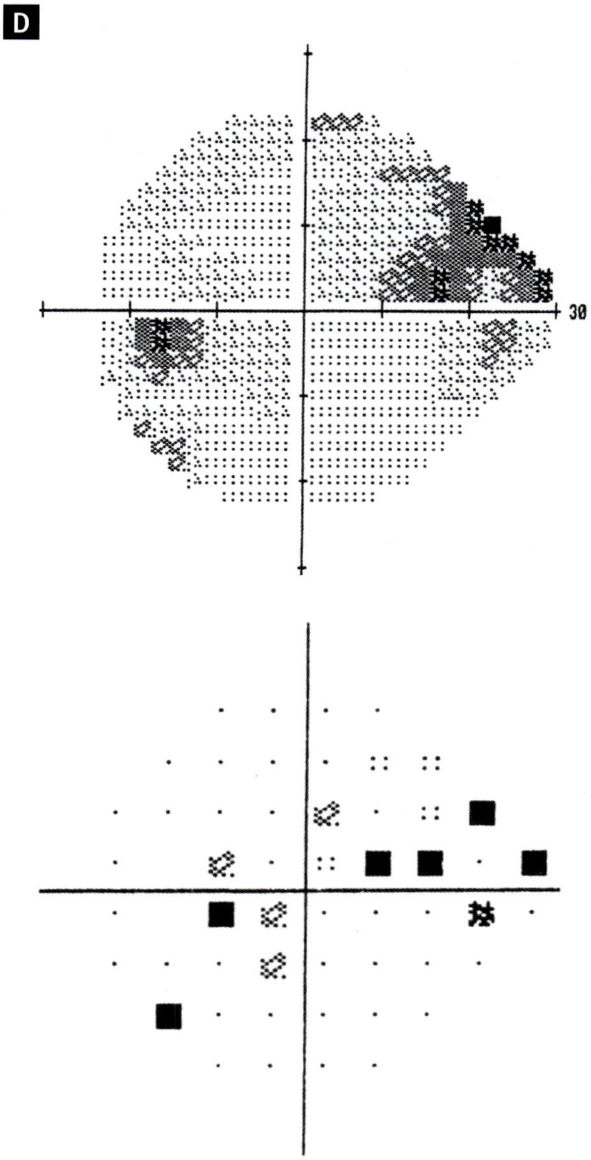

The other eye of the same patient (page 356). A. Optical Coherence Tomography shows a decrease of the mean nerve fibre layer thickness (39μm). B. Optic disc C/D ratio in the horizontal and vertical axis is 0.79. In patients with tilted optic discs there may be scotomas in the visual fields and a difficulty in cupping estimation. In this particular patient the detection of decreased nerve fiber layer thickness in Optical Coherence Tomography renders necessary the initiation of treatment. C. Scanning Laser Polarimetry shows a mild decrease of nerve fiber layer thickness in the superior quadrant. D. Visual fields show a small scotoma in the superior nasal quadrant (nasal step).

CHAPTER 15

LATEST ADVANCES IN OPTICAL COHERENCE TOMOGRAPHY

SERGIOS TALIANTZIS

Since its introduction in 1996, Optical Coherence Tomography technology has undergone multiple generations of improvement. The third generation commercial Optical Coherence Tomography instrument, was launched in 2002. It used a technique that is now generally referred to as Time Domain Optical Coherence Tomography, since an A-scan or depth profile is acquired by scanning a mirror in the reference arm as a function of time[1]. In this technique the reference arm of a Michelson interferometer is rapidly scanned over the cross-sectional imaging depth.

High-speed ultrahigh resolution Optical Coherence Tomography imaging technology using Fourier/spectral detection has several advantages, including improved image quality, resolution of 1 to 5 μm and up to 100-fold increased speed. In general, for a given acquisition time, high-speed imaging can increase the number of cross-sectional images acquired in a sequence to improve retinal coverage[2].

The acquired image, having almost 2 μm axial resolution and 2048 axial scans, is performed in 0.13 seconds. The higher resolution and greater number of transverse pixels in the high-speed ultra high-resolution Optical Coherence Tomography image improves the visualization of the internal retinal structures (figure 1).

Increased imaging speed enables the accurate topography of the optic nerve head to be presented, thus minimizing eye motion artifacts. In addition it

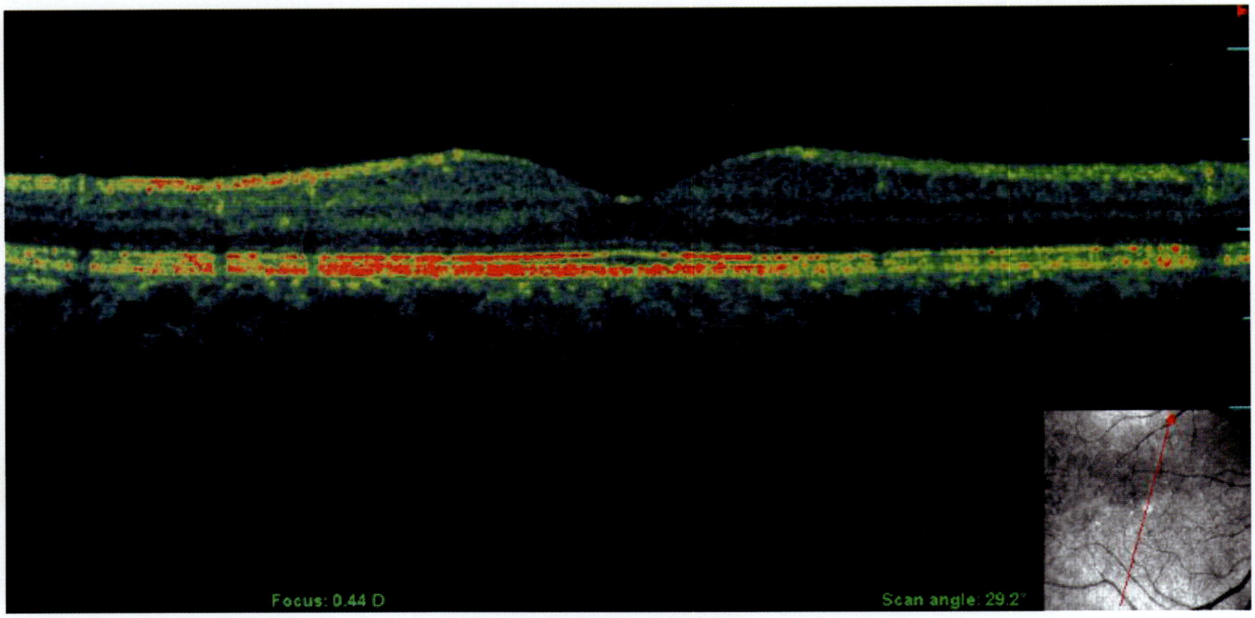

Fig. 1. Retinal structure scanned with Scanning Laser Opthalmoscopy Optical Coherence Tomography.

enables the acquisition of complete 3D datasets[3-6]. Fourier domain or spectral detection technique is a novel technique, that enables imaging speeds of ~25,000 axial scans per second, about 50 times faster than time-domain detection. Spectral/Fourier domain detection uses low-coherence interferometry to detect light echoes by using a spectrometer and a high-speed charge-coupled device camera to measure the interference spectrum.

Different echo time delays of light produce different frequencies of fringes in the interference spectrum. Therefore, axial scan information can be measured by taking the Fourier transform (a Fourier transform is a mathematical operation that extracts the frequency content of a signal). Spectral/Fourier domain detection essentially measures all echoes of light simultaneously rather than sequentially as in time-domain detection. Therefore, it enables a dramatic improvement in sensitivity and imaging speed. Because Optical Coherence Tomography with Spectral/Fourier domain detection can measure all echoes of light from different delays simultaneously, it has an enormous speed and sensitivity advantage compared to Optical Coherence Tomography using standard detection[7-10].

Several manufacturers have introduced new Optical Coherence Tomography systems to the market. A partial list of manufacturers of Optical Coherence Tomography systems based on Spectral/Fourier domain detection includes:

- Cirrus HD-Optical Coherence Tomography (Carl Zeiss Meditec).
- Spectralis Heidelberg Retina Analyzer + Optical Coherence Tomography (Heidelberg Engineering).
- Optical Coherence Tomography / Scanning Laser Ophthalmoscope (Ophthalmic Technologies).
- S Optical Coherence Tomography Copernicus (Optopol Technology).
- RTVue-100 (Optovue).
- 3D Optical Coherence Tomography-1000 (Topcon Medical Systems).

These instruments have similar specifications with axial image resolutions in the 5 to 7 μm range, transversal resolution in the 12 to 20 μm and acquisition speeds in the 20,000 to 40,000 axial scans per second range. All are based on Spectral/Fourier domain detection and all of the instruments have similar capabilities in terms of 3-D imaging. Differences are found in imaging protocols and analysis software. Each of these instruments promises to provide improved integration of clinical diagnostic imaging. Some combine diagnostic modalities such as fundus photography, laser angiography or scanning laser ophthalmoscopy with Optical Coherence Tomography scans; others allow the importing of infrared, autofluorescence, fluorescein angiography and indocyanine green angiography images for direct comparison with Optical Coherence Tomography images. The next generation of Optical Coherence Tomography has arrived along with dramatically increased image-acquisition speeds and the

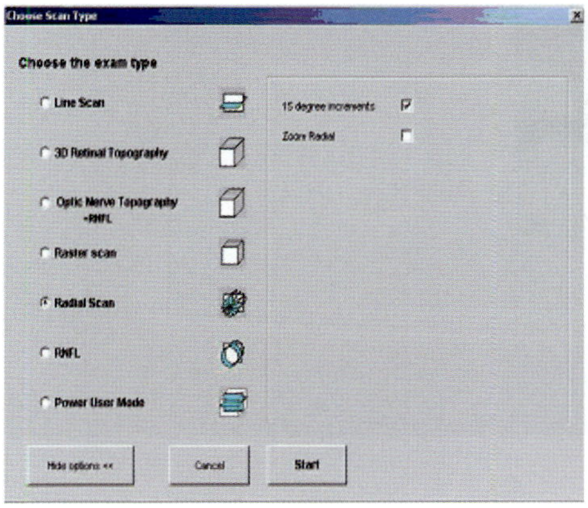

Fig. 2. Optical Coherence Tomography scanning modes

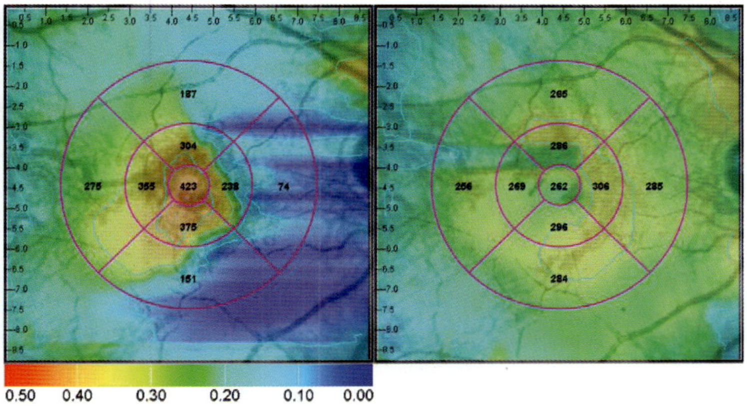

Fig. 3. 3D topography map "compare"

promise of improved diagnostics[11-14].

The Spectral Optical Coherence Tomography channel analyzes retinal structures by measuring the time delay of light that is backscattered from different micro-structural layers in the retina. It produces cross-sectional images (B-Scan) of the vitreoretinal interface and retina.

The user can select from the following Optical Coherence Tomography scanning modes: Line Scan (B-Scan) Optical Coherence Tomography, Raster Optical Coherence Tomography Line Scan, Radial Optical Coherence Tomography Line Scan, 3D Retinal Topography, Optic Nerve Topography and Circular retinal nerve fiber layer scan (figure 2).

In the B-scan Optical Coherence Tomography mode the image may be presented in different ways: either of the same size as the Optical Coherence Tomography image, side by side or of much smaller size, to allow most of the display resolution to be allocated to the B-scan Optical Coherence Tomography image.

Three-dimensional Retinal Topography Analyze after the 3D topographic captured dataset can be viewed and analyzed through a number of methods:

1) The "Analyze" 3D Topography displays a 3D Topographic Map with Retinal Thickness (measured between the vitreoretinal interface and the retinal pigment epithelium).

2) 3D Topography maps "compare": compares two topography examinations of the same patient of the same eye (figure 3).

3) 3D tomography – tomography explore: allows the user to view and assess the 3D dataset in different methods (figure 4) and can transform 3D topographic data display into a 3D tomographic data. It can also remove layers from the retina. The user can also generate C-scan images (Time Domain Only) from the 3-D tomographic map cutting through the 3D Topographic volume in a Coronal direction (figure 5).

4) 3D optic nerve head analysis. After 3D topographic dataset is captured and saved, it can be viewed and analyzed through several different methods.

Using analyze for the optic nerve the software will automatically measure the following parameters: disk area, cup area, rim area, cup/disk area ratio, mean cup depth, max cup depth.

The software can also automatically analyze the retinal nerve fiber layer thickness and volume of the region and data can be compared for changes over time (figure 6).

The compare and explore features can be used with the 3D Optic Nerve data in the same way as with the 3D Retinal Topography.

5) Retinal nerve fiber layer Thickness Map display. The retinal nerve fiber layer Thickness Map is displayed below the Optical Coherence Tomography image, (thickness indicated in microns), starting at the temporal point through the superior, nasal inferior and finishing back at the temporal point (figure7).

Using the new technology Spectral Domaine Optical Coherence Tomography various diseases are presented (figure 8).

The main commercial instruments of Spectral Domaine Optical Coherence Tomography and their characteristics are the following:

1. Cirrus HD-Optical Coherence Tomography by Carl

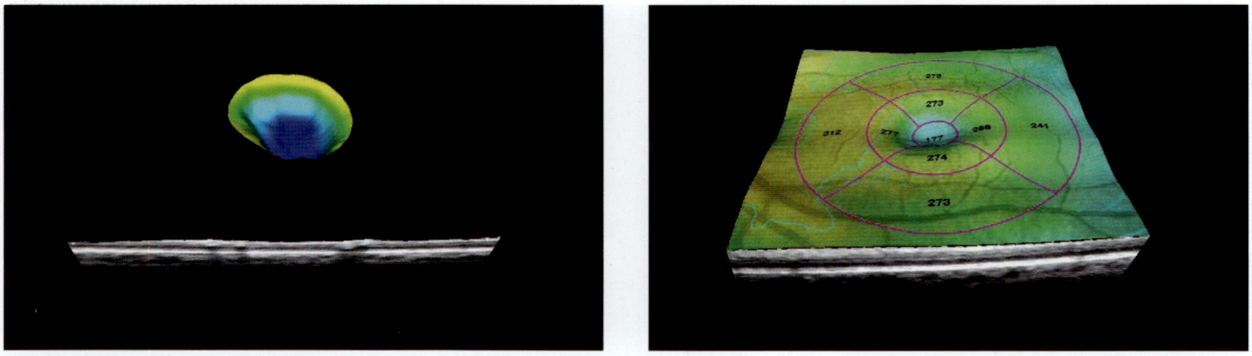

Fig. 4. 3D topography

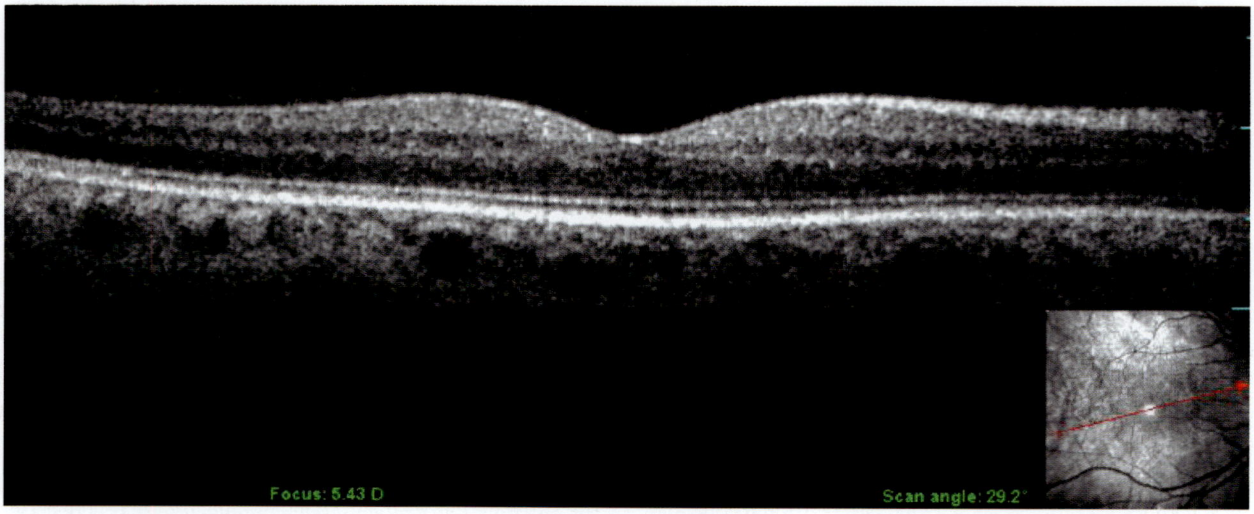

Fig. 5.

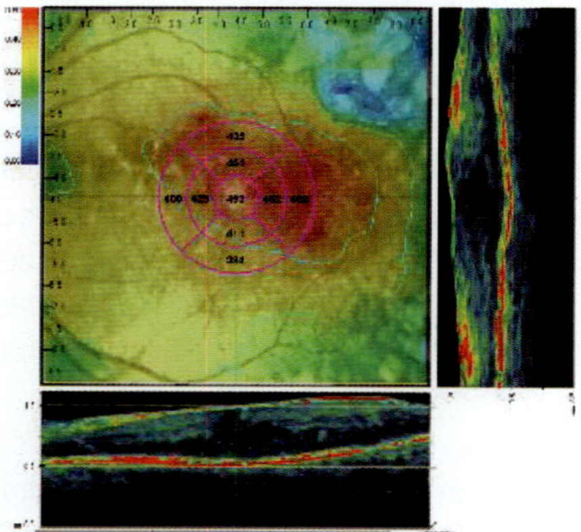

	Avg thick μ	Volume μL
Center	453	
Center circle	453	0.34
Superior inner	454	0.341
Temporal inner	462	0.364
Inferior inner	411	0.309
Nasal inner	420	0.328
Superior outer	435	0.595
Temporal outer	462	0.643
Inferior outer	384	0.528
Nasal outer	400	0.557
Totals	428	3.993

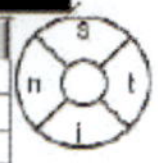

Fig. 6.

Zeiss Meditec provides axial cross-sectional and 3-D imaging and measurement of posterior ocular structures, including the retina, the retinal nerve fiber layer, the macula and the optic disc using an optical source of superluminescent diode.

2. RTVue-100 by Optovue provides complete nerve head analysis for glaucoma diagnosis in 0.35 seconds, full retinal, inner retinal and outer retinal thickness maps & metrics and internal limiting membrane and retinal pigment epithelium elevation maps and metrics.

3. Spectralis Family by Heidelberg Engineering (Spectralis Heidelberg Retina Analyzer + Optical Coherence Tomography and Spectralis IR + Optical Coherence Tomography) combines spectral Optical Coherence Tomography with angiography. Spectralis Optical Coherence Tomography offers two imaging modes (Spectral Domain-Optical Coherence Tomography and Infrared), while the Spectralis Heidelberg Retina Analyzer+Optical Coherence Tomography includes

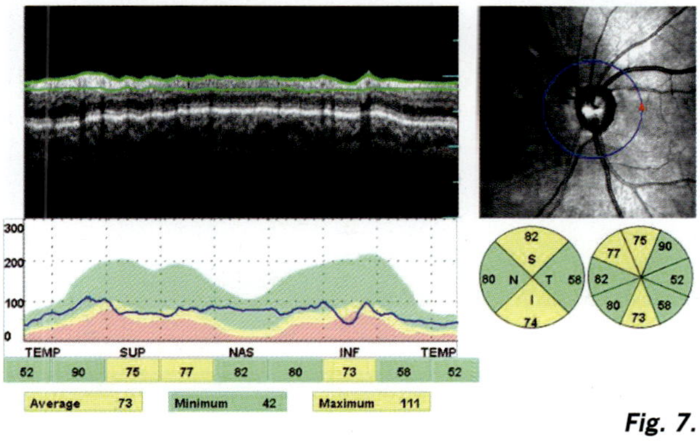

Fig. 7.

four additional imaging modes (autofluorescence, red free imaging, fluorescein angiography and ICG angiography).

4. Spectral Optical Coherence Tomography/Scanning Laser Ophthalmoscope by OTI uses a light generated from an infrared broadband Super Luminescent Diode. The confocal scanning ophthalmoscope and high-resolution Optical Coherence Tomography obtains images through the same optics for pixel-to-pixel correspondence with 3-D Optical Coherence Tomography images, retinal thickness, volume, area and topographic maps.

5. S Optical Coherence Tomography Copernicus by Reichert provides 3-D retinal imaging with mapping of retinal thickness, retinal nerve fiber layer and retinal pigment epithelium with capabilities of zooming, rotating, sectioning and surface reconstruction, 3-D optic nerve analysis with automated software for nerve measurement, including the nerve fiber layer, 3-D retinal nerve fiber layer thickness analysis and retinal pigment epithelium analysis and deformation maps.

6. 3D Optical Coherence Tomography-1000 by Topcon scans a large area with densely sampled data to ensure that the area of concern is captured. The software gives the opportunity for a direct comparison between the raster scans on the retinal image to the corresponding Optical Coherence Tomography tomographic layers. The accurate retinal registration permits subsequent scans of the same area to be repeated for better patient management.

It has similar interface with Topcon's IMAGEnet software and integration with other types of imaging (red-free, fluorescein, indocyanine green and autofluorescence). There is also the possibility for pinpoint registration between Optical Coherence Tomography data and fundus images for reliable and reproducible results, 3-D "virtual microscopic view" of the targeted area and true-Color 45° nonmydriatic retinal photo documentation. The axial resolution is 6 μm and the transverse less than 20 μm in tissue.

The examination speed is 18,000 A-scans per second.

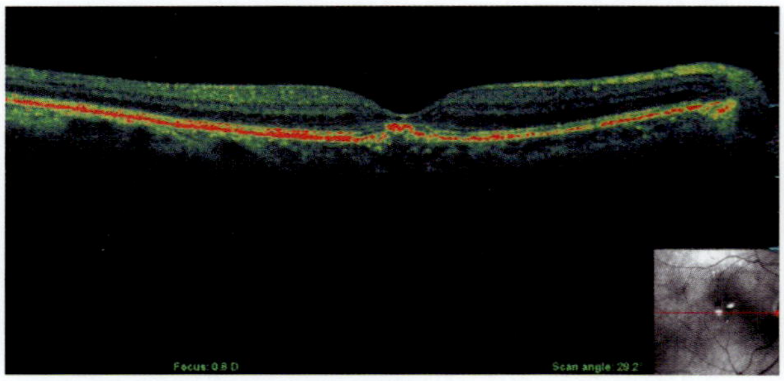

Drusen and retinal pigment epithelium atrophy

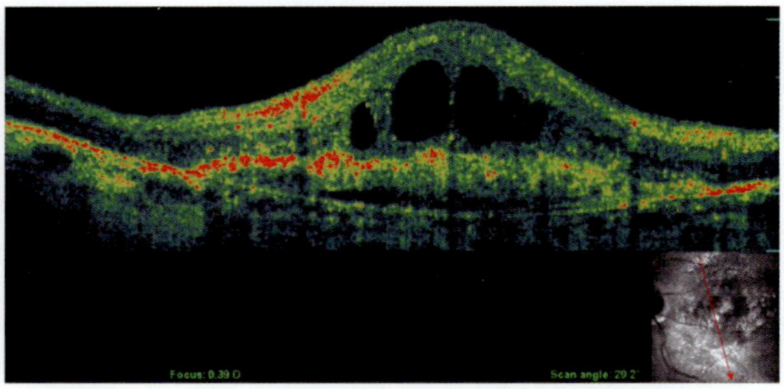

Wet age-related macular degeneration

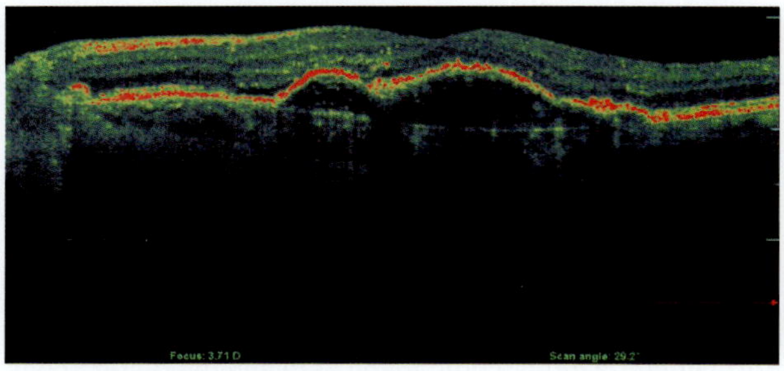

Pigment epithelium detachment

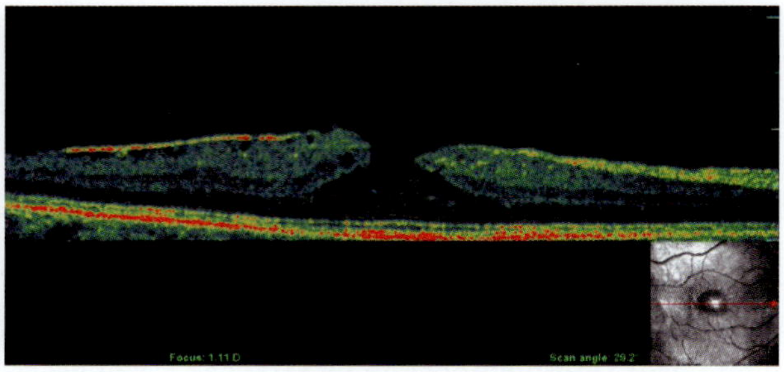

Macular pseudohole

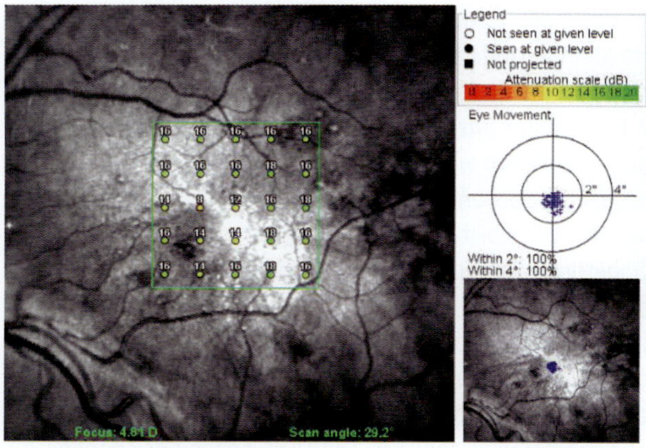

Microperimetry

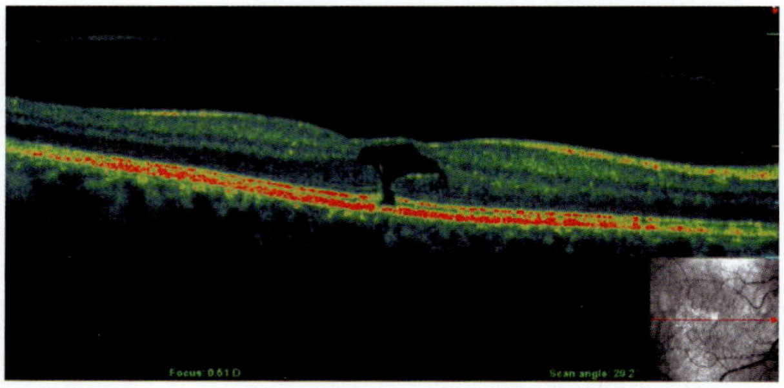

Impending macular hole

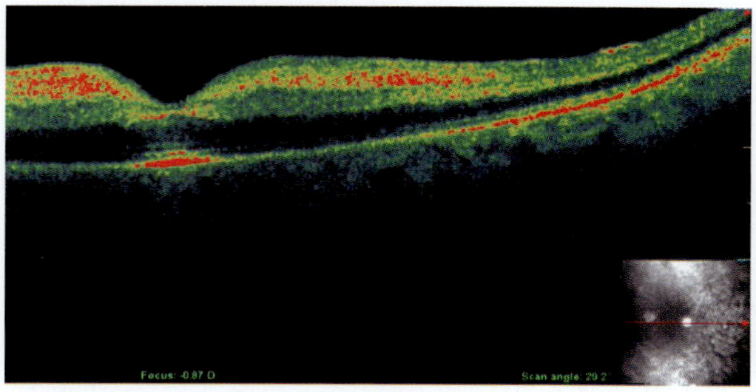

Retinal pigment epithelium lesion

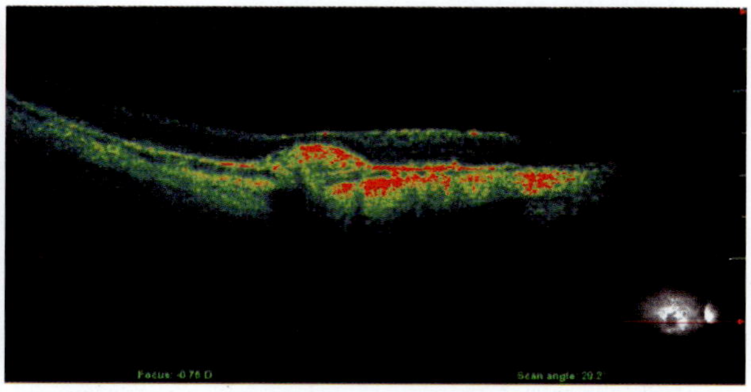

Choroidal neovascular membrane secondary to high myopia

Fig. 8

BIBLIOGRAPHY

1. Schuman JS, Puliafito CA, Fujimoto JG. Opt cal Coherence Tomography of Ocular Diseases. 2nd ed. Thorofare, NJ: SLACK Incorporated ; 2004.

2. Wojtkowski M, Srinivasan V, Fujimoto JG, et al. Three-dimensional retinal imaging with high-speed ultrahigh-resolution optical coherence tomography. Ophthalmology 2005;112(10):1734-1746.

3. Ko TH, Fujimoto JG, Duker JS et al. Comparison of ultrahigh and standard-resolution optical coherence tomography for imaging macular hole pathology and repair. Ophthalmology 2004;111(11):2033-2043.

4. Cense B, Nassif N, Chen TC, et al. ultrahigh resolution high-speed retinal imaging using spectral-domain optical coherence tomography. Optics Express 2004;12:2435-2447.

5. Nassif N, Cence B, Park BH, et al. In vivo human retinal imaging by ultrahigh-speed spectral domain optical coherence tomography. Opt Lett 2004;29(5):480-482.

6. Fercher AF, Drexler W, Hitzenberger CK. Optical coherence tomography. Principles and applications. Rep Prog Phys 2003; 66: 239-303.

7. Fercher AF, Hitzenberger CK, Kamp G, El-Zaiat SY. Measurement of Intraocular Distances by Backscattering Spectral Interferometry. Optics Communications 1995; 117: 43-48.

8. Hausler G, Lindner MW. Coherence Radar and Spectral Radar. New tools for dermatological diagnosis. J Biomed Opt 1998; 3: 21-31.

9. Choma MA, Sarunic MV, Yang C, Izatt JA. Sensitivity advantage of swept source and Fourier domain optical coherence tomography. Optics Express 2003; 11: 2183-2189.

10. De Boer JF, Cense B, Park BH, Pierce MC, Tearney GJ, Bouma BE. Improved signal to-noise ratio in spectral-domain compared with time-domain optical coherence tomography. Optics Letters 2003; 28: 2067-2069.

11. Leitgeb R, Hitzenberger CK, Fercher AF. Performance of Fourier domain vs. time domain optical coherence tomography. Optics Express 2003; 11: 889-894.

12. Mitsui T. Dynamic range of optical reflectometry with spectral interferometry. Jap J Appl Phys(Part 1 Regular Papers Short Notes & Review Papers) 1999; 38: 6133-6137.

13. De Boer JF, Cense B, Park BH, Pierce MC, Tearney GJ, Bouma BE. Improved signal to-noise ratio in spectral-domain compared with time-domain optical coherence tomography. Optics Letters 2003; 28: 2067-2069.

14. White BR. In vivo dynamic human retinal blood flow imaging using ultra-high-speed spectral domain optical Doppler tomography. Optics Express 2003; 11: 3490-3497.

INDEX

E

F

N

O

P

R

S

T

U

V

W